A TEXTBOOK OF CLINICAL PHARMACOLOGY

Fourth Edition

EDITED BY

James M Ritter
MA, DPhil, FRCP
Professor of Clinical Pharmacology, Guy's, King's and St Thomas's Medical Schools, London, UK

Lionel D Lewis
MA, MB BCh, MD, FRCP
Associate Professor of Medicine/Pharmacology and Toxicology, Dartmouth Medical School, Hanover, New Hampshire, USA

Timothy GK Mant
BSc, FFPM, FRCP
Medical Director, Guy's Drug Research Unit, Guy's Hospital, London, UK

ARNOLD

A member of the Hodder Headline Group
LONDON
Co-published in the United States of America
by Oxford University Press Inc., New York

First published in Great Britain in 1981
Second edition published in Great Britain in 1986
Third edition published in Great Britain in 1995
Fourth edition published in 1999 by
Arnold, a member of the Hodder Headline Group,
338 Euston Road, London NW1 3BH

http://www.arnoldpublishers.com

Co-published in the United States of America by
Oxford University Press Inc.,
198 Madison Avenue, New York, NY 10016
Oxford is a registered trademark of Oxford University Press

British Library Cataloguing in Publication Data
A catalogue record for this book is available from the British Library

Library of Congress Cataloging-in-Publication Data
A catalog record for this book is available from the Library of Congress

ISBN 0 340 70593 0

1 2 3 4 5 6 7 8 9 10

Commissioning Editor: Fiona Goodgame
Production Editor: Rada Radojicic
Production Controller: Iain McWilliams
Cover Design: Terry Griffiths

Typeset in 9.5/12pt Palatino by
J&L Composition Ltd, Filey, North Yorkshire
Printed and bound in Spain by Mateu Cromo SA

A TEXTBOOK OF CLINICAL PHARMACOLOGY

This book is dedicated to the memory of
Professor Howard Rogers

CONTENTS

FOREWORD

It is only four years since the last edition of this book was published but the rapid expansion of understanding of the processes involved in disease, particularly at the molecular level, has presented fresh therapeutic possibilities and new and novel drugs have been introduced.

The extensive revision and addition of new material has been achieved without undue increase in the size of the book. It still contains all the clinical pharmacology required by undergraduate medical students but is comprehensive enough to include accounts of the growing points of the subject, thus rendering it very useful for revision or reference by post-graduates and prescribing doctors.

Those working in pharmaceutical sciences are increasingly involved in the use of drugs. Pharmacists, in particular, and those in the pharmaceutical industry will find this book has an important place in their studies.

Nurses can already prescribe on a limited scale and their role in the therapeutic use of drugs is likely to expand. They are also ideally placed to note and record the effects, whether beneficial or adverse, of drug treatment: a copy of this book should be available in every school of nursing library.

In the overcrowded medical curriculum there is an ever-present danger that clinical pharmacology will be consigned to a very minor part of the teaching programme in spite of being the subject which underpins the prescribing of drugs – one of the major responsibilities of doctors, and one which becomes ever more complex.

Professor Ritter and his team have produced a text which will make a major contribution to the teaching and understanding of clinical pharmacology. Its popularity will continue and ensure that students are fully versed in the scientific background and its practical application to the use of drugs.

Professor JR Trounce

PREFACE

Clinical pharmacologists have special expertise and interest in the use of drugs in humans. Surgeons, obstetricians and physicians of every subspeciality prescribe drugs for their patients on a daily basis to prevent and treat illness. With the extraordinary increase in the therapeutic armamentarium over the last 50 years, there has been a parallel increase in the potential for iatrogenic disease. Understanding the principles of clinical pharmacology is essential for safe and effective therapeutic practice. This book is addressed primarily to medical students and junior doctors. Our aim has been to provide an account both of the general principles of the subject, and of how these are applied in the management of common clinical conditions.

The first section deals with general principles including pharmacodynamics, pharmacokinetics and the various factors that modify drug disposition and drug interactions. Recognition and monitoring of adverse effects and the introduction of new drugs are also discussed. We have deliberately avoided algebraic formulae, concentrating instead on the practical utility of concepts such as half-life, clearance and volume of distribution in deciding such things as dose interval or the need for a loading dose.

The second section of the text addresses the treatment of common diseases of major organ systems (nervous, cardiovascular, etc.) and of diseases that influence multiple systems (infectious diseases, cancer, clinical toxicology, immune disorders, etc.). Basic pathophysiology, which is essential to understanding the approach to treatment, is described briefly, followed by principles of management and an account of the most important drugs used. In discussing individual drugs, emphasis is given to clinical use and benefits, mechanisms of action, adverse effects, relevant pharmacokinetics, and contraindications and clinically important drug interactions. Special situations (e.g. the use of drugs at extremes of age, in pregnancy, or in patients with coexisting disease of major organ systems) are considered separately where relevant. We hope that this part of the book will be read by students undertaking clincal work as they encounter particular diseases and the drugs used to treat them, and that they will thereby develop a secure background in rational therapeutics. We would emphasize that learning clinical pharmacology can only be effective if it is accompanied by clinical experience because, despite initial impressions, this is a practical subject and, as in clinical medicine, the patient is the best teacher. In our experience, attempts to learn the subject in isolation from clinical work inevitably fail.

We hope that, in addition to medical students and junior doctors, this book will also be useful to pharmacists, nurses, scientists in the pharmaceutical industry and others with professional interests in therapeutics.

James M Ritter
Lionel D Lewis
Timothy GK Mant

ACKNOWLEDGEMENTS

We would like to thank many colleagues who have helped us with advice and criticism in the revision and updating of the fourth edition. Their expertise in many specialist areas has enabled us to emphasize those factors most relevant. This edition's Chapter on Anaesthetics and Muscle Relaxants was rewritten with much help from Dr Zahid Khan, Consultant in Intensive Care and Anaesthetics at the City Hospital, Birmingham. For their input into this edition and/or the previous edition we are, in particular, grateful to Professor John Trounce, Professor Roy Spector, Professor Alan Richens, Dr Dipti Amin, Dr Anne Dornhorst, Dr Michael Isaac, Dr Terry Gibson, Dr Paul Glue, Dr Mark Kinirons, Dr Jonathan Barker, Dr Patricia McElhatton, Dr Robin Stott, Mr David Calver, Dr Jas Gill, Dr John Henry, Dr Ronan Kelly, Dr Piotr Bajorek, Miss Susanna Gilmour-White, Dr Mark Edwards, Dr Michael Marsh, Mrs Joanna Tempowski. We would also like to thank the Guy's, St Thomas' and Lewisham Hospitals Formulary Committee for permission to publish their guide to the use of antibiotics in modified form.

PART I

GENERAL PRINCIPLES

CHAPTER ONE

INTRODUCTION *to* THERAPEUTICS

- Use of drugs
- Adverse effects and risk/benefit
- Drug history and therapeutic plan
- Formularies and restricted lists
- Scientific basis of use of drugs in humans

USE OF DRUGS

People consult a doctor to find out what (if anything) is wrong (the diagnosis), and what should be done about it (the treatment). If they are well, they may nevertheless want to know how future problems can be prevented. Depending on the diagnosis, treatment may consist of reassurance, physical therapy, surgery, radiotherapy, psychotherapy and so on. Drugs are very often either the primary therapy or an adjunct to another modality (e.g. the use of analgesic and anaesthetic drugs in patients undergoing surgery). Sometimes contact with the doctor is initiated because of a public health measure rather than because of symptoms of disease (e.g. through contact tracing from an index case with an infectious disease, or through a screening programme intended to identify individuals at increased risk of malignant or cardiovascular disease). Again drug treatment is sometimes needed, often as a supplement to advice regarding personal habits. Consequently, practising doctors of nearly all specialties use drugs extensively, and therefore need to understand something of the scientific basis on which their use is founded.

A century ago, physicians had at their disposal only a handful of effective drugs (e.g. morphia, quinine, ether, aspirin and digitalis leaf), and even these were used less than optimally. In the ensuing decades, potent new drugs (e.g. thiamine, insulin, sulphonamides and antibiotics, synthetic antimalarials, anticonvulsants, cortisol, diuretics, antipsychotics and antidepressants, antimetabolites and alkylating agents, contraceptives, beta-blockers, H_2-blockers, converting enzyme inhibitors, calcium-channel blockers, drugs that lower cholesterol, fibrinolytics and antivirals) have been introduced. New drugs are fundamental to advances in medicine, and the ingenuity of pharmaceutical chemists is continuing to pay dividends in terms of discovery of improved drugs and drugs for new indications. Indeed, with advances in genetic engineering and in basic understanding of chemical mediators in biological control systems (witnessed by the introduction of such products as genetically engineered hepatitis vaccine, erythropoietin and monoclonal antibodies directed against interleukins and their receptors, among others), to say nothing of the experimental use of gene therapy in genetic disorders such as adenine deaminase deficiency, familial hypercholesterolaemia and cystic fibrosis, it is likely that the pace of change will accelerate further during the next few years. Changes in therapeutics that will be seen by a physician newly qualified today will consequently be at least as great, and probably far greater, than those of the last 40 years. Medical students and doctors in training therefore need to learn something of the *principles* of therapeutics. These are discussed in the first part of this book, while systematic considerations and current approaches to treatment of common diseases are the subject of the second part, together with specifics relating to selected important therapeutic drugs.

Adverse effects and risk/benefit

Medicinal chemistry has contributed immeasurably to human health and happiness, but the alleviation of suffering brought about by effective drugs has not been achieved without a price. Consequently, these advances have been paralleled by a necessary change in philosophy of the medical profession, and somewhat later of the public, towards therapeutics. A physician in Osler's day could safely adhere to the Hippocratic principle 'first do no harm', because the opportunities for doing good were so limited. The discovery of new drugs has transformed this situation, but unfortunately only at the expense of very real risks of doing harm. This is particularly striking in the case of cancer chemotherapy, where great advances (e.g. cures of leukaemias, Hodgkin's disease and testicular carcinomas) have been achieved through a preparedness to accept a limited degree of containable harm to the patient in a tightly controlled setting, but similar considerations apply in other fields of medicine as well as oncology.

Indeed, almost all (if not all) effective drugs can have adverse effects, and therapeutic judgements based on risk/benefit ratios now permeate all fields of medicine, even if the arguments are seldom formalized and may not be rehearsed consciously. This is unfortunate – drugs are the physician's prime therapeutic tools, just as diathermy and the scalpel are those of the surgeon, and just as a misplaced scalpel can spell disaster, so can a thoughtless prescription. Some of the more colourful and dramatic instances of such catastrophes make for gruesome reading in the annual reports of the medical defence societies, but perhaps as important is the morbidity and expense caused by less dramatic but more common errors.

How are prescribing errors to be minimized? By combining *general* knowledge of the disease to be treated and of the drugs that may be effective for that disease with *specific* knowledge about the particular patient. Dukes and Swartz, in their valuable work *Responsibility for Drug-Induced Injury*, list eight basic duties of prescribers:

1. *restrictive use* – to take a proper decision that drug therapy is warranted rather than other therapy or to 'wait and see';
2. *careful choice* of an appropriate drug, dosage and scheme of treatment with due regard to the likely risk/benefit ratio, the alternatives available, and the patient's needs and susceptibilities;
3. *consultation and consent* – wherever possible the patient should be consulted about the proposed treatment, and should give informed consent to it;
4. *prescription and recording* – to prescribe appropriately and with care and to record what is prescribed;
5. *explanation* to the patient of how the treatment will be given and what his or her role in it will be;
6. *supervision* of the course of therapy, observing developments and adapting it as necessary;
7. *termination* of therapy in an appropriate manner when it is no longer needed;
8. *conformity* with the law relating to the prescribing and use of medicines.

The following should be considered when deciding on a therapeutic plan:

1. the patient's age;
2. the possibility of coexisting disease, especially renal impairment, liver disease and cardiac or respiratory failure;
3. the possibility of pregnancy now or during treatment;
4. the patient's drug history;
5. the best that can reasonably be hoped for in this individual patient.

Drug history and therapeutic plan

A reliable drug history involves questioning the patient (and sometimes the family, neighbours, other physicians, etc.) about a number of issues.

What prescription tablets, medicines, drops (for eye, nose or ear), contraceptives, creams, suppositories or pessaries are being taken? What over-the-counter remedies are being used? Has the patient suffered from drug-induced rashes or other allergies, or other serious reactions? Has the patient ever been treated for anything similar in the past, and if so with what, and did it do the job or were there any problems? Has the patient ever had an anaesthetic, and if so were there any problems? Have there ever been any serious drug reactions in a close family member, or other familial disorders?

Taking these specifics into account, a therapeutic plan is formulated. At this stage, it is crucial that the potential prescriber is both meticulous and humble, especially when dealing with a situation he or she does not encounter every day. Checking contraindications, special precautions and doses in a formulary such as the *British National Formulary* (BNF) is the minimum that is needed. Where practicable, the proposed therapeutic plan is discussed with the patient, including consideration of the various options available, the goals of treatment, possible adverse effects, their likelihood and measures to be taken if these arise. It is crucial that the patient understands what is intended, and that he or she is happy about the means proposed to achieve these ends. (This will not, of course, be possible in demented or delirious patients, or in some other severely ill individuals, where discussion will be with any available family members.) The risks of causing harm can be minimized in this way, while at the same time the likelihood is increased that the patient will comply with the treatment plan that is finally agreed upon.

If the therapeutic plan includes the use of drugs, a prescription must be written clearly and legibly, conforming to legal requirements. In general this should include the generic name of the drug, and the dose, frequency and duration of treatment, and be signed. In addition, it is wise to print the prescriber's name, address and telephone number in order to facilitate communication from the pharmacist should a query arise. Appropriate follow-up must be arranged. Unfortunately there are still patients who believe that chronic conditions such as severe hypertension are treated by a 'course' of tablets, only to represent months or years later with a stroke, heart attack or renal failure.

FORMULARIES AND RESTRICTED LISTS

Historically, formularies listed the multiple ingredients commonly prescribed as mixtures by physicians up until the Second World War. The perceived need for hospital formularies disappeared transiently when such mixtures were replaced by proprietary products of consistent quality prepared by the pharmaceutical industry. The *British National Formulary* (British Medical Association and Royal Pharmaceutical Society of Great Britain 1999) is updated regularly and contains information about all such preparations that are currently available in the UK. Because of the bewildering array of licensed products, many of which are alternatives to one another, many hospitals have reintroduced formularies that are essentially a restrictive list of the drugs stocked by the hospital pharmacy, from which doctors are encouraged to prescribe. The objectives of such formularies are to encourage rational prescribing, to simplify purchasing and storage of drugs, and to obtain the 'best buy' among alternative preparations. Such formularies have the advantage of encouraging consistency, and when decided with input from local consultant prescribers they are usually well accepted.

SCIENTIFIC BASIS OF USE OF DRUGS IN HUMANS

The scientific basis of our understanding of drug action is provided by the discipline of pharmacology. Clinical pharmacology is the branch of pharmacology that deals with the effects of drugs in humans. It entails the study of the interaction of drugs with their receptors, the transduction (second messenger) systems to which these are linked and the changes that they bring about in cells, organs and the whole organism. These processes ('what the drug does to the body') are sometimes grouped together as 'pharmacodynamics'. The predictive value of animal pharmacology and toxicology studies is limited. Species differences, and the fact that much *in vivo* animal pharmacology research is necessarily conducted in anaesthetized animals, make human studies absolutely essential. However, modern methods of molecular and cell biology are permitting expression of human genes, including those that code for receptors and key signal transduction elements, in non-human cells and in transgenic animals, and seem likely to revolutionize our knowledge of these areas within the next few years. Hopefully this will improve the yield of relevant information from preclinical pharmacology and toxicology studies before the introduction of drugs in humans.

It is important to appreciate that drug effects which are important in humans do not necessarily occur in other species. For example, one of the early beta-blocking drugs (practolol) had to be withdrawn because it has adverse effects on the eye, skin and peritoneum. However, it proved impossible to produce an animal model of these toxic actions. Consequently, when drugs are introduced into the treatment of humans after animal studies have demonstrated potentially useful actions, considerable uncertainties remain regarding effects (especially subjective effects that determine whether or not the drug is well tolerated) and dose–response relationships. Such early-phase human studies are usually conducted in healthy volunteers, except when near inevitable toxicity is anticipated, as is the case for many antineoplastic drugs.

Basic pharmacologists can study isolated preparations in which the concentration of drug in the microenvironment of the receptors can be controlled fairly precisely, but such preparations are often only stable for a few minutes or hours. In therapeutics, drugs are administered to the whole organism by a route that is as convenient and safe as possible for the patient (usually by mouth), often for periods of days, weeks or more. Consequently, the drug concentration in the vicinity of the receptors is usually unknown, and long-term effects involving alterations in receptor density or function or the activation or modulation of homeostatic control loops may be of overriding importance. The processes of absorption, distribution, metabolism and elimination ('what the body does to the drug') determine the drug concentration–time relationships at the receptors. These processes are sometimes collectively known as 'pharmacokinetics'. There is considerable inter-individual variation in these processes due to both inherited and acquired factors, notably disease of the organs responsible for drug metabolism and excretion. Prescribers therefore need to understand the principles of pharmacokinetics in order to plan a rational therapeutic regime. Pharmacokinetic principles are described in Chapter 3 from the point of view of a prescriber rather than of a scientist involved in drug development or studying drug metabolism. Genetic influences on pharmacodynamics and pharmacokinetics ('pharmacogenetics') are discussed in Chapter 14, effects of disease are addressed in Chapter 7, and the use of drugs in pregnancy and at extremes of age is discussed in Chapters 9, 10 and 11.

There are no entirely satisfactory animal models of most important human diseases (e.g. atheroma, the major cause of death in western societies). Consequently, the only way to ensure that a drug with promising pharmacological actions (e.g. a new drug that lowers plasma cholesterol levels) is effective in treating or preventing disease (e.g. hyperlipidaemia, coronary artery disease) is to perform a clinical trial. It is important for prescribing doctors to understand the strengths and limitations of such trials, the principles of which are described in Chapter 15. Prescribers can then evaluate critically and objectively papers published in the literature on the new drugs that will certainly be introduced during their professional lifetimes. Ignorance of the principles of clinical trials leaves the physician at the mercy of sources of information that are biased by commercial interests. Sources of up-to-date and unbiased information include Dollery's encyclopaedic *Therapeutic Drugs 2nd edn.*, (published by Churchill Livingstone in 1999), which is an invaluable source of reference. Publications such as the *Adverse Reaction Bulletin*, *Prescribers Journal* and the succinctly argued *Drug and Therapeutics Bulletin* provide up-to-date discussions of therapeutic issues of current importance.

Key points

- Drugs are prescribed by physicians of all specialties to diagnose, prevent, ameliorate and cure disease.
- This carries risks as well as benefits.
- Therapy is optimized by combining general knowledge of drugs with specific knowledge of a patient and their circumstances.
- Evidence of efficacy is generally based on clinical trials.
- Rational prescribing is encouraged by local formularies.

Case history

A general practitioner reviews the medication of an 86-year-old woman with hypertension and moderate dementia of the multi-infarct type, who is living in a nursing home. Her family used to visit daily, but she no longer recognizes them, and needs help with dressing, washing and feeding. Drugs include bendrofluazide, atenolol, atorvastatin, aspirin, thioridazine, imipramine, lactulose and senna. On examination she smells of urine and has several bruises on her head, but otherwise seems well cared for. She is calm, but looks pale and bewildered, and has a pulse of 48 beats/min regular, and blood pressure 162/96 mmHg lying and 122/76 mmHg standing, during which she becomes sweaty and distressed. Her rectum is loaded with hard stool, she is moderately demented, and she has generalized increased tone and increased reflexes in the left leg and an extensor plantar reflex on that side. A review of the notes indicates that imipramine was started as a trial 3 years previously. Urine culture showed only a light mixed growth. All of the medications were stopped and manual evacuation of faeces was performed. Stool was negative for occult blood and the full blood count was normal. Two weeks later the patient was brighter and more mobile. She remained incontinent of urine at night but no longer during the day, her heart rate was 76 beats/min and her blood pressure was 208/108 mmHg lying and standing.

Comment

It is seldom helpful to give drugs in order to prevent something that has already happened (in this case multi-infarct dementia), and any benefit in preventing further ischaemic events has to be balanced against the harm done by the polypharmacy. In this case, drug-related problems probably include postural hypotension (due to imipramine, bendrofluazide and thioridazine), reduced mobility (due to thioridazine), constipation (due to imipramine and thioridazine), urinary incontinence (due to bendrofluazide and drugs causing constipation) and bradycardia (due to atenolol). Despite her pallor, the patient was not bleeding into the gastrointestinal tract, but aspirin could have caused this.

Further reading

Dukes MNG, Swartz B. 1988: *Responsibility for drug-induced injury*. Amsterdam: Elsevier.

Weatherall, DJ. 1996: Scientific medicine and the art of healing. In Weatherall DJ, Ledingham JGG, Warrell DA (eds), *Oxford textbook of medicine*, 3rd edn. Oxford: Oxford University Press, 7–10.

CHAPTER TWO

MECHANISMS *of* DRUG ACTION (PHARMACODYNAMICS)

- Introduction
- Receptors and signal transduction
- Agonists
- Competitive antagonists
- Partial agonists
- Slow processes
- Non-receptor mechanisms

INTRODUCTION

Pharmacodynamics is the study of effects of drugs on biological processes. For example, studies of the time-course of the effect of a dose of warfarin on prothrombin time, or of ranitidine on gastric acid secretion or of atenolol on heart rate are described as pharmacodynamic studies. The term 'pharmacodynamics' implies a process that changes with time, but in practice studies that concentrate on the effect of a drug at a single time after administration (e.g. the effect of a defined dose of aspirin on bleeding time 24 h after the dose) are also referred to as pharmacodynamic studies. Many endogenous hormones, neurotransmitters and other mediators exert their effects as a result of high-affinity binding to specific macromolecular protein or glycoprotein receptors in plasma membranes or cell cytoplasm, and many therapeutically important drugs exert their effects by combining with these receptors and either mimicking the effect of the natural mediator (in which case they are called agonists) or blocking it (in which case they are termed antagonists). Examples include oestrogens (used in contraception and hormone replacement therapy) and anti-oestrogens (used in treating breast cancer), alpha- and beta-adrenoceptor agonists and antagonists (used in treating hypertension and other cardiovascular and respiratory diseases), opioids, benzodiazepines, antihistamines and others.

Not all drugs work via receptors for endogenous mediators, and many therapeutic drugs exert their effects by combining with an enzyme, transport protein or other cellular macromolecule (e.g. DNA) and interfering with its function. Examples include inhibitors of acetylcholinesterase (used to treat myasthenia gravis and to reverse the effects of neuromuscular-blocking drugs after anaesthesia), monoamine oxidase inhibitors (used in Parkinsonism and in some patients with depression) and cardiac glycosides such as digoxin which inhibit Na^+/K^+ adenosine triphosphatase (ATPase). Some authorities reserve the term 'receptor' exclusively for receptors of endogenous mediators. However, this restricted sense has not been generally adopted, and a broader definition of receptor is 'a macromolecule which is the primary site of action of a drug or naturally occurring substance, usually a smaller molecule, that binds to it'. This broader usage includes receptors for naturally occurring substances that do not have mediator functions, such as adhesion molecules and low-density lipoprotein (LDL). Some diseases are caused by abnormalities in receptors. For example, myasthenia gravis is an autoallergic disease caused by increased acetylcholine-receptor turnover secondary to cross-linking of adjacent nicotinic acetylcholine receptors at the neuromuscular junction by specific antibodies. Patients with familial hypercholesterolaemia lack functional LDL receptors and suffer from severe premature atheromatous disease as a result, and patients with X-linked nephrogenic diabetes insipidus have a mutation in the gene for the V_2 receptor which is the site of action of vasopressin (antidiuretic hormone) in the kidney, and consequently have impaired ability to form concentrated urine.

Whether the site of action of a drug is a receptor for an endogenous mediator or an enzyme or ion channel, the binding is usually highly specific, with precise steric recognition between the small molecular ligand and the binding site on its macromolecular target. The binding forces are usually a combination of several weak interactions – electrostatic, dipole–dipole, hydrogen bonding, van der Waals' forces and others. Occasionally, strong covalent bonds are formed, as in the acetylation of a serine residue in the active site of cyclo-oxygenase by aspirin (acetylsalicylic acid), which prevents subsequent binding of substrate as a result of steric hindrance, or the alkylation of bases in DNA by cytotoxic drugs such as phosphoramide mustard (the active metabolite of cyclophosphamide).

Most drugs produce graded dose-related effects which can be plotted as a dose–response curve. Such curves are often approximately hyperbolic (Figure 2.1a), and can be conveniently plotted on semi-logarithmic paper to give the familiar sigmoidal shape (Figure 2.1b). This method of plotting dose–response curves facilitates quantitative analysis (see below) of full agonists (which produce graded responses up to a maximum value), antagonists (which produce no response on their own, but reduce the response to an agonist) and partial agonists (which produce some response, but to a lower maximum value than that of a full agonist, and antagonize full agonists) (Figure 2.2). In the clinical situation, dose–response curves are influenced by many factors, including genetic as well as acquired sources of variation including age, weight, nutrition and other drugs as well as psychological and social factors that strongly influence compliance and placebo response.

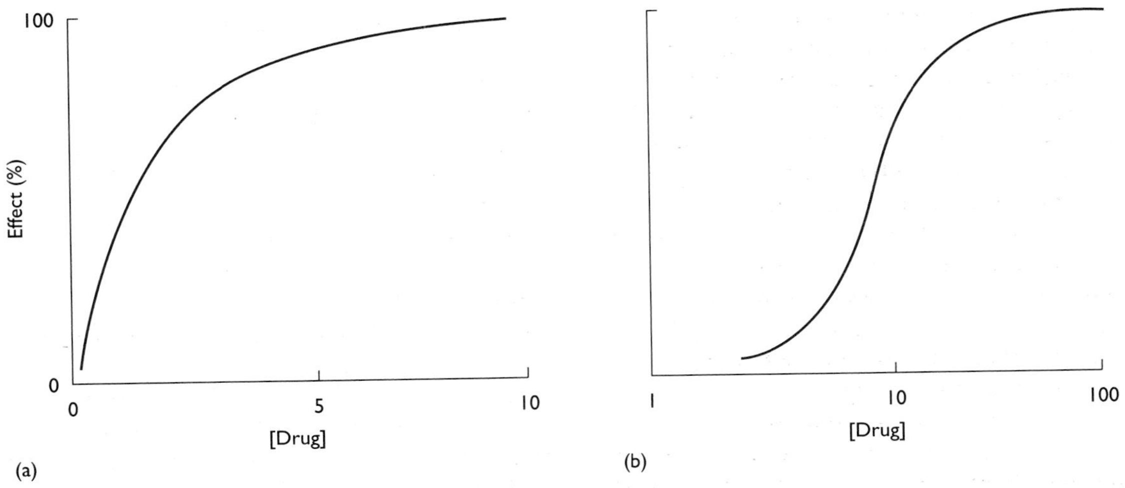

Figure 2.1: Dose-response curves plotted (a) arithmetically and (b) semi-logarithmically.

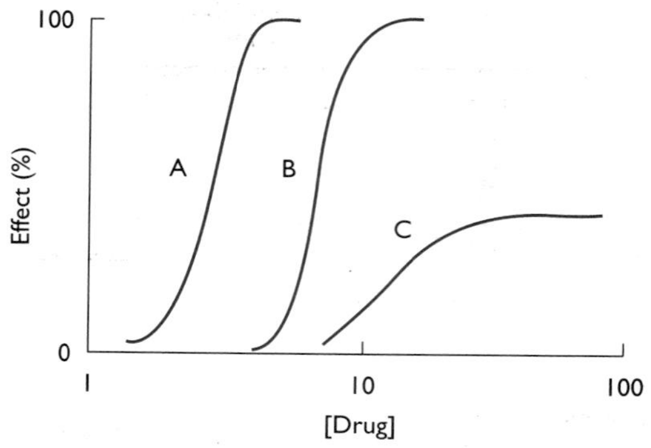

Figure 2.2: Dose-response curves of two full agonists (A,B) of different potency, and of partial agonist (C).

RECEPTORS AND SIGNAL TRANSDUCTION

Drugs are often potent (i.e. they produce effects at low concentration) and specific (i.e. small changes in structure lead to profound changes in potency, or cause a change from agonist to antagonist). High potency is a consequence of high affinity for specific macromolecular receptors. Receptors were originally classified by reference to the relative potencies of agonists and antagonists on preparations containing different receptors. A familiar example is the order of potency of isoprenaline > adrenaline > noradrenaline on tissues rich in β-receptors such as the heart contrasted with the reverse order in α-receptor-mediated responses such as vasoconstriction in resistance arteries supplying the skin. Quantitative potency data are best obtained from comparisons of different competitive antagonists, as explained below. Such data are supplemented, but not replaced, by radiolabelled ligand-binding studies. In this way, adrenoceptors were divided first into α and β, then subdivided into α_1/α_2 and β_1/β_2. Many other useful receptor classifications, including those of cholinoceptors, histamine receptors, serotonin receptors, benzodiazepine receptors, glutamate receptors and others have been proposed on a similar basis. Labelling with irreversible antagonists permitted receptor solubilization and purification using affinity chromatography. Partial sequencing of the amino-acid sequence then enabled oligonucleotide probes based on the deduced sequence to be used to extract the full-length DNA sequence coding for different receptors. As receptors are cloned and expressed in cells in culture, the original functional classifications have been supported and extended, and further developments are to be expected. Different receptor subtypes may be regarded as analogous to different forms of isoenzymes.

Receptors exist in four 'superfamilies' linked to distinct types of coupling mechanism (Figure. 2.3). Three families of receptor are located in the cell membrane, while the fourth is intracellular (e.g. steroid hormone and thyroxine receptors). In each of the three membrane families, hydrophobic α-helical regions form membrane-spanning domains. These link an extracellular binding domain with the effector domain. One family of receptors for fast neurotransmitters (e.g. glutamate, nicotinic acetylcholine receptors) is linked directly to a transmembrane ion channel. A second family of receptors for slow neurotransmitters and hormones (e.g. muscarinic acetylcholine receptors, β-adrenoceptors) is linked to an intracellular G-protein coupling domain. The third family is coupled directly to the catalytic domain of an enzyme on the inner membrane (e.g. insulin coupled to tyrosine kinase, atrial natriuretic hormone coupled to membrane-bound guanylyl cyclase). Precisely what distinguishes agonists from antagonists is not yet clear, but there have recently been great advances in understanding the events that link receptor activation with cellular response. These are termed signal transduction processes. They include the following.

1 Direct linkage to receptor-operated ion channels (e.g. for potassium or calcium ions). These processes operate rapidly (in the micro- to millisecond range), and their study has been greatly facilitated by the technique of patch clamping.
2 Linkage via guanosine triphosphate (GTP)-binding proteins (G-proteins) to adenylyl cyclase, which catalyzes the synthesis of cyclic adenosine monophosphate (cAMP), or to other enzymes that catalyze the synthesis of second messengers. Cyclic AMP is an intracellular second messenger whose actions are terminated by degradation by specific phosphodiesterase enzymes that are themselves targets of drug action. The G-proteins are heterotrimers (α, β

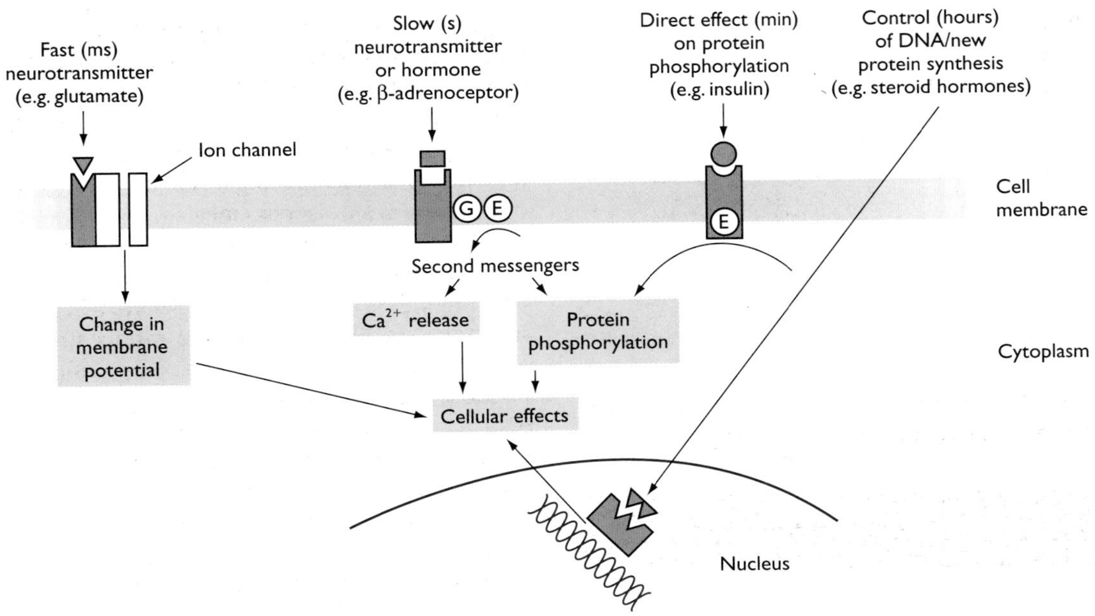

Figure 2.3: Receptors and signal transduction. G = G-protein; E = enzyme; Ca = calcium.

and γ subunits) with stimulatory or inhibitory α subunits (termed respectively α_s or α_i) that dissociate on combination of the receptor with agonist, and activate or inhibit the cyclase, operating on a time-scale ranging from seconds to minutes. An uncommon disease, pseudohypoparathyroidism, is caused by a genetic defect in the α_s subunit of the G-protein controlling adenylyl cyclase. Consequently, although the circulating concentration of parathyroid hormone is high, responses to it are blunted with reduced phosphate excretion by the kidney and skeletal abnormalities. Some endocrine disorders are caused by somatic mutations in genes encoding proteins in the cyclase/G-protein complex that result in the enzyme operating at 'full tilt' even in the absence of the hormonal agonist. Examples are an unusual form of hyperthyroidism due to hyperfunctioning adenomas in which the cells behave as though they are maximally stimulated by thyrotropin, and an unusual form of male sexual precocity in which Leydig cells in the testis behave as though they are maximally stimulated by luteinizing hormone.

3 Activation of one of several phospholipase enzymes. Phospholipase A_2 initiates the arachidonic acid cascade and also synthesis of lyso-PAF, which is the precursor of platelet-activating factor (PAF). Several of the eicosanoid products of arachidonic acid as well as PAF are believed to have intracellular messenger functions in addition to mediating actions via surface receptors on neighbouring cells. A specific phospholipase C attacks inositol phospholipid, liberating diacylglycerol, which diffuses in the lipid phase of cell membranes and activates membrane-bound protein kinase C. The highly polar second messenger 1,4,5-phosphatidyl inositol *bis*-phosphate (inositol trisphosphate, ITP) is formed simultaneously, diffuses through the cytoplasm and regulates release of calcium from intracellular stores and calcium entry via the plasma membrane.

4 Combination of drugs or hormones with cytoplasmic receptors is followed by combination via a DNA binding domain (containing zinc fingers) with a specific DNA receptor and derepression of transcription of messenger RNA with consequent new protein synthesis. Such effects (e.g. resulting from steroid receptor occupation) occur over a time course of minutes to hours.

AGONISTS

As explained above, it is useful to distinguish between drugs that act on receptors for endogenous mediators and those that do not, because only in the case of the former does it make sense to speak of agonists. For instance, it would be meaningless to talk of an agonist at the dihydrofolate reductase enzyme or at the voltage-dependent sodium channel, even though both of these are targets of drug action (e.g. of methotrexate or lignocaine, respectively), whereas it is useful to classify salbutamol as an agonist at the β_2-adrenoceptor. Agonists produce their effects by combining with and activating specific receptors for endogenous mediators. The process of activation depends on the signal transduction pathway to which the receptor is linked. The effect may be excitatory (e.g. adrenaline increases cardiac contractility) or inhibitory (e.g. dopamine relaxes renovascular smooth muscle, salbutamol relaxes airway smooth muscle). Agonists such as succinylcholine exert an apparently paradoxical inhibitory effect (neuromuscular blockade) by causing long-lasting depolarization at the neuromuscular junction, and hence inactivation of the voltage-dependent sodium channels that initiate the action potential.

Endogenous ligands have sometimes been discovered long *after* other drugs that act on their receptors. Endorphins and enkephalins (endogenous ligands of morphine receptors) were discovered many years after morphine, which is now recognized as an agonist at opioid receptors. Evidence is currently accumulating that membrane Na^+/K^+ ATPase is the receptor of an endogenous natriuretic hormone with ouabain-like properties, and there has been speculation about the possible existence of an endogenous agonist for voltage-dependent calcium channels, so views on drugs that act on these and other targets will continue to develop as their physiology is understood more completely.

COMPETITIVE ANTAGONISTS

Competitive antagonists combine with the same receptor as an agonist (e.g. ranitidine at histamine H_2-receptors), but fail to activate it, presumably because they do not provoke the conformational changes in the receptor that lead to activation of its signal transduction pathway. When combined with the receptor, they prevent access to it of its natural agonist/mediator. The complex between competitive antagonist and receptor is reversible. Consequently, in the presence of antagonist, a higher dose of agonist is needed to produce the same effect as in its absence. However, provided that the dose of agonist is increased sufficiently, a maximal effect can still be obtained, i.e. the antagonism is *surmountable*. The dose of agonist needed to produce the same effect in the presence of a fixed concentration of competitive antagonist as in its absence is a constant multiple known as the *dose ratio*. This results in the familiar parallel shift to the right of the log dose–response curve, since the addition of a constant length on a logarithmic scale corresponds to multiplication by a constant factor (Figure 2.4a). Examples of competitive antagonists include H_1 and H_2 antagonists, β-adrenoceptor antagonists and neuromuscular-blocking drugs such as pancuronium. By contrast, antagonists that do not combine with the same receptor (non-competitive antagonists), or drugs that combine irreversibly with their receptors (e.g. phenoxybenzamine, an irreversible α-receptor antagonist used in preparing patients with phaeochromocytoma for surgery), reduce the slope of the log dose–response curve and depress its maximum (Figure 2.4b).

The relationship between the concentration of a competitive antagonist [B], and the dose ratio (r) was worked out by Gaddum and by Schildt, and is as follows:

$$r - 1 = [B]/K_B$$

where K_B is the dissociation equilibrium constant of the reversible reaction of the antagonist with its receptor. K_B has units of concentration and is the concentration of antagonist needed to occupy half the receptors in the absence of agonist. The lower the value of K_B, the more potent is the drug. If

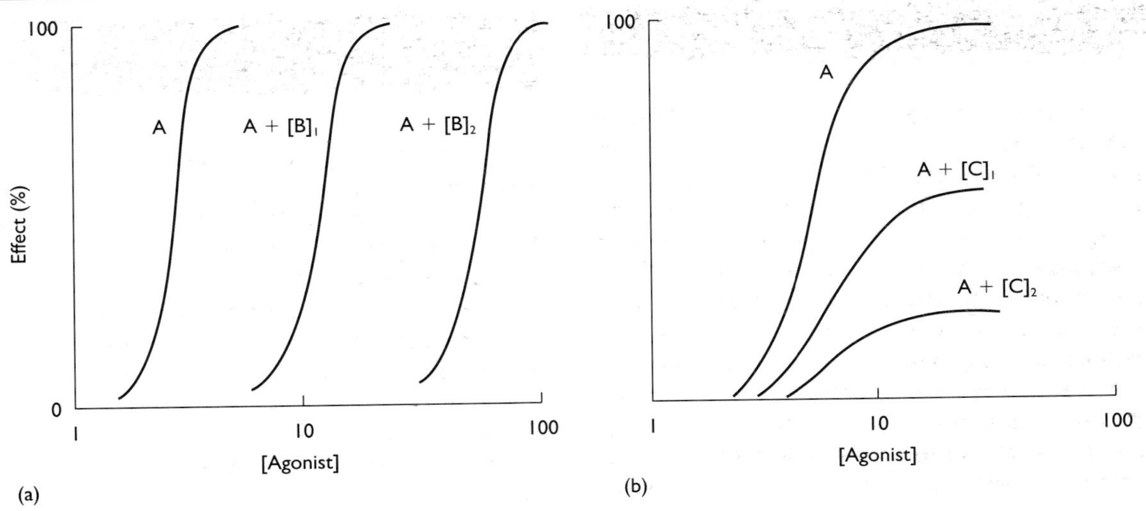

Figure 2.4: Drug antagonism. Control dose–response curves for an agonist A together with curves in the presence of (a) a competitive antagonist B and (b) a non-competitive antagonist C. Increasing concentrations of the competitive antagonist ([B]$_1$, [B]$_2$) cause a parallel shift to the right of the log dose–effect curve (a), while the non-competitive antagonist ([C]$_1$, [C]$_2$) flattens the curve and reduces its maximum (b).

several concentrations of a competitive antagonist are studied and the dose ratio is measured at each concentration, a plot of (r − 1) against [B] yields a $1/K_B$ (Figure 2.5a). Values of K_B estimated in this way often agree well with measurements of binding affinity using radiolabelled ligand, and are needed to confirm that high-affinity binding sites correspond to the receptor rather than to some other binding site such as a degradative enzyme or clearance

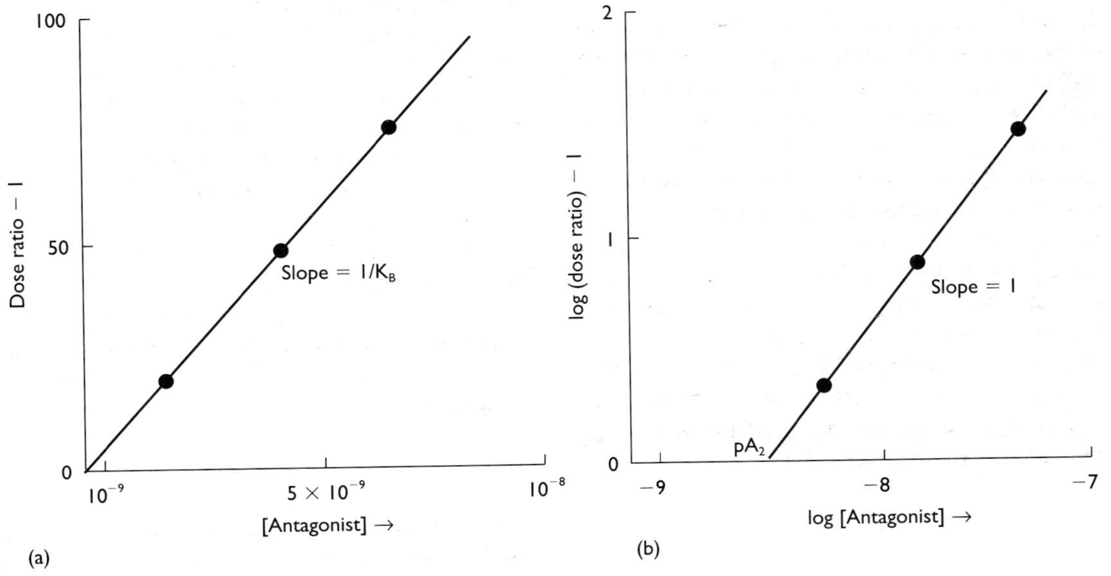

Figure 2.5: Competitive antagonism. (a) A plot of antagonist concentration vs. (dose ratio − 1) gives a straight line through the origin. (b) A log–log plot (a Schildt plot) gives a straight line of unit slope. The potency of the antagonist (pA$_2$) is determined from the intercept of the Schildt plot.

mechanism. Schildt pointed out that if $(r - 1)$ is plotted against [B] on log–log coordinates, a straight line results with a slope of unity and intercept $-\log K_B$, which he referred to as pA_2, by analogy with the logarithmic pH scale. The larger the numerical value of pA_2, the more potent is the drug. This kind of plot (known as a Schildt plot; Figure 2.5b) provides a means of quantifying the potencies of competitive antagonists. Such measurements provided the means of classifying and subdividing receptors in terms of the relative potencies of different antagonists.

Partial agonists

Some drugs combine with receptors and activate them, but are incapable of eliciting a maximal response, no matter how high their concentration may be. These are known as partial agonists, and are said to have low efficacy. Efficacy is a factor that can be ascribed a numerical value of zero for a competitive antagonist, one for a full agonist and a value between zero and one for a partial agonist, although this begs the question (for which there is currently no adequate answer) of what it is at the molecular level that determines whether or not a drug will activate a receptor having occupied it. Several partial agonists are used in therapeutics, including buprenorphine (a partial agonist at morphine μ-receptors) and oxprenolol and pindolol (partial agonists at β-adrenoceptors).

Full agonists are sometimes capable of eliciting a maximal response when only a small proportion of the receptors are occupied (a situation that is sometimes described by stating that there are 'spare receptors'), but this is not the case with partial agonists, where a substantial proportion of the receptors need to be occupied to cause a response. This has two consequences of potential therapeutic importance. First, partial agonists *antagonize* the effect of a full agonist, because most of the receptors are occupied with low-efficacy partial agonist with which the full agonist must compete. Thus a partial β-agonist such as pindolol itself raises heart rate modestly, but opposes any further increase in heart rate caused by a strong agonist such as noradrenaline. Consequently, exercise-induced increases in heart rate, which are mediated by increased sympathetic nerve output to the heart, are abolished or blunted. A second consequence of clinical importance is that it is more difficult to reverse the effects of a partial agonist such as buprenorphine with a competitive antagonist such as naloxone, than it would be to reverse the effects of a strong agonist such as morphine with the same antagonist. A larger fraction of the receptors is occupied by buprenorphine than by morphine, and a much higher concentration of naloxone is required to compete successfully and displace buprenorphine from the receptors.

Slow processes

Protracted exposure of receptors to agonists, as frequently occurs in therapeutic use as opposed to tissue bath experiments, can cause down-regulation or desensitization by one of several mechanisms. Desensitization is sometimes specific for a particular agonist (when it is referred to as homologous desensitization), or there may be cross-desensitization to different agonists (known as heterologous desensitization). Membrane receptors may become internalized and hence no longer accessible to drugs in the extracellular fluid. This occurs when low-density lipoprotein (LDL) particles are taken up via specific LDL receptors on hepatocytes. Alternatively, G-protein-mediated linkage between receptors and effector enzymes (e.g. adenylyl cyclase) may be disrupted. Since G-proteins link several distinct receptors to the same effector molecule, this can give rise to heterologous desensitization. Receptor desensitization is probably involved in the tolerance that occurs during prolonged administration of drugs such as morphine and the benzodiazepines (see Chapter 17 on hypnotics and Chapter 24 on control of pain).

Therapeutic effects sometimes depend on induction of tolerance, albeit rarely. For example, analogues of gonadotropin-releasing hormone (GnRH) such as buserelin are used to treat patients with disseminated prostate cancer. Gonadotropin-releasing hormone is released physiologically in a pulsatile manner. During continuous treatment with buserelin there is initial stimulation of luteinizing hormone (LH) and follicle-stimulating hormone (FSH) release, followed by receptor desensitization and suppression of LH and FSH release. This results in regression of the hormone-sensitive tumour. During the initial stages of treatment there is a risk of exacerbation of symptoms from tumour metastases, which can be prevented by use of an androgen receptor antagonist such as cyproterone acetate. Once tolerance to GnRH has developed, cyproterone acetate can be stopped, thereby avoiding the long-term side-effects of androgen-receptor blockade.

Conversely, reduced exposure of a cell or tissue to an agonist that is normally present results in increased receptor numbers and so-called up-regulation. Denervation supersensitivity to acetylcholine is a well-known example. Prolonged use of receptor-blocking drugs may produce an analogous effect. Up-regulation of receptors is important in some of the movement disorders caused by prolonged treatment with antipsychotic drugs (see Chapter 18). One example of clinical importance in some patients is increased β-adrenoceptor numbers following prolonged use of beta-blocking drugs such as atenolol. Abrupt drug withdrawal can lead to tachycardia and worsening angina in patients who are being treated for ischaemic heart disease. Whether receptor up-regulation also contributes to the withdrawal syndromes that occur on abrupt discontinuation of opiates, benzodiazepines, ethanol and anticonvulsants is not known.

NON-RECEPTOR MECHANISMS

In contrast to high-potency/high-selectivity drugs such as atropine or morphine, which combine with specific receptors, some drugs exert their effects via simple physical properties or chemical reactions due to their presence in some body compartment. Examples of medications that work in such ways include antacids (neutralization of gastric acid), the osmotic diuretic mannitol (increasing the osmolality of renal tubular fluid), and bulk and lubricating laxatives. These agents are of low potency and specificity, and hardly qualify as 'drugs' in the usual sense at all, although some of them are very useful medicines. Oxygen is an example of a highly specific therapeutic agent that is used in high concentrations (i.e. it is of low molar potency). It combines with a high-affinity binding site on a transport protein (haemoglobin) as well as dissolving in plasma, and works by promoting aerobic respiration in tissues. This is an example of a therapeutic agent of low potency but high specificity working through a non-receptor mechanism. Finally, metal chelating agents, which are used in the treatment of certain kinds of poisoning and of copper or iron overload in Wilson's disease or thalassaemia, are examples of drugs that exert their effects through interaction with small molecular species rather than with macromolecules, yet which possess significant specificity.

General anaesthetics are believed to act in or on membrane lipids. They have low molar potencies determined by their olive oil/water partition coefficients, and low specificity. Debate as to whether general anaesthetics may in fact after all act on specific receptors in hydrophobic regions of membrane proteins has recently been rekindled. Furthermore, some of the effects of ethanol (another drug sometimes used to exemplify non-receptor-mediated mechanisms) are partly

Key points

- Most drugs are potent and specific; they combine with receptors for endogenous mediators or with high affinity sites on enzymes or ion-transport mechanisms.
- There are four superfamilies of receptors; one is intracellular (e.g. steroid receptors) and three are membrane bound:
  - directly linked to ion channel (e.g. nicotinic acetylcholine receptor);
  - linked via G-proteins to an enzyme, often adenylyl cyclase (e.g. β_2-receptors);
  - directly coupled to the catalytic domain of an enzyme (eg. insulin)
- Many drugs work by antagonizing agonists. Drug antagonism can be:
  - competitive;
  - non-competitive;
  - physiological.
- Partial agonists produce an effect that is less than the maximum effect of a full agonist. They antagonize full agonists.
- Tolerance can be important during chronic administration of centrally acting drugs.

reversed by flumazenil, a benzodiazepine receptor antagonist. The distinction between receptor-mediated and non-receptor-mediated centrally acting drugs is thus currently somewhat blurred.

Case history

A young man is brought unconscious to the emergency room. He is unresponsive and hypoventilating, and he has needle tracks on his arms and pin-point pupils. Naloxone is administered intravenously and within 30 s the patient is fully awake and breathing normally. He is extremely abusive and leaves hospital having attempted to assault the doctor.

Comment

The clinical picture is of opioid narcotic overdose, and this was confirmed by the response to naloxone, a competitive antagonist of opioids at μ-receptors (see Chapter 24). It would have been wise to have restrained the patient before administering the naloxone, which can precipitate withdrawal symptoms. It is to be anticipated that he will again become comatose shortly after discharging himself, as naloxone is eliminated more rapidly than most opioids, so the agonist effect of the overdose will be reasserted as the concentration of the antagonist (naloxone) in the region of the receptors falls while the opioid agonist persists.

Further reading

Rang HP, Dale MM, Ritter JM. 1999: How drugs act: molecular aspects. In *Pharmacology*, 4th edn. Edinburgh: Churchill Livingstone, 19–46.

CHAPTER THREE

PHARMACOKINETICS

- Introduction
- Constant-rate infusion
- Single-bolus dose
- Repeated (multiple) dosing
- Deviations from the one-compartment model with first-order elimination

INTRODUCTION

By convention, pharmacokinetics is defined as the study of the time-course of drug absorption, distribution, metabolism and excretion, whereas the term pharmacodynamics refers to the corresponding pharmacological response. The magnitude of the pharmacological effect is usually directly dependent on the concentration of the drug (or an active metabolite) in the vicinity of the receptors, although there are a few exceptions in the form of 'hit-and-run' drugs that form irreversible bonds with their sites of action so that their effects outlast their presence at these sites (e.g. aspirin, omeprazole, alkylating agents and some monoamine oxidase inhibitors). Understanding pharmacokinetic principles combined with specific information regarding the pharmacokinetic profile of an individual drug facilitates appropriate use of the drug (e.g. route of administration, dose interval), and may to help explain therapeutic failure or toxicity (see Chapter 8). The limitations of this approach also need to be borne in mind. When pharmacokinetic parameters of a particular drug are looked up, it should be appreciated that these are derived from a limited and relatively homogeneous population, usually of healthy male volunteers. Age, genetic factors, disease (especially renal or hepatic disease) or the coadministration of other drugs can markedly alter these values in an individual patient.

In view of the complexity of the human body, it is inevitable that pharmacokinetic formulations must be based on drastically simplifying assumptions. Despite this, such formulations are often mathematically cumbrous, rendering the subject unintelligible to many clinicians. The object of this chapter is to introduce and explain some basic pharmacokinetic concepts by considering three clinical dosing situations, namely constant-rate intravenous infusion, bolus-dose injection and repeated dosing. For a more extended treatment the reader is recommended to consult *Clinical Pharmacokinetics; Consequences and Applications* by Rowland and Tozer.

Bulk flow in the bloodstream is very rapid, as is diffusion after drugs have traversed membranous barriers, so the rate-limiting step in drug distribution is usually the penetration of these barriers. This is determined mainly by the lipid solubility of the drug, highly polar water-soluble drugs being transferred slowly whereas highly lipid-soluble, non-polar drugs are transferred rapidly across the lipid-rich membranes of cells. A few polar drugs are transported rapidly by a different mechanism, namely by combination with a specific carrier. The simplest pharmacokinetic model considers the body to be a single well-stirred compartment in which an administered drug distributes homogeneously instantaneously, and from which it is eliminated. Many drugs are eliminated at a rate that is proportional to their concentration – 'first-order' elimination. A one-compartment model with first-order elimination often approximates the clinical situation surprisingly well once absorption and distribution have occurred. We shall start by considering this, and then describe some important deviations from it.

CONSTANT-RATE INFUSION

If a drug is administered intravenously into one arm via a syringe driven by a constant-rate infusion pump, and a series of blood samples are drawn from the contralateral arm for measurement of drug concentration, a plot of plasma concentration vs. time can be constructed (Figure 3.1). At time zero, just as the infusion is started, the plasma drug concentration is also zero, so the curve begins at the origin. The concentration then rises, rapidly at first and then more slowly until a plateau is approached that represents a steady state. At steady state the rate of input of drug to the body (as determined by the concentration of drug in the syringe and the setting of the infusion pump) is equal to the rate of elimination of drug from the body. The plasma drug concentration at plateau is called the steady-state concentration (C_{SS}). The steady-state concentration depends on the rate of drug infusion, and on the clearance of the drug from the body, such that the greater the infusion rate or the lower the clearance, the greater is C_{SS}. The clearance is the

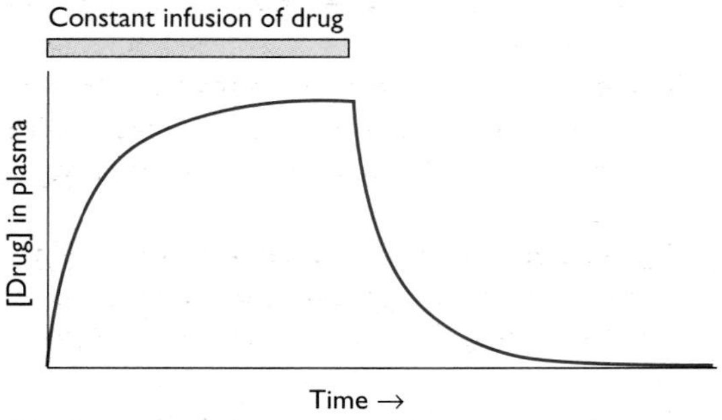

Figure 3.1: Plasma concentration of a drug during and after a constant intravenous infusion as indicated by the bar.

volume of plasma from which the drug is totally eliminated (i.e. cleared) per unit time. At steady state:

$$\text{administration rate} = \text{elimination rate}$$
$$\text{elimination rate} = C_{SS} \times \text{clearance}$$

so:

$$\text{clearance} = \text{administration rate}/C_{SS}$$

Consider an example. A drug is infused at 10 mg/min, and the plasma concentration rises to a steady-state value of 2 mg/mL. At steady state the rate of elimination is the same as the rate of input, i.e. 10 mg/min. Ten milligrams of drug are contained in 5 mL of plasma (since the concentration is 2 mg/mL), so 5 mL of plasma are cleared every minute (clearance = 5 mL/min).

Clearance is the best measure of the efficiency with which a drug is eliminated from the body, whether by renal excretion, metabolism or a combination of both. The concept will be familiar from physiology, where clearances of substances with particular properties are used as measures of physiologically important processes such as glomerular filtration rate, effective renal plasma flow or hepatic plasma flow. For instance, inulin (which is not metabolized, is filtered at the glomeruli but is neither reabsorbed from nor secreted into the renal tubules) is used in this way to estimate the glomerular filtration rate. In the case of therapeutic drugs, knowledge of the clearance in an individual patient helps the physician to adjust the dose accurately in such a way as to achieve a desired target steady-state concentration of drug in the patient's plasma, since:

$$\text{required administration rate} = \text{desired } C_{SS} \times \text{clearance}$$

This is useful in situations where therapy is guided by measurement of drug concentrations in plasma. The reason why clearance is not used more by clinicians is partly that these situations are fairly rare (see Chapter 8), and partly that chemical pathology laboratories often quote therapeutic ranges and report plasma concentrations of drugs in molar terms, whereas drug doses are usually expressed in units of mass. Consequently, one needs to know the molecular weight of the drug before one can use this method of calculating the rate of administration required to achieve a plasma concentration within the given therapeutic range.

When drug infusion is stopped, the plasma concentration declines again toward zero. The time taken for plasma concentration to halve is the half-life ($t_{\frac{1}{2}}$). A one-compartment model with first-order elimination predicts an exponential decline in concentration when the infusion is discontinued as shown in Figure 3.1. After a second half-life has elapsed, the concentration will have halved again (i.e. to 25% of the original concentration), and so on. The increase in drug concentration when the infusion is started is also exponential, being the inverse of the decay curve. This has a very important practical implication, namely that the half-life of a drug not only determines the time-course of its disappearance when administration is stopped, but also determines the time-course of its accumulation when administration is started. This will be discussed again when multiple dosing is considered.

The half-life is a very useful concept for the clinician, helping to determine a sensible dose interval, indicating the time over which drug accumulation occurs after starting a patient on a regular dose regimen, and helping to determine the advisability or otherwise of a loading dose as explained below. However, it is not a direct measure of drug elimination, since differences in $t_{\frac{1}{2}}$ can be caused either by differences in the efficiency of elimination (i.e. the clearance) or differences in another important parameter, namely the volume of distribution (V_d). Clearance and not $t_{\frac{1}{2}}$ must therefore be used when a measure of the efficiency with which a drug is eliminated is required.

SINGLE-BOLUS DOSE

The concept of apparent V_d can be readily understood in the context of the relationship between the size (mass) of a bolus dose and the plasma concentration that results. The volume of distribution is a multiplying factor with units of volume relating the amount of drug in the whole body to the plasma concentration, C_p (i.e. the amount of drug in the body = $C_p \times V_d$). Before addressing the biological situation, consider a very simple physical analogy. By definition, concentration (c) is equal to mass (m) divided by volume (v):

$$c = \frac{m}{v}$$

Thus if a known mass of an inert marker substance (say 300 mg) is dissolved in a glass beaker of water of unknown volume (v), v can be estimated by measuring the concentration of substance in a sample of solution. For instance, if the concentration is 0.1 mg/mL, we would calculate that v = 3000 mL ($v = m/c$). This is valid unless a fraction of the substance has become adsorbed on to the glass surface of the beaker, in which case the solution will be less concentrated than if all of the substance had been present dissolved in the water. If, say, 90% of the substance is adsorbed in this way, then the concentration in solution will be 0.01 mg/mL, and the volume will be correspondingly overestimated, as 30 000 mL in this example. Based on the mass of substance dissolved and the measured concentration, we might say that it is 'as if' the substance was dissolved in 30 L of water, whereas the real volume of water in the beaker is only 3 L.

Now consider the parallel situation in which a known mass of a drug (say 300 mg) is injected intravenously into a human. Suppose that distribution occurs instantaneously before any drug is eliminated, and that blood is sampled and the

Key points

- Pharmacokinetics deals with how drugs are handled by the body, and includes drug, absorption distribution metabolism and excretion.
- Clearance (Cl) is the volume of plasma from which a drug is eliminated (metabolism + excretion) per unit time.
- During constant IV infusion, the plasma drug concentration rises to a steady state (C) determined by the administration rate (A) and clearance (C_{ss} = A/Cl).
- The rate at which C_{ss} is approached as well as the rate of decline in plasma concentration when infusion is stopped are determined by the half-life ($t_{\frac{1}{2}}$).
- The volume of distribution (V_d) is an apparent volume that relates dose (D) to plasma concentration (C): it is 'as if' dose D mg was dissolved in V_d L to give a concentration of C mg/L.

concentration of drug measured in the plasma is 0.1 mg/mL. We could infer that it is 'as if' the drug has distributed in 3 L, and we would say that this is the apparent volume of distribution. If the measured plasma concentration was 0.01 mg/mL, we would say that the apparent volume of distribution was 30 L, and if the measured concentration was 0.001 mg/mL, the apparent volume of distribution would be 300 L.

What does volume of distribution mean? From these examples it is obvious that it is not necessarily the real volume of a body compartment, since it may be greater than the volume of the whole body. At the lower end, values of V_d are limited by the plasma volume (approximately 3 L in an adult). This is the smallest volume in which a drug could distribute following intravenous injection, but there is no theoretical upper limit on V_d, with very large values occurring when very little of the injected dose remains in the plasma, most being taken up into fat or bound to tissues.

In reality, processes of elimination begin as soon as the bolus dose (d) of drug is administered, the drug being cleared at a rate Cl_s (total systemic clearance). In practice, a series of blood samples are obtained at intervals starting shortly after administration of the dose. If the one-compartment, first-order elimination model holds, there is an exponential decline in plasma drug concentration, just as at the end of the constant rate infusion (Figure 3.2a). If the data are plotted on semi-logarithmic graph paper, with time on the abscissa, a straight line with a negative slope results (Figure 3.2b). Extrapolation back to zero time gives the concentration (c_0) that would have occurred at time zero, and this is used to calculate V_d:

$$V_d = \frac{d}{c_0}$$

Half-life can be read off the graph as the time between any point (concentration c_0) and the point at which the concentration c_t has decreased by 50%, i.e. $c_0/c_t = 2$. The slope of the line is the elimination rate constant, k_{el}:

$$k_{el} = \frac{Cl_s}{V_d}$$

$t_{\frac{1}{2}}$ and k_{el} are related as follows:

$$t_{\frac{1}{2}} = \frac{\ln 2}{k_{el}} = \frac{0.693}{k_{el}}$$

The volume of distribution is related partly to the characteristics of the drug, (e.g. lipid solubility) and partly to patient characteristics (e.g.body size, plasma protein concentration, body water and fat content). In general, highly lipid-soluble compounds that are able to penetrate cells and fatty tissues have a large V_d, whereas highly polar water-soluble compounds have a smaller V_d. The volume of distribution determines the peak plasma concentration after a bolus dose, so factors that influence V_d, such as body mass, need to be taken into account when deciding on dose (e.g. by expressing dose per kg body weight). In babies (see Chapter 10), not only is body mass small, but the body composition differs qualitatively from that in the adult, proportionately more body mass being accounted for by aqueous rather than fatty tissues. Thus the 'standard' starting dose expressed on a 'per kg body weight' basis of a polar drug such as gentamicin is higher in babies than in adults. Conversely, in elderly people fat accounts for a greater proportion of body mass than in young adults.

Knowing V_d (or having an estimate of it) tells the physician what peak plasma concentration can be expected following a bolus dose. It is also useful to know V_d when considering dialysis as a means of accelerating drug elimination in poisoned patients (see Chapter 53). Drugs with a

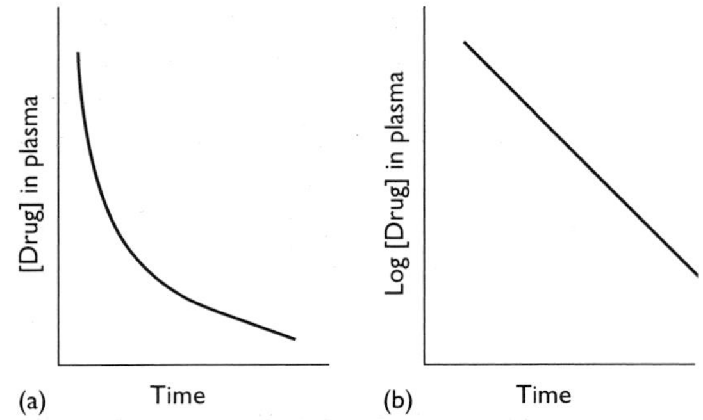

Figure 3.2: One-compartment model. Plasma concentration–time curve following a bolus dose of drug plotted (a) arithmetically and (b) semi-logarithmically. This drug fits a one-compartment model, i.e. its concentration falls exponentially with time.

large V_d (e.g. many tricyclic antidepressants) are unlikely to be removed efficiently by haemodialysis, especially if they are also highly bound by plasma protein, because only a small fraction of the total drug in the body is present in unbound form in the plasma, the fluid compartment accessible to the artificial kidney.

If both V_d and $t_{\frac{1}{2}}$ of a drug are known (or can be estimated) in an individual subject, they can be used to calculate the systemic clearance of the drug using the following expression:

$$Cl_s = 0.693 \times \frac{V_d}{t_{\frac{1}{2}}}$$

Note that clearance has units of volume/unit time (e.g. mL/min), V_d has units of volume (e.g. mL), $t_{\frac{1}{2}}$ has units of time (e.g. min) and 0.693 is a constant arising because $\ln -(0.5) = \ln 2 = 0.693$. This expression relates clearance to V_d and $t_{\frac{1}{2}}$, but unlike the steady-state situation referred to above, it only applies for a single-compartment model with first-order elimination kinetics.

Key points

- The 'one-compartment' model treats the body as a single well-stirred compartment. Immediately following a bolus dose D, the plasma concentration rises to a peak (C_0) theoretically equal to D/V_d and then declines exponentially.
- The rate constant of this process (k_{el}) is given by Cl/V_d. k_{el} is inversely related to $t_{\frac{1}{2}}$, which is given by $0.693/k_{el}$. Thus $Cl = 0.693 \times V_d/t_{\frac{1}{2}}$.
- Repeated bolus dosing gives rise to accumulation similar to that observed with constant-rate infusion, but with oscillations in plasma concentration rather than a smooth rise. The size of the oscillations is determined by the dose interval and by $t_{\frac{1}{2}}$. The steady state is approached (87.5%) after three half-lives have elapsed.

REPEATED (MULTIPLE) DOSING

If multiple doses of a drug are administered at intervals much greater than the half-life, little if any accumulation occurs (Figure 3.3a). Some drugs are used effectively in this way (e.g. penicillin to treat a mild infection by a susceptible organism). More often it is desirable to achieve a continuous finite plasma concentration. Figure 3.3b shows the plasma concentration–time curve that results when a constant dose of drug is administered as a bolus at intervals less than the half-life. It is apparent that the average concentration rises toward a plateau just as if the drug was being administered by constant-rate infusion. That is, after one half-life the average concentration is 50% of the plateau (steady-state) concentration, after two half-lives it is 75%, after three half-lives it is 87.5%, and after four half-lives it is 93.75%. However, unlike the constant-rate infusion situation, the actual plasma concentration at any time swings above or below the mean level. Increasing the dosing frequency smoothes out the peaks and troughs between doses, while decreasing the frequency has the opposite effect. If the peaks are too high, toxicity may result, while if the

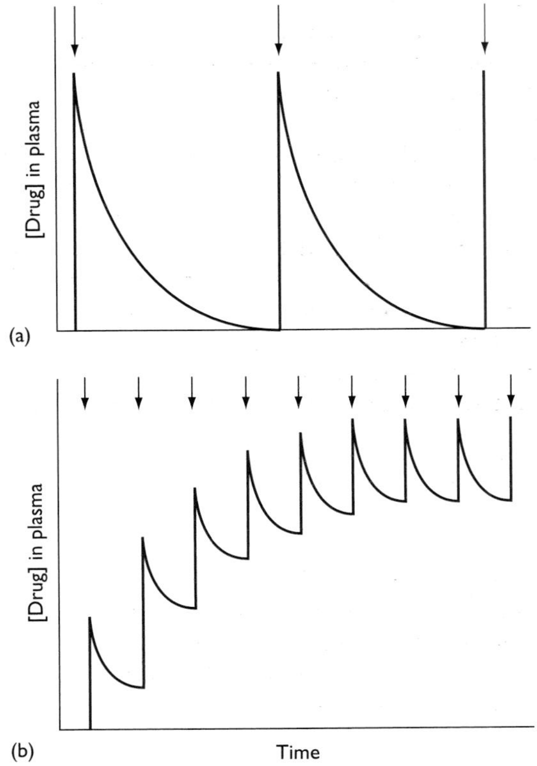

Figure 3.3: Repeated bolus dose injections (at arrows) at (a) intervals much greater than $t_{\frac{1}{2}}$ and (b) intervals less than $t_{\frac{1}{2}}$.

troughs are too low there may be a loss of efficacy. If a drug is administered once every half-life, the peak plasma concentration will be double the trough level. In practice, this amount of variation is acceptable in many therapeutic situations, so a dosing interval is often selected that is approximately equal to the half-life.

Knowing the half-life of a drug alerts the prescriber to the likely time-course over which it will accumulate. Drug excretion often declines with age (see Chapter 11), so that for a given dose higher plasma concentrations may be achieved in the elderly. A further pitfall is that several drugs have active metabolites that are eliminated more slowly than the parent drug. This is the case with several of the benzodiazepines, which have metabolites with half-lives of many days. Consequently, adverse effects such as memory impairment and ataxia, which may incorrectly be ascribed to ageing or disease, may make their appearance when the steady state is approached after several weeks of treatment, when four to five half-lives (of the active metabolite) have elapsed. Such effects only resolve slowly (over a similar time-course) when dosing is discontinued.

Knowing the half-life of a drug also helps the prescribing physician to decide whether or not to initiate treatment with a loading dose. For example, consider the use of digoxin (half-life approximately 40 h). This drug is usually prescribed once daily, resulting in a less than twofold variation in maximum and minimum plasma concentrations, and reaching > 90% of the mean steady-state concentration in approximately 1 week (i.e. four half-lives). In many clinical situations (e.g. a patient with atrial fibrillation and no evidence of heart failure) such a time-course is acceptable. In other cases (e.g. a patient with heart failure and a ventricular rate of 155 beats/min) a more rapid response can be achieved by using a loading dose.

However, this loading-dose strategy is not universally appropriate. Thus the rate-limiting step in achieving a desired therapeutic response may occur at or beyond the level of the receptor (i.e. the time-course of the response may be determined by pharmacodynamic rather than pharmacokinetic processes). Examples include the use of glucocorticoids in a patient with acute severe asthma, where latency is accounted for by processes of transcription and new protein synthesis subsequent to receptor occupancy (see Chapters 2 and 32), or initiation of warfarin treatment in a patient with deep vein thrombosis, where latency depends on clearance from the body of preformed vitamin K-dependent coagulation factors (see Chapter 29).

Deviations from the one-compartment model with first-order elimination

Two-compartment model

This is useful for understanding a situation that often occurs following an intravenous bolus dose. Instead of a simple exponential decline in plasma concentration as predicted by the one-compartment model, what is often actually observed is a biphasic decline (Figure 3.4). The two-compartment model (Figure 3.5) treats the body as a smaller central compartment and a larger peripheral compartment. Again, these compartments have no precise physiological or anatomical meaning, although the central compartment is assumed to consist of blood (from

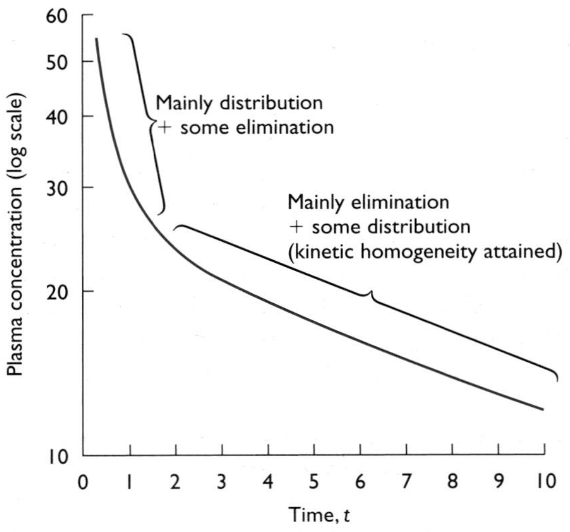

Figure 3.4: Two-compartment model. Plasma concentration-time curve (semi-logarithmic) following a bolus dose of a drug that fits a two-compartment model.

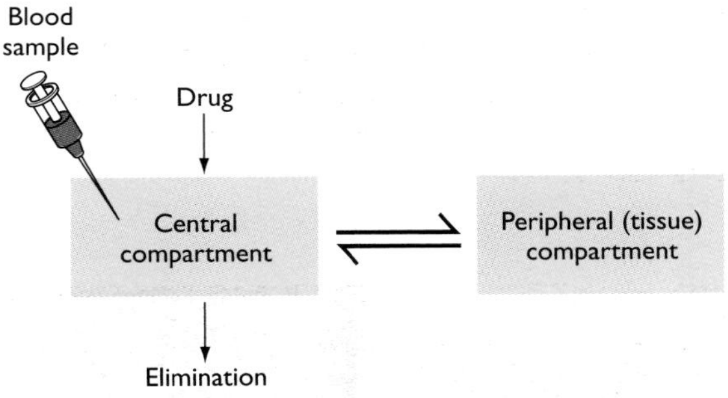

Figure 3.5: Schematic representation of a two-compartment model.

which samples are taken for analysis) with the extracellular spaces of some well-perfused tissues such as heart, lungs, liver and kidneys. The peripheral compartment consists of less well-perfused tissues such as muscle, skin and fat, into which drug permeates more slowly. Reversible transfer occurs between these two compartments depending on such factors as blood flow and affinity of tissues for the drug.

When a drug is instantaneously introduced (i.e. by intravenous injection), into the central compartment the drug concentration in the plasma falls biphasically. The initial rapid fall is called the α phase, and mainly reflects distribution from the central to the peripheral compartment, although elimination also starts from the moment when the drug enters the body. At some point in time a pseudodistribution equilibrium is attained between the central and peripheral compartments, when the ratio of drug in each compartment approaches a constant value which is maintained during the second slower phase of decline in blood concentration, which mainly reflects elimination. This second slower phase is called the β phase, and the corresponding $t_{\frac{1}{2}}$ is known as $t_{\frac{1}{2}\beta}$. This is the appropriate value for clinical use, such as estimation of need for loading dose, time to plateau, likely accumulation and time required for elimination.

For some drugs even the two-compartment model is insufficient to describe the observed plasma concentration–time curves. More complex models such as a three-compartment model with central and 'shallow' and 'deep' peripheral compartments have been used to describe the triphasic decline in the log plasma concentration vs. time curves of several drugs (e.g. amiodarone). However, these are algebraically unwieldy and seldom clinically useful, and will not be considered further here.

Non-linear ('dose-dependent') pharmacokinetics

Although many drugs are eliminated at a rate that is approximately proportional to their concentration (i.e. they obey 'first-order' kinetics), there are several therapeutically important exceptions. To understand how these arise, consider a drug that is eliminated by conversion to an inactive metabolite by an enzyme, and suppose that at high concentrations the enzyme becomes saturated. The drug concentration and reaction velocity will be related by the Michaelis–Menten equation (Figure 3.6). At low concentrations the rate is approximately linearly related to concentration (first-order kinetics), whereas at saturating concentrations the rate is independent of concentration (zero-order kinetics). Similar behaviour is anticipated when a drug is eliminated by a saturable transport process. In clinical practice, drugs that exhibit non-linear kinetics are the exception rather than the rule. This is because most drugs are used therapeutically at doses

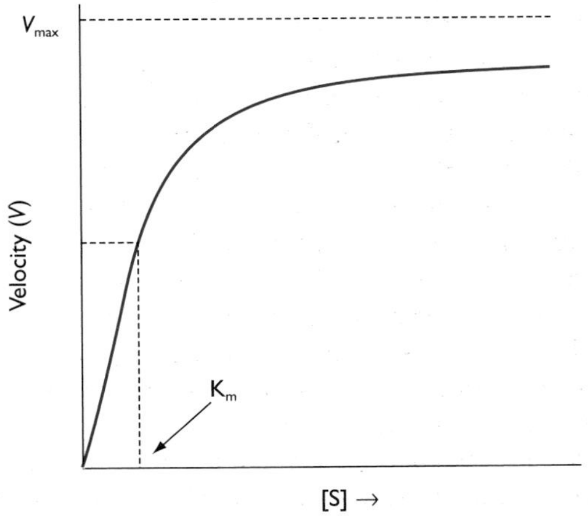

Figure 3.6: Michaelis–Menten relationship between the velocity (V) of an enzyme reaction and the substrate concentration ([S]). [S] at 50% V_{max} is equal to K_m, the Michaelis–Menten constant.

that give rise to concentrations that are well below the Michaelis constant (K_m, i.e. the concentration at which the rate of elimination is half maximal), and so operate on the lower, approximately linear, part of the Michaelis–Menten curve relating elimination velocity to plasma concentration.

Drugs that show non-linear kinetics in the therapeutic range include salicylate, heparin, phenytoin and ethanol. Some drugs (e.g. barbiturates) show non-linearity in the part of the toxic range that is encountered clinically. The implications of non-linear pharmacokinetics include the following.

1 The decline in concentration vs. time following a bolus dose of such a drug is not exponential. Instead, elimination begins slowly and accelerates as plasma concentration falls, as illustrated in Figure 3.7.
2 The time required to eliminate 50% of a dose, increases with increasing dose and the concept of a constant half-life is meaningless.
3 A relatively modest increase in dose of such a drug dramatically increases the amount of drug in the body once the drug-elimination process is saturated, as illustrated in Figure 3.8. This is very important clinically when using

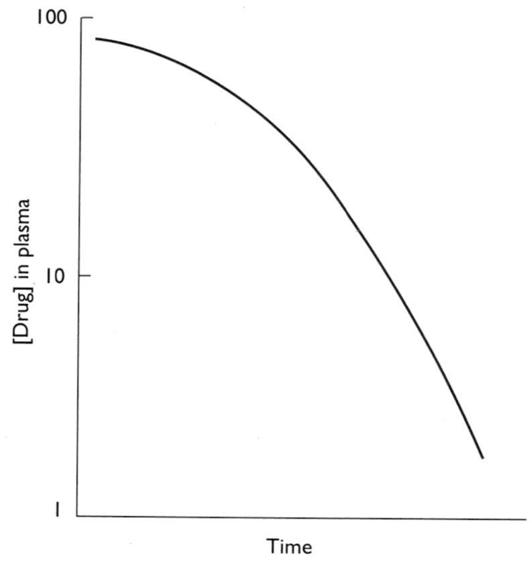

Figure 3.7: Non-linear kinetics: plasma concentration-time curve following administration of a bolus dose of a drug eliminated by Michaelis–Menten kinetics.

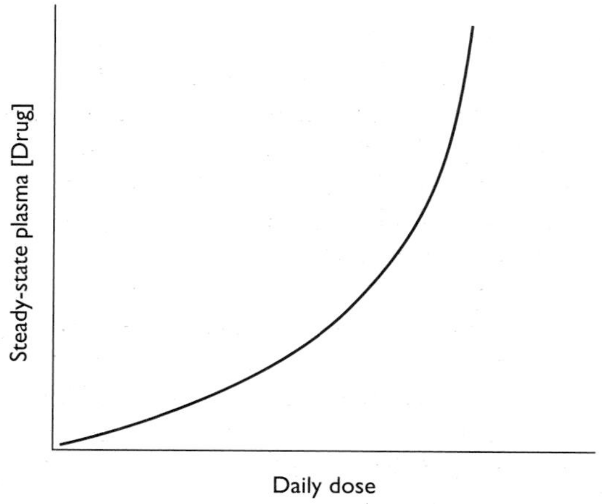

Figure 3.8: Non-linear kinetics: steady-state plasma concentration of a drug following repeated dosing as a function of dose.

plasma concentrations of a drug as a guide to dosing. Consider phenytoin, with a therapeutic range of 10–20 mg/L. If in a particular patient a dose of 200 mg/day is found to give a steady-state plasma concentration of 7.5 mg/L and phenytoin had linear kinetics, doubling the dose to 400 mg/day would double the steady-state plasma concentration to 15 mg/L, which is nicely within the therapeutic range. However, phenytoin does not have linear kinetics, so doubling the dose would actually cause a proportionately much greater increase in concentration and almost certainly precipitate toxicity. A much smaller dose increment is appropriate. Moreover, because of the decreased rate of elimination at higher plasma concentrations (i.e. because of the longer apparent $t_{\frac{1}{2}}$) the plateau is only attained after a longer time period than at the lower dose. In practice, dose increments of phenytoin should therefore be small (25–50 mg/day), and the plasma concentration should be checked 10–14 days after increasing the dose.

ENTEROHEPATIC CIRCULATION

Interpretation of plasma concentration–time curves is complicated when there is an enterohepatic circulation of the drug in question. This occurs

Key points

- *Two-compartment* model. Following a bolus dose, the plasma concentration falls bi-exponentially, instead of a single exponential as in the one-compartment model. The first (α) phase mainly represents distribution; the second (β) phase mainly represents elimination.
- *Non-linear ('dose-dependent') kinetics*. If the elimination process (e.g. drug-metabolizing enzyme) becomes saturated, the clearance rate falls. Consequently, increasing the dose causes a disproportionate increase in plasma concentration. Such drugs (e.g. phenytoin) are often difficult to use in clinical practice.

when drug (e.g. rifampicin, several oestrogens) is conjugated in the liver and conjugate is secreted in the bile but is then broken down by the intestinal flora, with regeneration of free drug that is reabsorbed from the gut. This can result in a second peak in plasma concentration following an intravenous bolus dose.

Case history

A young man develops idiopathic epilepsy and treatment is started with phenytoin, 200 mg daily, given as a single dose last thing at night. After a week, the patient's serum phenytoin concentration is 25 μmol/L. The dose is increased to 300 mg/day. One week later he is complaining of unsteadiness, there is nystagmus and the serum concentration is 125 μmol/L. The dose is reduced to 250 mg/day. The patient's symptoms improve and the serum phenytoin level falls to 60 μmol/L (within the therapeutic range).

Comment

Phenytoin shows dose-dependent kinetics; the serum concentration at the lower dose was below the therapeutic range, so the dose was increased. Despite the apparently modest increase (to 150% of the original dose), the plasma concentration rose disproportionately, causing symptoms and signs of toxicity (see Chapter 21).

FURTHER READING

Rowland M, Tozer TN. 1995: Therapeutic regimens. In *Clinical pharmacokinetics: concepts and applications*, 3rd edn. Baltimore, MD: Williams and Wilkins, 53–105.

CHAPTER FOUR

DRUG ABSORPTION *and* ROUTES *of* ADMINISTRATION

- Introduction
- Bioavailability, bioequivalence and generic vs. proprietary prescribing
- Prodrugs
- Routes of administration

INTRODUCTION

Drugs must cross several biological membranes to reach their sites of action. Drug absorption, and hence the possible routes by which a particular drug may usefully be administered in order to obtain a systemic effect, is determined by the rate and extent of penetration of such membranes. Conversely, drugs are sometimes used for their local effects, in which case systemic absorption from the site of application is a disadvantage. Most biological membranes are readily penetrated by lipid-soluble substances and low-molecular-weight lipid-insoluble molecules, whilst presenting a barrier to larger lipid-insoluble molecules. A simple model considers such membranes as a lipid barrier containing small aqueous channels. The most convenient route of drug administration for patients is usually by mouth, and absorption processes in the alimentary tract are among the best understood.

BIOAVAILABILITY, BIOEQUIVALENCE AND GENERIC VS. PROPRIETARY PRESCRIBING

Drugs must reach the systemic circulation if they are to exert a systemic effect. When administered other than intravenously, and specifically when administered by mouth, most drugs are absorbed incompletely (Figure 4.1). There are three reasons for this:

1 drug is inactivated within the gut lumen by gastric acid, digestive enzymes or bacteria;
2 absorption is incomplete; and
3 presystemic ('first-pass') metabolism occurs in the gut wall and liver.

If hepatic metabolism is rapid and extensive, nearly all of an absorbed dose may be cleared from the portal venous blood so that little or no drug is present in hepatic venous blood (i.e. the hepatic *extraction ratio* is nearly 100%), and little drug enters the systemic circulation. Together these processes account for the fact that the bioavailability of orally administered drugs (i.e. the extent to which the active component in a pharmaceutical product enters the systemic circulation in active form) is less than 100%. Drug absorption depends on the presence of drug in solution at the absorption site. Many factors in the manufacture of the dosage form influence its disintegration, dispersion and dissolution. Pharmaceutical factors are therefore important in determining bioavailability. Tablets and capsules are complex products, for in addition to the drug there are excipients, disintegrating agents, binders, diluents, lubricants and dyes, all of which

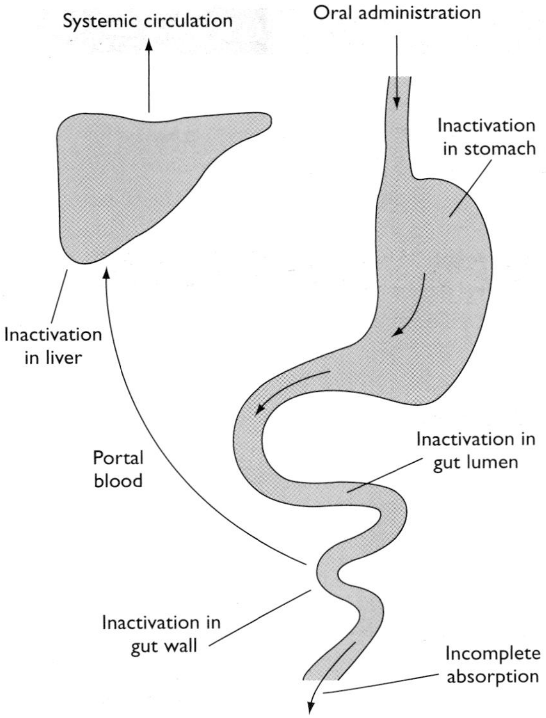

Figure 4.1: Drug absorption following oral administration may be incomplete for several reasons.

contribute to their performance as drug delivery systems, and influence bioavailability.

Differences in absorption from different preparations of the same drug occur, but it is important to distinguish statistically significant from clinically important differences in this regard. The former are common, whereas the latter are not. However, differences in bioavailability did account for an epidemic of anticonvulsant intoxication in Australia in 1968–1969. This was investigated in Brisbane, where affected patients were found to be taking one brand of phenytoin. It was shown that the excipient in the responsible phenytoin capsules was changed from calcium sulphate to lactose several months before the outbreak, and that this change increased phenytoin bioavailability, thereby precipitating toxicity.

Similarly, an apparently minor change in the manufacturing process of Lanoxin™ (a digoxin preparation made in the UK) resulted in reduced potency due to poor bioavailability, making this comparable with the potency of most other brands. Restoring the original manufacturing conditions restored potency but led to some confusion, and considerable variation occurred in blood levels recorded in patients who changed from 'old' to 'new' Lanoxin. These events drew attention to the non-equivalence of digoxin tablets available in the UK, and alerted physicians to the potential for toxicity due to treatment with different digoxin formulations. Improved manufacturing standards have now reduced these problems.

These examples raise the question of whether prescribing should be by generic name or by proprietary or brand name. When a new preparation is marketed in the UK it has a proprietary name supplied by the pharmaceutical company, and a non-proprietary (generic) name supplied by the *British Pharmacopoiea*. It is usually available only from the company that introduced it until the patent expires. After this, other companies can manufacture and market the product, sometimes under its generic name and sometimes under their own proprietary name. At this stage, hospital pharmacists usually shop around for the best buy. If a hospital doctor prescribes by proprietary name, the same drug produced by another company may be substituted. This saves considerable amounts of money. In contrast, if a general practitioner prescribes a proprietary product, the pharmacist must dispense that product even though it may cost more than the same drug made by another company. The attractions of generic prescribing in terms of minimizing costs are therefore obvious, but there are counterarguments, the strongest of which relates to the bioequivalence or otherwise of the proprietary product with its generic competitors. The formulation of a drug (i.e. excipients, etc.) differs between products, sometimes affecting bioavailability. This is a particular concern with slow-release or sustained-release preparations, or preparations to be administered by different routes (e.g. rectal vs. oral preparations). Drug regulatory bodies have strict criteria to assess whether such products can be licensed without the full supporting information that would be required for a completely new product (i.e. one based on a new chemical entity).

Absolute bioavailability is determined by measuring the area under the plasma concentration–time curve (AUC) following oral and intravenous administration (100% bioavailability). The area under the concentration–time curve represents the

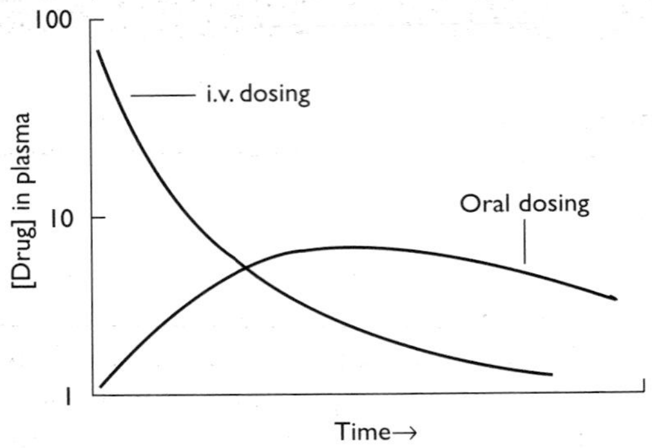

Figure 4.2: Oral vs. intravenous dosing: plasma concentrations–time curves following administration of a drug (I.V.) or by mouth (oral).

amount of drug absorbed, so a comparison of AUC after oral administration with AUC after intravenous administration expressed as a percentage gives the percentage bioavailability following oral administration (Figure 4.2). It will be noted that the absolute bioavailability of two drugs may be the same (i.e. the same AUC), but that the kinetics may be very different (e.g. one may have a much higher peak plasma concentration than the other, but a shorter duration). The rate at which a drug enters the body determines the onset of its pharmacological action, and also influences the intensity and sometimes the duration of its action, and is important in addition to the extent (completeness) of absorption.

The concept of bioavailability can also be criticized as implying a spurious precision and universality to the numerical value assigned. It must be appreciated that bioavailability will vary not only between groups of patients with different characteristics of age, gastrointestinal motility and pH, hepatic blood flow, and so on, but also that changes of these variables occur within an individual, so 'bioavailability' can vary from one occasion to another. However, doctors prescribing for patients need to be confident that different preparations (branded or generic) are sufficiently similar for their substitution to be unlikely to lead to clinically important alterations in outcome. Regulatory authorities have responded to this need by requiring companies who are seeking to introduce generic equivalents to products that are no longer protected by patent to present evidence

Key points

- Drugs must cross membranes to reach the systemic circulation, unless they are administered intravenously. This is determined by the lipid solubility of the drug and the area of membrane available for absorption, which is very large in the case of the ileum, because of the villi and microvilli. Sometimes polar drugs can be absorbed via specific transport processes (carriers).
- Even if absorption is complete, not all of the dose may reach the systemic circulation if the drug is metabolized in the wall of the intestine or in the liver, which can extract drug from the portal blood before it reaches the systemic circulation via the hepatic vein. This is called presystemic (or 'first-pass') metabolism.
- 'Bioavailability' describes the completeness of absorption into the systemic circulation. The amount of drug absorbed is determined by measuring the plasma concentration at intervals after dosing and integrating by estimating the area under the plasma concentration/time curve (AUC). This AUC is expressed as a percentage of the AUC when the drug is administered intravenously (100% absorption). 0% bioavailability implies that no drug enters the systemic circulation, whereas 100% bioavailability means that all of the dose is absorbed into the systemic circulation. Bioavailability may vary not only between different drugs and different pharmaceutical formulations of the same drug, but also from one individual to another, depending on factors such as dose, whether the dose is taken on an empty stomach, and the presence of gastrointestinal disease.
- The *rate* of absorption is also important (as well as the completeness), and is expressed as the time to peak plasma concentration (T_{mex}). Sometimes it is desirable to formulate drugs in slow-release preparations to permit once daily dosing and/or to avoid transient adverse effects corresponding to peak plasma concentrations. Substitution of one such preparation for another may give rise to clinical problems unless the preparations are 'bioequivalent'. Regulatory authorities may therefore require evidence of bioequivalence before licensing generic versions of existing products.
- Prodrugs are metabolized to pharmacologically active products. They provide an approach to improving absorption and distribution.

that their product behaves similarly to the one that is currently marketed. If evidence is presented that a new product can be treated as therapeutically equivalent to the current 'market leader' this is accepted as 'bioequivalence'. This does not imply that all possible pharmacokinetic parameters are identical between the two products, but that any such differences are unlikely to be of medical importance, and it is a useful regulatory concept, albeit one that is hard to define quantitatively in a general way (i.e. applying to different drugs).

It is impossible to give a universal answer to the generic vs. proprietary issue for prescribing doctors. However, substitution of generic for brand-name products seldom causes problems. In addition, brand names cause confusion by creating multiple alternatives to the approved name, and unlike many approved names they seldom reveal the pharmacological category of the drug (e.g. suffix -olol for beta-blockers, -statin for β-hydroxymethylglutaryl coenzyme A (HMGCoA) reductase inhibitors, -opril for converting-enzyme inhibitors, etc.).

PRODRUGS

One approach to improving absorption or distribution to a relatively inaccessible tissue (e.g. brain) is to modify the drug molecule chemically to form a compound that is better absorbed and from which active drug is liberated after absorption. Such modified drugs are termed prodrugs. Examples are shown in Table 4.1.

Table 4.1: Prodrugs

Prodrug	Product
Elanapril	Enalaprilat
Benorylate	Aspirin + paracetamol
Levodopa	Dopamine
Minoxidil	Minoxidil sulphate
Carbimazole	Methimazole

ROUTES OF ADMINISTRATION

ORAL ROUTE

For local effect

Oral drug administration may be used to produce local effects within the gastrointestinal tract. Examples include antacids, activated charcoal (given in some cases of poisoning to bind the toxic agent in the gut lumen), oral vancomycin (given to patients with pseudomembranous colitis to kill toxin-producing *Clostridium difficile* within the bowel), and sulphasalazine, which delivers 5-amino salicylic acid (5-ASA) to the colon, thereby prolonging remission in patients with ulcerative colitis. Sulphasalazine commonly causes adverse effects (5–55% of patients treated), ranging from trivial to severe. These are mainly attributable to the sulphapyridine moiety rather than the active 5-ASA, leading to the design of agents without a sulphur-based carrier. These include mesalazine and olsalazine, which have different mechanisms whereby the active 5-ASA is liberated. Mesalazine has a pH-dependent acrylic coat that degrades when the surrounding pH is greater than 7, as in the colon and distal part of the ileum. Olsalazine is a prodrug consisting of a dimer of two 5-ASA moieties joined by an azo bond that is cleaved by colonic bacteria. Olsalazine is superior to mesalazine in preventing relapses of ulcerative colitis, especially those which occur in the distal and sigmoid colon, presumably because it delivers 5-ASA more reliably than mesalazine to the distal colon.

Drugs that are not absorbed can have a systemic effect via an indirect action. Cholestyramine, a bile acid binding resin that lowers plasma concentrations of low-density lipoprotein cholesterol and reduces the risk of myocardial infarction in men with hypercholesterolaemia, is an example of this.

For systemic effects

Oral administration of drugs is safer and more convenient than injection. There are two main mechanisms of drug absorption by the gut.

Passive diffusion

This is the most important mechanism. Non-polar lipid-soluble agents are well absorbed from the gut, mainly from the small intestine, because of its enormous absorptive surface area. In the case of weak acids or weak bases, the non-ionized form of the drug is relatively fat soluble and thus diffuses easily. Absorption is therefore influenced by the *pK* of the drug and the pH at the absorption site. However, in practice the very large surface area of the small intestine is of overriding importance. For example, if salicylate (a weak acid) is given with propantheline (which slows gastric emptying) its absorption is retarded, whereas if it is given with metoclopramide (which speeds gastric emptying) its absorption is accelerated.

Active transport

This requires a specific, carrier-mediated, energy-consuming mechanism. Naturally occurring polar nutrients and aliments including sugars, amino acids and vitamins are absorbed by active or facilitated transport mechanisms. Drugs that are analogues of such molecules compete with these substrates and are transported via the carrier. Examples include L-dopa, methyldopa, some antimetabolites (such as methotrexate and 5-fluorouracil) and lithium (which competes with sodium ions for absorption).

Other factors that influence absorption from the gastrointestinal tract include the following:

1 *surgical interference with gastric function* – gastrectomy reduces absorption of drugs, including digoxin, levodopa, sulphonamides, ethambutol, ethionamide, iron and folic acid;
2 *disease of the gastrointestinal tract* (e.g. coeliac disease, cystic fibrosis) – the effects of such disease are unpredictable, but often surprisingly minor (see Chapter 7);
3 *the presence of food or other substances in the gut* – the timing of drug administration in relation to food can be important. Food and drink dilute the drug and can adsorb or otherwise complex with it. Food also influences the rate and/or extent of absorption by altering gastric emptying. Transient increases in hepatic portal blood flow, such as occur after a meal, may result in *greater* availability of drug by reducing presystemic hepatic metabolism. Plasma concentrations of propranolol and metoprolol are considerably higher when given with food, for this reason.
Conversely, most oral antibiotics should be given on an empty stomach to avoid impairment of absorption by food. Anthelmintics should also be taken similarly to maximize the concentration of drug to which the parasites are exposed. Indomethacin, levodopa, iron preparations, sodium valproate and other drugs that are likely to cause indigestion when given on an empty stomach should be taken with food;
4 *drug metabolism by intestinal flora* – this may affect drug absorption and activity. The examples of sulphasalazine and olsalazine have been described above. Sulphinpyrazone is converted to an active sulphide metabolite by bacteria in the colon. Alteration of bowel flora (e.g. by concomitant use of antibiotics) can interrupt enterohepatic recycling and result in loss of activity of the low oestrogen contraceptive pill (see Chapter 13 on drug interactions).

Prolonged action and sustained-release preparations

Some drugs with short elimination half-lives need to be administered at inconveniently short intervals, making compliance difficult for the patient. A drug with similar actions but a longer half-life may be substituted. Examples are terazosin or doxazosin (long-acting α_1-adrenoceptor antagonists) for prazosin, or amlodipine (a long-acting calcium-channel antagonist) for nifedipine. Where no such option exists, there are various pharmaceutical means of slowing absorption of a rapidly eliminated drug. The aim of such sustained-release preparations is to release a steady 'infusion' of drug into the gut lumen for absorption during transit through the small intestine. Reduced dosing frequency may improve compliance and, in the case of some drugs (e.g. carbamazepine, quinidine), may reduce adverse effects due to high peak plasma concentrations. Absorption of such preparations is likely to be incomplete, so it is especially important that bioavailability is established before their general introduction. Other problems associated with slow-release preparations include the following.

1 Because transit time through the small intestine is only about 6 h, prolongation of the dosage interval from 12 to 24 h is not reliably achieved.
2 If the gut lumen is narrowed or intestinal transit is slow, as in the elderly, there is a danger of high local drug concentrations causing mucosal damage. Osmosin™, an osmotically released formulation of indomethacin, had to be withdrawn because it caused bleeding and ulceration of the small intestine.
3 Overdose with sustained-release preparations is difficult to treat because large amounts of drug continue to be absorbed several hours after the tablets have left the stomach.
4 There is reduced flexibility of dosing, since sustained-release tablets should not be divided.
5 Expense.

BUCCAL AND SUBLINGUAL ROUTE

Drugs are administered to be retained in the mouth for local disorders of the pharynx or buccal mucosa such as aphthous ulcers (hydrocortisone lozenges or carbenoxelone gel) or thrush (nystatin lozenges).

Sublingual administration is an effective means of causing systemic effects, and has distinct advantages over oral administration (i.e. the drug to be swallowed) for drugs with pronounced presystemic metabolism, providing direct and rapid access to the systemic circulation, bypassing the intestine and liver. Glyceryl trinitrate and buprenorphine are given sublingually for this reason. Glycerine trinitrate is taken either as a sublingual tablet or as a spray. Sublingual administration provides short-term effects which can be terminated by swallowing the tablet. Tablets for buccal absorption provide more sustained plasma concentrations, and are held in one spot between the lip and the gum until they have dissolved.

RECTAL ROUTE

Drugs may be given rectally for their local effects (e.g. sulphasalazine or corticosteroid suppositories or retention enemas in the treatment of proctitis). Drugs are also absorbed when administered by this route, and are sometimes given rectally, a route of administration that is culturally more accepted in France and Italy than in the UK, for their systemic effects rather than their local actions. The following advantages have been claimed for the rectal route of administration.

1 Exposure to the acidity of the gastric juice and to digestive enzymes is avoided.
2 The portal circulation is partly bypassed, thereby reducing presystemic metabolism.
3 This route can be used in patients who are unable to swallow or who are vomiting.
4 Its duration of action may be prolonged.

Rectal diazepam is useful for controlling convulsions when it is impossible to establish venous access during status epilepticus (as is often the case in children). Metronidazole is well absorbed when administered rectally, and is less expensive than intravenous preparations. Rectal administration is occasionally used to ensure nocturnal absorption of drugs (e.g. indomethacin for the morning stiffness of rheumatoid arthritis), or when the drug is poorly absorbed when given by mouth (e.g. ergotamine during a migraine attack), but there are usually more reliable alternatives, and drugs that are given rectally can cause severe local irritation.

SKIN

Drugs are applied topically to treat skin diseases such as psoriasis or acne (see chapter 50). Systemic absorption can sometimes cause undesirable effects, for example in the case of potent glucocorticoids, especially if applied to large areas under occlusive dressings, but the application of drugs to skin can also be used to achieve a systemic therapeutic effect. The skin has evolved as an impermeable integument, so the problems of getting drugs through it are completely different from transport through an absorptive surface such as the gut. Factors affecting percutaneous drug absorption include the following:

1 *skin condition* – injury and disease affecting the stratum corneum result in shunts across the horny layer allowing greater penetration. The penetration of isotopically labelled hydrocortisone increases from 1–2% to 78–90% after removal of the stratum corneum by repeated stripping with cellophane tape;
2 *age* – infant skin is more permeable than adult skin;
3 *region* – skin sites differ in permeability (plantar < anterior forearm < scalp < scrotum < posterior auricular skin);
4 *hydration of the stratum corneum* – this is one of the most important factors, which increases the passage of all substances that penetrate skin. Under plastic-film occlusion (sometimes employed by dermatologists) the stratum corneum changes from a tissue normally containing very little water (10%) to one containing up to 50% water with increased permeability. Penetration of corticosteroids into the skin is increased up to 100-fold by occlusion, and systemic side-effects occur more commonly;
5 *vehicle* – little is known about the importance of the various substances which over the years have been empirically included in skin creams and ointments. The physical chemistry of these mixtures may be very complex and change during an application. For example, evaporation of water from an ointment may cause phase reversal from a suspension of oil in water to a suspension of water in oil, with resulting changes in the solubility and partitioning of drug within the ointment;
6 *physical properties of the drug* – as with other biological membranes, penetration of drugs through skin increases with increasing lipid solubility of the drug. When compounds are relatively insoluble, reduction of particle size in the cream or ointment enhances absorption, and solutions penetrate best of all. As expected, the rate of drug absorption increases as the drug concentration in the preparation is increased;
7 *surface area to which the drug is applied* – this is especially important when treating infants who have a relatively large surface area to volume ratio.

Transdermal absorption is sufficiently reliable to enable systemically active drugs (e.g. glyceryl trinitrate, oestradiol, hyoscine, nicotine) to be administered by this route in the form of patches to be applied to the skin. As with injection or buccal administration, transdermal administration bypasses presystemic metabolism in the gut wall or liver. Patients should be instucted to apply each dose to the same general anatomical area (e.g. chest for glyceryl trinitrate, buttock for oestradiol, behind the ear for hyoscine), but to a different spot for successive patches, to minimize local irritation. Patches are more expensive than alternative preparations, and are only justified if a particular patient markedly prefers them, or in some instances of poor compliance.

Gels or creams are sometimes rubbed into the skin overlying a tender muscle or joint. This may influence symptoms by the following:

1 placebo effect;
2 mechanical effects of rubbing/massage on underlying blood vessels and other structures;
3 a so-called 'counterirritant' effect, i.e. the relief of discomfort in a deep structure by stimulating pain fibres in the skin by some irritant such as capsaicin (the irritant from red pepper);
4 absorption of a non-steroidal anti-inflammatory drug such as piroxicam. Although small amounts of piroxicam are absorbed transdermally, this does not lead to higher concentrations in the underlying joint than elsewhere in the body, and the efficacy of such gels is not great.

LUNGS

Drugs, notably steroids, β_2-adrenoceptor agonists, muscarinic receptor antagonists and sodium cromoglycate, are inhaled as aerosols or particles for their local effects on bronchioles. Nebulized antibiotics are also sometimes used in children with cystic fibrosis and recurrent *Pseudomonas* infections. Drug absorption in these circumstances can give rise to unwanted systemic effects. Physical properties that limit systemic absorption are therefore desirable. For example, ipratropium is a quaternary ammonium ion analogue of atropine which is highly polar by virtue of the charged quaternary ammonium N^+ group, and is consequently poorly absorbed and has fewer atropine-like side-effects than would a more lipid-soluble muscarinic receptor-blocking drug. A large fraction of an 'inhaled' dose of salbutamol is in fact swallowed. However, the bioavailability of swallowed salbutamol is low due to inactivation by sulphation in the gut wall, so systemic effects such as tremor are minimized in comparison to effects on the bronchioles.

The lungs are ideally suited for absorption from the gas phase, since the total respiratory surface area is about 60 m^2, through which only 60 mL blood are percolating in the capillaries, thus presenting an enormous absorptive surface area. This is exploited in the case of volatile anaesthetics, as discussed in Chapter 23.

NOSE

Drugs such as steroids and sympathomimetic amines may be administered intranasally for their local effects on the nasal mucosa. Systemic absorption may result in undesirable effects, such as loss of control of blood pressure by antihypertensive medication, in such circumstances.

Nasal mucosal epithelium has remarkable and potentially very valuable absorptive properties, notably the capacity to absorb intact complex peptides that cannot be administered by mouth because they would be digested. This has opened up an area of therapeutics that was previously limited by the inconvenience of repeated injections. At present, drugs administered by this route include desmopressin (DDAVP – an analogue of antidiuretic hormone) for patients with diabetes insipidus and buserelin (an analogue of gonadotropin-releasing hormone) for patients with prostate cancer, but there is great interest in this area and every reason to hope for new indications for intranasal administration.

EYE, EAR AND VAGINA

Drugs are administered topically to these sites for their local effects (e.g. chloramphenicol eyedrops for purulent conjunctivitis, sodium bicarbonate eardrops for softening wax, and nystatin pessaries for treating *Candida* infections). Occasionally, they are absorbed in sufficient quantity to have undesirable systemic effects, such as worsening of asthma caused by timolol (a β-adrenoceptor antagonist) eyedrops given for open-angle glaucoma, or diarrhoea caused by a prostaglandin E_2 pessary administered to induce therapeutic abortion. However, such absorption is not sufficiently reliable to make use of these routes for therapeutic ends.

Systems have been developed to apply drugs locally using rate-controlling membranes. For example, the pilocarpine 'Ocusert' system for glaucoma is a flat, flexible, elliptical-shaped device consisting of a drug reservoir core containing pilocarpine enclosed in two outer plastic polymer membranes. These membranes give a zero-order release rate of pilocarpine, i.e. release is at a constant rate and does not decrease as the reservoir empties. The device is small enough to insert comfortably into the lower conjunctival sac, and can remain there releasing drug for several days. This may improve compliance, since the alternative is to use pilocarpine drops several times daily, and it also provides smoother control of intra-ocular pressure with a reduced total pilocarpine dosage.

INTRAMUSCULAR INJECTION

Lipid-soluble drugs diffuse freely through capillary walls and are well absorbed when administered intramuscularly. Polar drugs can also be absorbed rapidly, provided they are of low molecular weight. However, polar drugs of high molecular weight are only absorbed slowly, via the lymphatics.

The rate of absorption is also governed by the total surface area available for diffusion, and is increased when the solution is distributed throughout a large volume of muscle. Dispersion of the solution is enhanced by massage of the injection site. Transport away from the injection site is governed by muscle blood flow, and this varies from site to site (deltoid > vastus lateralis > gluteus maximus). Blood flow to muscle is increased by exercise and absorption rates are increased in all sites after exercise. Conversely, shock, heart failure or other conditions that decrease muscular blood flow reduce absorption.

The drug must be sufficiently water soluble to remain in solution at the injection site until absorption occurs. This is a problem for some drugs, including phenytoin, diazepam and digoxin, as crystallization and/or poor absorption occur when these are given by intramuscular injection, which should therefore be avoided. Slow absorption is useful in some circumstances where appreciable concentrations of drug are required for prolonged periods. For example, benzathine penicillin is a suspension for deep intramuscular injection of value in treating late latent syphilis which is caused by sensitive slowly dividing organisms (penicillin works by inhibiting bacterial cell wall synthesis in dividing organisms; see Chapter 42). Depot intramuscular injections are also used to improve compliance in psychiatric patients (e.g. the decanoate ester of fluphenazine which is slowly hydrolysed to release active free drug).

Intramuscular injection has a number of disadvantages:

1. pain – muscle is poorly innervated with pain fibres compared to skin, but distension with large volumes is painful, and injected volumes should usually be no greater than 5 mL;
2. sciatic nerve palsy following injection into the buttock – this is avoided by injecting into the upper outer gluteal quadrant;
3. sterile abscesses at the injection site (e.g. paraldehyde);
4. elevated serum creatine phosphokinase due to enzyme release from muscle can cause diagnostic confusion;
5. severe allergic reactions (e.g. anaphylaxis) may be protracted because there is no way of stopping absorption of the drug;
6. the intramuscular route is not always more effective or rapid than the oral route (e.g. for diazepam or chlordiazepoxide, oral administration requires a lower dose of drug and produces a given level of sedation more rapidly than intramuscular injection);
7. haematoma formation can occur, especially after fibrinolytic therapy.

Subcutaneous injection

This is influenced by the same factors that affect intramuscular injections. Cutaneous blood flow is lower than in muscle, and therefore absorption is slower. If the skin of a limb is injected, drug absorption is increased by exercise (one factor in exercise-induced hypoglycaemia in insulin-dependent diabetics). Absorption is retarded by immobilization, reduction of blood flow by a tourniquet and local cooling, all of which may be used to reduce absorption in wasp stings and snake bites.

Adrenaline incorporated into an injection reduces the absorption rate by causing vasoconstriction. Conversely, hyaluronidase increases it by spreading the injection more widely within subcutaneous tissues.

Sustained effects from subcutaneous injections are extremely important clinically, most notably in the treatment of insulin-dependent diabetics. Isophane insulin is a suspension of insulin with protamine often used to initiate twice daily regimes. Insulin zinc suspension (amorphous) has an intermediate duration of action, and insulin zinc suspension (crystalline) has a more prolonged duration of action.

Sustained effects have also been obtained from subcutaneous injections by using oily suspensions (e.g. in the past of vasopressin, now largely superceded by intranasal administration of desmopressin), or by implanting a compressed pellet of drug subcutaneously (e.g. oestrogen or testosterone for hormone replacement therapy).

Intravenous injection

This has the following advantages:

1. rapid action (e.g. frusemide in pulmonary oedema);
2. presystemic metabolism is avoided (e.g. glyceryl trinitrate infusion in patients with unstable angina);
3. intravenous injection is used for drugs that are not absorbed by mouth (e.g. gentamicin and heparin). It is also used for drugs that are too painful or toxic to be given intramuscularly (e.g. streptokinase or mustine). Mustine and other cytotoxic drugs must not be allowed to leak from the vein or considerable damage and pain will result;
4. intravenous infusion is easily controlled, enabling precise titration of drugs with short half-lives. This is essential for drugs such as sodium nitroprusside or epoprostenol (prostacyclin).

The chief drawbacks of intravenous administration are as follows:

1 once injected, drugs cannot be recalled;
2 very high drug levels result if the drug is given too rapidly – the right heart receives the highest concentration, possibly as a bolus, and drugs with arrhythmogenic potential such as phenytoin have caused fatal cardiac arrest when administered too rapidly by this route;
3 embolism of foreign particles or air, sepsis or thrombosis are all possible, especially in addicts self-administering drugs of abuse. Probably the greatest hazard during legitimate use is sepsis occurring via intravenous catheters in neutropenic, immunosuppressed or debilitated patients;
4 accidental extravascular injection or leakage of toxic drugs (e.g. doxorubicin and vincristine) produce severe local tissue necrosis;
5 inadvertent intra-arterial injection can cause arterial spasm and peripheral gangrene.

INTRATHECAL INJECTION

This route provides access to the central nervous system for drugs that are normally excluded by the blood–brain barrier. This inevitably involves very high risks of neurotoxicity, and this route should *never* be used without adequate training. (In the UK, junior doctors who have made mistakes of this kind have been held criminally as well as professionally negligent.) The possibility of causing death or permanent neurological disability is such that extra care must be taken in checking that both the drug and the dose are correct. Examples of drugs used in this way include methotrexate (to eliminate malignant cells from the central nervous system in childhood leukaemias) and local anaesthetics (e.g. bupivacaine) or opiates (e.g. morphine) administered by an anaesthetist to produce spinal anaesthesia. (More commonly anaesthetists use the much safer extradural route to administer local anaesthetic drugs to produce regional analgesia without depressing respiration, e.g. in women during labour.) Aminoglycosides are sometimes administered by neurosurgeons via a cisternal reservoir to patients with Gram-negative infections of the

Key points

- Oral – generally safe and convenient.
- Buccal/sublingual – circumvents presystemic metabolism.
- Rectal – useful in patients who are vomiting.
- Transdermal – limited utility, avoids presystemic metabolism.
- Lungs – volatile anaesthetics.
- Nasal – useful absorption of some peptides (e.g. DDAVP; see Chapter 41).
- Intramuscular – useful in some urgent situations (e.g. behavioural emergencies).
- Subcutaneous – useful for insulin and heparin in particular.
- Intravenous – useful in emergencies for most rapid and predictable action, but too rapid administration is potentially very dangerous, as a high concentration reaches the heart as a bolus.
- Intrathecal – specialized use by anaesthetists.

Case history

The health visitor is concerned about an 8-month-old girl who is failing to grow. The child's mother tells you that she has been well apart from a recurrent nappy rash, but on examination there are features of Cushing's syndrome. On further enquiry the mother tells you that she has been applying clobetasone, which she had been prescribed herself for eczema, to the baby's napkin area. There is no biochemical evidence of endogenous over-production of glucocorticoids. The mother stops using the clobetasone cream on her daughter, on your advice. The features of Cushing's syndrome regress and growth returns to normal.

Comment

Clobetasone is an extremely potent steroid (see Chapter 50). It is prescribed for its topical effect but can penetrate skin, especially of an infant. The amount prescribed that is appropriate for an adult would readily cover a large fraction of an infant's body surface area. If plastic pants are used around the nappy this may increase penetration through the skin (just like an occlusive dressing, which is often deliberately used to increase the potency of topical steroids; see Chapter 50), leading to excessive absorption and systemic effects as in this case.

brain. The antispasmodic baclofen is sometimes administered by this route.

Penicillin used to be administered intrathecally to patients with pneumococcal meningitis, because of the belief that it penetrated the blood–brain barrier inadequately. However, when the meninges are inflamed (as in meningitis), high-dose intravenous penicillin results in adequate concentrations in the cerebrospinal fluid. Intravenous penicillin should now always be used for meningitis, since penicillin is a predictable neurotoxin (it was formerly used to produce an animal model of seizures), and seizures, encephalopathy and death have been caused by injecting a dose intrathecally that would have been appropriate for intravenous administration.

FURTHER READING

Fix JA. 1996: Strategies for delivery of peptides utilizing absorption-enhancing agents. *Journal of Pharmaceutical Sciences* **85**:1282–5.

Mathiovitz E, Jacobs JS, Jong NS *et al*. 1997: Biologically erodable microspheres as potential oral drug delivery systems. *Nature* **386**:410-14.

Rowland M, Tozer TN. 1995: Absorption and distribution Kinetics. In *Clinical pharmacokinetics: concepts and applications*, 3rd edn. Baltimore, MD: Williams and Wilkins, 11–50.

Rowland M, Tozer TN. 1995: Absorption. In *Clinical pharmacokinetics: concepts and applications*, 3rd edn. Baltimore, MD: Williams and Wilkins, 119–36.

Rowland M, Tozer TN. 1995: Distribution. In *Clinical pharmacokinetics: concepts and applications*, 3rd edn. Baltimore, MD: Williams and Wilkins, 137–55.

CHAPTER FIVE

DRUG METABOLISM

- Introduction
- Phase I metabolism
- Metabolism of drugs by intestinal organisms
- Phase II metabolism (conjugation reactions)
- Enzyme induction
- Enzyme inhibition
- Presystemic metabolism ('first-pass' effect)

INTRODUCTION

Drug metabolism is a complex and important part of biochemical pharmacology. There are considerable species variations in drug metabolism and, at least until recently, the subject has been hindered by limited availability of human tissue. Much of our present understanding derives from analytical studies of drugs and metabolites in plasma or urine from human volunteers. The aim of this chapter is to introduce some of the basic principles of drug metabolism.

The pharmacological activity of many drugs is reduced or abolished by enzymic processes, and drug metabolism is one of the main mechanisms by which drugs are inactivated. Examples include oxidation of phenytoin and of alcohol. However, not all metabolic processes result in inactivation, and drug activity is sometimes *increased* by metabolism, as in activation of prodrugs (e.g. decarboxylation of levodopa to dopamine in central neurones, and conversion of enalapril to its active metabolite enalaprilat).

The formation of polar metabolites from a non-polar drug permits efficient urinary excretion (see Chapter 6). However, some metabolic transformations result in active compounds with a longer half-life than the parent drug (e.g. diazepam has a half-life of 20–50 h, whereas its pharmacologically active metabolite desmethyldiazepam has a plasma half-life of approximately 100 h). Delayed effects that manifest many days after starting regular treatment with such drugs can be caused by the accumulation of such long-lived metabolites.

It is convenient to divide drug metabolism into two phases (I and II) (Figure 5.1) which sometimes, but not always, occur sequentially. Phase I reactions involve a metabolic modification of the drug (commonly oxidation, reduction or hydrolysis). Products of phase I reactions may be either pharmacologically active or inactive. Phase II reactions are synthetic conjugation reactions between the drug and a second molecule (or between a phase I metabolite of a drug and a second molecule). The products have increased polarity compared to the parent drugs and are therefore more readily excreted in the urine (or,

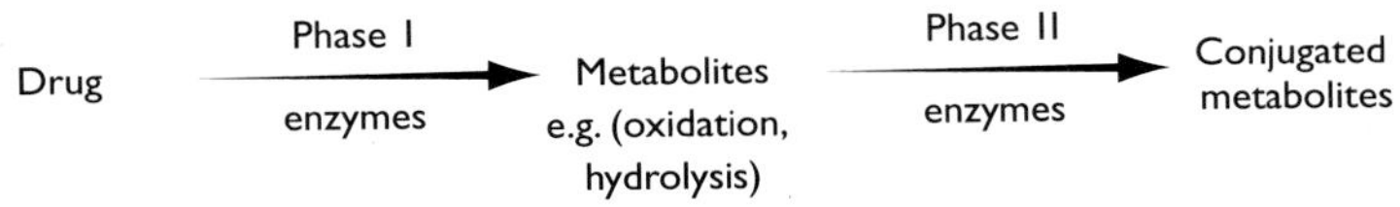

Figure 5.1: Phase I and II of drug metabolism.

less often, in the bile), and they are usually – but not always – pharmacologically inactive. Molecules or groups involved in conjugation reactions include glucuronic acid, glycine, glutamine, sulphate and acetate.

PHASE I METABOLISM

The liver is the most important site of drug metabolism. Hepatocyte endoplasmic reticulum is particularly important, but the cytosol and mitochondria are also involved in phase I reactions.

ENDOPLASMIC RETICULUM

Hepatic smooth endoplasmic reticulum contains enzyme systems that metabolize foreign substances ('xenobiotics', i.e. drugs as well as pesticides, fertilizers and other chemicals that may contaminate human food supplies). Centrifugation of hepatic homogenates yields a microsomal fraction that is rich in endoplasmic reticulum, and is used to study these metabolic processes, which include oxidation, reduction and hydrolysis.

Oxidation

Microsomal oxidation causes aromatic or aliphatic hydroxylation, deamination, dealkylation or S-oxidation. These reactions all involve reduced nicotinamide adenine dinucleotide phosphate (NADP), molecular oxygen, mixed function oxidase and one or more of a group of cytochrome P_{450} haemoproteins. Cytochrome P_{450} (so named because it reacts with carbon monoxide to yield a pink (P) complex with an absorption peak at 450 nm) acts as a terminal oxidase in the oxidation reaction. Such reactions are generally rather non-specific with regard to substrate, in contrast to many enzyme-catalysed reactions, although cytochrome P_{450} exists in several distinct isoenzyme forms, each with a different, albeit often overlapping, pattern of substrate preferences (Table 5.1).

Modern pharmacology owes much to the study of plant-derived products (alkaloids), and it may be that it was of selective advantage to be able to detoxify a range of such plant poisons. The most versatile mechanism for doing so, namely the cytochrome P_{450} system, may have evolved from other cytochromes and cytochrome P_{450} enzyme systems involved in the oxidative biosynthesis of mediators or other biochemically important intermediates. For example, synthase enzymes involved in the oxidation of arachidonic acid to prostaglandins and thromboxanes are cytochrome P_{450} enzymes with distinct specificities.

Reduction

Reduction requires reduced NADP-cytochrome c reductase or reduced NAD-cytochrome b_5 reductase. Chloramphenicol is reduced by NADH and a nitroreductase in the liver by this mechanism.

Hydrolysis

Pethidine is de-esterified to meperidinic acid by hepatic membrane-bound esterase activity.

NON-ENDOPLASMIC RETICULUM DRUG METABOLISM

Oxidation

Oxidation of alcohol to acetaldehyde and of chloral to trichlorethanol is catalysed by a cytosolic enzyme ('alcohol dehydrogenase') whose substrates also include vitamin A and the aldehyde retinene. Diamine oxidase (DAO) and monoamine oxidase (MAO) are membrane-bound mitochondrial enzymes that oxidatively deaminate primary amines to aldehydes (further oxidized to carboxylic acids) or ketones. Monoamine oxidase occurs in liver, kidney, intestine and nervous tissue, and its substrates include catecholamines (dopamine, noradrenaline and adrenaline), tyramine, phenylephrine and tryptophan derivatives (5-hydroxytryptamine and tryptamine). Diamine oxidase has a substrate specificity overlapping that of MAO, and is involved in histamine metabolism. Oxidation of purines by xanthine oxidase (e.g. of 6-mercaptopurine to inactive 6-thiouric acid) is non-microsomal.

Reduction

This includes, for example, enzymic reduction of double bonds, e.g. methadone, naloxone.

Table 5.1: Cytochrome P_{450} isoenzymes commonly involved in drug metabolism with representative drug substrates and their specific inhibitors and inducers

Enzyme	Substrate	Inhibitor	Inducer
Cytochrome $P_{450\ 1A2}$	Caffeine Theophylline Warfarin	Cimetidine Fluvoxamine	Smoking Cruciferous vegetables
**Cytochrome $P_{450\ 2A6}$	Coumarin		
**Cytochrome $P_{450\ 2C9}$	Losartan Naproxen Phenytoin Warfarin	Fluconazole Sulphenazole	Barbiturates Rifampicin
**Cytochrome $P_{450\ 2C19}$	Diazepam Moclobamide Omeprazole Proguanil	Fluoxetine Ketoconazole	
**Cytochrome $P_{450\ 2D6}$	Codeine (Opioids) Dextromethorphan Haloperidol Metoprolol Mexilitine Nortryptiline Propafenone	Cimetidine Fluoxetine Quinidine	
Cytochrome $P_{450\ 2E1}$	Chlormezanone Halothane Paracetamol Theophylline	Diethyldithio-carbamate	Ethanol Isoniazid
Cytochrome $P_{450\ 3A4}$	Amiodarone Astemizole Cyclosporin Hydrocortisone (& other steroids) Lignocaine Lovastatin Midazolam Nifedipine Tamoxifen Tacrolimus Terfenadine Vincristine	Cimetidine Diltiazem Erythromycin (and other macrolides) Gestodene Grapefruit juice Itraconazole Ketoconazole Saquinavir Ritonavir Verapamil	Barbiturates Carbamazepine Dexamethasone Rifampicin

** = Known genetic polymorphisms
Approximate % of drugs used therapeutically metabolized by each isoenzyme:
Cytochrome $P_{450\ 3A4}$ = 58%; cytochrome $P_{450\ 2D6}$ = 20%; cytochrome $P_{450\ 2C}$ = 18%; cytochrome $P_{450\ 1A2}$ = 2%; cytochrome $P_{450\ 2E1}$ = 2%

Hydrolysis

Esterases catalyse hydrolytic reactions, including cleavage of suxamethonium by plasma cholinesterase, an enzyme that exhibits pharmacogenetic variation (see Chapter 14), as well as hydrolysis of aspirin (acetylsalicylic acid) to salicylate, of enalapril to enalaprilat and of many other drugs.

Metabolism of drugs by intestinal organisms

This is important for drugs undergoing entero-hepatic circulation. For example, oestradiol,which is excreted in bile as a glucuronide conjugate, loses glucuronic acid by microbial activity so that free drug is available for reabsorption via the terminal ileum, only a small proportion (approximately 7%) being excreted in the faeces under normal circumstances, although this can increase if gastrointestinal disease or concurrent antibiotic use alters the intestinal flora.

Phase II metabolism (conjugation reactions)

Glucuronidation

Conjugations between glucuronic acid and carboxyl groups are involved in the metabolism of bilirubin, salicylate and lorazepam.

Some patients inherit a deficiency of glucuronide formation that presents clinically as a non-haemolytic jaundice due to excess unconjugated bilirubin (Crigler–Najjar syndrome). Drugs that are normally conjugated in this way aggravate the jaundice in such patients.

O-glucuronides formed by reaction with a hydroxyl group of the drug result in an ether glucuronide. This occurs with morphine, paracetamol and chloramphenicol.

Amino acid reactions

Glycine and glutamine are the amino acids chiefly involved in conjugation reactions in humans. Glycine forms conjugates with nicotinic acid and salicylate, whilst glutamine forms conjugates with *p*-aminosalicylate. Hepatocellular damage depletes the intracellular pool of these amino acids, thus restricting this pathway. Amino acid conjugation is also reduced in the newborn.

Acetylation

Acetate derived from acetyl coenzyme A conjugates with several drugs, including isoniazid, hydralazine and procainamide (see Chapter 14 for a discussion in polymorphic variation in drug acetylation). Acetylating activity resides in the cytosol and is widely distributed, occurring in leucocytes and gastrointestinal cells as well as in the liver, in which it is present in reticulo-endothelial rather than parenchymal cells.

Methylation

Methylation proceeds by a pathway involving S-adenosyl methionine as methyl donor to drugs with free amino, hydroxyl or thiol groups. Catechol O-methyltransferase is an example of such a methylating enzyme, and is of physiological as well as pharmacological importance. It is present in the cytosol, and catalyses the transfer of a methyl group to catecholamines, inactivating noradrenaline, dopamine and adrenaline. Phenylethanolamine N-methyltransferase is also important in catecholamine metabolism. It methylates the terminal $-NH_2$ residue of noradrenaline to form adrenaline in the adrenal medulla. It also acts on exogenous amines, including phenylethanolamine and phenylephrine. It is induced by glucocorticoids, and its presence in high activity in the adrenal medulla reflects the anatomical arrangement of the blood supply to the medulla which comes from the adrenal cortex and consequently contains very high concentrations of corticosteroids.

Sulphation

Sulphation of hydroxyl (alcoholic or phenolic) and amine groups occurs in the cytosol via an active sulphate compound, 3′-phosphoadenosine 5′-phosphosulphate (PAPS). This system forms sulphates such as heparin and chondroitin sulphate under physiological conditions. Sulphotransferases produce ethereal sulphates from several oestrogens and androgens, from 3-hydroxycoumarin (a phase I metabolite of warfarin) and from chloramphenicol. There are a number of

S-transferases in the liver, with different specificities.

Mercapturic acid formation

Mercapturic acid formation via reaction with cysteine in glutathione (a tripeptide) is a relatively unusual pathway. However, it is very important in *paracetamol overdose*, when the usual pathway of paracetamol elimination is overwhelmed, with resulting production of a highly toxic metabolite (N-acetylbenzoquinone imine, NABQI). NABQI is detoxified by conjugation with reduced glutathione, and the availability of this is critical in determining the clinical outcome. Seriously poisoned patients are therefore treated with thiol donors such as acetyl cysteine or methionine to increase the endogenous supply of reduced glutathione (see Chapter 53).

Glutathione conjugates

Naphthalene and some sulphonamides also form conjugates with glutathione. One endogenous function of glutathione conjugation is formation of a sulphidopeptide leukotriene, leukotriene (LT) C_4. This is formed by conjugation of glutathione with LTA_4, analogous to a phase II reaction. LTA_4 is an epoxide which is synthesized from arachidonic acid by a 'phase I' type oxidation reaction catalysed by a lipoxygenase enzyme. LTC_4, together with its dipeptide product LTD_4, comprise the activity once known as slow-reacting substance of anaphylaxis, and these leukotrienes are believed to play a role as bronchoconstrictor mediators in anaphylaxis and possibly in asthma (see Chapter 32).

Enzyme induction

Enzyme induction (Table 5.1) is a process in which there is enhanced enzyme activity because of increased enzyme synthesis (or, less often, reduced enzyme breakdown). This increased enzyme activity is sometimes accompanied by hypertrophy of the endoplasmic reticulum. There is a rise in cytochrome P_{450} content and increased cytochrome P_{450} reductase activity. The size of the liver and hepatic blood flow also increase.

There is much inter-individual variability in the degree of induction produced by a given agent, part of which is inherited.

Studies of induction suggest selectivity. For example, rifampicin selectively increases N-demethylation of antipyrine relative to its 4-hydroxylation and 3-methylhydroxylation. Exogenous inducing agents include not only drugs but also halogenated insecticides (particularly chlorophenothane – DDT – and gamma-benzene hexachloride), herbicides, polycyclic aromatic hydrocarbons, dyes, food preservatives, nicotine and alcohol. A practical consequence of enzyme induction is that if two or more drugs are given simultaneously, then one substance that is an inducing agent accelerates the metabolism of other drugs (see Chapter 13 for a discussion of the practical consequences of this). Substrates of induced drug-metabolizing enzymes include pollutants, carcinogens and normal body constituents (e.g. steroids, bilirubin, thyroxine and fat-soluble vitamins), in addition to drugs.

Tests for enzyme induction

The level of induction of liver enzymes can be assessed by measuring the clearance of a drug such as antipyrene on other probe substrates such as debrisoquine, although this is seldom indicated clinically. The erythrocyte breath test or the urinary ratio of 6-β-hydroxycortisol/cortisol have also been used. It is unlikely that a single test will ever be totally adequate, since the mixed function oxidase system is so complex that at any one time the activity of some enzymes may be increased and that of others reduced.

Enzymes in cells (e.g. fibroblasts and lymphocytes) and tissues other than liver are also capable of undergoing induction.

Induction of drug metabolism is a model of variable expression of a constant genetic constitution. It is important in drug elimination and also in several other biological processes, including adaptation to extrauterine life, which involves a series of biochemical changes, delay in which is hazardous to the infant. Many of the mediators of such changes are hormones, including glucocorticoids, thyroxine and glucagon.

Neonates fail to form glucuronide conjugates because of immaturity of hepatic glucuronyl transferase. Chloramphenicol conjugation (and hence excretion) is impaired, rendering neonates at risk of 'grey baby' syndrome if they are treated with chloramphenicol. Defective bilirubin conjugation increases the risk of accumulation of unconjugated lipid-soluble bilirubin that can enter the brain, staining the basal ganglia ('kernicterus') and causing choreoathetosis. Another important consequence of immature enzyme systems in premature infants is a low level of lung surfactant and consequent respiratory distress. Administration of glucocorticoids as enzyme inducers to the mothers of certain high-risk babies before delivery reduces the likelihood of this hazard.

Enzyme inhibition

Several drugs, including monoamine oxidase inhibitors, allopurinol, methotrexate, converting-enzyme inhibitors, non-steroidal anti-inflammatory drugs and many others, exert their therapeutic effects by enzyme inhibition. Quite apart from such direct actions, inhibition of drug metabolism by a concurrently administered drug (Table 5.1) can lead to drug accumulation and toxicity. For example, cimetidine, which owes its therapeutic action to antagonism at the histamine H_2-receptor, inhibits drug metabolism by the cytochrome P_{450} system and therefore potentiates the actions of quite unrelated drugs such as warfarin (see Chapter 13). However, this kind of clinically important enzyme inhibition is, less common than enzyme induction.

The specificity of enzyme inhibition is sometimes incomplete. For example, disulfiram, which is used to encourage abstinence in alcoholics, owes its therapeutic effect to inhibition of oxidation of acetaldehyde formed from ethanol, but it also prolongs the half-life of antipyrine and raises the steady-state plasma concentrations of warfarin and phenytoin in patients receiving these drugs. The mechanism of these last two interactions is unknown, but presumably results from inhibition of microsomal drug metabolism. Warfarin and phenytoin compete with one another for metabolism, coadministration resulting in elevation of plasma steady-state concentrations of both drugs. Chloramphenicol is a non-competitive inhibitor of microsomal enzymes and inhibits phenytoin, tolbutamide and chlorpropamide metabolism.

Presystemic metabolism ('first-pass' effect)

The metabolism of some drugs is markedly dependent on the route of administration. Following oral administration, drugs gain access to the systemic circulation via the portal vein, so the entire absorbed dose is exposed first to the intestinal wall and then to the liver before gaining access to the rest of the body. A considerably smaller fraction of the absorbed dose goes through gut and liver in subsequent passes because of distribution to other tissues and drug elimination by other routes.

If a drug is subject to a high hepatic clearance (i.e. it is rapidly metabolized by the liver), a substantial fraction will be extracted from the portal blood and metabolized before it reaches the systemic circulation. This is known as presystemic metabolism.

The route of administation and presystemic metabolism markedly influence the pattern of drug metabolism. For example, when salbutamol is given to asthmatic subjects, the ratio of unchanged drug to metabolite in the urine is 2:1 after intravenous administration, but 1:2 after an oral dose. When lignocaine is given orally, the concentrations of the major primary metabolite monoethyl glycine xylidide (MEGX) are comparable to those of lignocaine itself, whereas after a single intravenous dose, MEGX concentrations are about 15–20% of those of lignocaine. Propranolol undergoes substantial hepatic presystemic metabolism, and small doses given orally are completely metabolized before they reach the systematic circulation. After intravenous administration the area under the plasma concentration–time curve is proportional to the dose administered and passes through the origin, (Figure 5.2). After oral administration the relationship, although linear, does not pass through the origin and there is a threshold dose below which measurable concentrations of propranolol are not detectable in systemic venous plasma. In patients with portocaval anastomoses

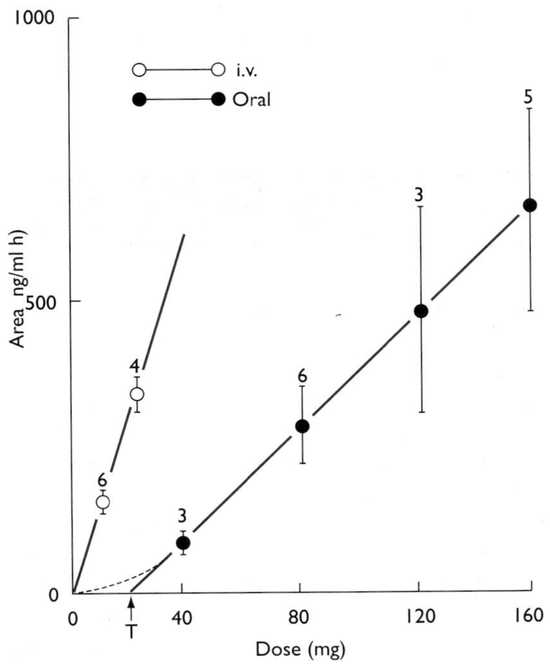

Figure 5.2: Area under blood concentration–time curve after oral (•) and intravenous (o) administration of propanolol to humans in various doses. T′ is the apparent threshold for propanolol following oral administration (Reproduced from Shand DG and Rangno RE 1972: *Pharmacology* **7**, 159 with permission of S Karger AG, Basle.)

bypassing the liver, hepatic presystemic metabolism is bypassed, so very small doses are needed compared to the usual oral dose.

Presystemic metabolism is not limited to the liver, since the gastrointestinal mucosa also metabolizes drugs such as salbutamol, levodopa, chlorpromazine cyclosporin before they enter hepatic portal blood. Pronounced first-pass metabolism by either the gastrointestinal mucosa (e.g. salbutamol, levodopa) or liver (e.g. glyceryl trinitrate, morphine, naloxone) necessitates high oral doses by comparison with the intravenous route. Alternative routes of drug delivery (e.g. rectal, buccal, sublingual, inhalation or transdermal routes) partly or completely bypass presystemic elimination (see Chapter 4).

Drugs that undergo extensive presystemic metabolism usually exhibit pronounced inter-individual variability in drug disposition. This results in highly variable responses to therapy, and is one of the major difficulties in their clinical use. Variability in first-pass metabolism results from the following:

1 genetic variation – for example, the bioavailability of hydralazine is about twofold greater in slow compared to fast acetylators. Presystemic hydroxylation of debrisoquine, metoprolol and encainide also depends on a genetic polymorphism;
2 induction or inhibition of metabolic enzymes;
3 food increases liver blood flow and can *increase* the bioavailability of drugs such as propranolol, metoprolol and hydralazine by increasing the amount of drug presented to the liver in unit time above the threshold for complete hepatic extraction;
4 drugs that increase liver blood flow have similar effects to food – for example, hydralazine

Key points

- There are two phases of drug metabolism. Phase I metabolism introduces a reactive group into a molecule, usually by oxidation, by a microsomal system present in the liver. Cytochrome P_{450}, a family of haemoproteins with many distinct isoenzyme forms, is critical to many phase I reactions.
- Products of phase I metabolism may be pharmacologically active as well as being chemically reactive. They can cause toxic effects as they are produced in the liver.
- Phase II reactions involve conjugation (e.g. glucuronidation).
- Products of phase II metabolism are polar and can therefore be excreted efficiently by the kidneys. Unlike the products of phase I metabolism, they are nearly always pharmacologically inactive.
- Phase I and phase II reactions often (but not invariably) occur in sequence, the conjugation reaction involving the reactive group inserted by the phase I oxidation.
- Cytochrome P_{450} enzymes can be induced by several drugs and dietary constituents (e.g. carbamazepine, alcohol, brussels sprouts).
- Cytochrome P_{450} enzymes are also inhibited by drugs (e.g. cimetidine, several antibiotics) and dietary constituents (e.g. grapefruit).
- Induction or inhibition of the cytochrome P_{450} system are important causes of drug interactions (see Chapter 13).

Case history

A 32-year-old woman is brought to the hospital emergency room by her sister, having swallowed an unknown number of paracetamol tablets washed down with vodka 6 h previously, after a row with her partner. She is a known alcoholic. Apart from signs of intoxication, examination is unremarkable. Plasma paracetamol concentration is 100 mg/L. Following discussion with the Resident Medical Officer/Poisons Information Service, it is decided to administer acetylcysteine.

Comment

In paracetamol overdose, the usual pathway of elimination is overwhelmed and a highly toxic product (N-acetyl benzoquinone imine, known as "NABQI") is formed by cytochrome P_{450} metabolism. A plasma paracetamol concentration of of 100 mg/L 6 h after ingestion would not usually require treatment, but in this alcoholic woman the liver enzymes will have been induced, so the threshold for active treatment is lowered (see Chapter 53). Acetylcysteine is a specific antidote, as it increases reduced glutathione which conjugates NABQI within hepatocytes.

increases propranolol bioavailability by approximately one-third, whereas drugs that reduce liver blood flow (e.g. β-adrenoceptor antagonists) reduce it;

5 non-linear first-pass kinetics are common (e.g. hydralazine, propranolol, 5-fluorouracil) – increasing the dose disproportionately increases bioavailability, so the fraction of the dose of such a drug that reaches the systemic circulation depends dramatically on dose. When low doses of aspirin are given orally, little or no acetyl salicylic acid reaches the systemic circulation, and acetylation of cyclo-oxygenase is limited to portal venous tissues and to circulating elements such as platelets. Larger doses result in appreciable systemic concentrations of aspirin, as well as its metabolite salicylate;

6 liver disease increases the bioavailability of some drugs with extensive first-pass extraction, (e.g. chlormethiazole and pethidine).

Further reading

Boobis AR, Edwards RJ, Adams DA, Davies DS. 1996: Dissecting the function of P_{450}. *British Journal of Clinical Pharmacology* **42**, 81–9.

Halpert JR. 1995: Structural basis of selective P_{450} inhibition. *Annual Review of Pharmacology and Toxicology* **35**, 29–53.

Nelson DR, Koymans L, Kamataki T. 1996: P_{450} superfamily: update on new sequences, gene mapping, accession numbers and nomenclature. *Pharmacogenetics* **6**, 1–42.

Park BK, Kitteringham NR, Pirmohamed M, Tucker GT. 1996: Relevance of induction of human drug-metabolising enzymes: pharmacological and toxicological implications. *British Journal of Clinical Pharmacology* **41**, 477–91.

CHAPTER SIX

RENAL EXCRETION *of* DRUGS

INTRODUCTION

The kidneys are involved to some degree in the elimination of virtually every drug or drug metabolite. Whether or not renal elimination is the major or only a minor contributor to total body clearance of any particular drug is largely determined by its polarity. The kidneys receive 20% of the cardiac output, and in a healthy young adult about 130 mL/min of protein-free filtrate is formed at the glomeruli. Only 1–2 mL of this filtrate finally appears in the urine. Consequently, non-polar lipid-soluble drugs are very efficiently reabsorbed down the >100-fold concentration gradient that is generated between tubular and interstitial fluids.

Non-polar drugs often have a large volume of distribution (due to partition into fat), so only a small fraction of drug in the body at any time is present in plasma where it is accessible to glomerular filtration or secretion into the tubules. Elimination of non-polar drugs therefore usually depends on metabolic conversion in the liver or intestine to more polar metabolites, which are then excreted in the urine. Polar substances are eliminated efficiently by the kidneys, because they are not freely diffusible across the tubular membrane and so remain in the urine despite the concentration gradient favouring back-diffusion into interstitial fluid. Renal elimination of polar drugs or drug metabolites is influenced by several processes that alter the drug concentration in the tubular fluid. Depending on which of these predominates, the renal clearance of a drug may be either an important or a trivial component in its overall elimination.

GLOMERULAR FILTRATION

The glomerular filtrate contains similar concentrations of low-molecular-weight solutes to plasma. In contrast, molecules with a molecular weight of ≥ 66 000 (including plasma proteins and drug–protein complexes) do not pass the glomerulus. Accordingly, only free drug passes into the filtrate. Renal impairment (see Chapter 7) predictably reduces the elimination of drugs that depend on glomerular filtration for their clearance (e.g. digoxin, aminoglycoside antibiotics). Drugs that are highly bound to albumin in plasma are not efficiently filtered, because only the free fraction is able to diffuse down its concentration gradient into the glomerular fluid, and this has little effect on the total (bound plus free) concentration of drug in plasma in the glomerular capillaries.

Proximal tubular secretion

There are mechanisms for active secretion of both acids and bases into the tubular fluid in the proximal segment. These are relatively non-specific in their structural requirements, and share some of the characteristics of transport systems in the intestine. The organic acid transport mechanism excretes hippuric acid, endogenous phenols, sulphates and glucuronides, as well as acidic drugs such as probenecid, penicillin and some sulphonamides. For some acidic drugs (e.g. benzylpenicillin) virtually all of the drug is excreted in this way. Para-aminohippuric acid (PAH) is excreted so efficiently by this mechanism that at appropriate concentrations it is completely extracted from the renal plasma in a single pass (i.e. during intravenous infusion of PAH its concentration in renal venous blood is zero). Clearance of PAH is therefore limited by the rate at which it is delivered to the kidney, i.e. renal blood flow. Consequently PAH clearance is used as a non-invasive measure of renal blood (or, more strictly, renal plasma) flow.

The organic base transport mechanism contributes to the elimination of basic drugs (e.g. quinidine, cimetidine) from the body.

Each mechanism is characterized by a maximal rate of transport for a given drug, so the process is theoretically saturable, although this maximum is rarely reached in practice. Because secretion of free drug occurs up a concentration gradient from peritubular fluid into the lumen, the equilibrium between unbound and bound drug in plasma can be disturbed, with bound drug dissociating from protein-binding sites. Unlike glomerular filtration, tubular secretion can therefore eliminate drugs efficiently even if they are highly protein bound. Competitive effects can occur between drugs carried on these systems. Thus probenecid, a weak acid, competitively inhibits the tubular secretion of the penicillins and methotrexate, whilst cimetidine competes with quinidine for the basic drug transport system.

Passive distal tubular reabsorption

The renal tubule behaves like a lipid barrier separating the high drug concentration in the tubular lumen and the lower concentration in the interstitial fluid and plasma. Reabsorption of drug down its concentration gradient therefore occurs by passive diffusion. To traverse the lipid membrane of the tubule, the drug must be lipid soluble, so that for highly lipid-soluble drugs such as griseofulvin, reabsorption is so effective that its renal clearance is virtually zero. Conversely, polar substances, such as mannitol, are too water soluble to be absorbed, and are eliminated virtually without reabsorption.

Tubular reabsorption is influenced by urine flow rate. Diuresis increases the renal clearance of drugs that are passively reabsorbed, since the concentration gradient is reduced. Diuresis may be induced deliberately in order to increase drug elimination during treatment of overdose.

Reabsorption of drugs that are weak acids (AH) or bases (B) depends upon the pH of the tubular fluid, because this determines the fraction of acid or base in the charged, polar form and the fraction in the uncharged non-polar lipid-soluble form. For acidic drugs, the more alkaline the urine, the greater the renal clearance, and vice versa for basic drugs, since:

$$AH \rightleftharpoons A^- + H^+$$

and

$$B + H^+ \rightleftharpoons BH^+$$

Thus high pH (alkaline conditions) favours A^-, the charged form of the weak acid which remains in the tubular fluid and is excreted in the urine, while low pH (acid conditions) favours BH^+, the charged form of the base. This is utilized in treating overdose with aspirin (a weak acid) by causing an alkaline urine, thereby accelerating elimination of salicylate (see Chapter 53).

The extent to which urinary pH affects renal excretion of weak acids and bases depends quantitatively upon the pK_a of the drug. Relatively strong acids or bases are essentially completely ionized (and therefore lipid insoluble) over the entire range of physiological urine pH, and so undergo little passive reabsorption. The critical range of pK_a values for pH-dependent excretion is about 3.0–6.5 for acids and 7.5–10.5 for bases.

Urinary pH may also influence the fraction of the total dose which is excreted unchanged. Thus about 57% of a dose of amphetamine is excreted unchanged (i.e. as the parent drug rather than as a metabolite) in acid urine (pH 4.5–5.6), compared to about 7% in subjects with alkaline urine (pH 7.1–8.0). Administration of amphetamines with sodium bicarbonate has been used illicitly by athletes to enhance the pharmacological effects of the drug on performance, as well as to make its detection by urinary screening tests more difficult. The extent to which urinary pH changes alter the rate of drug elimination naturally depends on the contribution that renal clearance makes to the total drug clearance from the body.

Key points

- The kidney cannot excrete non-polar substances efficiently, since these diffuse back into blood as the urine is concentrated. Consequently, the kidney excretes polar drugs and/or the polar metabolites of non-polar compounds.
- Renal impairment reduces the elimination of drugs that depend on glomerular filtration, so the dose of drugs such as digoxin must be reduced, or the dose interval (e.g. between doses of aminoglycoside) must be increased, to avoid toxicity.
- There are specific secretory mechanisms for organic acids and organic bases in the proximal tubules which lead to the efficient clearance of weak acids such as penicillin and weak bases such as cimetidine. Competition for these carriers can cause drug interactions, although less commonly than induction or inhibition of cytochrome P_{450}.
- Passive reabsorption limits the efficiency with which the kidney eliminates drugs. Weak acids are best eliminated in an alkaline urine (which favours the charged form, A^-), whereas weak bases are best eliminated in an acid urine (which favours the charged form, BH^+).
- The urine may be deliberately alkalinized by infusing sodium bicarbonate intravenously in the management of overdose with weak acids such as aspirin (see Chapter 53), to increase elimination of salicylate.
- Lithium ions are actively reabsorbed in the proximal tubule by the same system that normally reabsorbs sodium, so salt depletion (which causes increased proximal tubular sodium ion reabsorption) causes lithium toxicity unless the dose of lithium is reduced.

Case history

A house officer (HO) sees a 53-year-old woman in the emergency room with a 6-hour history of fevers, chills, loin pain and dysuria. She looks very ill, with a temperature of 39.5°C, blood pressure of 80/60mm Hg and right loin tenderness. The white blood cell count is raised at 15 000, and there are numerous white cells and rods in the urine. Serum creatinine is normal at 90 μmol/L. The HO wants to start treatment with aminoglycoside antibiotic pending the availability of a bed on the intensive-care unit. Despite the normal level creatinine level, he is concerned that the dose may need to be adjusted and calls the Resident Medical Officer for advice.

Comment

The HO is right to be concerned. The patient is hypotensive and will be perfusing her kidneys poorly. Serum creatinine may be normal in *acute* renal failure. It is important to obtain an adequate peak concentration to combat her presumed Gram-negative septicaemia. It would therefore be appropriate to start treatment with the normal dose. This will achieve the usual peak concentration (since the volume of distribution will be similar to that in a healthy person). However, the *next* dose should not normally be given until an urgent blood level has been obtained so that the dose interval may be appropriately prolonged if renal failure does indeed supervene.

ACTIVE TUBULAR REABSORPTION

This is a relatively minor process in the case of most therapeutic drugs. Uric acid is reabsorbed by an active transport system which is inhibited by uricosuric drugs such as probenecid and sulphinpyrazone. Lithium, riboflavine and fluoride also undergo active tubular reabsorption. Conditions in which sodium reabsorption is enhanced, notably salt depletion, predispose to lithium intoxication.

FURTHER READING

Rowland M, Tozer TN. 1995: Elimination in *Clinical pharmacokinetics: concepts and applications*, 3rd edn. Baltimore, MD: Williams and Wilkins, 156–83.

CHAPTER SEVEN

EFFECTS *of* DISEASE *on* DRUG DISPOSITION

- Introduction
- Gastrointestinal disease
- Cardiac failure
- Renal disease
- Liver disease
- Thyroid disease

INTRODUCTION

Several common disorders influence the way in which the body handles drugs. It is important that the possibility of such disorder is borne in mind before prescribing a course of therapy. Gastrointestinal, cardiac, renal, liver and thyroid disorders all influence pharmacokinetics, and individualization of therapy is important in patients with such disturbances. Most of this chapter is devoted to their influence on pharmacokinetics, with a few additional comments regarding the influences of disease on pharmacodynamics.

GASTROINTESTINAL DISEASE

Gastrointestinal disease alters the absorption of orally administered drugs, and prescribers need to bear in mind that therapeutic failure may be a consequence of this. Alternative routes of administration (see Chapter 4) may be appropriate in such circumstances.

GASTRIC EMPTYING

Gastric emptying is an important determinant of the rate and sometimes also the extent of drug absorption (see Chapter 4). Several pathological factors alter gastric emptying (Table 7.1). However, there is little detailed information about the effect of these on drug absorption. Absorption of aspirin (even when administered as a solution) is delayed in migraine attacks, and a more rapid effect can be achieved by administering it with metoclopramide, which increases gastric emptying. Pyloric stenosis results in impaired absorption of paracetamol and doubtless also of other drugs.

SMALL INTESTINAL DISEASE

The very large surface area of small intestine available for drug absorption provides a substantial

Table 7.1: Pathological factors influencing the rate of gastric emptying

Decreased rate	Increased rate
Trauma	Duodenal ulcer
Pain (including myocardial infarction, acute abdomen)	Gastroenterostomy
Labour	Coeliac disease
Migraine	
Myxoedema	
Raised intracranial pressure	
Intestinal obstruction	
Gastric ulcer	

functional reserve, so extensive disease may be present without a clinically important reduction in drug absorption occurring. Despite the destruction of villi and microvilli in coeliac disease, with a consequent reduction in the area available for drug absorption, most orally active drugs are effective when administered by mouth in the usual dose. Crohn's disease typically affects the terminal ileum (in contrast to coeliac disease, which affects the jejunum), but may involve any part of the small or large intestine. Absorption of clindamycin and of sulphamethoxazole *increases* in Crohn's disease, peak concentrations of the latter being approximately three times those in healthy controls. Absorption of trimethoprim is slightly reduced, and hypothetically the change in the ratio of the two components of co-trimoxazole (sulphamethoxazole/trimethoprim) could influence the efficacy of this combination. In practice, trimethoprim as a single agent is now preferred in most clinical situations in any event, so this is unlikely to be a problem, except possibly when co-trimoxazole is used in patients infected with *Pneumocystis carinii*.

Pancreatic disease

Pancreatic disease can produce steatorrhoea and reduce absorption of highly lipophilic molecules, including the fat-soluble vitamins. Significant reductions in the absorption of cephalexin have been demonstrated in cystic fibrosis, necessitating increased doses in such patients.

Cardiac failure

Cardiac failure affects pharmacokinetics in several ways, although the clinical importance of some of them has yet to be established. In practice, the most important thing is for the prescriber to be alert to the possibility that therapeutic failure is due to malabsorption, and to appreciate that the risk of toxicity is increased by reduced clearance. Consequently, it is essential to monitor each patient's response to therapy and to individualize therapy accordingly. The following pharmacokinetic phenomena may be abnormal in patients with heart failure.

Absorption

Malabsorption of many substances, including drugs, can occur in cardiac failure because of mucosal oedema. In addition, reduced gastrointestinal blood flow due to low cardiac output can reduce drug absorption. Splanchnic vasoconstriction accompanies cardiac failure as an adaptive response redistributing blood to more vital organs, and exacerbates any problem with drug absorption. Other secondary changes in gastrointestinal motility, secretion, altered pH, and so on, presumably also affect drug absorption adversely. However, reliable data on the effects of cardiac failure on drug absorption are limited. The absorption of thiazide diuretics (e.g. hydrochlorothiazide) is reduced by 30–40% in such patients. The total availability of loop diuretics (e.g. frusemide, bumetanide) is not affected by heart failure, but absorption of frusemide is delayed, and there is a marked blunting of its diuretic effect, which does not occur if it is administered intravenously.

Distribution

Drug distribution is altered by cardiac failure. The apparent volume of distribution (V_d) of quinine and quinidine in patients with congestive cardiac failure is approximately one-third of normal. Usual doses can therefore result in elevated plasma concentrations, producing toxicity. The volume of distribution of lignocaine is also reduced by approximately 25% in heart failure, with corresponding increases in plasma concentrations. The decreased volume of distribution in patients with heart failure is probably caused by decreased tissue perfusion, and perhaps in part by an alteration in the partition of drugs such as lignocaine between blood and tissue components. The distribution volume of frusemide, which is largely confined to the vascular compartment, is little changed in heart failure.

Tissue injury during myocardial infarction causes a rise in erythrocyte sedimentation rate (ESR) and in the plasma concentration of acute-phase reaction proteins. Acute-phase proteins include α_1-acid glycoprotein, which binds to many basic drugs (e.g. chlorpromazine, many β-adrenoceptor antagonists). Thus acute myocardial infarction is associated with increased binding of such drugs, and perhaps with reduced efficacy. A decrease in free disopyramide concentration of approximately 50% has been documented over the first 5 days following myocardial infarction, and similar but less marked changes have been reported for lignocaine. The clinical significance of such changes is uncertain.

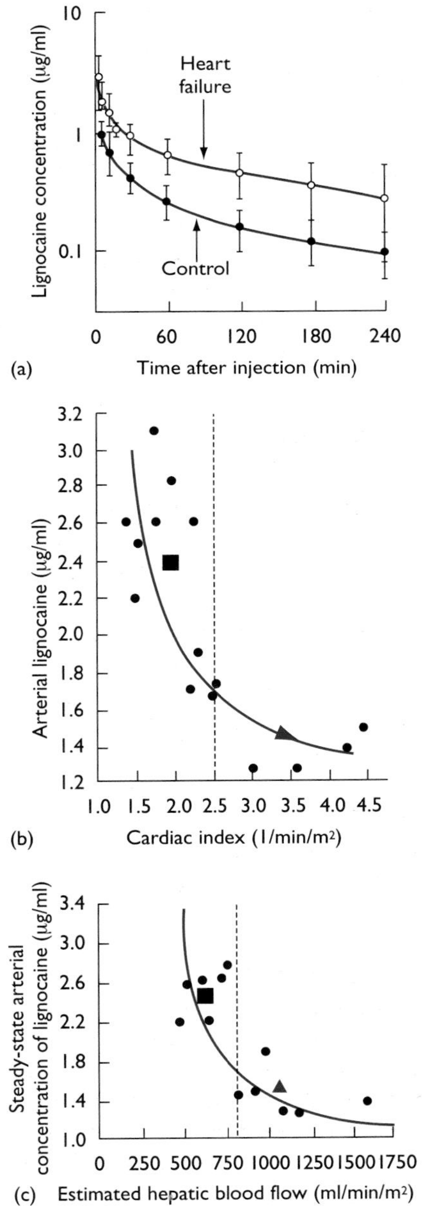

Elimination

Elimination of several drugs by the liver and/or kidneys is diminished in heart failure. Decreased hepatic perfusion accompanies reduced cardiac output. Drugs such as lignocaine with an extraction ratio of >70% show perfusion-limited clearance, and steady-state levels are inversely related to cardiac output (Figure 7.1). The terminal half-lives of lignocaine and its two pharmacologically active metabolites monoethylglycinexylidide (MEGX) and glycinexylidide (GX) are prolonged in patients following myocardial infarction. During lignocaine infusion the steady-state concentrations are almost 50% higher in patients with cardiac failure than in healthy volunteers. The potential for lignocaine toxicity in heart failure is further increased by the accumulation of MEGX and GX, which have cardiodepressant and convulsant properties.

Similar decreases in elimination occur with other drugs with high hepatic extraction ratios. Theophylline clearance is decreased and its half-life is doubled in patients with cardiac failure and pulmonary oedema, although inter-patient variability is wide relative to these kinetic changes. If a patient with chronic stable heart failure also has severe reversible asthmatic bronchospasm, and aminophylline is used in its treatment, the above considerations indicate that the patient should receive a normal loading dose, but that plasma drug concentrations will subsequently need to be

Figure 7.1: (a) Mean values (and standard deviations) of plasma lignocaine concentrations in seven heart failure patients and controls following a 50-mg intravenous bolus. (b) Relationship between arterial lignocaine level and cardiac index (dotted vertical line is lower limit of normal cardiac index, square is mean for low cardiac index patients, triangle is mean for patients with normal cardiac index). (c) Relationship of steady-state arterial lignocaine level following 50-mg bolus and infusion of 40 mg/kg/min (vertical line is lower limit of normal hepatic blood flow, square is mean for patients with low hepatic blood flow, triangle is mean for patients with normal flow). (Reproduced from (a) Thompson PD *et al.* 1971: *American Heart Journal* **82**, 417; (b & c) Stenson RE *et al.* 1971: *Circulation* **43**, 205. With permission of the American Heart Association Inc.).

monitored especially closely in view of the possibility of excessive accumulation.

The metabolic capacity of the liver is also reduced in heart failure both by tissue hypoxia and by hepatocellular damage from hepatic congestion. Liver biopsy samples from patients with heart failure have reduced drug-metabolizing activity.

Heart failure reduces renal elimination of drugs because of reduced glomerular filtration, predisposing to toxicity from drugs such as aminoglycosides and digoxin that are eliminated by this route.

RENAL DISEASE

RENAL IMPAIRMENT

Renal excretion is a major route of elimination for many drugs, as described in Chapter 6, and drugs and their metabolites excreted predominantly by the kidneys accumulate in renal failure. In addition to this self-evident effect on elimination, renal disease also affects other pharmacokinetic parameters (i.e. drug absorption, distribution and metabolism) in more subtle ways.

Absorption

Gastric pH increases in chronic renal failure because urea is cleaved, yielding ammonia which buffers acid in the stomach. This reduces the absorption of ferrous sulphate, and possibly also of other drugs. Nephrotic syndrome is sometimes associated with resistance to oral diuretics, and malabsorption of loop diuretics through the oedematous intestine may contribute to this.

Distribution

Renal impairment causes accumulation of several acidic substances that compete with drugs for binding sites on albumin and other plasma proteins. Although this alters the pharmacokinetics of many drugs, it is seldom clinically important. Phenytoin is an exception, because therapy is guided by plasma concentration and routine analytical methods detect total (bound and free) drug. In renal impairment, protein binding is reduced, so for any measured phenytoin concentration, free (active) drug is increased compared to a subject with normal renal function and the same measured total concentration. The therapeutic range therefore has to be adjusted to lower values in patients with renal impairment, as otherwise doses will be selected that cause toxicity.

Tissue binding of digoxin is reduced in patients with impaired renal function, resulting in a lower volume of distribution than in healthy subjects. A smaller loading dose of digoxin is therefore appropriate in such patients, although the effect of reduced glomerular filtration on digoxin clearance is even more important, necessitating a reduced maintenance dose as decribed below.

The blood–brain barrier is more permeable in uraemia. This can result in increased access of drugs to the central nervous system, an effect that is believed to contribute to the increased incidence of confusion caused by cimetidine in patients with renal failure.

Metabolism

Metabolism of several drugs is reduced in renal failure. These include acyclovir and metaclopramide, non-renal clearance of which is reduced in patients with uraemia. Conversion of sulindac to its active sulphide metabolite is also impaired in renal failure. However these effects are probably of minor practical importance.

Renal excretion

Glomerular filtration and tubular secretion of drugs usually fall *pari passu* in patients with renal impairment. The decline in drug excretion is directly related to glomerular filtration rate (GFR). Some measure or estimate of GFR is therefore essential when deciding on an appropriate dose regimen for patients with impaired renal function. Radioisotope (e.g. chromium-EGTA) or inulin clearance measurement of GFR is seldom feasible in acute situations. The measurement of endogenous creatinine clearance requires accurate urine collection, which is often far from easy in ill, confused and incontinent patients. Furthermore, it is often not safe to delay treatment until the collection is complete and a result is available.

Estimation of GFR from a single plasma measurement therefore has much to commend it. Blood urea is virtually useless as an index of renal drug elimination, because it is influenced by protein intake and metabolism, liver function, state of hydration, urine flow and other factors. However, plasma creatinine adjusted for body weight, age and sex is more helpful, and is usually adequate for clinical purposes provided that its limitations are appreciated. Glomerular filtration rate declines predictably and substantially with age, but the plasma creatinine concentration usually remains in the 'normal' range because creatinine production also declines in the elderly secondary to reduced muscle mass. Figure 7.2 shows a nomogram for estimation of creatinine clearance given plasma creatinine, age, sex and body weight.

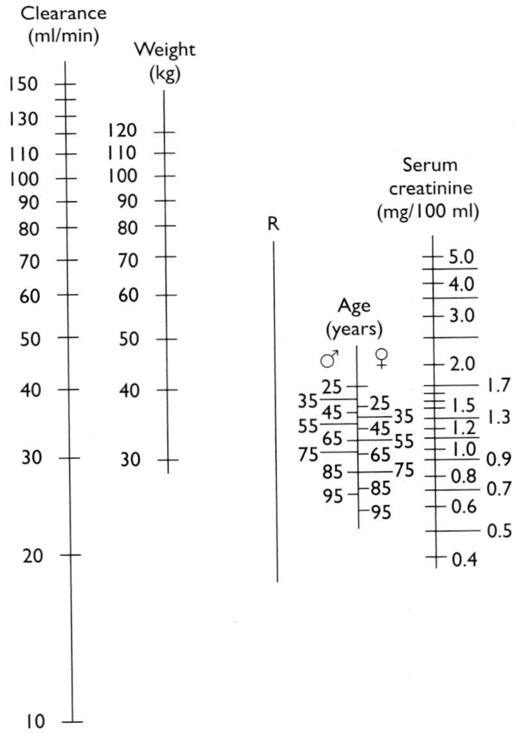

Figure 7.2: Nomogram for rapid evaluation of endogenous creatinine clearance – with a ruler joining weight to age. Keep ruler at crossing point on R, then move the right-hand side of the ruler to the appropriate serum creatinine value and read off clearance from the left-hand scale. (Reproduced with permission from Siersbaek-Nielson K *et al.* 1971: *Lancet* **1** 1133.) © The Lancet Ltd.

Alternatively, some formula such as a modification of that of Cockcroft and Gault is used:

$$\text{creatinine clearance (mL/min)} = \frac{1.2 \times [140 - \text{age (years)}] \times \text{weight (kg)}}{\text{plasma creatinine } (\mu\text{M})}$$

Estimated creatinine clearance is used to adjust the dose regimen for drugs with a low therapeutic index that are eliminated mainly by renal excretion.

The main limitation of plasma creatinine as a means of estimating GFR is in acute renal failure. Plasma creatinine reflects renal function accurately in *chronic* renal failure unless severe, but only increases after an acute reduction in renal function after a lag of several days. Plasma creatinine would be normal immediately after bilateral nephrectomy, even though GFR was zero. A normal creatinine level therefore does *not* mean that usual doses can be assumed to be safe in a patient who may have suffered an *acute* renal insult, such as an episode of severe hypotension during septicaemia, injury or other such conditions.

Adjustment of dose regimens in patients with renal impairment must be considered for drugs for which there is >50% elimination by renal excretion. *The British National Formulary* tabulates drugs to be avoided or used with caution in patients with renal failure. Common examples are shown in Table 7.2.

Detailed recommendations on dosage reduction can be found in textbooks of nephrology. These are useful for getting treatment under way but, although precise, such recommendations are inevitably based only on the effects of reduced renal function on drug elimination in 'average' populations. Individual variation is substantial, and therapeutic monitoring of efficacy, toxicity

Table 7.2: Examples of drugs to be used with especial caution or avoided in renal failure

Aminoglycosides	Captopril
Digoxin	Enalapril
Lithium	Allopurinol
Amphotericin B	Atenolol
Metformin	Ciprofloxacin
Ethambutol	Trimethoprim
Azathioprine	Methotrexate

and sometimes of drug concentrations is essential in patients with impaired renal function.

There are two ways of reducing the total dose to compensate for impaired renal function. Either each dose can be reduced, or the interval between each dose can be lengthened. The latter method is useful when a drug must achieve some threshold concentration to produce its desired effect, but does not need to remain at this level throughout the dose interval. This is the case with aminoglycoside antibiotics. Therapy with these drugs is appropriately monitored by measuring 'peak' levels (in blood sampled at a fixed brief interval after dosing, sufficient to permit at least partial tissue distribution), which indicate whether the dose is large enough to achieve a therapeutic plasma concentration, and 'trough' levels immediately before the next dose (see Chapter 4). If the peak level is satisfactory but the trough level is higher than desired (i.e. toxicity is present or imminent), the dose is not reduced but the interval between doses is increased.

Renal haemodynamics

Patients with mild renal impairment depend on vasodilator prostaglandin biosynthesis to preserve renal blood flow and GFR. The same is true of patients with heart failure, nephrotic syndrome, cirrhosis or ascites. Such patients develop acute reversible renal impairment, often accompanied by salt and water retention and hypertension if treated with non-steroidal anti-inflammatory drugs (NSAIDs), because these inhibit cyclo-oxygenase and hence the synthesis of vasodilator prostaglandins, notably prostaglandin I_2 (prostacyclin) and prostaglandin E_2. Sulindac is a partial exception because it inhibits cyclo-oxygenase less in kidneys than in other tissues, although this specificity is incomplete and dose dependent.

Converting-enzyme inhibitors (e.g. captopril, enalapril) can also cause reversible renal failure due to altered renal haemodynamics. This occurs predictably in patients with bilateral renal artery stenosis or with renal artery stenosis involving a single functioning kidney. The explanation is that in such patients GFR is preserved in the face of the fixed proximal obstruction by angiotensin-II-mediated efferent arteriolar vasoconstriction. Inhibition of converting enzyme disables this homeostatic mechanism and precipitates renal failure.

Nephrotic syndrome

The plasma albumin concentration in patients with nephrotic syndrome is low, resulting in increased fluctuations of free drug concentration following each dose. This could cause adverse effects, although in practice this is seldom clinically important. The high albumin concentration in tubular fluid contributes to the resistance to diuretics that sometimes accompanies nephrotic syndrome. This is because both loop diuretics and thiazides act on ion-transport processes in the luminal membranes of tubular cells. Protein binding of such diuretics within the tubular lumen therefore reduces the concentration of free (active) drug in tubular fluid in contact with the ion transporters on which they act.

Prescribing for patients with renal disease

1 Consider the possibility of renal impairment before drugs are prescribed.
2 Check how drugs are eliminated before prescribing them. If non-renal elimination accounts for less than 50% of total elimination, then dose reduction will probably be necessary.
3 Monitor therapeutic and adverse effects and, where appropriate, drug concentrations in plasma.
4 Use potentially nephrotoxic drugs (e.g. aminoglycosides, NSAIDs, converting enzyme inhibitors), with special care.

Once a potential problem has been identified, there are a number of handbooks, of which the *British National Formulary* is the most concise, simple and accessible, that provide guidelines for dose adjustment in patients with renal impairment. These are useful approximations to get treatment under way, but the mathematical precision of some of the more elaborate tables of recommendations is illusory, and must not lull the inexperienced into a false sense of security – they do *not* permit a full 'course' of treatment to be prescribed safely. The patient must be monitored and their treatment modified in the light of individual responses.

Liver disease

The liver is the main site of drug metabolism (see Chapter 5). Liver disease causes multiple pathophysiological disturbances and unpredictable effects on drug handling. The precise aetiology of the disease is only of limited relevance, the end stage in chronic liver disease being similar in many conditions, with a combination of hepatocyte necrosis and fibrosis. Direct portal tract to hepatic vein shunts develop, resulting in reduced presentation of hepatic portal blood to hepatocytes. Vascular resistance within the liver increases, producing portal hypertension and opening up extrahepatic collaterals between the portal and systemic circulations. Initially, hepatic regeneration compensates for cell loss, but with continuing damage hepatic function is compromised. This is reflected in decreased protein synthesis and reduced serum albumin and coagulation factors.

Attempts to correlate changes in the pharmacokinetics of drugs with tests for derangement of liver function have been unsuccessful, in contrast to the successful use of plasma creatinine in renal impairment. In chronic liver disease, serum albumin is the most useful index of hepatic drug-metabolizing activity, possibly because a low albumin level reflects depressed synthesis of hepatic proteins, including those involved in drug metabolism. Prothrombin time also shows a moderate correlation with drug clearance by the liver. However, in neither case has a continuous relationship been demonstrated, and such indices of hepatic function serve mainly to distinguish the severely affected from the milder cases. Indocyanine green, antipyrine and lignocaine have also proved of little value as markers of hepatic function, although lignocaine is currently undergoing re-evaluation in this regard.

Currently, therefore, empiricism coupled with an awareness of an increased likelihood of adverse drug effects and close clinical monitoring is the best way to approach a patient with liver disease. Drugs should be used only if absolutely necessary, and the risks should be weighed against any potential advantage. If possible, drugs that are eliminated by routes other than the liver should be employed. Some of the effects of liver disease on pharmacokinetics are described here, and some empirical 'rules' with regard to prescribing for patients with liver disease are laid out below.

Pharmacokinetic factors that are affected in liver disease include the absorption, distribution and metabolism of drugs.

Absorption

Absorption of drugs is altered in liver disease because portal hypertension and hypoalbuminaemia cause mucosal oedema. Portal/systemic anastomoses allow the passage of orally administered drug directly into the systemic circulation, bypassing hepatic presystemic metabolism and markedly increasing the bioavailability of drugs such as propranolol and chlormethiazole, which must therefore be started in low doses in such patients and titrated according to effect.

Distribution

Drug distribution is altered in liver disease. Reduced plasma albumin levels reduce plasma protein binding. This is also influenced by bilirubin and other endogenous substances that accumulate in liver disease and may displace drugs from binding sites (as in renal failure). The free fraction of tolbutamide is increased by 115% in cirrhosis, and that of phenytoin is increased by up to 40%. It is particularly important to appreciate this when plasma concentrations of phenytoin are being used to monitor therapy, as unless the therapeutic range is adjusted downward, toxicity will be induced, as explained above in the section on drug distribution in renal disease.

Reduced plasma protein binding increases the apparent V_d if other factors remain unchanged. Increased V_d of several drugs (e.g. diazepam, lignocaine, theophylline) is indeed observed in patients with liver disease. Increased V_d partly or completely explains the observed changes in $t_{\frac{1}{2}}$ of such drugs in patients with liver disease, invalidating the interpretation of much early work where this was not appreciated. Disease-induced alterations in clearance and V_d often act in opposite directions with regard to their effect on $t_{\frac{1}{2}}$, probably accounting for inconsistencies in studies where $t_{\frac{1}{2}}$ was the only pharmacokinetic parameter estimated. Data on $t_{\frac{1}{2}}$ in isolation provide little information about the extent of changes in metabolism or drug distribution which result from liver disease.

METABOLISM

Cytochrome P_{450} is reduced in patients with very severe liver disease, but drug metabolism is surprisingly little impaired in patients with moderate to severe disease. There is a poor correlation between microsomal enzyme activity from liver biopsy specimens *in vitro* and drug clearance measurements *in vivo*. Even in very severe disease, the metabolism of different drugs is not affected to the same extent. It is therefore hazardous to extrapolate from knowledge of the handling of one drug to effects on another in an individual patient with liver disease. A possible explanation for this heterogeneity lies in the multiple forms of cytochrome P_{450}, some of which act on different substrates, and which may be affected differently by hepatocellular dysfunction.

PRESCRIBING FOR PATIENTS WITH LIVER DISEASE

1 Risks must be weighed against any possible benefit, and drugs should only be prescribed if the risk/benefit is judged to be favourable.
2 If possible, use drugs that are eliminated by routes other than the liver.
3 Response and adverse effects (and occasionally drug concentrations) must be monitored closely, and therapy adjusted accordingly.
4 Sedative and analgesic drugs are common precipitants of hepatic coma, probably because of a combination of pharmacokinetic and pharmacodynamic alterations, and should be avoided if possible.
5 Predictable hepatotoxins (e.g. cytotoxic drugs) should only be used for the strongest of indications, and then only with close clinical and biochemical monitoring.
6 Drugs that are known to cause idiosyncratic liver disease (e.g. isoniazid, phenytoin, methyldopa) are not necessarily contraindicated in stable chronic disease, as there is no evidence of an increased susceptibility to further damage. Oral contraceptives are not advisable if there is active liver disease or a history of jaundice of pregnancy, but need not be withheld after recovery from acute hepatitis.
7 Constipation favours bacterial production of false neurotransmitter amines in the bowel, and drugs that cause constipation (e.g. verapamil, tricyclic antidepressants) should be avoided if possible in patients at risk of hepatic encephalopathy.
8 *Drugs that inhibit catabolism of such amines (e.g. monoamine oxidase inhibitors) also provoke coma and should be avoided.*
9 Kaliuretic drugs (e.g. thiazide or loop diuretics) also provoke encephalopathy, and potassium-sparing drugs such as spironolactone or amiloride are often preferable.
10 Fluid overload and ascites are exacerbated by drugs that cause sodium retention (e.g. indomethacin, glucocorticoids, stilboestrol or carbenoxolone) and those containing sodium (e.g. sodium-containing antacids and high-dose carbenicillin).
11 Avoid drugs that interfere with haemostasis (e.g. aspirin, anticoagulants and fibrinolytics) whenever possible, because of the increased risk of bleeding, especially if varices are suspected.

THYROID DISEASE

Thyroid dysfunction affects drug disposition partly as a result of effects on drug metabolism and partly via changes in renal elimination. The existing data refer to only a few drugs, but it is prudent to anticipate the possibility of increased sensitivity of hypothyroid patients to many drugs when prescribing. Information is available for the following drugs.

DIGOXIN

It has been known for many years that myxoedematous patients are extremely sensitive to digoxin, whereas unusually high doses are required to control the ventricular rate in thyrotoxic atrial fibrillation. In general, hyperthyroid patients have lower plasma digoxin concentrations and hypothyroid patients have higher plasma concentrations than euthyroid patients on the same dose. There is no significant difference in half-life between these groups, and a difference in V_d has been postulated to explain the alteration of plasma concentration with thyroid activity. Changes in renal function which occur with changes in thyroid status complicate this interpretation. Glomerular filtration rate is increased in thyrotoxicosis and decreased in myxoedema. These changes in renal function influence elimination, and the reduced plasma levels of digoxin correlate closely with the increased creatinine clearance in thyrotoxicosis. In addition, enhanced biliary clearance, digoxin malabsorption due to intestinal hurry and increased hepatic metabolism have all been postulated as factors contributing to the insensitivity of thyrotoxic patients to cardiac glycosides.

Anticoagulants

Oral anticoagulants produce an exaggerated prolongation of prothrombin time in hyperthyroid patients. This is due to increased metabolic breakdown of vitamin K-dependent clotting factors, rather than to changes in drug kinetics.

Glucocorticoids

Glucocorticoids are metabolized by hepatic mixed-function oxidases which are influenced by thyroid status. In hyperthyroidism there is increased cortisol production and a reduced cortisol half-life, the converse being true in myxoedema.

Thyroxine

The normal half-life of thyroxine (6–7 days) is reduced to 3–4 days by hyperthyroidism and prolonged to 9–10 days by hypothyroidism. This is of considerable clinical importance when deciding on an appropriate interval at which to increase the dose of thyroxine in patients treated for myxoedema, especially if they have coincident ischaemic heart disease which would be

Key points

Disease profoundly influences the response to many drugs by altering pharmacokinetics and/or pharmacodynamics.

- Gastrointestinal disease:
  - (a) diseases that alter gastric emptying influence the response to oral drugs (e.g. migraine reduces gastric emptying, limiting the effectiveness of analgesics);
  - (b) ileum/pancreas – relatively minor effects.
- Heart failure:
  - (a) absorption of drugs (e.g. frusemide) is reduced as a result of splanchnic hypoperfusion;
  - (b) elimination of drugs that are removed very efficiently by the liver (e.g. lignocaine) is reduced as a result of reduced hepatic blood flow, predisposing to toxicity;
  - (c) tissue hypoperfusion increases the risk of lactic acidosis with metformin (cor pulmonale especially predisposes to this because of hypoxia).
- Renal disease:
  - (a) chronic renal failure – as well as reduced excretion, drug absorption, distribution and metabolism may also be altered. Serum creatinine concentration provides a useful index of the need for dose adjustment in chronic renal failure;
  - (b) nephrotic syndrome leads to altered drug distribution because of altered binding to albumin and altered therapeutic range of concentrations for drugs that are extensively bound to albumin (e.g. some anticonvulsants). Albumin in tubular fluid binds diuretics and causes diuretic resistance. Glomerular filtration rate is preserved in nephrotic syndrome by compensatory increased prostaglandin synthesis so, NSAIDs (see Chapter 25) can precipitate renal failure.
- Liver disease – as well as effects on drug metabolism, absorption and distribution may also be altered because of portal systemic shunting, hypoalbuminaemia and ascites. There is no simple biochemical marker (analogous to serum creatinine in chronic renal failure) to guide dose adjustment in liver disease, and a cautious "trial-and-error" approach is used.
- Thyroid disease:
  - (a) hypothyroidism increases sensitivity to digoxin and opioids;
  - (b) hyperthyroidism increases sensitivity to warfarin and reduces sensitivity to digoxin.

Case history

A 57-year-old alcoholic is admitted to hospital because of gross ascites and peripheral oedema. He looks chronically unwell, is jaundiced, and has spider naevi and gynaecomastia. His liver and spleen are not palpable in the presence of marked ascites. Serum chemistries reveal hypoalbuminuria, sodium 132 mmol/L, potassium 3.5 mmol/L, creatinine 105 μmol/L, and international normalized ratio (INR) is increased at 1.8. The patient is treated with frusemide and his fluid intake is restricted. Over the next 5 days he loses 10.5 kg, but you are called to see him because he has become confused and unwell. On examination he is drowsy and has asterixis ('liver flap'). His blood pressure is 100/54 mmHg with a postural drop. His serum potassium is 2.6 mmol/L, creatinine has increased to 138 μmol/L and the urea concentration has increased disproportionately.

Comment

It is a mistake to try to eliminate ascites too rapidly in patients with cirrhosis. In this case, in addition to prerenal renal failure, the patient has developed profound hypokalaemia, which is commonly caused by frusemide in a patient with secondary hyperaldosteronism with a poor diet. The hypokalaemia has precipitated hepatic encephalopathy. It would have been better to have initiated treatment with spironolactone to inhibit his endogenous aldosterone. Great caution will be needed in starting such treatment now that the patient's renal function has deteriorated, and serum potassium levels must be monitored closely.

exacerbated if an excessive steady-state thyroxine level was achieved.

Antithyroid drugs

The half-life of propylthiouracil and methimazole is prolonged in hypothyroidism and shortened in hyperthyroidism. These values return to normal on attainment of the euthyroid state, probably because of altered hepatic metabolism.

Opiates

Patients with hypothyroidism are exceptionally sensitive to opioid analgesics, which cause profound respiratory depression in this setting.

Further reading

Carmichael DJS. 1998 Handling of drugs in kidney disease. In Davison AM, Cameron JS, Grünfeld J-P *et al.* (eds), *Oxford textbook of clinical nephrology* 2nd edn. Oxford: Oxford University Press, 2659–78.

Rowland M, Tozer TN. 1995: Disease. In *Clinical pharmacokinetics: concepts and applications*, 3rd edn. Baltimore, MD Williams and Wilkins, 248–66.

CHAPTER EIGHT

THERAPEUTIC DRUG MONITORING

- Introduction
- Role of drug monitoring in therapeutics
- Pharmacokinetic factors and drug response
- Practical aspects
- Drugs for which therapeutic drug monitoring is used

INTRODUCTION

The large inter-patient variability in responses to drugs results from two main sources:

1 pharmacokinetic variability in absorption, distribution, metabolism or elimination;
2 pharmacodynamic variability in sensitivity at or beyond receptors, due to acquired differences (e.g. age, obesity or effects of disease such as hypothyroidism or myasthenia gravis) or inherited disease (e.g. glucose-6-phosphate dehydrogenase deficiency).

Measurement of drug concentrations in the blood or plasma allows evaluation of the relative importance of these two sources of variation, and in some instances facilitates adjustment of dosage to produce the desired response. Monitoring of drug therapy by clinical response has been used for many years and, where applicable, is more valuable than complex methods of drug analysis. Pharmacodynamic measures of response include clinical or laboratory measurements such as relief of pain in response to an analgesic, arterial blood pressure in patients with hypertension, peak expiratory flow rate in patients with asthma, bactericidal activity of plasma from a patient treated with antibiotics for bacterial endocarditis, or international normalized ratio (INR) in patients treated with oral anticoagulants. There is no place for routine estimation of plasma concentrations of drugs that achieve adequate concentrations in all patients without causing toxicity following a standard dose.

ROLE OF DRUG MONITORING IN THERAPEUTICS

Monitoring drug concentrations to assist in the therapy of an individual patient is sometimes a useful supplement to clinical monitoring. Determination of concentrations of drugs in plasma can also be useful in other ways (e.g. management of overdose, see below). Accurate and convenient assay methods are necessary. Measurements of drug concentrations in plasma are most useful when:

1 A direct relationship exists between the drug (or drug metabolite) concentration in plasma or other accessible biological fluid and pharmacological or toxic effect, i.e. a therapeutic range of plasma concentrations has been established. In contrast, drugs with irreversible or 'hit-and-run' actions (e.g. some monoamine oxidase inhibitors or alkylating agents) are generally unsuited to this approach. The development of tolerance to drug action also restricts the usefulness of plasma concentrations;

2 the effect cannot readily be assessed by clinical observation. This is particularly so when the clinical end point is 'quantal' (e.g. a *grand mal* seizure), and there is no satisfactory intermediate end point which is a continuous variable (such as blood pressure or INR). Plasma concentration is a useful indirect continuous variable whereby therapy can be adjusted to optimize efficacy and minimize toxicity in some such cases;

3 inter-individual variability in plasma drug concentrations from the same dose is large and unpredictable (e.g. phenytoin);

4 there is a low therapeutic index (i.e. ratio of toxic concentration/effective concentration is < 2). Drugs with a narrow 'therapeutic window' are particularly suitable for plasma concentration monitoring. Measurement of drug concentrations helps when several drugs are being given concurrently and serious interactions are anticipated;

5 it is sometimes useful to check that replacement treatment is adequate and not excessive, and in some situations, such as treatment of hypothyroidism, measuring the concentration in plasma of thyroxine, for example, may be the most appropriate way of doing this. In other situations the response to therapy is best monitored by a measure of drug effect (i.e. a pharmacodynamic measure). Examples include the rise in reticulocyte count and haematocrit in patients with Addisonian pernicious anaemia treated with vitamin B_{12}, or those with iron deficiency treated with ferrous sulphate;

6 there are circumstances in which compliance with therapy with drugs such as theophylline, phenytoin or carbamazepine needs to be checked;

7 there are some cases of poisoning (e.g. with paracetamol or aspirin) in which knowledge of the plasma concentration can be invaluable in deciding on the need for active measures such as the use of specific antidotes.

PHARMACOKINETIC FACTORS AND DRUG RESPONSE

Pharmacokinetic factors can influence the relationship between plasma drug concentration and response. For example, the rate of change of plasma concentration determines pharmacological responses to some drugs, including alcohol, amphetamine and barbiturates. There is a close relationship between pharmacological effects of amphetamine and the initial rate of entry of the drug into the circulation, but not the peak plasma level or the area under the plasma concentration–time curve (AUC).

PRACTICAL ASPECTS

Drug distribution and active metabolite formation influence the relationship between plasma drug concentration and effect, as may alterations of homeostatic mechanisms. A constant tissue to plasma drug concentration ratio only occurs during the terminal β-phase of elimination. Measurements should therefore be made when enough time has elapsed after a dose for this to have been established. Greater care is therefore required in the timing and labelling of specimens for drug concentration determination than is the case for 'routine' chemical pathology specimens. Usually during repeated dosing a sample is taken just before the next dose to assess the 'trough' concentration, and a sample may also be taken at some specified time after dosing (depending on the drug) to determine the 'peak' level.

Given this information, the laboratory should be able to produce useful information. Useful advice on the interpretation of this information is sometimes available from a local therapeutic drug-monitoring service such as is provided by some clinical pharmacology and/or clinical pharmacy departments. In general, the cost of measuring drug levels is greater than for clinical chemical estimations, and to use expensive facilities to produce 'numbers' resulting from analysis of samples taken at random from patients described only by name or number is meaningless and misleading, as well as being a waste of money.

Analytical techniques of high specificity (often relying on high-performance liquid chromatography or radioimmunoassay) avoid the pitfalls of several of the older spectrophotometric methods for drugs such as theophylline which were influenced by inactive metabolites. Drugs administered concomitantly may interfere with assays. For example, some laboratories assay antibiotics by a microbiological assay, and if the patient is given a second antibiotic concurrently, the results are rendered meaningless. The clinician should always be aware of the possibility of error in laboratory data. Experience with quality-control monitoring of anticonvulsant analyses performed by laboratories both in the UK and in the USA have revealed that repeated analyses of a reference sample can produce some startlingly different results. The most important principle for the clinician is that plasma drug concentrations must always be interpreted in the context of the patient's clinical state.

Few prospective studies have been made of the effects of using therapeutic drug-monitoring services on the quality of patient care. A retrospective survey conducted at the Massachusetts General Hospital showed that before the use of digoxin monitoring 13.9% of all patients receiving digoxin showed evidence of toxicity, and that this figure fell to 5.9% following the introduction of monitoring.

DRUGS FOR WHICH THERAPEUTIC DRUG MONITORING IS USED

Table 8.1 lists those drugs which may be monitored therapeutically.

Table 8.1: Therapeutically monitored drugs

Drug	Therapeutic range
Digoxin	0.8–2 μg/L (1–2.6 nmol/L)
Lithium	0.4–1 mmol/L
Aminoglycoside antibiotics	Various*
Phenytoin	10–20 mg/L (40–80 μmol/L)
Methotrexate	Not applicable†
Theophylline	5–20 mg/L (28–110 μmol/L)
Cyclosporin	50–200 μg/L
Some anti-arrhythmic drugs	Various

* Peak and trough levels are needed – see text.

† Monitoring must be performed to prevent toxicity: plasma concentrations of > 5 μmol/L 24 h after dosing usually require high-dose leucovorin to prevent serious bone-marrow/gut toxicity.

1 *Digoxin* (therapeutic range 0.8–2 μg/L, 1–2.6 nmol/L) and other cardiac glycosides – measuring the plasma concentration can help as a guide to individualizing therapy, and may also be a useful adjunct in cases of suspected toxicity or poor compliance.
2 *Lithium* – plasma concentrations in samples obtained 12 h after dosing of 0.4–1 mmol/L are usually regarded as therapeutic, although a lower range of 0.4–0.8 mmol/L has also been recommended mania prophylaxis.
3 *Aminoglycoside antibiotics* – for gentamicin, peak concentrations measured 30 min after dosing of 7–10 mg/L are usually effective against sensitive organisms, and trough levels, measured immediately before a dose, of 1–2 mg/L reduce the risk of toxicity; for amikacin and netilmycin, the desirable peak concentration is 4–12 mg/L, with a trough value of ≤ 4 mg/L; for tobramycin, the desirable peak is 4–5 mg/L, with a trough of ≤ 2 mg/L.
4 *Phenytoin* (normal therapeutic range 10–20 mg/L, 40–80 μmol/L) and some other anticonvulsants including *carbamazepine* (approximate therapeutic range 5–10 mg/L, 20–40 μmol/L). When using the steady-state plasma concentration of phenytoin as a guide to dose adjustment, it is important to be aware of the non-linear nature of its pharmacokinetics, and of the possible effects of concurrent renal or hepatic disease or of pregnancy on its distribution.
5 *Methotrexate* does not have a clear concentration–effect relationship, the duration of exposure of neoplastic cells to the drug being at least as important as concentration, although plasma concentrations of <10 nmol/L are unlikely to achieve antineoplastic effects. However, plasma concentration is an important predictor of toxicity, and concentrations of > 5 μmol/L 24 h after a dose or 100 nmol/L 48 h after dosing usually require high-dose folinic acid (leucovorin) to prevent severe toxicity to gastrointestinal tract and bone marrow.

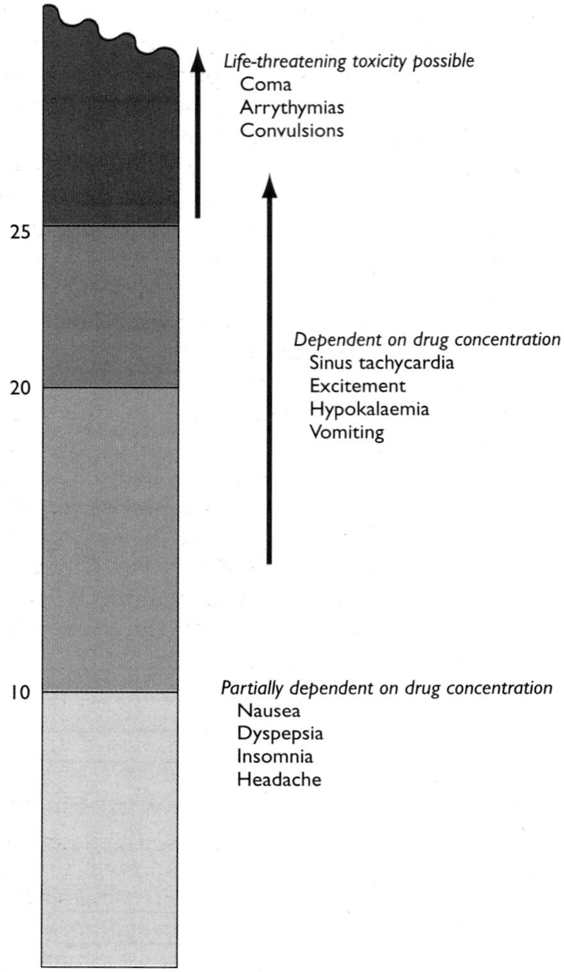

Figure 8.1: Theophylline plasma concentrations (mg/L). Note that there is a wide variation in the incidence and severity of adverse effects. (Adapted from Mant T, Henry J and Cochrane G in Henry J, Volans G (eds), *ABC of Poisoning. Part 1: Drugs*. London: British Medical Journal.)

6 *Theophylline* is an effective drug with a narrow therapeutic index (Figure 8.1), and many factors influence its clearance (Figure 8.2). Measurement of plasma theophylline concentration can help to minimize toxicity, which can be severe (e.g. unheralded cardiac arrhythmias or seizures). A therapeutic range of 5–20 mg/L is quoted. This is rather an oversimplification, and plasma concentrations of 15–20 mg/L are associated with severe toxicity in neonates due to decreased protein binding and accumulation

Key points

- Determining the plasma concentrations of drugs in order to adjust therapy is referred to as therapeutic drug monitoring (TDM). It has distinct but limited applications.
- TDM permits dose individualization and is useful when there is a clear relationship between plasma concentration and pharmacological or toxic effects.
- The timing of blood samples in relation to dosing is crucial. For aminoglycosides, samples are obtained for measurement of peak and trough levels. To guide chronic therapy (e.g. with anticonvulsants), sufficient time must elapse after starting treatment or changing dose for the steady state to have been achieved, before sampling.
- Drugs which may usefully be monitored in this way include digoxin, lithium, aminoglycosides, several anticonvulsants, methotrexate, theophylline, several anti-arrhythmic drugs (including amiodarone) and cyclosporin.
- Individualization of dosage using TDM permits the effectiveness of these drugs to be maximized while minimizing their potential toxicity.

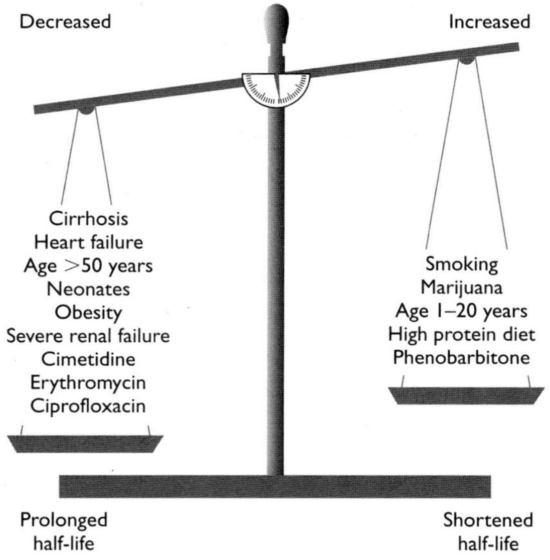

Figure 8.2: Theophylline clearance. (Adapted from Mant T, Henry J and Cochrane G) in Henry J, Volans G (eds), *ABC of Poisoning. Part 1: Drugs*. London: British Medical Journal.)

Case history

A 35 year old asthmatic is admitted to hospital at 6 o'clock in the morning because of a severe attack of asthma. She has been treated with salbutamol and beclomethasone inhalers supplemented by a modified-release preparation of theophylline, 300 mg at night. She has clinical evidence of a severe attack, and does not improve with nebulized salbutamol and oxygen. Treatment with intravenous aminophylline is considered.

Comment

Aminophylline is a soluble preparation of theophylline (mixed with ethyenediamine), which has a role in patients with life-threatening asthma. However, it is essential to have rapid access to an analytical service to measure blood aminophylline concentrations if this drug is to be used safely, especially in this situation where the blood concentration of aminophylline resulting from the modified-release preparation that the patient took the night before admission must be determined before starting treatment. Aminophylline toxicity (including seizures and potentially fatal cardiac arrhythmias) can result if the dose is not individualized in relation to plasma concentration.

of caffeine, to which theophylline is methylated in neonates but not in older children.

7 Therapeutic ranges of plasma concentrations of several *anti-arrhythmic drugs* (e.g. lignocaine) have been established with reasonable confidence. *Amiodarone*, an effective anti-arrhythmic drug, is difficult to use because of its extremely long plasma half-life and significant toxicities. The therapeutic range of plasma amiodarone concentrations for ventricular arrhythmias (1.0–2.5 mg/L) is higher than that needed for atrial arrhythmias (0.5–1.5 mg/L). It is not useful to measure the plasma concentrations of other anti-arrhythmic drugs routinely, dose adjustment being made on clinical grounds. However, plasma concentration determination can be helpful if there is unexpected therapeutic failure or unexpected toxicity.

8 *Cyclosporin* – careful pharmacokinetic monitoring of this uniquely valuable but toxic immunosuppressant is essential. Trough plasma concentrations in the range 50–200 μg/L are usually recommended during maintenance treatment. Compliance is a particular problem in children, and deterioration in renal function can reflect either graft rejection due to inadequate cyclosporin concentration or toxicity from excessive concentrations.

FURTHER READING

Aronson JK, White NJ. 1996 Monitoring drug therapy. In Weatherall DJ, Ledingham JGG, Warrell DA (eds), *Oxford textbook of medicine*, 3rd edn. Oxford: Oxford University Press, 1260–1.

Aronson JK, Hardman M, Reynolds DJM. 1993: *ABC of monitoring drug therapy*. London: BMJ Publications.

CHAPTER NINE

DRUGS *in* PREGNANCY

- Introduction
- Harmful effects on the fetus
- Recognition of teratogenic drugs
- Pharmacokinetics in pregnancy
- Prescribing in pregnancy
- Non-therapeutic drugs

INTRODUCTION

The use of drugs in pregnancy is complicated by the potential for harmful effects on the growing fetus, altered maternal physiology and the paucity and difficulties of research in this field.

Key points

- There is potential for harmful effects on the growing fetus.
- Because of human variation, subtle effects may be virtually impossible to identify.
- There is altered maternal physiology.
- There is notable paucity of and difficulties in research in this area.
- Assume all drugs are harmful until proven otherwise.

HARMFUL EFFECTS ON THE FETUS

Because experience with many drugs in pregnancy is severely limited, it should be assumed that all drugs are potentially harmful until sufficient data exist to indicate otherwise. 'Social' drugs (alcohol and cigarette smoking) are definitely damaging and their use should be discouraged.

In the placenta, maternal blood is separated from fetal blood by a cellular membrane. The diffusion path is longer in early pregnancy than in late pregnancy. Most drugs with a molecular weight of less than 1000 can cross the placenta. This is usually by passive diffusion down the concentration gradient, but can occasionally involve active transport. The rate of diffusion depends firstly on the concentration of free drug (i.e. non-protein bound) on each side of the membrane, and secondly on the lipid solubility of the drug, which is determined in part by the degree of ionization. Diffusion occurs if the drug is in the unionized state. Placental function is also modified by changes in blood flow, and drugs which reduce placental blood flow can reduce birth weight. This may be the mechanism which causes the small reduction in birth weight following treatment of the mother with beta-blockers in pregnancy. Early in embryonic development, exogenous substances accumulate in the neuroectoderm. The blood–brain barrier to diffusion is not developed until the second half of pregnancy, and the susceptibility of the central nervous system (CNS) to developmental toxins may be partly related to this. The human placenta possesses multiple enzymes that are primarily involved with endogenous steroid metabolism, but which may also contribute to drug metabolism and clearance.

Key points

- A cellular membrane separates the maternal and fetal blood.
- Most drugs cross the placenta by passive diffusion.
- Placental function is modified by changes in blood flow.
- There are multiple placental enzymes, primarily involved with endogenous steroid metabolism, which may also contribute to drug metabolism.

The stage of gestation influences the effects of drugs on the fetus. It is convenient to divide pregnancy into four stages, namely fertilization and implantation (< 17 days), the organogenesis/embryonic stage (17–57 days), the fetogenic stage and delivery.

Fertilization and implantation

Animal studies suggest that interference with the fetus before 17 days gestation causes abortion, i.e. if pregnancy continues the fetus is unharmed.

Organogenesis/embryonic stage

At this stage the fetus is differentiating to form major organs, and this is the critical period for teratogenesis. Teratogens cause deviations or abnormalities in the development of the embryo that are compatible with prenatal life and are observable postnatally. Drugs that interfere with this process can cause gross structural defects (e.g. thalidomide phocomelia).

Some drugs are confirmed teratogens (Table 9.1), but for many the evidence is inconclusive. Thalidomide was unusual in the way in which a very small dose of the drug given on only one or two occasions between the fourth and seventh weeks of pregnancy produced serious malformations. Despite its wide use, it was nearly 4 years before these adverse effects were recognized.

Table 9.1: Some drugs that are definitely teratogenic in humans

Thalidomide	Androgens
Cytotoxic agents	Progestogens
Alcohol	Danozol
Warfarin	Diethylstilboestrol
Retinoids	Radioisotopes
Most anticonvulsants	Some live vaccines
Ribavarin	Lithium

Fetogenic stage

In this stage the fetus undergoes further development and maturation. Even after organogenesis is almost complete, drugs can still have significant adverse effects on fetal growth and development.

- ACE inhibitors cause fetal and neonatal renal dysfunction.
- Drugs used to treat maternal hyperthyroidism can cause fetal and neonatal hypothyroidism.
- Tetracycline antibiotics inhibit growth of fetal bones and stain teeth.
- Aminoglycosides cause fetal VIIIth nerve damage.
- Opioids and cocaine taken regularly during pregnancy can lead to fetal drug dependency.
- Warfarin can cause fetal intracerebral bleeding.
- Beta-blockers may cause intrauterine growth restriction when used in pregnancy, but are considered safe in the third trimester.
- Indomethacin, a potent inhibitor of prostaglandin synthesis, is used under specialist supervision to assist closure of patent ductus arteriosus in premature infants.

Delivery

Some drugs given late in pregnancy or during delivery may cause particular problems. Pethidine, administered as an analgesic can cause fetal apnoea (which is reversed with naloxone). Anaesthetic agents given during Caesarean section may transiently depress neurological, respiratory and muscular functions. Warfarin given in

Key points

- Fertilization and implantation < 17 days.
- Organogenesis/embryonic stage 17–57 days.
- Fetogenic stage.
- Delivery.

late pregnancy causes a haemostasis defect in the baby, and predisposes to cerebral haemorrhage during delivery.

The male

Although it is generally considered that sperm cells damaged by drug effects will not result in fertilization, the manufacturers of griseofulvin, the antifungal agent, advise men not to father children during or for 6 months after treatment. Finasteride, an anti-androgen used in the treatment of benign prostatic hyperplasia, is secreted in semen, and may be teratogenic to male fetuses.

Recognition of teratogenic drugs

The incidence of serious congenital abnormality is about 2% of all births, and a small but unknown fraction of these are due to drugs. The background incidence of major malformations rises to almost 5% by the age of 5 years. Two principal problems face those who are trying to determine whether a drug is teratogenic when it is used to treat disease in humans.

1 Many drugs produce birth defects when given experimentally in large doses to pregnant animals. This does not necessarily mean that they are teratogenic in humans at therapeutic doses. Indeed, the metabolism and kinetics of drugs at high doses in other species is so different from that in humans as to limit seriously the relevance of such studies.
2 Fetal defects are common (2%). Consequently, if the incidence of drug-induced abnormalities is low, a very large number of cases has to be observed to define a significant increase above this background level. Effects on the fetus may take several years to become clinically manifest. For example, diethylstilboestrol was widely used in the late 1940s to prevent miscarriages and preterm births, despite little evidence of efficacy. In 1971 an association was reported between adenocarcinoma of the vagina in girls in their late teens whose mothers had been given diethylstilboestrol during the pregnancy. Exposure to stilboestrol *in utero* has also been associated with a T-shaped uterus and other structural abnormalities of the genital tract, and increased rates of ectopic pregnancy and premature labour.

The tragedy of thalidomide, and the sinister delayed presentation of diethylstilboestrol toxicity, illustrate the absolute necessity for meticulous data analysis of drug administration in pregnancy – assessing the efficacy and both short- and long-term side-effects on both mother and fetus – before the introduction of any new treatment can be recommended during pregnancy when acceptable alternatives are available.

Key points

- The background incidence of serious congenital abnormality recognized at birth is approximately 2%, and at 5 years it is nearly 5%.
- Environmental and genetic factors can influence a drug's effect.
- Maternal disease can affect the fetus.
- Studies of large doses in pregnant animals are of doubtful relevance.
- Effects may be delayed (e.g. diethylstilboestrol).
- Meticulous data collection is required for drugs administered during pregnancy and outcome, including long-term follow-up. At present the Committee on Safety of Medicines (CSM) requests records of all drugs administered to a mother who bears an abnormal fetus. More complete (but with inherent practical difficulties) data collection by the CSM, the National Teratology Information Services, the pharmaceutical industry and drug information agencies on all prescriptions during pregnancy will require long-term follow-up of offspring.

Pharmacokinetics in pregnancy

Ethical and practical considerations make pharmacokinetic studies in pregnancy difficult. However, there is no evidence that pregnancy changes the pharmacological response, and known differences in drug effects are usually explained by altered pharmacokinetics.

Absorption

Gastric emptying and small intestinal motility are reduced. This is of little consequence unless rapid drug action is required. Vomiting associated with pregnancy may make oral drug administration impractical.

Distribution

During pregnancy the blood volume increases by one-third, with expansion in plasma volume (from 2.5 to 4 L at term) being disproportionate to expansion in red cell mass, so that haematocrit falls. There is also an increase in body water due to a larger extravascular volume and changes in the uterus and breasts.

Oedema, which at least one-third of women experience during pregnancy, may add up to 8 L to the volume of extracellular water. For water-soluble drugs (which usually have a relatively small volume of distribution) this increases the apparent volume of distribution and, although clearance is unaltered, their half-life is prolonged. During pregnancy, the plasma protein concentration falls and there is increased competition for binding sites due to competition by endogenous ligands such as increased hormone levels. These factors alter the total amount of bound drug and the apparent volume of distribution. However, the concentration of free drug usually remains unaltered, because a greater volume of distribution of free drug is accompanied by increased clearance of free drug. Thus in practice these changes are rarely of pharmacological significance. However, they may cause confusion in monitoring of plasma drug levels, since this usually measures total (rather than free) drug concentrations.

Metabolism

Metabolism of drugs by the pregnant liver is increased, largely due to enzyme induction, perhaps by raised hormone levels. Liver blood flow does not change. This may lead to an increased rate of elimination of those drugs (e.g. theophylline), for which enzyme activity rather than liver blood flow is the main determinant of elimination rate.

Renal excretion

Excretion of drugs via the kidney increases because renal plasma flow almost doubles and the glomerular filtration rate increases by two-thirds during pregnancy. This has been documented for digoxin, lithium, ampicillin, cephalexin and gentamicin.

Key points

Known differences in drug effects can usually be explained by altered pharmacokinetics. Increased volume of distribution, hepatic metabolism and renal excretion all tend to reduce drug concentration. Decreased plasma albumin levels increase the ratio of free drug in plasma

Prescribing in pregnancy

The prescription of drugs to a pregnant woman is a balance between possible adverse drug effects on the fetus and the risk to mother and fetus of leaving maternal disease inadequately treated. Effects on the human fetus cannot be reliably predicted from animal studies – hence one should prescribe drugs for which there is experience of safety over many years in preference to new or untried drugs. The smallest effective dose should be used. The fetus is most sensitive to adverse drug effects during the first trimester. It has been estimated that nearly half of all pregnancies in the UK are unplanned, and that most women do not present to a doctor until 5–7 weeks after conception. Thus all women of childbearing potential should be assumed to be pregnant until it has been proved otherwise.

Delayed toxicity is a sinister problem (e.g. diethylstilboestrol), and if the teratogenic effect of thalidomide had not produced such an unusual congenital abnormality, namely phocomelia, its detection might have been delayed further. If drugs (or environmental toxins) have more subtle effects on the fetus, (e.g. a minor reduction in intelligence) or cause an increased incidence of a common disease (e.g. atopy), these effects may never be detected. Many publications demand careful prospective controlled clinical trials, but the ethics and practicalities of such studies often make their demands unrealistic. A more rational approach is for drug regulatory bodies, the pharmaceutical industry and drug information agencies to collaborate closely and internationally to collate all information concerning drug use in pregnancy (whether inadvertent or planned) and associate these with outcome not only of the fetus but also of the adult. This will require significant investment of time and money as well as considerable encouragement to doctors and midwives to complete the endless forms. For now, all who prescribe drugs must be aware of the potential hazard to pregnant women and judge each case on its individual merit. To do this, doctors must have rapid access to clear information on the experience of drug use in pregnancy and the morbidity/mortality of untreated disease. A rational decision can then be made as to which if any drug therapy is necessary. Doctors have a responsibility to warn patients of the risks of over-the-counter medicines, smoking and alcohol abuse in pregnancy.

Key points

Prescribing in pregnancy is a balance between the risk of adverse drug effects on the fetus and the risk of leaving maternal disease untreated. The effects on the human fetus are not reliably predicted by animal experiments. However, untreated maternal disease may cause morbidity and/or mortality to mother and/or fetus.

Therefore:

- minimize prescribing;
- use 'tried and tested' drugs whenever possible in preference to new agents;
- use the smallest effective dose;
- remember that the fetus is most sensitive in the first trimester;
- consider pregnancy in all women of childbearing potential;
- discuss the potential risks of taking or withholding therapy with the patient;
- seek guidance on the use of drugs in pregnancy in the *British National Formulary*, Drug Information Services, National Teratology Information Service (NTIS);
- warn the patient about the risks of smoking, alcohol, over-the-counter drugs and drugs of abuse.

Guidance on the use of drugs for a selection of conditions is summarized below. If in doubt, consult the *British National Formulary*, appendix 4 (which is appropriately conservative). Information about the safety of drugs in pregnancy can also be obtained from The National Teratology Information Service (Tel 0191 232 1525).

ANTIMICROBIAL DRUGS

Antimicrobial drugs are commonly prescribed during pregnancy. The safest antibiotics in pregnancy are the penicillins and cephalosporins. Trimethoprim is a theoretical teratogen as it is a folic acid antagonist. The aminoglycosides can cause ototoxicity. There is minimal experience in pregnancy with the fluroquinolones (e.g ciprofloxacin), and they should be avoided. Erythromycin is probably safe. Metronidazole is a teratogen in animals, but there is no evidence of teratogenicity in humans, and its benefit in serious anaerobic sepsis probably outweighs any risks. Unless there is a life-threatening infection in the mother, antiviral agents should be avoided in pregnancy. Falciparum malaria (see Chapter 46) has an especially high mortality rate in late pregnancy. Fortunately, the standard regimens of intravenous and oral quinine are safe in pregnancy.

ANALGESICS

Opioids cross the placenta. This is particularly relevant in the management of labour when the use of opioids such as pethidine depresses the fetal respiratory centre and can inhibit the start of normal respiration. If the mother is dependent on opioids, the fetus can experience opioid withdrawal syndrome during and after delivery, which can be fatal. In neonates the chief withdrawal symptoms are tremor, irritability, diarrhoea and vomiting. Chlorpromazine is commonly used to treat this withdrawal state. Paracetamol is preferred to aspirin when mild analgesia is required. In cases where a systemic anti-inflammatory action is required (e.g. in rheumatoid arthritis), ibuprofen is the drug of choice. Non-steroidal anti-inflammatory drugs can cause constriction of the ductus arteriosus. Occasionally this may be used to therapeutic benefit.

Anaesthesia

Anaesthesia in pregnancy is a very specialist area and should only be undertaken by experienced anaesthetists. Local anaesthetics used for regional anaesthesia readily cross the placenta. However, when used in epidural anaesthesia the drug remains largely confined to the epidural space. Pregnant women are at increased risk of aspiration. Although commonly used, pethidine frequently causes vomiting and may also lead to neonatal respiratory depression. Metoclopramide should be used in preference to prochlorperazine (which has an anti-analgesic effect when combined with pethidine), and naloxone (an opioid antagonist) must always be available. Respiratory depression in the newborn is not usually a problem with modern general anaesthetics currently in use in Caesarean section. Several studies have shown an increased incidence of spontaneous abortions in mothers who have had general anaesthesia during pregnancy, although a causal relationship is not proven, and in most circumstances failure to operate would have dramatically increased the risk to mother and fetus.

Anti-emetics

Nausea and vomiting are common in early pregnancy, but are usually self-limiting, and ideally should be managed with reassurance and non-drug strategies such as small frequent meals, avoiding large volumes of fluid, and raising the head of the bed. If symptoms are prolonged or severe, drug treatment may be effective. Meclozine and cyclizine are commonly used, although both have been weakly associated with an increased risk of congenital malformations. Metoclopramide is considered to be safe and efficacious in labour and before anaesthesia in late pregnancy, but its routine use in early pregnancy cannot be recommended because of the lack of controlled data, and the significant incidence of dystonic reactions in young women.

Dyspepsia and constipation

The high incidence of dyspepsia due to gastro-oesophageal reflux in the second and third trimesters is probably related to the reduction in lower oesophageal sphincter pressure. Non-drug treatment (reassurance, small frequent meals and advice on posture) should be pursued in the first instance, particularly in the first trimester. Fortunately, most cases occur later in pregnancy when non-absorbable antacids such as alginates should be used. In late pregnancy metoclopromide is particularly effective as it increases lower oesophageal sphincter pressure. H_2-receptor blockers should not be used for non-ulcer dyspepsia in this setting. Constipation should be managed with dietary advice. Stimulant laxatives may be uterotonic and should be avoided if possible.

Peptic ulceration

Antacids may relieve symptoms. Cimetidine and Ranitidine have been widely prescribed in pregnancy without obvious damage to the fetus. There is inadequate safety data on the use of omeprazole in pregnancy. Sucralphate has been recommended for use in pregnancy in the USA, and this is rational as it is not systemically absorbed. Misoprostol, a prostaglandin which stimulates the uterus, is contraindicated because it causes abortion.

Anticonvulsants

Epilepsy in pregnancy can lead to fetal and maternal morbidity/mortality through convulsions, whilst all of the anticonvulsants used have been associated with teratogenic effects, (e.g. phenytoin is associated with cleft palate and congenital heart disease). However, there is no doubt that the benefits of good seizure control outweigh the drug-induced teratogenic risk. Thorough explanation to the mother, ideally before a planned pregnancy, is essential, and it must be emphasized that the majority (> 90%) of epileptic mothers have normal babies. (The usual risk of fetal malformation is about 2%, and in epileptic mothers it is up to 10%.) In view of the association of spina bifida with sodium valproate and carbamazepine therapy, it is often recommended that the standard dose of folic acid should be increased to 4–5 mg daily. Both of these anticonvulsants cause hypospadias. As in non-pregnant epilepsy, single-drug therapy is preferable. Plasma concentration monitoring is particularly relevant for phenytoin, because the decrease in plasma protein binding and the increase in hepatic metabolism may cause considerable changes in the plasma concentration of free (active) drug. As always, the guide to the correct dose is freedom from fits and absence of toxicity. Owing to the changes in plasma protein binding, it is generally recommended that the therapeutic range is 5–15 mg/L, whereas in the non-pregnant state it is 10–20 mg/L. This is only a rough guide, as protein binding varies.

Carbamazepine, phenytoinoe and phenobarbitone have been implicated in neonatal haemorrhage secondary to effects on vitamin K-dependent clotting factors. Hence the *British National Formulary* recommends predelivery vitamin K for the mother and post-delivery vitamin K for the neonate.

Magnesium sulphate is the treatment of choice for the prevention and control of eclamptic seizures.

Key points

- Epilepsy in pregnancy can lead to increased fetal and maternal morbidity/mortality.
- All anticonvulsants are teratogens.
- The benefits of good seizure control *outweigh* drug-induced teratogenic risk.
- Give a full explanation to the mother (preferably before pregnancy): most epileptic mothers (> 90%) have normal babies.
- Advise an increase in the standard dose of folic acid up to 12 weeks.
- Make a referral to the neurologist and obstetrician.
- If epilepsy is well controlled, do not change therapy.
- Monitor plasma concentrations (levels tend to fall, and note that the bound:unbound ratio changes); the guide to the correct dose is freedom from fits and absence of toxicity.
- An early ultrasound scan at 12 weeks may detect gross neural-tube defects.
- Detailed ultrasound scan and α-fetoprotein at 16–18 weeks should be considered.
- *The British National Formulary* recommends vitamin K predelivery for mothers (and post-delivery to neonate) on carbamazepine, phenytoin or phenobarbitone.

ANTICOAGULATION

Warfarin has been associated with nasal hypoplasia and chondrodysplasia when given in the first trimester, and with CNS abnormalities after administration in later pregnancy, as well as a high incidence of haemorrhagic complications towards the end of pregnancy. Neonatal haemorrhage is difficult to prevent because of the immature enzymes in fetal liver and the low stores of vitamin K. Heparin, which does not cross the placenta, is the anticoagulant of choice in pregnancy, although chronic use can cause maternal osteoporosis and thrombocytopenia (see Chapter 29). Low-molecular-weight heparins are probably as safe and effective as unfractionated heparin. A longer duration of action allows once daily administration, whereas unfractionated heparin is administered twice daily in most prophylactic regimens. Women on long-term oral anticoagulants should be warned that these drugs are likely to affect the fetus in early pregnancy. Subcutaneous heparin (usually self-administered) must be substituted for warfarin as soon as possible, and well before the critical period of 6–9 weeks' gestation.

Key points

- Pregnancy is associated with a hypercoagulable state.
- Warfarin has been associated with nasal hypoplasia and chondrodysplasia in the first trimester, and with CNS abnormalities in late pregnancy, as well as haemorrhagic complications.
- Heparin does not cross the placenta, but chronic use is associated with an increased risk of maternal osteoporosis and thrombocytopenia. Daily (or bd) subcutaneous injections are needed. Low-molecular-weight heparins may be preferable.
- There is no ideal regimen. *Seek specialist advice.* Possible regime: first trimester, heparin; second trimester, warfarin; third trimester, heparin.

Subcutaneous heparin can be continued throughout pregnancy but, due to the risk of maternal osteoporosis and thrombocytopenia, warfarin may be considered as an alternative during the second trimester, changing back to heparin at 36 weeks. Patients with prosthetic heart valves present a special problem, and in these patients, despite the risks to the fetus, warfarin is often given up to 36 weeks. The prothrombin time/international normalized ratio (INR) (warfarin) or activated partial thromboplastin time (APTT) (heparin) should be monitored closely.

Cardiovascular drugs

Hypertension in pregnancy (see Chapter 27) can normally be managed with either methyldopa which has the most extensive safety record in pregnancy, or labetalol, although beta-blockers may cause intrauterine growth retardation when used in the first two trimesters. Parenteral hydralazine is useful for lowering blood pressure in pre-eclampsia. Diuretics should not be started to treat hypertension in pregnancy, although some American authorities now continue thiazide diuretics in women with essential hypertension who are already stabilized on these drugs. Modified-release preparations of nifedipine are also used for hypertension in pregnancy, but angiotensin-converting enzyme inhibitors must be avoided.

Hormones

Progestogens, particularly synthetic ones, can masculinize the female fetus. There is no evidence that this occurs with the small amount of progestogen (or oestrogen) present in the oral contraceptive – the risk applies to large doses. Corticosteroids do not appear to give rise to any serious problems when given via inhalation or in short courses. Transient suppression of the fetal hypothalamic–pituitary–adrenal axis has been reported. Rarely, cleft palate and congenital cataract have been linked with steroids in pregnancy, but the benefit of treatment usually outweighs any such risk. Iodine and antithyroid drugs cross the placenta and can cause hypothyroidism and goitre. Management of hyperthyroidism during pregnancy is discussed in Chapter 37.

Tranquillizers and antidepressants

Benzodiazepines accumulate in the tissues and are slowly eliminated by the neonate, resulting in prolonged hypotonia ('floppy baby'), subnormal temperatures (hypothermia), periodic cessation of respiration and poor sucking. There is no evidence that the phenothiazines, tricyclic antidepressants or fluoxetine are teratogenic. Lithium can cause fetal goitre and possible cardiovascular abnormalities.

Non-therapeutic drugs

Excessive ethanol consumption is associated with spontaneous abortion, craniofacial abnormalities, mental retardation, congenital heart disease and impaired growth. Even moderate alcohol intake may adversely affect the baby – the risk of having an abnormal child is about 10% in mothers drinking 30–60 mL ethanol per day, rising to 40% in chronic alcoholics. Fetal alcohol syndrome describes the distinct pattern of abnormal morphogenesis and central nervous system dysfunction in children whose mothers were chronic alcoholics, and this syndrome is a leading cause of mental retardation. After birth the characteristic craniofacial malformations diminish, but microcephaly and to a lesser degree short stature persist. Cigarette smoking is associated with spontaneous abortion, premature delivery, small babies, increased perinatal mortality and a higher incidence of sudden infant death syndrome (cot death). Cocaine causes vasoconstriction of placental vessels. There is a high incidence of low birth weight, congenital abnormalities and, in particular, delayed neurological and behavioural development.

Case history

A 20-year-old female medical student attended her GP requesting a course of Septrin® (co-trimoxazole) for cystitis. On taking the history, her GP learned that the patient had noticed increased urinary frequency over the last 3 days. She had had two previous episodes of lower urinary tract infection (UTI), confirmed on laboratory testing, which started with urinary frequency and resolved with Septrin®. She was uncertain as to the date of her last menstrual bleed, but said it was about 6 weeks earlier. She did not think she was at risk of pregnancy as her periods had been irregular since stopping the oral contraceptive 1 year previously due to fears about thrombosis, and her boyfriend used a condom. Physical examination, which did not include a vaginal examination, was normal. Urinalysis was 1+ positive for blood and a trace of protein.

Question

Why should the GP *not* prescribe co-trimoxazole for this patient?

Answer

Until proven otherwise, it should be assumed that this woman is pregnant. Co-trimoxazole (a combination of sulphamethoxazole and trimethoprim) has been superseded by trimethoprim alone as a useful drug in lower urinary tract infection. The sulphamethoxazole does not add significant antibacterial advantage in lower UTI, but does have sulphonamide-associated side-effects, including the rare but life-threatening Stevens–Johnson syndrome. Both sulphamethoxazole and trimethoprim inhibit folate synthesis and are theoretical teratogens. If pregnancy is confirmed (urinary frequency is an early symptom of pregnancy in some women, due to a progesterone effect) and if the patient has a lower UTI confirmed by pyuria and bacteria on microscopy whilst awaiting culture and sensitivity results, amoxycillin is the treatment of choice. Alternatives include an oral cephalosporin or nitrofurantoin. *Note that lower urinary tract infection in pregnancy can rapidly progress to acute pyelonephritis.*

Further reading

Anon. 1996: Preconception, pregnancy and prescribing. *Drugs and Therapeutics Bulletin* **34**, 25–7.

Koren G, Pastuszak A, Ito S. 1998: Drugs in pregnancy. *New England Journal of Medicine* **338**, 1128–36.

Rubin PC. 1998: Drug treatment during pregnancy. *British Medical Journal* **317**, 1503–6.

Further information for health professionals

National Teratology Information Service
Regional Drug and Therapeutics Centre
Wolfson Unit
Clarement Place
Newcastle upon Tyne
NE1 4LP

Telephone: 0191 232 1525

CHAPTER TEN

DRUGS *in* INFANTS *and* CHILDREN

- Introduction
- Pharmacokinetics
- Pharmacodynamics
- Breast-feeding
- Practical aspects of prescribing
- Research

INTRODUCTION

Children cannot be regarded as miniature adults in terms of drug response, due to differences in body constitution, drug absorption and elimination, and sensitivity to adverse reactions.

PHARMACOKINETICS

ABSORPTION

Reduced gastric acidity in neonates results in greater oral absorption of certain antibiotics (e.g. amoxycillin). The rate of gastric emptying is very variable during the neonatal period, and may be delayed by disease such as respiratory distress syndrome and congenital heart disease. To ensure that adequate blood concentrations reach the systemic circulation in the sick neonate, it is common practice to use intravenous preparations. The major practical difference in young children is the more frequent use of oral liquid preparations, resulting in less accurate dosing and a more rapid rate of absorption (although minimal difference in bioavailability). This can be significant for drugs with a close correlation between high peak plasma concentration and adverse effects, or low trough concentration and lack of efficacy (e.g. carbamazepine and theophylline). Infant skin is thin, and percutaneous absorption is increased relative to that in adults. Hence systemic absorption of corticosteroids from local preparations may be increased, and can cause toxicity if these drugs are used extensively.

DISTRIBUTION

Body fat content is relatively low in children, leading to a lower volume of distribution of fat-soluble drugs (e.g. diazepam) in babies. Plasma protein binding of drugs is reduced in neonates due to a lower plasma albumin concentration and altered binding properties of albumin and globulin. This is not generally of clinical significance although the risk of kernicterus caused by displacement of bilirubin from albumin by sulphonamides (see Chapter 12) is well recognized. The blood–brain barrier is more permeable in neonates and young children, leading to an increased risk of central nervous system (CNS) adverse effects.

METABOLISM

At birth the hepatic microsomal enzyme system (see chapter 5) is relatively immature (particularly in the preterm infant), but after the first 4 weeks it matures rapidly. Chloramphenicol can produce 'grey baby syndrome' in neonates due to high plasma levels secondary to inefficient glucuronidation. Drugs administered to the mother can induce neonatal enzyme activity(e.g. barbiturates). In children there is evidence that aspirin metabolism is relatively impaired, whilst phenobarbitone metabolism is increased. This may be because of induction of hepatic enzyme activity, or because the ratio of the weight of the liver to body weight is up to 50% higher than in adults.

Excretion

All renal mechanisms (filtration, secretion and reabsorption) are reduced in babies, and renal excretion of drugs is relatively reduced in the newborn. Glomerular filtration rate (GFR) increases rapidly during the first 4 weeks of life, with consequent changes in the rate of drug elimination (Table 10.1).

Key points

Prevalance of chronic illness in children requiring drug therapy

- 1 in 8 children have asthma;
- 1 in 250 children have epilepsy;
- 1 in 750 children have diabetes mellitus.

Key points

At birth, renal and hepatic function are less efficient than in adulthood. Drug effects may be prolonged and accumulation may occur. These factors are exaggerated in the premature infant.

Table 10.1: Changes in rate of drug elimination with development

Stage of development	Plasma half-life of genetamicin
Premature infant	
< 48 h old	18
5–22 days old	6
Normal infant	
1–4 weeks old	3
Adult	2

Pharmacodynamics

Documented evidence of differences in receptor sensitivity in children is lacking, and the apparently paradoxical effects of some drugs (e.g. hyperkinesia with phenobarbitone, sedation of hyperactive children with amphetamine) are as yet unexplained.

Breast-feeding

Breast-feeding can lead to toxicity in the infant if the drug enters the milk in pharmacological quantities. The milk concentration of some drugs (e.g. iodides) may exceed the maternal plasma concentration, but the total dose delivered to the baby is usually very small. However, drugs in breast milk may cause hypersensitivity reactions even in very low doses. Virtually all drugs that reach the maternal systemic circulation will enter breast milk, especially lipid-soluble unionized low-molecular-weight drugs. Milk is weakly acidic, so drugs that are weak bases are concentrated in breast milk by trapping of the charged form of the drug (compare with renal elimination; see Chapter 6). However, the resulting dose administered to the fetus in breast milk is usually clinically insignificant, although some drugs are contraindicated (Table

Table 10.2: Some drugs to be avoided during breast-feeding

Vitamin A/retinoid analogues (e.g. etretinate)
Amiodarone
Aspirin
Stimulant laxatives
Benzodiazepines
Chloramphenicol
Ciprofloxacin
Cocaine
Combined oral contraceptives
Cyclosporin
Cytotoxics
Ergotamine
Octreotide
Sulphonylureas
Thiazide diuretics

10.2), and breast-feeding should cease during treatment if there is no safer alternative.

The infant should be monitored if β-adrenoceptor antagonists, carbimazole, corticosteroids or lithium are prescribed to the mother. β-adrenoceptor antagonists rarely cause significant bradycardia. Carbimazole should be prescribed at its lowest effective dose to reduce the risk of hypothyroidism in the neonate/infant. In high doses, corticosteroids can affect the infant's adrenal function and lithium may cause intoxication. There is a theoretical risk of Reyes' syndrome if aspirin is prescribed to the breast-feeding mother. Warfarin is not containdicated during breast-feeding. Bromocriptine and diuretics suppress lactation, but their adverse effects outweigh their benefits in women who choose not to breast-feed. Metronidazole gives milk an unpleasant taste.

Practical aspects of prescribing

Compliance and route of administration

Sick neonates will usually require intravenous drug administration. Accurate dosage and attention to fluid balance are essential. Sophisticated syringe pumps with awareness of 'dead space' associated with the apparatus are necessary.

Children under the age of 5 years may have difficulty swallowing even small tablets, and hence oral preparations which taste pleasant are often necessary to improve compliance. Liquid preparations are given by means of a graduated syringe. However, chronic use of sucrose-containing elixirs encourages tooth cavities and gingivitis. Moreover, the dyes and colourings used may induce hypersensitivity.

Pressurized aerosols (e.g. salbutamol inhaler, see Chapter 32) are usually only practicable in children over the age of 10 years, as co-ordinated deep inspiration is required unless a device such as a spacer is used. Spacers can be combined with a face mask from early infancy. Likewise, nebulizers may be used to enhance local therapeutic effect and reduce systemic toxicity.

Only in unusual circumstances, i.e. extensive areas of application (especially to inflamed or broken skin), or in infants, does systemic absorption of drugs (e.g. steroids, neomycin) become significant following topical application to the skin.

Intramuscular injection should only be used when absolutely necessary. Intravenous therapy is less painful, but skill is required to cannulate infants' veins (and a confident colleague to keep the target still!). Children find intravenous infusions uncomfortable and restrictive. Rectal administration (see Chapter 4) is a convenient alternative, (e.g. metronidazole to prevent/treat anaerobic infections). Rectal diazepam is particularly valuable in the treatment of status epilepticus when intravenous access is often difficult. Rectal diazepam may also be administered by parents. Rectal administration should also be considered if the child is vomiting.

Paramount to ensuring compliance is full communication with the child's parents and teachers. This should include information not only on how to administer the drug, but also on why it is being prescribed, for how long the treatment should continue and whether any adverse effects are likely.

Case history

A 2-year-old epileptic child is seen in the Accident and Emergency Department. He has been fitting for at least 15 min. The casualty officer is unable to cannulate a vein to administer intravenous diazepam. The more experienced medical staff are dealing with emergencies elsewhere in the hospital.

Question
Name two drugs, and their route of administration, with which the casualty officer may terminate the convulsions.

Answer
Rectal diazepam solution.
Intramuscular paraldehdyde.

Dosage

Even after adjustment of dose according to surface area, calculation of the correct dose must consider the relatively large volume of distribution of polar drugs in the first 4 months of life, the immature microsomal enzymes and reduced renal function. The *British National Formulary* and specialist paediatric textbooks and formularies provide appropriate guidelines and must be consulted by physicians who are not familiar with prescribing to infants and children.

Adverse effects

With a few notable exceptions, drugs in children generally have a similar adverse effect profile to those in adults. Of particular significance is the potential of chronic corticosteroid use, including high-dose inhaled corticosteroids, to inhibit growth. Aspirin is avoided in children under 12 years (except in specific indications) due to an association with Reye's syndrome, a rare but often fatal illness of unknown aetiology consisting of hepatic necrosis and encephalopathy, often in the aftermath of a viral illness. Tetracyclines are deposited in growing bone and teeth, causing staining and occasionally dental hypoplasia, and should not be given to children. Fluoroquinolone antibacterial drugs may damage growing cartilage. Dystonias with metoclopramide and hepatic failure with sodium valproate occur relatively more frequently in children.

Case history

A 14-year-old boy with a history of exercise-induced asthma, for which he uses salbutamol PRN (on average 2 puffs twice daily and before exercise) is seen by his GP because of malaise and nocturnal cough. On examination he has a mild fever (38°C), bilateral swollen cervical lymph nodes and bilateral wheeze. Ampicillin is prescribed for a respiratory tract infection. The next day the boy develops a widespread maculopapular rash.

Question 1

What is the cause of the rash?

Question 2

What is the likely cause of the nocturnal cough, and how may this be treated?

Answer 1

Ampicillin rash in infectious mononucleosis (glandular fever).

Answer 2

Poorly controlled asthma. Regular inhaled corticosteroid or cromoglycate.

Research

Research in paediatric clinical pharmacology is limited. Not only is there concern about the potential for adverse effects of new drugs on those who are growing and developing mentally but there are also considerable ethical problems encountered in research involving individuals who are too young to give informed consent. New drugs are often given to children for the first time only when no alternative is available or when unacceptable side-effects have been encountered in a particular individual with established drugs. For these reasons, pharmaceutical companies seldom seek to license their products for use in children. When drugs are prescribed to children that are not licensed for use in this age group it is important to make careful records of both efficacy and possible adverse effects. Parents should be informed of any unlicensed use of drugs in their children.

Further reading

Rylance GW. 1994: Prescribing for infants and children. In Fealey J (ed.) *New drugs*, 3rd edn. London: BMJ Publications.

Rylance GW, Armstrong D. 1997: Adverse drug events in children. *Adverse Drug Reaction Bulletin* **184**, 699–702.

Paediatric Formulary, 5th edn. (revised 1999). Guy's, St. Thomas' and Lewisham Hospitals.

CHAPTER ELEVEN

DRUGS *in the* ELDERLY

- Introduction
- Pharmacokinetic changes
- Pharmacodynamic changes
- Compliance in the elderly
- Effect of drugs on some major organ systems in the elderly
- Practical aspects of prescribing for the elderly
- Research

INTRODUCTION

The proportion of elderly people in the population is increasing steadily in economically developed countries. The elderly are subject to a variety of complaints, many of which are chronic and incapacitating, and so they receive a great deal of drug treatment. Elderly people represent some 12% of the population of the UK, but consume about one-third of the National Health Service's drug expenditure. Adverse drug reactions become more common with increasing age. In one study, 11.8% of patients aged 41–50 years experienced adverse reactions to drugs, but this increased to 25% in patients over 80 years of age. There are several reasons for this.

1 Elderly people take more drugs. In one survey in general practice, 87% of patients over 75 years of age were on regular drug therapy, with 34% taking three to four different drugs daily. The most commonly prescribed drugs were diuretics (34% of patients), analgesics (27%), tranquillizers and antidepressants (24%), hypnotics (22%) and digoxin (20%). All of these are associated with a high incidence of important adverse effects.
2 Pharmacokinetics change with increasing age and concomitant disease, leading to higher plasma concentrations of drugs and increased liability to side-effects (see below).
3 Homeostatic mechanisms become less effective with advancing age, so individuals are less able to compensate for adverse effects such as unsteadiness or postural hypotension.
4 The central nervous system becomes more sensitive to the actions of sedative drugs.
5 Increasing age produces changes in the immune response that can cause an increased liability to allergic reactions.

PHARMACOKINETIC CHANGES

ABSORPTION

Iron, xylose, galactose, calcium and thiamine absorption are reduced in old people. Most drugs are absorbed by simple diffusion down the concentration gradient, and this is not impaired by age. Intestinal blood flow is reduced by up to 50% in the elderly, and gastric motility is increased, probably due to the tendency towards reduced acid secretion in the old. However, unless gastrointestinal pathology is present, it appears that age *per se* does not affect drug absorption to a large extent.

Distribution

Ageing is associated with loss of weight and lean body mass, and with an increased ratio of fat to muscle and body water. This enlarges the volume of distribution of fat-soluble drugs such as diazepam and lignocaine, whereas the distribution of polar drugs such as digoxin is reduced compared to that in younger adults. When the dosage of a drug is critical, it is important to make suitable adjustment for body weight. Changes in plasma proteins also occur with ageing, especially if the latter is associated with chronic disease and malnutrition with a fall in albumin and a rise in gamma-globulin concentrations.

Hepatic metabolism

There is a decrease in the rate of hepatic clearance of some but not all drugs with advancing age. Many early studies depended on demonstrating a prolonged plasma half-life (Figure 11.1), which could be secondary to an increased apparent volume of distribution rather than reduced metabolism. Changes in clearance with age should be documented to confirm that ageing reduces drug metabolism. The reduced rate of clearance of long-half-life benzodiazepines has important clinical consequences, as when these are prescribed for prolonged periods, slow accumulation of drug (and active metabolites) may lead to adverse effects whose onset may occur days or weeks after initiating therapy. Consequently, confusion or memory impairment may be falsely attributed to ageing rather than to adverse drug effects.

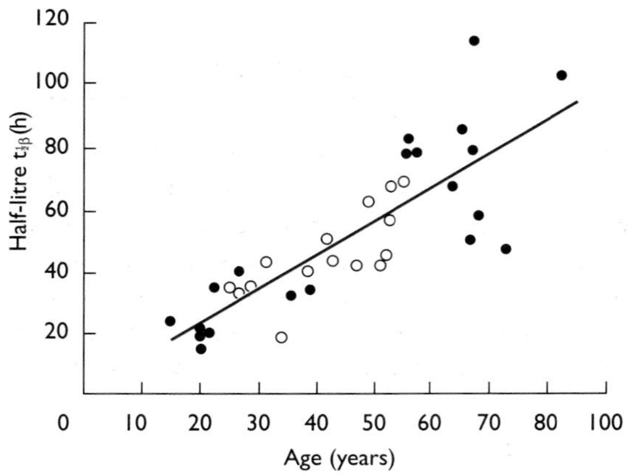

Figure 11.1: Relationship between diazepam half-life and age in 33 normal individuals. Non-smokers (●); Smokers (○). (Reproduced from Klotz U *et al.* 1975: *Journal of Clinical Investigation* **55** 347.)

Renal excretion

Probably the most important cause of drug accumulation in the elderly is declining renal function. In healthy individuals aged over 80 years the glomerular filtration rate is < 60–70 mL/min, and renal disorders associated with advancing years (e.g. prostatic hypertrophy) further reduce renal function. The glomerular filtration rate falls at a rate of approximately 1 mL/min/1.73 m^2 each year after the age of 20 years. It is important to appreciate that, although glomerular filtration rate declines with age, *this is not adequately reflected by serum creatinine*, which can remain within the range defined as 'normal' for a younger adult population despite a marked decline in renal function. This is related to the lower endogenous production of creatinine in the elderly secondary to their reduced muscle mass.

Tubular function also declines with age. These changes are reflected in the increasing plasma creatinine and urea concentrations with age. A number of dosage rules and nomograms are based on creatinine clearance (see Chapter 7). Drugs that are mainly excreted via the kidney are likely to accumulate in patients in their seventies and eighties if given in doses suitable for young adults. Examples of drugs which may require reduced dosage in the elderly secondary to reduced renal excretion and/or hepatic clearance are listed in Table 11.1.

Key points

Pharmacokinetic changes in the elderly include:

- Absorption of iron, calcium and thiamine is reduced.
- There is an increased volume of distribution of fat-soluble drugs (e.g. diazepam).
- There is a decreased volume of distribution of polar drugs (e.g. digoxin).
- There is reduced hepatic clearance of long-half-life benzodiazepines.
- Declining renal function is the most important cause of drug accumulation.

Table 11.1: Examples of drugs requiring dose adjustment in the elderly

Aminoglycosides (e.g. gentamicin)
Atenolol
Cimetidine
Diazepam
Digoxin
Non-steroidal anti-inflammatory drugs
Oral hypoglycaemic agents
Warfarin

Pharmacodynamic changes

Evidence that the elderly are intrinsically more sensitive to drugs than the young is scarce. However, the sensitivity of the elderly to benzodiazepines as measured by psychometric tests is increased, and their effects last longer than in the young. It is common clinical experience that benzodiazepines given to the elderly at hypnotic doses used for the young can produce prolonged daytime confusion even after single doses. The incidence of confusion associated with cimetidine is increased in the elderly. Other drugs may expose physiological defects that are a normal concomitant of ageing. Postural hypotension can occur in healthy elderly people, and the increased incidence of postural hypotension from drugs such as phenothiazines, β-adrenoceptor antagonists, tricyclic antidepressants and diuretics in elderly patients is not surprising. The increase in heart rate produced by isoprenaline is diminished in older patients, suggesting that the sensitivity of the β-receptor response mechanism decreases with age. Clotting factor synthesis by the liver is reduced in the elderly, and old people often require lower warfarin doses for effective anticoagulation than younger adults.

Key points

Pharmacodynamic changes in the elderly include:

- increased sensitivity to CNS effects (e.g. benzodiazepines, cimetidine);
- increased incidence of postural hypotension (e.g. phenothiazines, beta-blockers, tricyclic antidepressants, diuretics);
- reduced clotting factor synthesis, reduced warfarin for anticoagulation;
- increased toxicity from NSAIDs;
- increased incidence of allergic reactions to drugs.

Compliance in the elderly

Young adult patients frequently fail to take their medicines as instructed even when they have diseases such as tuberculosis, where there should be considerable motivation towards compliance. Non-compliance is even more common (possibly about 60%) in elderly people. This may be due either to a failure of memory or to not understanding how the drug should be taken. In addition, patients may have previously prescribed drugs in the medicine cupboard which they take from time to time. It is therefore essential that the drug regimen is kept simple and explained carefully. There is scope for improved methods of packaging so that over- or under-dosage is prevented. Multiple drug regimens must be avoided if possible. Not only will such regimens confuse the patient, but they increase the risk of interactions (see Chapter 13).

Effect of drugs on some major organ systems in the elderly

Central nervous system

Cerebral function in old people is easily disturbed, resulting in disorientation and confusion. Drugs are one of the factors that contribute to this state; sedatives and hypnotics can easily precipitate a loss of awareness and clouding of consciousness. Over-vigorous attempts to lower blood pressure may produce cerebral ischaemia and confusion.

Night sedation

The elderly do not sleep as well as the young. They sleep for a shorter time, their sleep is more likely to be broken and they are more easily aroused. This is quite normal, and old people should not have the expectations of the young so far as sleep is concerned. Before hypnotics are commenced, other possible factors should be considered and treated if possible. These include the following:

1 pain, which may be due to such causes as arthritis;
2 constipation – the discomfort of a loaded rectum;
3 urinary frequency;
4 depression;
5 anxiety;
6 left ventricular failure;
7 dementia.

A little more exercise may help, and 'catnapping' in the day should be reduced to a minimum.

The prescription of hypnotics (see Chapter 17) should be minimized in the elderly.

Tranquillizers

Restlessness and agitated depression are common in old people and are associated with dementia. These states can be ameliorated by phenothiazines (e.g. thioridazine) (see Chapter 18). However, they are associated with a high incidence of adverse events in this age group.

Of particular importance are the following:

1 the development of Parkinsonian symptoms, particularly slowness and rigidity, may be a problem and may require lowering the dose or stopping the drug. Concurrent use of anti-Parkinsonian drugs (e.g. muscarinic antagonists) is associated with a high incidence of adverse effects in this age group (e.g. urinary retention). The elderly are more prone to Parkinsonian syndromes and tardive dyskinesia than are young people;
2 postural hypotension;
3 hypothermia.

Antidepressants

Although depression is common in old age and may indeed need drug treatment, it should be remembered that the tricyclic antidepressants (see Chapter 19) can cause constipation, urinary retention and glaucoma (all due to their parasympathetic blocking action), and also drowsiness, confusion, postural hypotension and cardiac arrhythmias. The possibility that depression could result from a drug used in the treatment of another disease (e.g. a β-adrenoreceptor antagonist) should be remembered. Tricyclic antidepressants can produce worthwhile remissions of depression but should be started at very low dosage, (e.g. amitriptyline, 25 mg *nocte*), and only cautiously increased in dose.

Lofepramine is an alternative which has fewer of the anticholinergic side-effects that are particularly troublesome in this age group.

Selective 5-hydroxytryptamine reuptake inhibitors (e.g. fluoxetine) are as effective as the tricyclics and have a distinct side-effect profile (see Chapter 19). They are generally well tolerated by the elderly. However, they are more expensive than tricyclic antidepressants.

Anti-Parkinsonian drugs

The anticholinergic group of anti-Parkinsonian drugs (e.g. benzhexol, orphenadrine) quite often cause side-effects in the elderly. Urinary retention is common in men. Glaucoma may be precipitated or aggravated and confusion may occur with quite small doses. Levodopa can be effective, but it is particularly important to start with a small dose. Levodopa, 100 mg, and carbidopa, 10 mg (co-careldopa), is a suitable initial dose and can be increased gradually as needed. In patients with dementia the use of anticholinergics, levodopa or amantidine may produce adverse cerebral stimulation and/or hallucinations, leading to decompensation of cerebral functioning, with excitement and inability to cope.

CARDIOVASCULAR SYSTEM

Hypertension

There is excellent evidence that treating hypertension in the elderly reduces both morbidity and mortality. Treatment of hypertension in the elderly is discussed in Chapter 27.

Digoxin

Digoxin toxicity is common in the elderly because of the decreased renal elimination and reduced apparent volume of distribution. Confusion, nausea and vomiting, altered vision and an acute abdominal syndrome resembling mesenteric artery obstruction are all more common features of digoxin toxicity in the old than in the young. Hypokalaemia due to decreased potassium intake (potassium-rich foods are often expensive), faulty homeostatic mechanisms resulting in increased renal loss and the concomitant use of diuretics is commoner in the old, and is a contributory factor in some patients. Digoxin is sometimes prescribed when there is no indication for it (e.g. for an irregular pulse which is due to multiple ectopic beats rather than atrial fibrillation). At other times the indications for initiation of treatment are correct but the situation is never reviewed. In one series of geriatric patients on digoxin the drug was withdrawn in 78% of cases without detrimental effects.

Diuretics

Diuretics are more likely to cause adverse effects (e.g. postural hypotension, glucose intolerance and electrolyte disturbances) in elderly patients. Too vigorous a diuresis may result in urinary retention in an old man with an enlarged prostate, and necessitate bladder catheterization with its attendant risks. Brisk diuresis in patients with mental impairment or reduced mobility can result in incontinence. For many patients a thiazide diuretic such as bendrofluazide is adequate. Loop diuretics such as frusemide should be used in acute heart failure or in the lowest effective dose for maintenance treatment of chronic heart failure. Clinically important hypokalaemia is uncommon with low doses of diuretics, but plasma potassium should be checked after starting treatment. If clinically important hypokalaemia develops, a thiazide plus potassium-retaining diuretic (amiloride or triamterene) can be considered, but there is a risk of hyperkalaemia due to renal impairment, especially if angiotensin-converting enzyme (ACE) inhibitors are given together with the diuretic for hypertension or heart failure. Thiazide-induced gout and glucose intolerance are important side-effects. Non-steroidal anti-inflammatory drugs antagonize some of the therapeutic effects of diuretics.

Ischaemic heart disease

See Chapter 28.

Angiotensin-converting enzyme inhibitors

This group of drugs plays an important part in the treatment of chronic heart failure as well as hypertension (see Chapters 27 and 30), and is effective and usually well tolerated in the elderly. However, hypotension, hyperkalaemia and renal failure are more common in this age group. The possibility of renal artery stenosis should be born in mind and serum creatinine levels checked before and after starting treatment. Potassium-retaining diuretics should be stopped and plasma potassium levels monitored.

Oral hypoglycaemic agents

Diabetes is common in the elderly, and many patients are treated with oral hypoglycaemic drugs. It is best for elderly patients to be managed with diet if at all possible, and to use drugs only to relieve symptoms of hyperglycaemia. Chlorpropamide (half-life 36 h) can cause prolonged hypoglycaemia and is specifically contraindicated in this age group, glibenclamide should also be avoided. Shorter-acting drugs (e.g. gliclazide; see Chapter 36) are preferred.

Antibiotics

Antibiotics do not usually cause undue problems in old age so long as the decline in renal function is remembered when an aminoglycoside or tetracycline is used. Amoxycillin and ampicillin are the commonest causes of drug rashes in the elderly.

Non-steroidal anti-inflammatory drugs (NSAIDs)

The elderly are particularly susceptible to NSAID-induced peptic ulceration, gastrointestinal impair-

Case history

An 80-year-old retired publican was referred with 'congestive cardiac failure and acute retention of urine'. His wife said his symptoms of ankle swelling and breathlessness had gradually increased over a period of 6 months despite the GP doubling the water tablet (co-amilozide) which he was taking for high blood pressure. Over the previous week he had become mildly confused and restless at night, for which the GP had prescribed thioridazine. His other medication included ketoprofen for osteoarthritis and frequent magnesium trisilicate mixture for indigestion. He had been getting up nearly 10 times most nights for a year to pass urine. During the day he passed small amounts of urine often. Over the previous 24 h he had been unable to pass urine. His wife thought most of his problems were due to the fact that he drank two pints of beer each day since his retirement 7 years previously.

On physical examination he was clinically anaemic but not cyanosed. Findings were consistent with congestive cardiac failure. His bladder was palpable up to his umbilicus. Rectal examination revealed an enlarged, symmetrical prostate and black tarry faeces. Fundoscopy revealed a grade II hypertensive retinopathy.

Initial laboratory results revealed that the patient had acute on chronic renal failure, dangerously high potassium levels (7.6 mmol/L) and anaemia (Hb 7.4 g/dL). Emergency treatment included calcium chloride, dextrose and insulin, urinary catheterization, frusemide and haemodialysis. Gastroscopy revealed a bleeding gastric ulcer. The patient was discharged 2 weeks later, when he was symptomatically well. His discharge medication consisted of regular doxazosin and ranitidine, and paracetamol prn.

Question

Describe how each of this patient's drugs prescribed before admission may have contributed to his clinical condition.

Answer

Co-amilozide – hyperkalaemia – amiloride, exacerbation of prostatic symptoms – thiazide

Thioridazine – urinary retention

Ketoprofen – gastric ulcer, antagonism of thiazide diuretic, salt retention, possibly interstitial nephritis

Magnesium triosilicate mixture – additional sodium load (6 mmol Na^{+}/10 mL)

Comment

Iatrogenic disease due to multiple drug therapy is common in the elderly. The use of amiloride in renal impairment leads to hyperkalaemia. This patient's confusion and restlessness were most probably related to his renal failure. Thioridazine may mask some of the symptoms/signs and delay treatment of the reversible organic disease. The analgesic of choice in osteoarthritis is paracetamol, due to its much better tolerance than NSAID. The sodium content of some antacids can adversely affect cardiac and renal failure.

ment and fluid retention. NSAIDs are frequently prescribed inappropriately for osteoarthritis before physical and functional interventions and oral paracetamol have been adequately utilized. If an NSAID is required as adjunctive therapy, the lowest effective dose should be used. Ibuprofen is probably the NSAID of choice in terms of minimizing gastrointestinal side-effects. Misoprostol should be considered as prophylaxis against upper gastrointestinal complications in those most at risk. Ranitidine is commonly prescribed to prevent duodenal ulceration and dyspepsia.

PRACTICAL ASPECTS OF PRESCRIBING FOR THE ELDERLY

Improper prescription of drugs is a common cause of morbidity in elderly people. Common-sense rules for prescribing have been suggested (and do not apply only to the elderly).

1 Take a full drug history (see Chapter 1), which should include any adverse reactions and use of over-the-counter drugs.
2 Know the pharmacological action of the drug employed.
3 Use the lowest effective dose.
4 Use the fewest possible number of drugs the patient needs.
5 Drugs should not be used to treat symptoms without first discovering the cause of the symptoms (i.e. first diagnosis, then treatment).
6 Drugs should not be withheld because of old age, but it should be remembered that there is no cure for old age either.

7 A drug should not be continued if it is no longer necessary.
8 Do not use a drug if the symptoms it causes are worse than those it is intended to relieve.
9 It is seldom sensible to treat the side-effects of one drug by prescribing another.

In the elderly it is often important to pay attention to matters such as the formulation of the drug to be used – many old people tolerate elixirs and liquid medicines better than tablets or capsules. Supervision of drug taking may be necessary, as an old person with a serious physical or mental disability cannot be expected to comply with any but the simplest drug regimen. Containers require especially clear labelling, and should be easy to open – child-proof containers are often also grandparent-proof!

RESEARCH

Despite their disproportionate consumption of medicines, the elderly are often under-represented in clinical trials. This may result in the data being extrapolated to an elderly population inappropriately, or the exclusion of elderly patients from new treatments from which they might benefit. It is essential that, both during a drug's development and after it has been licensed, subgroup analysis of elderly populations is carefully examined both for efficacy and for predisposition to adverse effects.

Case history

A previously mentally alert and well-orientated 90-year-old woman became acutely confused two nights after hospital admission for bronchial asthma which, on the basis of peak flow and blood gases, had responded well to inhaled salbutamol and oral prednisolone. Her other medication was cimetidine (for dyspepsia), digoxin (for an isolated episode of atrial fibrillation 2 years earlier) and nitrazepam (for night sedation).

Question

Which drugs may be related to the acute confusion?

Answer

Prednisolone, cimetidine, digoxin and nitrazepam.

Comment

If an H_2-antagonist is necessary, ranitidine is preferred in the elderly. It is likely that the patient no longer requires digoxin (which accumulates in the elderly). Benzodiazepines should not be used for sedation in elderly (or young) asthmatics. They may also accumulate in the elderly. The elderly tend to be more sensitive to adverse drug effects on the CNS.

FURTHER READING

Anon. 1998: Symposium: care of elderly people. *Prescribers Journal* **348**, 197–264.

Montamat SC, Cusack BJ, Vestal RE. 1989: Management of drug therapy – the elderly. *New England Journal of Medicine* **321**, 303–9.

Rochon Gurwitz. 1995: Drug therapy. *Lancet* **346**, 32–6.

Royal College of Physicians 1997: *Medication for older people*. London: Royal College of Physicians.

Swift C. 1994: Prescribing for the elderly. In *New drugs*, 3rd edn. London: BMJ Publications.

CHAPTER TWELVE

ADVERSE DRUG REACTIONS

- Introduction
- Adverse drug reaction monitoring/surveillance (pharmacovigilance)
- Allergic adverse drug reactions
- Examples of allergic and other adverse drug reactions
- Identification of the drug at fault
- Prevention of allergic drug reactions

INTRODUCTION

Adverse drug reactions are unwanted effects caused by normal therapeutic doses. Drugs are great mimics of disease, and adverse drug reactions present with diverse clinical signs and symptoms. The classification proposed by Rawlins and Thompson (1977) divides reactions into type A and type B (Table 12.1).

Type A reactions, which constitute the great majority of adverse drug reactions, are usually a consequence of the drug's main pharmacological effect (e.g. bleeding from warfarin) or a low therapeutic index (e.g. nausea from digoxin), and they are therefore predictable. They are dose-related and usually mild, although they may be serious or even fatal (e.g. intracranial bleeding from warfarin). Such reactions are usually due to incorrect dosage (too much or for too long), for the individual patient or to disordered pharmacokinetics, usually impaired drug elimination. The term 'side-effects' is often applied to minor type A reactions.

Type B ('idiosyncratic') reactions are not predictable from the drug's main pharmacological action, are not dose-related and are severe, with a considerable mortality. The underlying pathophysiology of type B reactions is poorly if at all understood, and often has a genetic or immunological basis. Type B reactions occur infrequently (1:1 000–1:10 000 treated subjects being typical).

Adverse drug reactions due to specific drug–drug interactions are considered in Chapter 13. Three further minor categories of adverse drug reaction have been proposed:

1 *type C* – continuous reactions due to long-term drug use (e.g. neuroleptic-related tardive dyskinesia or analgesic nephropathy);
2 *type D* – delayed reactions (e.g. alkylating

Table 12.1: Some examples of type A and type B reactions

Drug	Type A reaction	Type B
Chlorpromazine	Sedation	Cholestatic jaundice
Naproxen	Gastrointestinal haemorrhage	Agranulocytosis
Phenytoin	Ataxia	Hepatitis, lymphadenopathy
Thiazides	Hypokalaemia	Thrombocytopenia
Quinine	Tinnitus	Thrombocytopenia
Warfarin	Bleeding	Breast necrosis

agents leading to carcinogenesis, or retinoid-associated teratogenesis);

3 *type E* end-of-use reactions such as adrenocortical insufficiency following withdrawal of corticosteroids, or withdrawal syndromes following discontinuation of treatment with clonidine, benzodiazepines, tricyclic antidepressants or β-adrenoreceptor antagonists.

There are between 30 000 and 40 000 medicinal products available directly or on prescription in the UK. A recent survey suggested that approximately 80% of adults take some kind of medication during any 2–week period. Exposure to drugs in the population is thus substantial, and the incidence of adverse reactions must be viewed in this context. Type A reactions are believed to be responsible for up to 3% of acute hospital admissions and 2–3% of consultations in general practice. In hospital, clinically significant adverse reactions are estimated to complicate 10–20% of all admissions, prolonging hospital stay and causing suffering and an appreciable number of fatalities, as well as wasting resources. They are most frequent and severe in neonates, the elderly, women, patients with hepatic or renal disease, and individuals with a history of previous adverse drug reactions. Adverse drug reactions often occur early in therapy (during the first 1–10 days). The drugs most commonly implicated are digoxin, antimicrobials, diuretics, potassium salt replacements, analgesics, sedatives and major tranquillizers, insulin, aspirin, glucocorticosteroids, antihypertensives and warfarin.

Factors involved in the aetiology of adverse drug reactions can be classified as shown in Table 12.2.

Key points

- *Type A reaction* – an extension of the pharmacology of the drug, dose related, and accounts for most adverse reactions (e.g β-adrenoreceptor antagonist-induced bradycardia or AV- block).
- *Type B reaction* – idiosyncratic reaction to the drug, not dose related, rare but severe (e.g. chloramphenicol-induced aplastic anaemia).
- Other types of drug reaction (much rarer):
  type C reaction – continuous reactions due to long-term use; analgesic nephropathy;
  type D reaction – delayed reactions of carcinogenesis or teratogenesis;
  type E reaction – drug withdrawal reactions (e.g. benzodiazepines).

Table 12.2: Factors involved in adverse drug reactions

Patient factors	
Intrinsic	*Extrinsic*
Age – neonatal, infant and elderly	Environment – sun
Sex – hormonal environment	Xenobiotics (e.g. drugs, herbicides)
Genetic abnormalities (e.g. enzyme or receptor polymorphisms)	Malnutrition
Previous adverse drug reactions, allergy, atopy	
Presence of organ dysfunction – disease	
Personality and habits – alcoholic, drug addict, nicotine, compliance	
Prescriber factors	
Incorrect drug or drug combination	
Incorrect route of administration	
Incorrect dose	
Incorrect duration of therapy	
Drug factors	
Drug–drug interactions (see Chapter 13)	
Pharmaceutical – batch problems, shelf-life, incorrect dispensing	

Adverse drug reaction monitoring/surveillance pharmacovigilance

The evaluation of drug safety is complex, and there are many methods for monitoring adverse drug reactions. Each of these has its own advantages and shortcomings, and no single system can offer the absolute security that public opinion expects. The ideal method would identify adverse drug reactions with a high degree of sensitivity and specificity and respond rapidly. It would detect rare but severe adverse drug reactions, but would not be overwhelmed by common ones, the incidence of which it would quantify together with predisposing factors. Continued surveillance is mandatory after a new drug has been marketed, as it is inevitable that the preliminary testing of medicines in humans during drug development, although excluding many ill effects, cannot identify uncommon adverse effects. A variety of early detection methods have been introduced to identify adverse drug reactions as swiftly as possible.

Phase I/II/III trials

Early (phase I/II) trials (see Chapter 15) are important for assessing the tolerability and dose–response relationship of new therapeutic agents. However, these studies are, very insensitive at detecting adverse reactions because they are performed on relatively few subjects (perhaps 200–300). This is illustrated by the failure to detect the serious toxicity of several drugs (e.g. practolol, benoxaprofen, temofloxacin, felbamate, dexfenfluramine and fenfluramine, troglitazone) before marketing. However, phase III clinical trials can establish the incidence of common adverse reactions and relate this to therapeutic benefit. Analysis of the reasons given for dropping out of phase III trials is particularly valuable in establishing whether common events such as headache, constipation, lethargy or male sexual dysfunction are truly drug related. The Medical Research Council Mild Hypertension Study unexpectedly identified impotence as being more commonly associated with thiazide diuretics than with placebo or β-adrenoreceptor antagonist therapy in this way. Table 12.3 illustrates how difficult it is to detect adverse drug reactions with 95% confidence, even when there is no background incidence and the diagnostic accuracy is 100%. (This 'easiest-case' scenario approximates to the actual situation with thalidomide teratogenicity – spontaneous phocomelia is almost unknown, and the condition is almost unmistakable. It is sobering to consider that an estimated 10 000 malformed babies were born world-wide before thalidomide was withdrawn.) Regulatory authorities may act after three or more documented events.

The problem of adverse drug reaction recognition is much greater if the reaction resembles spontaneous disease in the population, such that physicians are unlikely to attribute the reaction to drug exposure. The numbers of patients that must be exposed to enable such reactions to be detected are probably greater than those quoted in Table 12.3 by more than one or two orders of magnitude.

Yellow card scheme and post-marketing surveillance

Untoward effects that have not been detected in clinical trials become apparent when the drug is used on a wider scale. Case reports in the litera-

Table 12.3: Numbers of subjects that would need to be exposed in order to detect adverse drug reactions

Expected frequency of the adverse effect	Approximate number of patients required to be exposed For 1 event	For 3 events
1 in 100	300	650
1 in 1000	3000	6500
1 in 10 000	30 000	65 000

ture, which may often stimulate further reports, remain the most sensitive means of detecting rare but serious and unusual adverse effects. In the UK, a Register of Adverse Reactions was started in 1964. The Committee on Safety of Medicines (CSM) and the Medicines Control Agency (MCA) operate a system of spontaneous reporting on pre-paid yellow postcards. Doctors and dentists are asked to report adverse events which they consider to be due to drugs. Pharmacists have also recently been asked to contribute to this reporting system. The yellow card scheme consists of three stages:

1 collection of data;
2 analysis of data;
3 feedback to physicians.

Such methods of surveillance are useful, but under-reporting is a major limitation. Probably fewer than 10% of appropriate adverse reactions are reported. This may be due partly to confusion about what events to report, and partly to difficulty in recognizing the possible relationship of a drug to an adverse event, especially when the patient has been taking several drugs. A further problem is that, as explained above, if the drug increases the incidence of a common disorder (e.g. gall-bladder disease), the change in incidence must be very large to be detectable. Doctors are inefficient at detecting adverse reactions to drugs, and those reactions that are reported are in general the obvious or previously described and well-known ones. Several initiatives are currently in progress to attempt to improve this situation by both education and involvement of specially trained pharmacists in and outside hospitals.

The CSM introduced a system of high vigilance for newly marketed drugs. Any newly marketed drug has on its data sheet and its entry in the *British National Formulary* a black triangle for its first 2 years on the general market. This conveys to the prescriber that any unexpected event occurring in a patient prescribed this drug should be reported by the yellow card system. The pharmaceutical company marketing a new drug is also responsible for obtaining accurate reports on all patients treated up to an agreed number. This scheme was successful in the case of benoxaprofen, an anti-inflammatory analgesic. Following its release, there were spontaneous reports to the CSM of photosensitivity and onycholysis. Further reports appeared in the elderly, in whom its half-life is prolonged, of cholestatic jaundice and hepatorenal failure, which was fatal in eight cases. Benoxaprofen was subsequently taken off the market when 3 500 adverse drug reaction reports were received with 61 fatalities. The yellow card/black triangle scheme was also instrumental in the early identification of urticaria and cough as adverse effects of angiotensin-converting enzyme inhibitors. Although potentially the population under study by this system consists of all the patients using a drug, in fact under-reporting yields a population that is not uniformly sampled. Such data can be unrepresentative and hence difficult to work with statistically. This accounts for the paucity of accurate incidence data for adverse drug reactions.

Systems such as the yellow card scheme are relatively inexpensive and easy to manage, and facilitate ongoing monitoring of all drugs, all consumers and all types of adverse reaction. Reports from the drug regulatory bodies of 22 countries are collated by the World Health Organization (WHO) Unit of Drug Evaluation and Monitoring in Geneva. Rapid access to reports from other countries should be of great value in detecting rare adverse reactions, although the same reservations apply to this register as apply to national systems. In addition, this database could reveal geographical differences in the pattern of untoward drug effects.

Prescription event monitoring

Successful studies have been conducted by the Drug Surveillance Research Unit at the University of Southampton using prescription event monitoring. Prescriptions for certain drugs are identified by the prescriptions pricing office in Edinburgh. These are followed up and the prescribing doctor is asked to fill in a simple questionnaire recording any medical event from the patient notes. This has the advantage that the prescriber does not have to judge causality between the event and the drug. This scheme identified a new event associated with enalapril, i.e. deafness, in 19 of 12 500 cases. This is in excess of an expected five patients developing deafness in the general population, and requires further investigation, but it highlights the potential usefulness of the approach as well as one of its main limitations, namely the absence of a control goup.

Case–control studies

The great difficulty in detecting rare adverse drug effects is that, as discussed above, a very large number of patients have to be monitored in order to detect an effect. An alternative approach is to identify patients with a disorder which it is postulated could be caused by an adverse reaction to a drug, and to compare the frequency of exposure to possible aetiological agents with a control group. A prior suspicion (hypothesis) must exist to prompt the setting up of such a study – examples are the possible connection between irradiation or environmental pollution and certain malignancies, especially where they are observed in clusters. Artefacts can occur as a result of unrecognized bias from faulty selection of patients and controls, and the approach remains controversial among epidemiologists, public health physicians and statisticians. Despite this, there is really no practicable alternative for investigating a biologically plausible hypothesis relating to a disease which is so uncommon that it is unlikely to be represented even in large trial or cohort populations. The method has had some apparent successes, including the linking of stilboestrol with vaginal adenocarcinoma and of lincomycin with pseudomembranous colitis and, recently, the association between fenoterol use and an increased number of deaths in asthmatics. In its simplest form it is really an extension of the idea of the alert doctor, but with the considerable amount of data now available in such studies as the Boston Drug Surveillance Program (see below), it should be possible to use this method on a wider scale and in a more sophisticated manner.

Patient questionnaires

Self-administered questionnaires have limitations, especially in relation to selective recall bias. They have been used for out-patients attending hypertension and diabetic clinics, and have detected previously unsuspected adverse effects, (e.g. headache and weakness in the legs as effects of metformin). They have also been used to show an absence of effects, (e.g. that propranolol is not associated with any of the eye symptoms caused by practolol).

Intensive monitoring

Several hospital-based intensive monitoring programmes are currently in progress. The Aberdeen–Dundee system abstracts data from some 70 000 hospital admissions each year, storing these on a computer file before analysis. The Boston Collaborative Drug Surveillance Program (BCDSP), involving selected hospitals in several countries, is even more comprehensive. In the BCDSP all patients admitted to specially designated general wards are included in the analysis. Specially trained personnel obtain the following information from hospital patients and records:

1. background information (i.e. age, weight, height, etc.);
2. patient's medical history;
3. patient's drug exposure;
4. recognized side-effects of drugs;
5. outcome of treatment and changes in laboratory tests during hospital admission.

A unique feature of comprehensive drug-monitoring systems lies in their potential to follow up and investigate adverse reactions suggested by less sophisticated detection systems, or by isolated case reports in medical journals. Furthermore, the frequency of side-effects can be determined more cheaply than by a specially mounted trial to investigate a simple adverse effect. Thus, for example, the risk of developing a rash with ampicillin was found to be around 7% both by clinical trial and by the BCDSP, which can quantify such associations almost automatically from data on its files. New adverse reactions or drug interactions are sought by multiple correlation analysis of the data. Thus, when an unexpected relationship arises, such as the 20% incidence of gastrointestinal bleeding in severely ill patients treated with ethnacrynic acid compared to 4.3% among similar patients treated with other diuretics, this cannot be attributed to bias arising from awareness of the hypothesis during data collection, since the data were collected before the hypothesis was proposed. Conversely, there is a possibility of chance associations arising from multiple comparisons ('type I' statisical error), and such associations must be reviewed critically before accepting a causal link. It is possible to identify predisposing risk factors. In the association between ethacrynic acid and gastrointestinal bleeding these were female sex, a high blood urea concentration, previous heparin administration and intravenous administration of the drug. An important aspect of this type of approach is that *lack* of clinically important associations can also be investigated. Thus no significant association between aspirin and renal disease was found, whereas long-term aspirin consumption is associated with a decreased incidence of myocardial infarction, an association which has been shown to be of therapeutic importance in randomized clinical trials (see Chapter 28). There are plans to extend intensive drug monitoring to cover other areas of medical practice.

However, in terms of new but uncommon adverse reactions, the numbers of patients undergoing intensive monitoring while taking a particular drug will inevitably be too small for the effect to be detectable. Such monitoring can therefore only provide information about relatively common, early reactions to drugs used under hospital conditions. Patients are not in hospital long enough for detection of delayed effects, which are among the reactions least likely to be recognized as such even by an astute clinician.

MONITORING FROM NATIONAL STATISTICS

A great deal of information is available from death certificates, hospital discharge diagnoses and similar records. From these data it may be possible to detect a change in disease trends and relate this to drug therapy. Perhaps the best-known example of this is the increased death rate in young asthmatics noted in the mid-1960s, which was associated with overuse of bronchodilator inhalers containing non-specific β-adrenoreceptor agonists (e.g. adrenaline and/or isoprenaline). Although relatively inexpensive, the shortcomings of this method are obvious, particularly in diseases with an appreciable mortality, since large numbers of patients must suffer before the change is detectable. Data interpretation is particularly difficult when hospital discharges are used as a source of information, since discharge diagnosis is often provisional or incomplete, and may be revised during follow-up.

RECORD LINKAGE

Record linkage is under investigation as a method of monitoring adverse drug reactions. The basic idea is that records from different sources (e.g. general practice and hospital records, pharmacy records, dental records, certificated cause of death, parents' records and those of their children, and so on) are linked and analysed. Such linkage could be particularly useful when seeking really long-term ill effects of drugs (or other factors), such as the possible increased occurrence of malignancy or of mental retardation in individuals whose mothers had received drugs during pregnancy. Analysis of data is becoming more sophisticated with the use of computers to store information, but one must know what information is worth storing, and ask the correct questions, in order to avoid the situation of 'garbage in–garbage out'!

Various types of inquiry can be made, including the following:

1 follow-up of cohorts of individuals who have received selected drugs, to determine adverse reactions attributable to the drug. This approach is of most value when a drug is already suspected of producing some particular effect, and is not particularly suited to the discovery of unexpected adverse effects. A defect is the absence of a control group;
2 follow-up of patients with specific diseases, rather than those treated with specific drugs, is sometimes easier to carry out because most clinicians categorize their patients under disease rather than under treatment. Thus it is possible to investigate adverse reactions to anticonvulsant drugs by selecting the records of epileptics. One of the largest disease-oriented systems is that of the USA Perinatal Study, which received data on drug exposure and fetal outcome from over 50 000 consecutive pregnancies. From this, evidence has been obtained linking malformations and maternal exposure to phenytoin.

Key points

- Rare (and often severe) adverse drug events may not be detected in early drug development but only defined in the first few years post marketing (phase IV of drug development).
- Be aware of and participate in the Committee on Safety of Medicines (CSM) *yellow card system* for reporting suspected adverse drug reactions.
- Use of any recently marketed drug which is identifed with a *black triangle* on its data sheet or in the *British National Formulary* indicates the need to be particularly suspicious about adverse drug reactions and to report any suspected adverse drug reaction via the yellow card system.
- *Constant vigilance by physicians for drug-induced disease, particularly for new drugs, but also for more established agents, is needed.*

Feedback

There is no point in collecting vast amounts of data on adverse reactions unless they are analysed and important information is reported back to prescribing doctors. In addition to articles in the medical press, the Committee on Safety of Medicines 'Current Problems in Pharmacovigilance' series deals with important and recently identified adverse drug reactions. If an acute and serious problem is recognized, doctors will usually receive notification from the CSM, and often from the pharmaceutical company marketing the product.

Allergic adverse drug reactions

Immune mechanisms are involved in a number of adverse effects caused by drugs (see Chapter 49). The development of allergy implies previous exposure to the drug or to some closely related substance. Most drugs are of low molecular weight (< 1 000 daltons) and thus are not antigenic. However, they can combine with substances of high molecular weight, usually proteins, to form an antigenic hapten conjugate.

The factors that determine the development of allergy to a drug are not fully understood. Some drugs (e.g. penicillin) are more likely to cause allergic reactions than others, and type I (immediate anaphylactic) reactions are more common in patients with a history of atopy. A correlation between allergic reactions involving immunoglobulin E (IgE) and human leucocyte antigen (HLA) serotypes has been reported, so genetic factors may also be important. There is some evidence that drug allergies are more common in older people, in women, and in those with a previous history of drug reaction. However, this may, merely represent increased frequencies of drug exposure in these groups, and prevalence figures (expressed relative to the appropriate denominator) are currently unavailable.

Types of allergy

Drugs cause a variety of allergic responses (Figure 12.1), and sometimes a single drug can be responsible for more than one type of allergic response.

Type I reactions

Type I reactions (e.g. β-lactams, penicillins and cephalosporins) are due to the production of reaginic (IgE) antibodies. The antigen–antibody reaction on the surface of mast cells causes degranulation and release of pharmacologically active substances. It commonly occurs with foreign serum or penicillin, but may also occur with streptomycin and some local anasthetics. With penicillin it is believed that the penicilloyl moiety of the penicillin molecule is responsible for the production of antibodies. Treatment of anaphylactic shock is discussed in Chapter 49.

Type II reactions

These are due to antibodies of class IgG and IgM which, on contact with antibodies on the surface of cells, are able to fix complement, causing cell lysis (e.g. penicillin or cephalosporins and methyldopa causing Coombs' positive haemolytic anaemia.

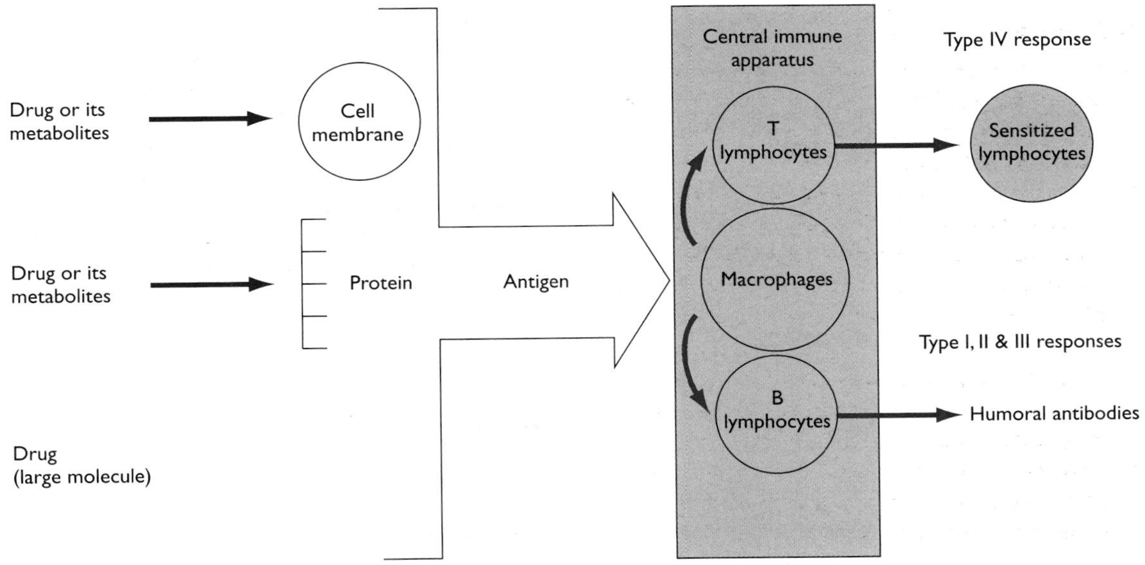

Figure 12.1 The immune response to drugs.

Type III immune complex arthus reactions

Circulating immune complexes can produce several clinical allergic states, including serum sickness and immune complex glomerulonephritis, and a syndrome resembling systemic lupus erythematosus. The onset of serum sickness is delayed for several days until the symptoms – fever, urticaria, arthropathy, lymphadenopathy and eosinophilia – develop. Proteinuria frequently occurs. Recovery takes a few days. Examples of causative agents include foreign serum, penicillin, sulphonamides, streptomycin and propylthiouracil. Amiodarone lung and hydralazine-induced systemic lupus syndrome are also possibly mediated by immune complex-related mechanisms, although these reactions are less well understood.

Type IV delayed hypersensitivity reactions

Type IV reactions are delayed hypersensitivity reactions, the classical example of which is contact dermatitis (e.g. to topical antibiotics such as penicillin or neomycin). The mechanism here is that the drug applied to the skin forms an antigenic conjugate with dermal proteins, stimulating formation of sensitized T-lymphocytes in the regional lymph nodes, with a resultant rash if the drug is applied again. Drug photosensitivity is due to a photochemical combination between the drug (e.g. tetracycline, amiodarone, chlorpromazine) and dermal protein. Delayed sensitivity can also result from the systemic administration of drugs.

Key points

Classification of immune-mediated adverse drug reactions

- *Type I* – urticaria or anaphylaxis due to the production of IgE against drug bound to mast cells, leading to massive release of mast-cell mediators locally or systemically (e.g. ampicillin skin allergy or anaphylaxis).
- *Type II* – IgG and IgM antibodies to drug which, on contact with antibodies on the cell surface, cause cell lysis by complement fixation (e.g. penicillin – haemolytic anaemia, quinidine – thrombocytopenia).
- *Type III* – circulating immune complexes produced by drug and antibody to drug deposit in organs, causing drug fever, urticaria, rash, lymphadenopathy, glomerulonephritis – often with eosinophilia (e.g. co-trimoxazole, β-lactams).
- *Type IV* – delayed-type hypersensitivity due to drug forming an antigenic conjugate with dermal proteins and sensitized T-cells reacting to drug, causing a rash (e.g. topical antibiotics).

Examples of allergic and other adverse drug reactions

Adverse drug reactions can be manifested in any organ system, or involve multiple organ systems, and in extraordinarily diverse forms. Specific instances are dealt with throughout this book. Some examples to illustrate the diversity of adverse drug reactions are given here.

Rashes

These are common manifestations of drug reactions. A number of immune and non-immune mechanisms may be involved which produce many different types of rash (Table 12.4).

Lymphadenopathy

Lymph-node enlargement can result from taking drugs (e.g. phenytoin). The mechanism involved is not known, but allergic factors may be involved. The reaction may be confused with a lymphoma, and inquiry about chronic drug-taking or drug abuse is important in patients with lymphadenopathy of unknown cause.

Blood dyscrasias

Thrombocytopenia, anaemia (aplastic, iron deficiency, macrocytic, haemolytic) and agranulocytosis can all be caused by drugs.

Thrombocytopenia can occur with many drugs, and in many but not all instances it is direct suppression of the megakaryocytes rather than immune processes which is important. Some of the drugs which most commonly cause thrombocytopenia include the following:

Table 12.4: Skin reactions to some commonly used drugs (continued opposite)

	Acne	Alopecia	Bullous	Epidermal necrolysis	Erythema multiforme	Erythema nodosa	Exfoliative dermatitis
Anticonvulsants	+			+	+	+	+
Barbiturates			+	+		+	+
Beta-blockers							
Chlorpropamide					+		+
Codeine						+	
Cytotoxics		+					
Gold							+
Griseofluvin							
Halides	+		+		+	+	+
Penicillins			+	+	+	+	+
Phenolphthalein			+		+		+
Phenothiazines					+		+
Phenylbutazone				+			+
Salicylates			+		+	+	
Steroids	+						
Streptomycin							
Sulphonamides				+	+	+	+
Tetracyclines				+			+
Thiazides					+	+	
Thioracils		+				+	

- thiazides;
- quinidine, quinine;
- heparin;
- sulphonamides;
- gold salts;
- most cytotoxic agents.

Haemolytic anaemia can be caused by a number of drugs, and sometimes immune mechanisms are responsible. Glucose-6-phosphate dehydrogenase deficiency (see Chapter 14) predisposes to non-immune haemolysis (e.g. to primaquine). Immune mechanisms include the following:

1 combination of the drug with the red-cell membrane, with the conjugate acting as an antigen. This has been shown to occur with penicillin-induced haemolysis, and may also occur with chlorpromazine, and sulphonamides;
2 alteration of the red-cell membrane by the drug so that it becomes autoimmunogenic. This may happen with methyldopa, and a direct positive Coombs' test develops in about 20% of patients who have been treated with this drug for more than 1 year. Haemolysis only actually occurs in a small proportion of cases. Similar changes can take place with levodopa, mefenamic acid and beta-lactam antibiotics;
3 causing non-specific binding of plasma protein to red cells, and thus causing haemolysis. This is believed to occur with cephalosporins.

Aplastic anaemia as an isolated entity is not common, but may occur either in isolation or as part of a general depression of bone-marrow activity (pancytopenia). Examples include chloramphenicol and (commonly and predictably) cytotoxic drugs.

Agranulocytosis can be caused by many drugs. Several different mechanisms are implicated, and it is not known whether allergy plays a part. The drugs most frequently implicated include the following:

- most cytotoxic drugs;
- antithyroid drugs;

Fixed	Lichenoid	Lupus erythematosus	Morbilliform	Nails	Photosensitivity	Porphyria	Purpura	Urticaria	Psoriasiform
		+	+					+	
+			+			+		+	
	+	+							+
								+	
			+	+			+		
+	+		+				+		
		+			+	+			
							+	+	
+							+	+	
+			+	+	+			+	
							+		
+		+							
+								+	
							+		
			+					+	
+		+			+		+	+	
+				+	+		+	+	
	+		+		+		+		
			+					+	

- sulphonamides and sulphonylureas (e.g. tolbutamide);
- antidepressants (especially mianserin; see Chapter 19) and antipsychotics (e.g. phenothiazines and clozapine);
- anti-epileptic drugs (e.g. carbamazepine and felbamate).

Systemic lupus erythematosus

Several drugs (including procainamide, isoniazid, hydralazine, chlorpromazine and anticonvulsants) produce a syndrome that resembles systemic lupus together with a positive antinuclear factor test. The development of this is closely related to dose, and in the case of hydralazine it also depends on the rate of acetylation of the drug, which is genetically controlled (see Chapter 14). There is some evidence that the drugs act as haptens, combining with DNA and forming antigens. Symptoms usually disappear when the drug is stopped, but recovery may be slow.

Vasculitis

Both acute and chronic vasculitis can result from taking drugs, and may have an allergic basis. Acute vasculitis with purpura and renal involvement occurs with penicillins, sulphonamides and penicillamine. A more chronic form can occur with phenytoin.

Renal dysfunction

All clinical expressions of renal disease can be caused by drugs, and common culprits are non-steroidal anti-inflammatory drugs and angiotensin-converting enzyme inhibitors (which cause functional and usually reversible renal failure in susceptible patients; see Chapters 25 and 27). Nephrotic syndrome results from several drugs (e.g. penicillamine, high-dose captopril, gold salts) which cause various immune-mediated glomerular injuries. Interstitial nephritis can be caused by several drugs, including non-steroidal anti-inflammatory drugs and penicillins, especially methicillin. Aminoglycoside antibiotics and vancomycin cause direct tubular toxicity. Many drugs cause electrolyte or acid–base disturbances via their predictable direct or indirect effects on renal electrolyte excretion (e.g. hypokalaemia and hypomagnaesemia from loop diuretics, hyperkalaemia from potassium-sparing diuretics, converting enzyme inhibitors and angiotensin II antagonists, proximal renal tubular acidosis from carbonic anhydrase inhibitors), and some cause unpredictable toxic effects on acid–base balance (e.g. distal renal tubular acidosis from amphotericin). Obstructive uropathy can be caused by uric acid crystals consequent on initiation of chemotherapy in patients with haematological malignancy, and – rarely – poorly soluble drugs such as sulphonamides, methotrexate or indinavir can themselves cause clinical problems consequent upon crystalluria.

Other reactions

Fever is a common manifestation of drug allergy, and should be remembered in patients with fever of unknown cause.

Liver damage (hepatitis with or without obstructive features) as a side-effect of drugs is important. It may be insidious, leading slowly to end-stage cirrhosis (e.g. during chronic treatment with methotrexate) or acute and fulminant (as in some cases of isoniazid, halothane or phenytoin hepatitis). Chlorpromazine or erythromycin may cause liver involvement characterized by raised alkaline phosphatase and bilirubin ('obstructive' pattern). Gallstones (and mechanical obstruction) can be caused by fibrates and other lipid-lowering drugs (see Chapter 26), and by octreotide, a somatostatin analogue used to treat a variety of enteropancreatic tumours, including carcinoid syndrome and VIPomas* (see Chapter 41). Immune mechanisms are implicated in some forms of hepatic injury by drugs, but are seldom solely responsible.

* VIP = vasoactive intestinal polypeptide.

Identification of the drug at fault

It is often difficult to decide whether a clinical event is drug related, and even when this is probable, it may be difficult to determine which drug is responsible, as patients are often taking more than one. One or more of several possible approaches may be appropriate.

1 A careful drug history is essential, but may be inconclusive because, although allergy to a drug implies previous exposure, the antigen may have occurred in foods (e.g. antibiotics are often fed to livestock and drug residues remain in the flesh), in drug mixtures or in some casual manner.
2 Provocation tests – which involve giving a very small amount of the suspected drug and seeing whether a reaction ensues. The commonest method is skin testing, where a drug is applied as a patch, or is pricked or scratched into the skin or injected intradermally. Unfortunately, prick and scratch testing is less useful for assessing the systemic reaction to drugs than it is for the more usual atopic antigens (e.g. pollens), and both false-positive and false-negative results can occur. Intradermal injection can provoke serious systemic anaphylaxis, and fatalities have been recorded. Patch testing is safe, and is useful for the diagnosis of contact sensitivity, but does not reflect systemic reactions. It may also itself cause allergy. Provocation tests can also involve giving small doses of the drug by inhalation, by mouth or parenterally, and should only be undertaken under expert guidance, after obtaining informed consent, and with full resuscitation facilities available.
3 Serological testing is rarely helpful, as the demonstration of circulating antibodies does not mean that they are necessarily the cause of the symptoms.
4 Sensitized lymphocytes – the demonstration of transformation occurring when lymphocytes are exposed to a drug suggests that they are T-lymphocytes sensitized to the drug, but interpretation of the results can be difficult in a clinical context. In this type of reaction the hapten itself will often provoke lymphocyte transformation, as well as the conjugate.
5 Often it is necessary to stop all of the drugs that a patient is taking and reintroduce them one by one until the drug at fault is discovered. This should only be done if the reaction is not serious, or if the drug is essential and no chemically unrelated alternative is available. Drug allergies should be recorded in the case-notes and the patient informed of the risks involved in taking the drug again.

Key points

How to attempt to define the drug causing the adverse drug reaction

- Define the likely causality of the effect of therapy by asking the following questions. Did the reaction and its time-course fit with the duration of suspected drug treatment and known adverse effects? Did the adverse effect disappear on drug withdrawal and, if rechallenged with the drug, reappear? Were other potential causes excluded?
- Provocation testing with skin testing – intradermal tests are neither very sensitive nor specific.
- Test the patient's serum for anti-drug antibodies, or test the reaction of the patient's lymphocytes *in vitro* to the drug and/or drug metabolite if appropriate.
- Consider stopping all drugs and reintroducing essential ones sequentially.
- Carefully document and highlight the adverse drug reaction and the most likely culprit in the case-notes

Prevention of allergic drug reactions

Although it is probably not possible to avoid allergic drug reactions altogether, the following measures can decrease the incidence.

1 Taking a drug history is essential whenever drug treatment is anticipated, particularly with antibiotics and other drugs with a high allergy potential. A history of atopy, although not excluding the use of drugs, should make one wary.
2 Drugs given orally are less likely to cause

Case history

A 73-year-old man develops severe shoulder pain and is diagnosed as having a frozen shoulder, for which he is prescribed a course of physiotherapy and given naproxen, 250 mg twice daily, by his local community practitioner. His practitioner knows him well and recalls he has normal renal function for his age. When he attends for review about 3 weeks later, he is complaining of tiredness and has noted reduced urine frequency. Over the past few days he has also developed arthralgias and a maculopapular rash on his trunk and limbs. His practitioner does a full blood count, erythrocyte sedimentation rate (ESR), serum chemistries, and urinalysis and urine microscopy. His full blood count shows an eosinophilia, his urinalysis shows 2+ protein and urine microscopy reveals eosinophuria. His creatinine level has risen from a previous value of 110 μmol/L to 280 μmol/L and his urea level is 20.5 mM; electrolytes are normal.

Question 1

If this is an adverse drug reaction, what type of reaction is it and what is the diagnosis?

Question 2

What is the best management plan, and should this patient ever receive naproxen again?

Answer 1

The patient has developed an acute interstitial nephritis, probably secondary to the recent introduction of naproxen treatment. This is a well-recognized syndrome, with the clinical features that the patient displays in this case, which is induced by many NSAIDs, particularly in the elderly. This is a type B adverse drug reaction which has an immune pathophysiology that is probably a combination of type III and type IV hypersensitivity reactions.

Answer 2

Discontinuation of the offending agent is vital, and this is sometimes sufficient to produce a return to baseline levels of renal function and the disappearance of systemic symptoms of fever and the rash. Recovery may possibly be accelerated and further renal toxicity minimized by a short (5–7 days) course of oral glucocorticosteroids, while monitoring renal function. The offending agent should not be used again in this patient unless the benefits of using it vastly outweigh the risks associated with its use in a serious illness.

severe allergic reactions than those given by injection.

3 Prophylactic skin testing is not usually practicable, and a negative test does not exclude the possibility of an allergic reaction. However, such testing may, be appropriate in cases where a suspect drug is potentially life-saving and there is no equally effective alternative. It probably reduces the risk of anaphylaxis if not of other less severe reactions.

4 Desensitization (hyposensitization) should only be used when continued use of the drug is essential. It involves giving a very small dose of the drug and increasing the dose at regular intervals, sometimes under cover of a glucorticosteroid and β_2-adrenoreceptor agonist. An antihistamine may be added if a drug reaction occurs, and equipment for resuscitation and therapy of anaphylactic shock must be close at hand. It is often successful, although the mechanism by which it is achieved is not fully understood.

FURTHER READING

Committee on Safety of Medicines and the Medicine Control Agency *Current Problems in Pharmacovigilance*. London: Committee on Safety of Medicines and the Medicine Control Agency. (Students are advised to monitor this publication for ongoing and future adverse reactions.)

Davies DM. 1991: *Textbook of adverse drug reactions*, 4th edn. Oxford: Oxford University Press.

Dukes MNG. 1992: *Meyler's side-effects of drugs. Vol. 12.* Amsterdam: Elsevier (see also companion volumes *'Side-Effects of Drugs Annuals'*, published annually since 1977).

Gross FH, Inman WHW. 1977: *Drug monitoring*. London: Academic Press.

Rawlins MD, Thompson JW. 1977: *Pathogenesis of adverse drug reactions*, 2nd edn. Oxford: Oxford University Press.

CHAPTER THIRTEEN

DRUG INTERACTIONS

- Introduction
- Useful interactions
- Trivial interactions
- Harmful interactions

INTRODUCTION

Drug interaction is the modification of the action of one drug by another as a result of one or more of three different kinds of mechanism:

1 pharmaceutical
2 pharmacodynamic
3 pharmacokinetic

Drug interaction is important because, whereas judicious use of more than one drug at a time can greatly benefit patients, adverse interactions are not uncommon, and may be catastrophic, yet are often avoidable. Multiple drug use ('polypharmacy') is extremely common, so the potential for drug interaction is enormous. One study showed that on average 14 drugs were prescribed to medical in-patients per admission (one patient received 36 different drugs). This undesirable state of affairs is likely to get worse, for several reasons.

1 Many drugs are not curative, but rather they ameliorate chronic conditions such as cardiac failure, arthritis, etc. The populations of western countries are ageing, so these diseases are progressively more likely to coexist within elderly individuals.
2 It is all too easy to enter an iatrogenic spiral in which a drug (often given for uncertain or inadequate reasons) results in an adverse effect that is countered by the introduction of another drug, and so on. Prescribers should heed the moral of the nursery rhyme about the old lady who swallowed a fly! Hospital admission provides an opportunity to review the medications that patients are receiving, to ensure that the overall regimen is rational.

Out-patients also often receive several drugs, sometimes supplemented by proprietary over-the-counter medicines, drugs supplied by friends and relatives, or drugs prescribed by other doctors without reference to the patient's own practitioner. The greater the number of drugs prescribed, the more likely things are to go wrong (Figure 13.1).

Drug interactions can be useful, of no consequence, or harmful.

USEFUL INTERACTIONS

INCREASED EFFECT

Drugs can be used in combination to enhance their effectiveness. Disease is often caused by complex processes, and drugs that influence different components of the disease mechanism may

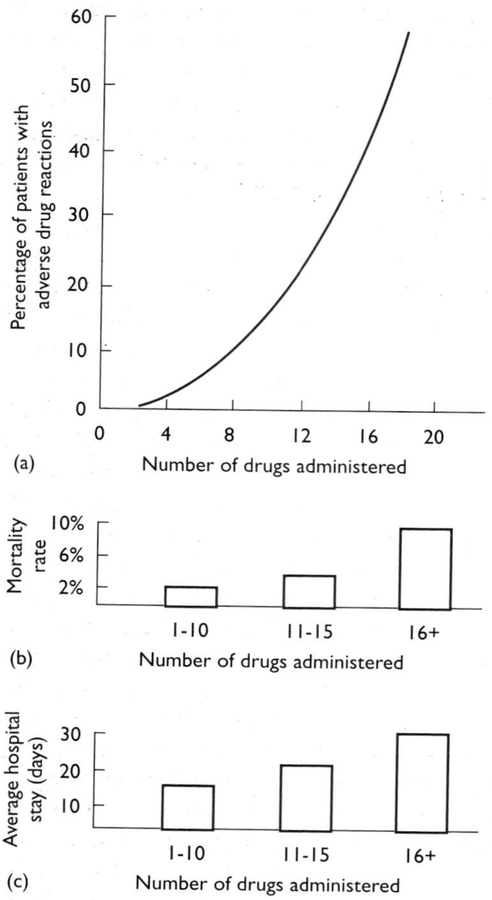

Figure 13.1: Relationship of number of drugs administered to (a) adverse drug reactions, (b) mortality rate and (c) average duration of hospital stay. (Reproduced by permission of the *British Medical Journal* from Smith JW et al. 1966 *Annals of Internal Medicine* **65** 631.)

have additive effects. Myocardial infarction is usually caused by white thrombus forming on a ruptured atheromatous plaque in a coronary artery. Such thrombi consist of fibrin and platelet aggregates, and the ISIS II study showed that streptokinase (a fibrinolytic drug) and aspirin (which inhibits platelet function) each improve outcome in patients with myocardial infarction, and that the combination of aspirin with streptokinase has an additive effect. Other examples include the use of a β_2 agonist with a glucocorticoid in the treatment of asthma (to cause bronchodilation and suppress inflammation, respectively), use of an H_2-antagonist with an antacid in acid peptic disease (to reduce acid secretion and buffer gastric fluid), use of a muscarinic antagonist with L-dopa in treating Parkinson's disease, and so on.

Combinations of antimicrobial drugs may be required when treating chronic infections, to prevent the selection of drug-resistant organisms. Tuberculosis is the best example of a disease whose successful treatment requires this approach, usually employing combinations that include isoniazid, rifampicin and pyrazinamide. Sometimes micro-organisms acquire drug resistance via synthesis of an enzyme that degrades antibiotic (e.g. penicillinase-producing staphylococci). This can sometimes be countered by using a combination of the antibiotic with an inhibitor of the enzyme. For example, co-amoxiclav is a combination of clavulanic acid, an inhibitor of penicillinase, with amoxycillin, a semisynthetic penicillin. Clavulinic acid has no antibacterial activity on its own, but by inhibiting penicillinase makes the combination effective against organisms that would be resistant to amoxycillin alone by reason of penicillinase production. These include most *Staphylococcus aureus* as well as a fraction of Gram-negative organisms such as *Escherichia coli, Haemophilus influenzae, Klebsiella* and some anaerobes. Imipenem, a broad-spectrum thienamycin β-lactam antibiotic, active against many Gram-positive and Gram-negative aerobic and anaerobic organisms, is partly inactivated by a dipeptidase in the kidney. This is overcome by administering imipenem in combination with cilastin, a specific renal dipeptidase inhibitor. This results in more prolonged plasma concentrations of imipenem.

Some combinations of drugs have a more than additive effect ('synergy'). Several antibacterial combinations are synergistic, including sulphamethoxazole with trimethoprim (co-trimoxazole). Each component acts on the folate pathway, but at different points. The combination is more effective than either component alone when tested against many micro-organisms *in vitro*. However, in clinical practice, trimethoprim is as effective as co-trimoxazole in many common infections (e.g. urinary tract infection), lacks sulphonamide-related toxicity and is less expensive. Nevertheless, co-trimoxazole is useful in special circumstances, especially in the treatment of *Pneumocystis carinii*. Aminoglycoside antibiotics synergize usefully with penicillin in some cases of enterococcal endocarditis. It is probable that several drugs used in cancer chemotherapy are mutually synergistic.

Therapeutic effects of drugs are often limited by the activation of a physiological control loop, particularly in the case of cardiovascular drugs. The use of a low dose of a second drug that interrupts this negative feedback may therefore enhance effectiveness substantially. Examples include the combination of a converting enzyme inhibitor (to block the renin–angiotensin system) with a diuretic (the effect of which is limited by activation of the renin–angiotensin system), or of a β-hydroxymethylglutaryl coenzyme A (HMG-CoA) reductase inhibitor (to block cholesterol biosynthesis) with a bile acid-binding resin (which on its own has a limited effect due to increased hepatic cholesterol biosynthesis).

Sometimes a drug is in such short supply as to make it worthwhile to use a second drug to interfere with its elimination. Historically this was the case when penicillin was introduced. Probenecid, which inhibits its secretion into the renal tubules, was used to maximize the effect of small doses of the drug. It is still used occasionally to prolong the action of penicillin-related antibiotics in single-dose treatment of sexually transmitted disease where non-compliance with multiple-dose treatment may have serious individual and public health consequences. Zidovudine is active against human immunodeficiency virus, but is expensive. It undergoes glucuronidation and is then eliminated into the urine by tubular secretion. Probenecid blocks glucuronidation of zidovudine and impairs its secretion into tubular fluid in the kidney, offering the intriguing possibility that combining these drugs might permit a reduced dose frequency and lower cost, without loss of efficacy. However, the safety of such a combination has yet to be evaluated thoroughly, and the occurrence of fever and rashes has limited long-term use of this combination.

MINIMIZE SIDE-EFFECTS

There are many situations, including moderate hypertension and heart failure, where low doses of two drugs may be better tolerated as well as more effective than larger doses of a single agent. To some extent this is the result of disabling physiological control mechanisms, as discussed above. Sometimes drugs with similar therapeutic effects have opposing undesirable metabolic effects, which can to some extent cancel out when the drugs are used together. The combination of a loop diuretic (e.g. frusemide) with a potassium-sparing diuretic (e.g. amiloride) provides an example of this principle, and such drug combinations are useful when hypokalaemia is clinically important, (e.g. when digoxin is needed to control atrial fibrillation in a patient with heart failure).

Predictable adverse effects can sometimes be averted by the use of drug combinations. Isoniazid neuropathy is caused by pyridoxine deficiency, and is prevented by the prophylactic use of pyridoxine. When desired and adverse effects of a drug are mediated by different receptors, it may be possible to block the adverse effects without losing effectiveness. Cholinesterase inhibitors improve strength in patients with myasthenia gravis because they increase the concentration of acetylcholine at the nicotinic receptors of the neuromuscular junction. Excessive doses cause diarrhoea, salivation and abdominal pain as a result of increased activation of muscarinic receptors, and these effects can be prevented by an atropine-like drug. A drug that inhibits the metabolism of another drug can be used to minimize adverse effects. An important instance is the combination of a peripheral dopa decarboxylase inhibitor (e.g. carbidopa or benserazide) with L-dopa. Carbidopa permits an equivalent therapeutic effect to be achieved with a lower dose of L-dopa than is needed when it is used as a single agent, while reducing dose-related peripheral side-effects of nausea and vomiting (see Chapter 18).

BLOCK ACUTELY AN UNWANTED (TOXIC) EFFECT

Reversal of the effect of one drug by another may be desirable, as for example when an anaesthetist uses a cholinesterase inhibitor to reverse neuromuscular blockade, or when antidotes such as naloxone or Fab fragments of digoxin antibodies are used to treat specific types of poisoning (see Chapter 53). Prevention of toxic effects may depend on binding the drug or its receptor, as in the above examples or, less directly, on influencing the metabolic pathways responsible for drug elimination, as in the use of acetyl cysteine in patients poisoned with paracetamol, or of sodium thiosulphate in cases of cyanide poisoning. The choice of the most appropriate antagonist depends on the urgency of the clinical situation. For instance, in a patient receiving warfarin, in whom the prothrombin time is excessively prolonged and who has some gastrointestinal bleeding but is haemodynamically stable, the use of vitamin K to compete with the warfarin and permit resynthesis of functional coagulation factors may be indicated. By contrast, were the same patient to be bleeding intracranially, the use of fresh plasma or factor concentrates would be required to reverse the effect of the warfarin noncompetitively and immediately.

TRIVIAL INTERACTIONS

Many of the interactions described in large compendia are based on animal or *in vitro* experiments, the results of which cannot be extrapolated uncritically to the clinical situation. Many such potential interactions are of no practical consequence. This is especially true of drugs with shallow dose–response curves, and of interactions that depend on competition for non-receptor binding sites.

SHALLOW DOSE–RESPONSE CURVES

Interactions are only likely to be clinically important when there is a steep dose–response curve and a narrow therapeutic window between minimum effective dose and minimum toxic dose of one or both interacting drugs. This is often not the case. For example, penicillin, when used in most ordinary clinical situations, is so non-toxic that the usual dose is more than adequate for therapeutic efficacy, yet far below that which would cause dose-related toxicity. Consequently, a second drug that interacts with penicillin is unlikely to cause either toxicity or loss of efficacy.

PLASMA AND TISSUE BINDING SITE INTERACTIONS

One large group of potential drug interactions that are seldom, if ever, clinically important, consists of drugs that displace one another from binding sites on plasma albumin or within tissues. This is a common occurrence, and can readily be demonstrated in plasma or solutions of albumin *in vitro*. However, the simple expectation that the displacing drug will increase the effects of the displaced drug by increasing its free (unbound) concentration is, seldom evident in clinical practice. This is because drug clearance (renal or metabolic) also depends directly on the concentration of free drug. Consider a patient receiving a regular maintenance dose of a drug. When a second displacing drug is commenced, the free concentration of the first drug rises only transiently before increased renal or hepatic elimination reduces total (bound plus free) drug, and restores the free concentration to that which prevailed before the second drug was started. Consequently, any increased effect of the displaced drug is transient, and is seldom important in practice, although it must be taken into account if therapy is being guided by measurements of plasma drug concentrations, as most such determinations are of total rather than free concentration (see Chapter 8). An exception, where a transient increase in free concentration of a circulating substance (albeit not a drug) can have devastating consequences, is provided by bilirubin in premature babies with severe jaundice, whose ability to metabolize bile pigments is immature. Unconjugated bilirubin is bound by plasma albumin, and injudicious treatment with drugs such as sulphonamides that displace it from these binding sites may permit diffusion of free bilirubin across the immature blood–brain barrier, consequent staining of and damage to basal ganglia (kernicterus) and subsequent choreoathetosis in the child.

Instances where clinically important consequences do occur on introducing a drug that displaces another from tissue-binding sites are in fact often due to additional actions of the second drug on *elimination* of the first. For instance, quinidine displaces digoxin from tissue-binding sites, and can cause digoxin toxicity, but only because it simultaneously reduces the renal clearance of digoxin by a separate mechanism. Phenylbutazone displaces warfarin from binding sites on albumin, and can cause excessive prolongation of the prothrombin time and bleeding, but only because it also inhibits the metabolism of the active isomer of warfarin, causing this to accumulate at the expense of the inactive isomer. Indomethacin also displaces warfarin from binding sites on albumin, but does not inhibit its metabolism and does not further prolong prothrombin time in patients treated with warfarin, although it can cause bleeding by causing peptic ulceration and interfering with platelet function.

HARMFUL INTERACTIONS

It is impossible to memorize reliably even the examples contained in this chapter, and prescribers should have access to suitable references (e.g. the *British National Formulary*) to check on potentially harmful interactions. There are certain drugs with steep dose–response curves and serious dose-related toxicities for which drug interactions are especially liable to cause harm, and where special caution is required with concurrent therapy. These include the following:

- anticoagulants;
- anticonvulsants;
- cytotoxic drugs;
- digoxin and other anti-arrhythmic drugs;
- monoamine oxidase inhibitors;
- oral hypoglycaemic agents;
- xanthine alkaloids (e.g. theophylline).

The frequency and consequences of an adverse interaction when two drugs are used together are seldom known precisely. Every time a doctor prescribes a drug or drug combination, he or she is in effect performing an experiment on that particular patient. Every individual has a peculiar set of characteristics that determine their response to therapy. When potentially interacting drugs are prescribed, adverse effects are probable but not inevitable.

RISK OF ADVERSE DRUG INTERACTIONS

In the Boston Collaborative Drug Surveillance Program, 234 of 3600 (about 7%) adverse drug reactions in acute-care hospitals were identified as being due to drug interactions. In a smaller study in a chronic-care setting the prevalence of adverse interactions was much higher (22%), probably because of the more frequent use of multiple drugs in elderly patients with multiple pathologies. The same problems exist for the detection of drug interactions as for adverse drug reactions. In particular, it is possible that the frequency of such interactions is underestimated due to attribution of poor therapeutic outcome to progression of underlying disease in settings where data are not being compared quantitatively. For example, graft rejection following renal transplantation is not uncommon. Historically, it took several years for nephrologists to appreciate that epileptic patients suffered much greater rejection rates than did non-epileptic subjects. These adverse events proved to be due to an interaction between anticonvulsant medication and immunosuppressant therapy, which was rendered ineffective because of increased drug metabolism. In future, a better understanding of the potential mechanisms of such interactions should lead to their prediction and prevention by study in early-phase drug evaluation.

SEVERITY OF ADVERSE DRUG INTERACTIONS

The manifestations of adverse drug interactions are diverse, including unwanted pregnancy (from failure of the contraceptive pill due to concomitant medication), hypertensive stroke (from hypertensive crisis in patients on monoamine oxidase inhibitors), gastrointestinal and other haemorrhage (from use of aspirin with warfarin), cardiac arrhythmias (e.g. secondary to interactions leading to electrolyte disturbance) and blood dyscrasias (e.g. from interactions between allopurinol and azathioprine). Adverse interactions can be severe as well as mild in intensity. In one study, 9 of 27 fatal drug reactions were caused by drug interactions.

Key points

- Drug interactions may be clinically useful, trivial or adverse.
- Useful interactions include those that enable efficacy to be maximized, such as the addition of a converting-enzyme inhibitor to a thiazide diuretic in a patient with hypertension inadequately controlled on diuretic alone (see Chapter 27). They may also enable toxic effects to be minimized, as in the use of pyridoxine to prevent neuropathy in malnourished patients treated with isoniazid for tuberculosis, and may prevent the emergence of resistant organisms (e.g. multi-drug regimens for treating tuberculosis, see Chapter 43).
- Many interactions that occur *in vitro* (e.g.competition for albumin) are unimportant *in vivo* because displacement of drug from binding sites leads to increased elimination by metabolism or excretion and hence to a new steady state where the total concentration of displaced drug in plasma is reduced, but the concentration of active, free (unbound) drug is the same as before the interacting drug was introduced. Interactions involving drugs with a wide safety margin (e.g. penicillin) are also seldom clinically important.
- Adverse drug interactions are not uncommon, and can have profound consequences, including death from hyperkalaemia and other causes of cardiac arrhythmia, unwanted pregnancy, transplanted organ rejection, etc.

Adverse interactions grouped by mechanism

Pharmaceutical interactions

These consist of incompatibilities that result in precipitation or inactivation when drugs are mixed. Drugs should not be added to blood or (usually) to blood products, and it is essential to check before making additions to infusions of crystalloid or dextrose solutions. Specific examples are listed in Table 13.1. Drugs may also interact physically or chemically in the lumen of the gut (e.g. tetracycline with iron or aluminum, and cholestyramine with digoxin or warfarin).

Pharmacodynamic interactions

These are the commonest drug interactions in clinical practice. Most of them have a simple mechanism consisting of summation or opposition of the effects of drugs with similar or opposing actions initiated by combination with different receptors. Since this type of interaction depends broadly on the effect of a drug, rather than on its specific chemical structure, such interactions are nonspecific. Drowsiness caused by an H_1–blocking antihistamine and by alcohol provides an example. It occurs to a greater or lesser degree with *all* H_1–blockers irrespective of the chemical structure of the particular drug used. Patients must be warned of the dangers of consuming alcohol concurrently when such antihistamines are prescribed, especially if they drive or operate machinery. Non-steroidal anti-inflammatory agents and antihypertensive drugs provide another clinically important example. Many, if not all, antihypertensive drugs (including beta-blockers, diuretics and converting-enzyme inhibitors) are rendered substantially less effective by concurrent use of most non-steroidal anti-inflammatory drugs, irrespective of the chemical group to which they belong. The interaction is probably due to inhibition of biosynthesis of vasodilator prostaglandins in the kidney.

Table 13.1: Interactions outside the body

Mixture	Result
Thiopentone + suxamethonium	Precipitation
Diazepam + infusion fluids	Precipitation
Phenytoin + infusion fluids	Precipitation
Soluble insulin + protamine zinc insulin	Reduced effect of soluble insulin
Heparin + hydrocortisone	Inactivation of heparin
Kanamycin + hydrocortisone	Inactivation of kanamycin
Penicillin + hydrocortisone	Inactivation of penicillin

Drugs with negative inotropic effects can precipitate heart failure, and this is especially true when negative inotropes with different mechanisms are used in combination. Cardiac status and route of administration are critical. Thus beta-blockers and calcium-channel blockers, which may be safely given together by mouth in many patients with uncomplicated hypertension or angina pectoris, precipitate heart failure, which may be fatal, if used sequentially intravenously in patients with supraventricular tachycardia.

Warfarin interferes with haemostasis by inhibiting the coagulation cascade, whereas aspirin influences haemostasis by inhibiting platelet function. Aspirin also predisposes to gastric bleeding by direct irritation and by inhibition of prostaglandin E_2 biosynthesis in the gastric mucosa. There is therefore the potential for serious adverse interaction between them. Patients anticoagulated with warfarin should be warned to avoid aspirin (outside of tightly monitored clinical trials specifically exploring this combination), as well as the many proprietary medicines that contain aspirin (e.g. Alka-Seltzer™, Lemsip™, Beecham's Powders™).

In some instances, important interactions occur between drugs acting at a common receptor. These interactions are generally useful when used deliberately – for example, the use of naloxone to reverse opiate intoxication, or less directly the reversal of muscular relaxation by tubocurarine by the local increase in acetylcholine caused by cholinesterase inhibition with neostigmine mentioned above. Such actions at a common receptor, or at least on a common receptor-initiated pathway, may occasionally underlie undesirable interactions. A possible example is drowsiness caused by concurrent use of alcohol and benzodiazepines. These drugs probably act on a common pathway as flumazenil, a benzodiazepine antagonist, also partly reverses the sedation caused by alcohol.

One potentially important type of pharmacodynamic drug interaction involves the interruption of physiological control loops. This was mentioned above as a desirable means of increasing efficacy in certain circumstances (e.g. diuretics with converting-enzyme inhibitors in treating hypertension). However, there are also situations in which such control mechanisms are vital, and their disablement is fraught with hazard. The use of beta-blocking drugs in patients with insulin-requiring diabetes is such a case, as these patients may depend on sensations initiated by activation of β-receptors to warn them of impending hypoglycaemic coma.

Alterations in fluid and electrolyte balance represent an important source of pharmacodynamic drug interactions (see Table 13.2). Combined use of diuretics with actions at different parts of the nephron (e.g. metolazone and frusemide) is valuable in the treatment of resistant oedema, but without close monitoring of plasma urea levels, such combinations readily cause excessive intravascular fluid depletion and prerenal renal failure (see Chapter 35). Thiazide and loop diuretics commonly cause mild hypokalaemia, which is usually of no consequence. However, the binding of digoxin to plasma membrane Na^+/K^+ adenosine triphosphatase (ATPase), and hence its toxicity, is increased when the extracellular potassium concentration is low. Concurrent use of such diuretics therefore increases the risk of digoxin toxicity. β_2-Agonists such as salbutamol also reduce the plasma potassium concentration, especially when used intravenously. Conversely, potassium-sparing diuretics

Table 13.2: Interactions secondary to drug-induced alterations of fluid and electrolyte balance

Primary drug	Interacting drug effect	Result of interaction
Digoxin	Diuretic-induced hypokalaemia	Digoxin toxicity
Lignocaine	Diuretic-induced hypokalaemia	Antagonism of anti-arrhythmic effects
Diuretics	NSAID-induced salt and water retention	Antagonism of diuretic effects
Tubocurarine	Diuretic-induced hypokalaemia	Prolonged paralysis
Lithium	Thiazide-induced reduction in renal clearance	Raised plasma lithium
Angiotensin-converting enzyme inhibitor	Potassium chloride and/or potassium-retaining diuretic-induced hyperkalaemia	Severe hyperkalaemia

NSAID 5 non-steroidal anti-inflammatory drug.

may cause hyperkalaemia if combined with potassium supplements and/or converting-enzyme inhibitors (which reduce circulating aldosterone), especially in patients with renal impairment. Hyperkalaemia is one of the commonest causes of fatal adverse drug reactions.

Pharmacokinetic interactions

ABSORPTION

In addition to direct interaction within the gut lumen, drugs that increase or reduce the rate of gastric emptying (e.g. metoclopramide or propantheline, respectively) can alter the rate or completeness of absorption of a second drug, particularly if this has low bioavailability. More importantly, drugs can interfere with the enterohepatic recirculation of other drugs. Failure of oral contraception (particularly low-dose oestrogen preparations) can result from concurrent use of antibiotics, due to this mechanism. Many different antibiotics have been implicated, although trimethoprim and co-trimoxazole are believed to be exceptions. Phenytoin reduces the effectiveness of cyclosporin A by an uncertain mechanism, possibly by reducing its absorption.

DISTRIBUTION

As explained above, interactions that involve only mutual competition for inert protein- or tissue-binding sites seldom, if ever, give rise to clinically important effects. Examples of complex interactions where competition for binding sites occurs in conjunction with reduced clearance are mentioned in the section below on renal elimination. Effects on specific transport mechanisms may prevent drugs from reaching their site of action on receptors, or else prolong their effect due to slow removal from the vicinity of receptors. Tricyclic antidepressants block high-affinity amine-uptake sites on presynaptic sympathetic nerve terminals, preventing the effect of adrenergic neurone-blocking drugs, and prolonging the action of amines such as noradrenaline and phenylephrine, whose action at the postsynaptic receptors is usually terminated by such uptake.

METABOLISM

Decreased efficacy can result from enzyme induction by a second agent (Table 13.3). Historically, barbiturates were clinically the most important enzyme inducers, but with the decline in their use, other anticonvulsants, notably carbamazepine and the antituberculous drug rifampicin, are now the commonest cause of such interactions. These necessitate special care in concurrent therapy with warfarin, phenytoin, oral contraceptives, glucocorticoids or cyclosporin.

Withdrawal of an inducing agent during continued administration of a second drug can result in a *slow* decline in enzyme activity, with emergence of delayed toxicity from the second drug due to what is no longer an appropriate dose. For example, a patient receiving warfarin may be admitted to hospital for an intercurrent event and receive treatment with a drug that induces the form of cytochrome P_{450} that metabolizes warfarin. During the hospital stay, the dose of warfarin therefore has to be increased in order to maintain measurements of international normalized ratio (INR) within the therapeutic range. The intercurrent problem is resolved, the inducing drug discontinued and the patient discharged while taking the larger dose of warfarin. If the INR is not checked frequently, bleeding may result from an excessive effect of warfarin days or weeks after discharge from hospital, as the effect of the enzyme inducer gradually wears off.

Inhibition of drug metabolism may also produce toxicity (Table 13.4). The time-course of such

Table 13.3: Interactions due to enzyme induction

Primary drug	Inducing agent	Effect of interaction
Warfarin	Barbiturates Alcohol Rifampicin	Decreased anticoagulation
Oral contraceptives	Rifampicin	Pregnancy
Prednisolone/cyclosporin	Anticonvulsants	Reduced immunosuppression (graft rejection)
Theophylline	Smoking	Decreased plasma theophylline

Table 13.4: Interactions due to enzyme inhibition

Primary drug	Inhibiting drug	Effect of interaction
Phenytoin	Isoniazid Cimetidine Chloramphenicol	Phenytoin intoxication
Warfarin	Allopurinol Metronidazole Phenylbutazone Co-trimoxazole	Haemorrhage
Azathioprine, 6MP	Allopurinol	Bone-marrow suppression
Pethidine	MAOI	Prolonged sedation
Theophylline	Cimetidine Erythromycin	Theophylline toxicity
Terfenadine	Erythromycin Ketoconazole	Ventricular tachycardia

MAOI = monoamine oxidase inhibitor, 6MP = 6-mercaptopurine.

interactions is often shorter than for enzyme induction, since it depends merely on the attainment of a sufficiently high concentration of the inhibiting drug at the metabolic site. Xanthine oxidase is responsible for inactivation of 6–mercaptopurine, itself a metabolite of azathioprine. Allopurinol markedly potentiates these drugs by inhibiting xanthine oxidase. Xanthine alkaloids (e.g. theophylline) are *not* inactivated by xanthine oxidase, but rather by a form of cytochrome P_{450}. Theophylline has serious (sometimes fatal) dose-related toxicities, and clinically important interactions occur with inhibitors of the cytochrome P_{450} system, notably cimetidine, ciprofloxacin and erythromycin. Asthmatic patients are often admitted to hospital with severe attacks of airflow obstruction precipitated by chest infections, so an awareness of these interactions before commencing antibiotic treatment is essential if aminophylline is to be administered as well. Erythromycin also inhibits cyclosporin A metabolism, and can cause severe toxicity.

Enzyme inhibition also accounts for clinically important interactions with phenytoin (isoniazid, cimetidine, chloramphenicol and sulphonamides have all been implicated) and with warfarin (where cimetidine, the sulphonamides and phenylbutazone are all important, and stereoselective inhibition of the isomers of warfarin is a complicating factor). Non-selective monoamine oxidase inhibitors (e.g. phenelzine) potentiate the action of indirectly acting amines such as tyramine, which is present in a wide variety of fermented products (Camembert and other soft cheeses, yeast extract and Chianti wine, among others) and in a number of drugs, including pethidine.

Clinically important impairment of drug metabolism may also result indirectly from haemodynamic effects rather than enzyme inhibition. Lignocaine is metabolized in the liver, and the hepatic extraction ratio is high. Consequently, any drug that reduces hepatic blood flow (e.g. a negative inotrope) will reduce hepatic clearance of lignocaine and cause it to accumulate. This accounts for the increased lignocaine concentration and toxicity that is caused by beta-blocking drugs. This is important following myocardial infarction, when beta-blockers are administered despite diminished myocardial reserve, and lignocaine is used to prevent recurrence of ventricular arrhythmias.

EXCRETION

Many drugs share a common transport mechanism in the proximal tubules (see Chapter 6), and can mutually reduce one another's excretion by competition (Table 13.5). The effect of probenecid on penicillin elimination was mentioned above, and sulphinpyrazone has a similar action. Aspirin and non-steroidal anti-inflammatory drugs inhibit secretion of methotrexate into urine, as well as displacing it from protein-binding sites, and can cause methotrexate toxicity. Most diuretics reduce

Table 13.5: Competitive interactions for renal tubular transport

Primary drug	Competing drug	Effect of interaction
Penicillin	Probenecid	Increased penicillin blood level
Methotrexate	Salicylates Sulphonamides	Bone-marrow suppression
Salicylate	Probenecid	Salicylate toxicity
Indomethacin	Probenecid	Indomethacin toxicity
Chlorpropamide	Phenylbutazone	Hypoglycaemia
Digoxin	Spironolactone Amiodarone Verapamil	Increased plasma digoxin

Key points

- There are three main types of adverse interaction:
  pharmaceutical;
  pharmacodynamic;
  pharmacokinetic.
- Pharmaceutical interactions are due to *in vitro* incompatabilities, and they occur outside the body (e.g. when drugs are mixed in a bag of intravenous solution, or in the port of an intravenous cannula).
- Pharmacodynamic interactions between drugs with a similar effect (e.g. drugs that cause drowsiness) are common. In principle they should be easy to anticipate, but they can cause serious problems, (e.g. if a driver fails to account for the interaction between an antihistamine and alcohol).
- Pharmacokinetic interactions are much more difficult to anticipate. They occur when one drug influences the way in which another is handled by the body:
  (a) *absorption* (e.g. broad-spectrum antibiotics interfere with enterohepatic recirculation of oestrogens and can cause failure of oral contraception);
  (b) *distribution* – competition for binding sites seldom causes problems on its own but, if combined with an effect on elimination (e.g. amiodarone/digoxin or NSAID/methotrexate), serious toxicity may ensue;
  (c) *metabolism* – many serious interactions stem from enzyme induction or inhibition. Important inducing agents include alcohol, rifampicin, rifabutin and anticonvulsants. Common inhibitors include many antibacterial drugs (e.g. isoniazid, chloramphenicol, macrolides, co-trimoxazole), cimetidine, allopurinol.
  (d) *excretion* (e.g. diuretics lead to increased reabsorption of lithium, reducing its clearance and predisposing to lithium accumulation and toxicity).

sodium absorption in the loop of Henlé or the distal tubule (see Chapter 35). This leads indirectly to increased proximal tubular reabsorption of monovalent cations via a homeostatic control loop. Increased proximal tubular reabsorption of lithium ions in patients treated with lithium salts can cause lithium accumulation and potentially fatal toxicity. Digoxin secretion is reduced by spironolactone, quinidine, verapamil and amiodarone, all of which can precipitate digoxin toxicity as a consequence, although several of these interactions are complex in mechanism, involving displacement from tissue binding sites in addition to reduced digoxin elimination.

Changes in urinary pH alter the excretion of drugs that are weak acids or bases, and administration of systemic alkalinizing or acidifying agents or carbonic anhydrase inhibitors changes the concentrations of these drugs in plasma and urine (e.g. the excretion of salicylate and of phenobarbitone is increased in an alkaline urine). Such effects are seldom clinically significant, although they are sometimes of value in the management of overdose to increase drug elimination (see Chapter 53).

Case history

A 64-year-old Indian man was admitted to hospital with miliary tuberculosis. In the past he had had a mitral valve replaced, and he had been on warfarin ever since. Treatment was commenced with isoniazid, rifampicin and pyrazinamide, and the INR was closely monitored in anticipation of increased warfarin requirements. He was discharged after several weeks with the INR in the therapeutic range on a much increased dose of warfarin. Rifampicin was subsequently discontinued. Two weeks later the patient was again admitted, this time drowsy and complaining of headache after mildly bumping his head on a locker. His pupils were unequal and the INR was > 5.0. Fresh frozen plasma was administered and neurosurgical advice was obtained.

Comment

This patient's warfarin requirement increased during treatment with rifampicin because of enzyme induction, and the dose of warfarin was increased to maintain anticoagulation. When rifampicin was stopped, enzyme induction gradually receded, but the dose of warfarin was not readjusted. Consequently, the patient became over-anticoagulated and developed a subdural haemotama in response to mild trauma. Replacment of clotting factors (present in fresh frozen plasma) is the quickest way to reverse the effect of warfarin overdose (see Chapter 29).

FURTHER READING

British Medical Association and Royal Pharmaceutical Society of Great Britain. 1998: *British National Formulary*. London: Medical Association and Royal Pharmaceutical Society of Great Britian. (Appendix 1 provides an up-to-date and succinct alphabetical list of interacting drugs, highlighting interactions that are potentially hazardous.)

Karalleidde L, Henry J. 1998: *Handbook of drug interactions*. London: Edward Arnold.

Stockley I. 1991: *Drug interactions*, 2nd edn. Oxford: Blackwell Scientific Publications.

CHAPTER FOURTEEN

PHARMACOGENETICS

- Introduction
- Mendelian traits that influence drug metabolism
- Inherited traits that influence drug action
- Inherited diseases that predispose to drug toxicity
- Polygenic influences on drug action

INTRODUCTION

Drug responses vary greatly between individuals. Such differences are due to genetic as well as environmental effects on drug absorption, distribution, metabolism or excretion (pharmacokinetics) and on receptor or post-receptor sensitivity (pharmacodynamics). In addition, several instances of adverse reactions to drugs that had originally been attributed to idiosyncratic or immunological mechanisms have been explained in terms of genetically determined variation in the activity of enzymes involved in detoxification, or of other abnormal proteins (e.g. variants of haemoglobin) that render an individual especially susceptible to some adverse reaction (e.g. haemolysis). The study of variation in drug responses under hereditary control is known as pharmacogenetics. Pharmacogenetic variation is sometimes due to the actions of a single mutant gene (as in genetic polymorphism, or Mendelian disorders that exhibit discontinuous variation). Tables 14.1 and 14.2 show examples of disorders that influence drug metabolism and drug response, respectively. Alternatively, pharmacogenetic variation can result from polygenic influences. There is currently great interest in the possibility that, by screening the DNA in an individual blood sample, it will be possible to select a drug that will be effective without causing adverse effects. Such individualized therapy could revolutionize therapeutics in the not too distant future.

MENDELIAN TRAITS THAT INFLUENCE DRUG METABOLISM

Abnormal sensitivity to a drug may be the result of an inborn error of its metabolism. Inheritance may be autosomal recessive, and such disorders are rare, although they are important because they may have severe consequences. However, there are also dominant patterns of inheritance that lead to much more common variations within the population. Genetic polymorphism is a type of variation in which individuals with sharply distinct characteristics coexist as healthy members of a population. It is probable that balanced polymorphism, when a substantial fraction of a population differs from the remainder in such a way over many generations, results when heterozygotes experience some selective advantage. Balanced polymorphisms of enzymes that are involved in drug metabolism are not uncommon, although the selective advantage conferred by heterozygosity is unknown.

ACETYLATOR STATUS

Administration of identical doses (per kg body weight) of isoniazid (INH), an antituberculous drug, to individuals in a population results in great variation in blood concentrations. A distribution histogram of such concentrations shows two distinct groups (i.e. a 'bimodal' distribution; Figure 14.1).

Table 14.1: Variations in drug metabolism due to genetic polymorphism

Pharmacogenetic variation	Mechanism	Inheritance	Occurrence	Drugs involved
Rapid-acetylator status	Increased hepatic N-acetyltransferase	Autosomal dominant	40% whites	Isoniazid; hydralazine; some sulphonamides; phenelzine; dapsone; procainamide
Suxamethonium sensitivity	Several types of abnormal plasma pseudocholinesterase	Autosomal recessive	Most common form 1: 2500	Suxamethonium
Defective hydroxylation of debrisoquine	Functionally defective cytochrome P_{450} 2D6	Autosomal recessive	8% Britons; 1% Saudi Arabians; 30% Chinese	Debrisoquine; metoprolol; nortriptyline
Ethanol sensitivity	Relatively low rate of alcohol metabolism	Usual in some ethnic groups	Orientals	Alcohol

Table 14.2: Variations in drug metabolism due to genetic polymorphism

Pharmacogenetic variation	Mechanism	Inheritance	Occurrence	Drugs involved
G6PD deficiency, favism, drug-induced haemolytic anaemia	80 distinct forms of G6PD	X-linked incomplete codominant	10 000 000 affected world-wide	Many – including 8-aminoquinolines, antimicrobials and minor analgesics (see text, Table 48.3)
Steroid-induced raised intra-ocular pressure	Unknown	Autosomal recessive (heterozygotes show some response)	5% white population	Glucocorticosteroids
Methaemoglobinaemia: drug-induced haemolysis	Methaemoglobin reductase deficiency	Autosomal recessive (heterozygotes show some response)	1:100 are heterozygotes	Same drugs as for G6PD deficiency
Malignant hyperthermia with muscular rigidity	Unknown	Autosomal dominant	1:20 000 of population	Some anaesthetics, especially halothane Suxamethonium
Acute intermittent porphyria: exacerbation induced by drugs	Increased activity of d-amino levulinic synthetase secondary to defective porphyrin synthesis	Autosomal dominant	Acute intermittent type 15:1 000 000 in Sweden; Porphyria cutanea tarda 1:100 in Afrikaaners	Barbiturates, chloral, chloroquine, ethanol, sulphonamides, phenytoin, griseofulvin and many others)

G6PD = glucose-6-phosphate dehydrogenase.

INH is metabolized in the liver by acetylation. Individuals who acetylate the drug more rapidly because of a greater hepatic enzyme activity achieve lower concentrations of INH in their blood following a standard dose than do slow acetylators. Acetylator status is conveniently measured using dapsone as the test drug by measuring the ratio of monoacetyldapsone to dapsone following a test dose.

Slow and rapid acetylator status are inherited in a simple Mendelian manner. Heterozygotes as well as homozygotes are rapid acetylators because rapid metabolism is an autosomal dominant. Around 55–60% of Europeans are slow acetylators and 40–45% are rapid acetylators. The rapid acetylator phenotype is most common in Eskimos and Japanese (95%), and rarest among some Mediterranean Jews (20%).

INH toxicity, in the form of peripheral neuropathy, most commonly occurs in slow acetylators, whilst slower response and higher risk of relapse of infection are more frequent in rapid acetylators, particularly when the drug is not given daily, but twice weekly. In addition, slow acetylators are more likely to show phenytoin toxicity when this drug is given with INH, because the latter inhibits hepatic microsomal hydroxylation of phenytoin. Isoniazid hepatitis *may* be more common among rapid acetylators, but the data are conflicting.

Acetylator status affects other drugs (e.g. procainamide, hydralazine) that are inactivated by acetylation. Steady-state plasma concentrations are higher in slow acetylators during chronic dosing with these drugs. Approximately 40% of patients treated with procainamide for 6 months or longer develop antinuclear antibodies. Slow acetylators are more likely to develop such antibodies than rapid acetylators (Figure 14.2), and more slow acetylators develop procainamide-induced lupus erythematosus. Similarly, lower doses of hydralazine are needed to control hypertension in slow acetylators (Figure 14.3), and in these individuals high doses (>200 mg/day) are more likely to lead to production of antinuclear antibodies and lupus syndrome.

Sulphasalazine is acetylated, and treatment of ulcerative colitis with this drug causes mild haemolysis in some patients, particularly those who are slow acetylators.

Acetylation may also detoxify carcinogens. The incidence of bladder cancer in men exposed to arylamines whilst employed in the dyestuffs industry is higher in slow acetylators, although there is no clear association of acetylator phenotype with sporadic bladder cancer.

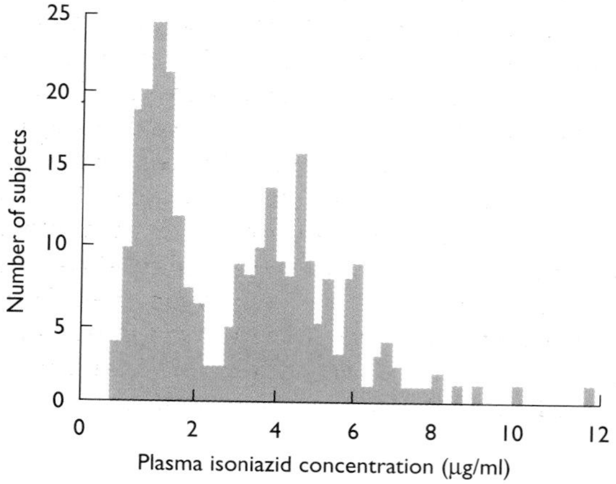

Figure 14.1 Plasma isoniazid concentrations in 483 subjects 6 h after oral isoniazid (9.8 mg/kg). Acetylator polymorphism produces a bimodal distribution into fast and slow acetylators. (Reproduced from Evans DAP *et al.* 1960: *British Medical Journal* **2**, 485, by permission of the Editor.)

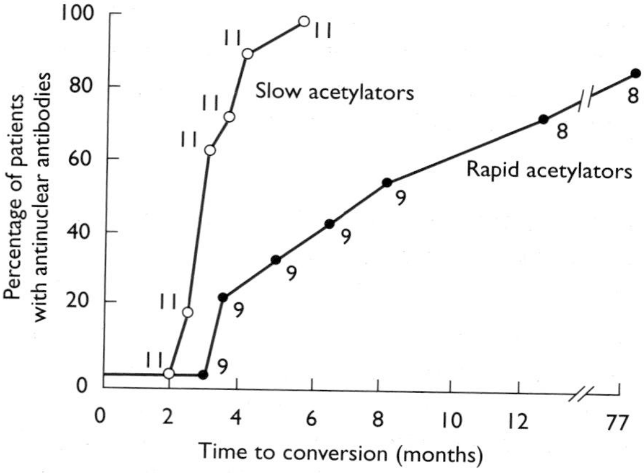

Figure 14.2: Development of procainamide-induced antinuclear antibody in slow acetylators (○) and rapid acetylators (●) with time. Number of patients shown at each point. (Reproduced from Woosley RL *et al.* 1978: *New England Journal of Medicine*; **298**, 1157, with permission.)

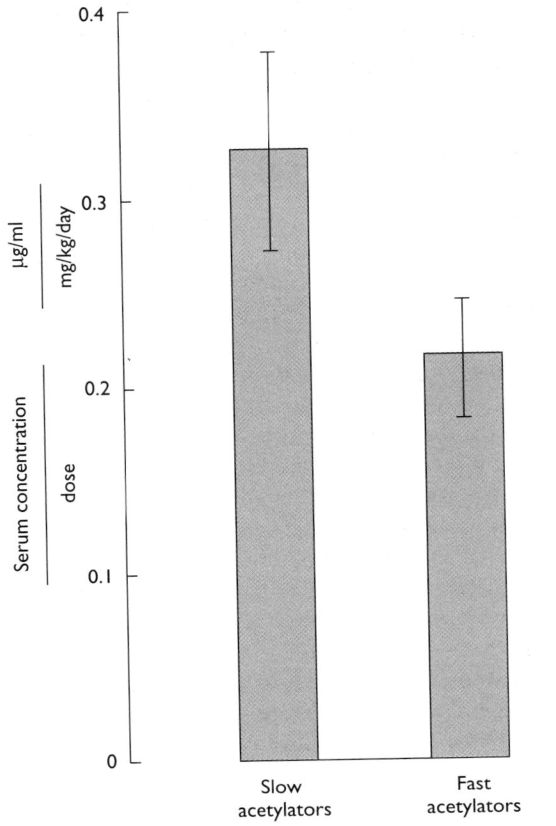

Figure 14.3: Relationship between acetylator status and dose-normalized serum hydralazine concentration (i.e. serum concentration corrected for variable daily dose). Serum concentrations were measured 1–2 h after oral hydralazine doses of 25–100 mg in 24 slow and 11 fast acetylators. (Reproduced from Koch-Weser J 1974: *Medical Clinics of North America* **58**, 1027.)

Debrisoquine hydroxylation via cytochrome $P_{450\ 2D6}$

4–Hydroxylation of debrisoquine (an adrenergic neurone-blocking drug was used in the past to treat hypertension) is deficient in about 8% of the UK population (Table 14.1). Hydroxylation polymorphisms explain several clinical phenomena:

- debrisoquine – excessive hypotension (in poor metabolizers);
- codeine – weak analgesic (in poor metabolizers);
- nortriptyline – headache and confusion (in poor metabolizers).

Several other drugs (e.g. metoprolol, propranolol, timolol, dextromethorphan) exhibit oxidation polymorphism associated with debrisoquine-linked defective metabolism. Other genetic polymorphism on the cytochrome P_{450} system include cytochrome $P_{450\ 2C9}$, cytochrome $P_{450\ 2C19}$ and cytochrome $P_{450\ 2A6}$ enzyme activity (see Table 5.1).

Tolbutamide metabolism – cytochrome $P_{450\ 2C9}$ polymorphism

This pharmacogenetic variant was described after the finding of a ninefold variation in the inter-individual rate of tolbutamide elimination. Inactivation of this sulphonylurea oral hypoglycaemic drug is largely genetically determined, by autosomal transmission. The primary site of genetic control is at the level of oxidation to hydroxytolbutamide by cytochrome $P_{450\ 2C9}$. The clinical implication is that a fixed-dose regime should not be applied indiscriminately. This is due to a polymorphism in cytochrome $P_{450\ 2C9}$, with 1:500 patients being slow metabolizers.

Sulphoxidation

Sulphoxidation displays polymorphism. There is an approximately 100–fold difference between individuals with regard to the amount of sulphoxide metabolites in the urine following a dose of carbocysteine. Sulphoxidation is inherited autosomally and is incompletely recessive. It is apparently independent of the nitrogen oxidation ('debrisoquine') system. It is not yet known whether this genotype controls oxidation of other sulphur-containing drugs (e.g. phenothiazines, thioxanthines), but an association has been demonstrated between impaired sulphoxidation and an increased incidence of adverse reactions to penicillamine therapy for rheumatoid arthritis.

Alcohol dehydrogenase

Not all enzyme variants have clinical effects. Alcohol dehydrogenase in human liver exists as an atypical variant with a specific activity about five times higher than the normal enzyme. This occurs in approximately 20% of Londoners. Despite the high specific activity of the atypical enzyme, alcohol oxidation *in vivo* is no higher than normal in individuals possessing this variant, because alcohol dehydrogenase is not the rate-limiting step in ethanol elimination.

Suxamethonium sensitivity

The usual response to a single intravenous dose of suxamethonium is muscular paralysis for about 6 min. The effect is brief because suxamethonium is rapidly hydrolysed by plasma pseudocholinesterase. Occasional individuals show a much more prolonged response and may remain paralysed and require artificial ventilation for 2 h or longer. This results from the presence of an aberrant form of plasma cholinesterase. The commonest variant which causes suxamethonium sensitivity occurs at a frequency of around 1 in 2500. Heterozygotes are unaffected carriers and represent about 4% of the population.

Inherited traits that influence drug action

Familial hypercholesterolaemia

Familial hypercholesterolaemia (FH) is an autosomal disease in which the ability to synthesize receptors for low-density lipoprotein (LDL) is impaired. Low-density-lipoprotein receptors are needed for hepatic uptake of LDL, and individuals with FH consequently have very high circulating concentrations of LDL, and suffer from atheromatous disease at a young age. Homozygotes completely lack the ability to synthesize LDL receptors, and may suffer from coronary artery disease in childhood, whereas the much commoner heterozygotes have intermediate numbers of receptors between homozygotes and healthy individuals, and commonly suffer from coronary disease in young adulthood. β-Hydroxy-β-methylglutaryl coenzyme A (HMGCoA) reductase inhibitors (an important class of drug for lowering circulating cholesterol levels) function largely by indirectly increasing the number of hepatic LDL receptors. Such drugs are especially valuable for treating heterozygotes with FH, because they restore hepatic LDL receptors towards normal in such individuals by increasing their synthesis. In contrast, they are relatively ineffective in homozygotes because such individuals entirely lack the genetic material needed for LDL-receptor synthesis.

Glucocorticoid-induced raised intra-ocular pressure

In some individuals, steroid eyedrops (e.g. 0.1% dexamethasone) cause a reversible increase in intra-ocular pressure. This response is inherited in a simple Mendelian manner. Populations can be divided into individuals who produce little or no (<5 mmHg) rise in pressure, those whose pressure rises by 5–15 mmHg and those with a rise of >15 mmHg. The clinical importance of this has been determined by observing the risk of developing open-angle (simple) glaucoma in individuals with the various allelic pairs. Heterozygotes have an 18-fold higher risk of developing glaucoma compared to individuals who are homozygous for low-pressure response to steroids, whilst homozygotes for high-pressure response have 101 times the risk of those who are homozygous for low-pressure response. Furthermore, steroid eyedrops precipitate glaucoma in some such individuals.

Warfarin resistance

This has been observed in very few pedigrees in humans, but has become common in rats, where the selective advantage is obvious (warfarin has been widely used as a rat poison).

Angiotensin-converting enzyme gene polymorphism

There is a genetic polymorphism involving the angiotensin-converting enzyme (ACE) gene. This involves a deletion in a flanking region of DNA that controls the activity of the gene. The double-deletion genotype may be an independent risk factor for coronary artery disease, especially in individuals who lack other conventional risk factors (e.g. hypertension or hypercholesterolaemia). If this is confirmed, it suggests the possibility of using drugs that act on the renin–angiotensin system (such as ACE inhibitors) in genetically defined individuals at high risk of heart disease.

INHERITED DISEASES THAT PREDISPOSE TO DRUG TOXICITY

GLUCOSE-6-PHOSPHATE DEHYDROGENASE DEFICIENCY

Glucose-6-phosphatase dehydrogenase (G6PD) catalyses the formation of reduced nicotinamide adenine dinucleotide phosphate (NADPH), which maintains glutathione in its reduced form (Figure 14.4). The gene for G6PD is located on the X-chromosome, so deficiency of this enzyme is inherited in a sex-linked manner. Glucose-6–phosphate dehydrogenase deficiency is common, especially in Mediterranean peoples, those of African or Indian descent and in the Far East. Reduced enzyme activity results in methaemoglobinaemia and haemolysis when red cells are exposed to oxidizing agents (e.g. as a result of ingestion of broad beans (*Vicia fava*), naphthalene or one of several drugs).

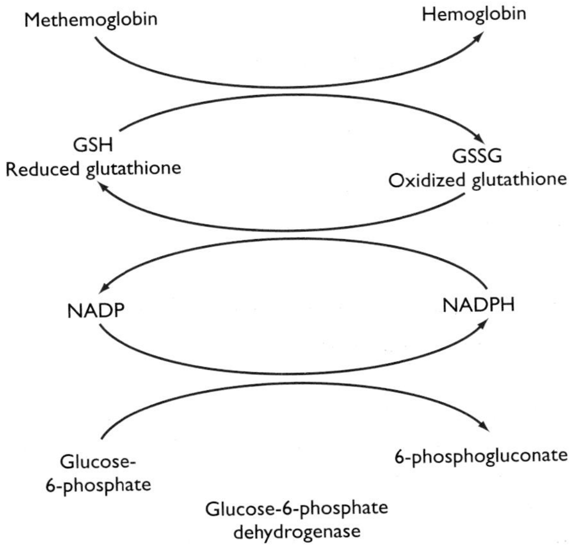

Figure 14.4 Site of glucose-6-phosphate dehydrogenase deficiency.

There are over 80 distinct variants of G6PD, but not all of them produce haemolysis. The lower the activity of the enzyme, the more severe is the clinical disease. The following drugs (see also Table 48.3) can produce haemolysis in such patients:

1. analgesics – aspirin;
2. antimalarials – primaquine, quinacrine, quinine;
3. antibacterials – sulphonamides, sulphones, nitrofurantoin, chloramphenicol;
4. miscellaneous – quinidine, probenecid, vitamin K.

Patients with G6PD deficiency treated with an 8–aminoquinoline (e.g. primaquine) should spend at least the first few days in hospital under supervision. If acute severe haemolysis occurs, primaquine may have to be withdrawn and blood transfusion may be needed. Cortisol, 100–200 mg, is given intravenously and the urine is alkalinized to reduce the likelihood of deposition of acid haematin in the renal tubules.

The high incidence of this condition in some areas is attributed to a balanced polymorphism, i.e. to a selective advantage conferred on heterozygotes. It is postulated that this selective advantage is due to a protective effect of partial enzyme deficiency against falciparum malaria. This is supported by the observation that in Sardinia there is a positive correlation between genes for both thalassaemia and G6PD deficiency and previous malarial endemicity. Resistance may arise because parasites survive less well in enzyme-deficient cells, due to the fact that these are more rapidly removed from the circulation.

Several other enzymic defects in the glutathione-generating system have been discovered which lead to haemolysis when oxidizing drugs are taken.

METHAEMOGLOBINAEMIA

Several compounds oxidize haemoglobin to methaemoglobin, including nitrates, nitrites, chlorates, sulphonamides, sulphones, nitrobenzenes, nitrotoluenes and anilines. In certain haemoglobin variants (e.g. HbM, HbH), the oxidized (methaemoglobin) form is not readily converted back into reduced, functional haemoglobin. Exposure to the above substances causes methaemoglobinaemia in individuals with these haemoglobin variants.

Similarly, nitrites, chlorates, dapsone and primaquine can cause cyanosis in patients with a deficiency of NADH-methaemoglobin reductase.

Other haemoglobin variants

Hb Zurich causes acute haemolytic reactions when sulphonamides are administered. HbH is a relatively common variant in the East (1 in 300 births in Bangkok). Oxidants cause acute haemolysis in homozygotes, similar to that which occurs in patients with G6PD deficiency.

Malignant hyperthermia

This is a rare but potentially fatal complication of general anaesthesia. The causative agent is usually halothane or suxamethonium. Sufferers exhibit a rapid rise in temperature and (usually) increasing muscular rigidity, tachycardia, sweating, cyanosis and rapid respiration. There are several forms, one of the commoner ones (characterized by halothane-induced rigidity) being inherited as a Mendelian dominant. The frequency of this phenotype is 1:20 000.

Several separate underlying muscle diseases predispose to malignant hyperthermia, including myopathies and myotonia congenita. Serum creatine phosphokinase is sometimes elevated in such individuals, but a more accurate prediction of susceptibility can be made by muscle biopsy. Muscle from affected individuals is abnormally sensitive to caffeine *in vitro*, responding with a strong contraction to low concentrations. (Pharmacological doses of caffeine release calcium from intracellular stores and cause contraction even in normal muscle at sufficiently high concentration.) Affected muscle responds similarly to halothane or suxamethonium.

Acute porphyrias

This group of diseases includes acute intermittent porphyria, variegate porphyria and hereditary coproporphyria. In all three varieties acute illness is precipitated by drugs because of inherited enzyme deficiencies in the pathway of haem synthesis (Figure 14.5). Drugs do not precipitate acute attacks in porphyria cutanea tarda, a non-acute porphyria, although this condition is aggravated by alcohol, oestrogens, iron and polychlorinated aromatic compounds.

Drug-induced exacerbations of acute porphyria (neurological, psychiatric, cardiovascular and gastrointestinal disturbances that are occasionally fatal) are accompanied by increased urinary excretion of 5–aminolevulinic acid (ALA) and porphobilinogen. An extraordinarily wide array of drugs can cause such exacerbations. Most of the drugs that have been incriminated are enzyme inducers that raise hepatic ALA synthetase levels. These drugs include phenytoin, sulphonylureas, ethanol, griseofulvin, sulphonamides, sex hormones, methyldopa, imipramine, theophylline, rifampicin, pyrazinamide and chloramphenicol. Often a single dose of one drug of this type can precipitate an acute episode, but in some patients repeated doses are necessary to provoke a reaction.

These patients used to fare considerably better *before* the therapeutic advances of the twentieth century, and it behoves clinicians to consider the possibility of this diagnosis and, having made it, to minimize drug treatment and seek specialist advice before prescribing *any* medication. A useful list of drugs that are unsafe for use in acute porphyrias is included in the *British National Formulary*.

Down's syndrome

Children with trisomy 21 exhibit excessive sensitivity to antimuscarinic drugs.

Gout

Some forms of gout are inherited in an autosomal-dominant manner. In other cases there is evidence of polygenic inheritance. Gout is aggravated by the following:

1 ethanol – this is metabolized by oxidation and simultaneous formation of NADH from NAD^+. NADH favours conversion of pyruvate to lactate, which impairs renal excretion of urate;

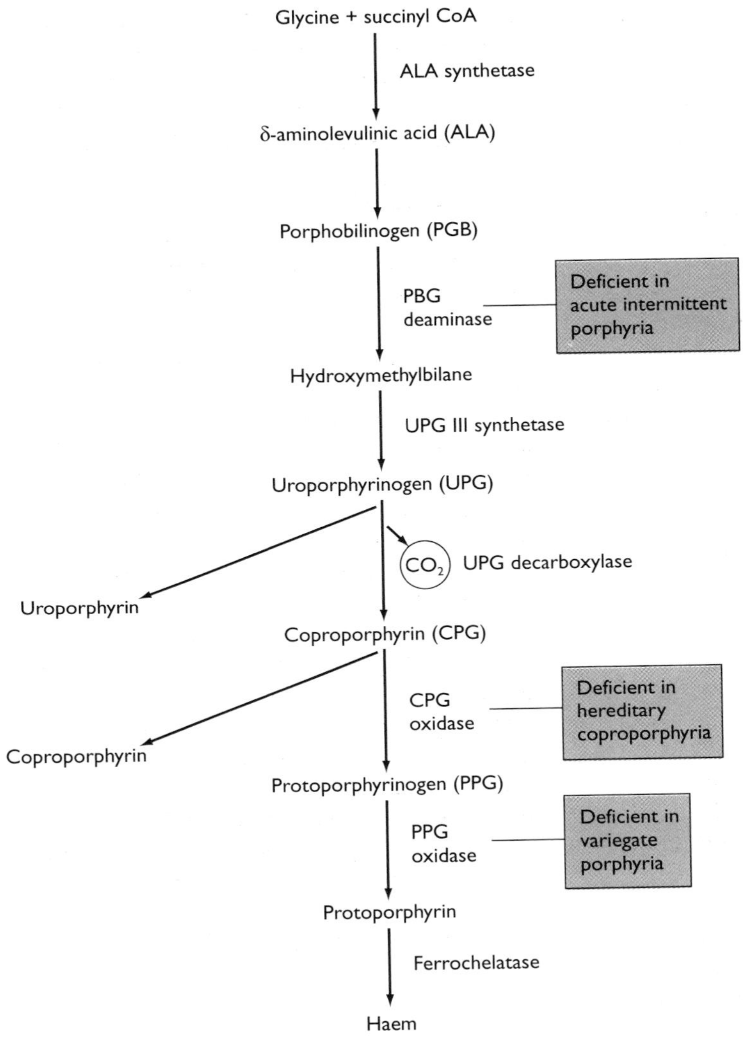

Figure 14.5 Porphyrin metabolism, showing sites of enzyme deficiency in the porphyrins.

2 diuretics – (both thiazides and loop diuretics). These reduce renal excretion of uric acid, and consequently increase the plasma urate concentration. As a result they precipitate gout in susceptible individuals;
3 allopurinol – this reduces the frequency of acute gouty attacks by inhibiting xanthine oxidase, which converts xanthine to uric acid. Allopurinol also inhibits total synthesis of purines. In a small number of patients (<1%) with reduced hypoxanthine–guanine phosphoribosyltransferase (HGPRT) activity, this second action of allopurinol does not operate, and the drug can (rarely) cause xanthine renal stones to form in such individuals. Activation of 6–mercaptopurine and azathioprine, which are purine antimetabolites, depends on HGPRT. Consequently, the therapeutic effects of these drugs are not obtained in patients who lack this enzyme (e.g. children with Lesch–Nyhan syndrome).

GILBERT'S DISEASE

This is a benign chronic form of hyperbilirubinaemia caused by an inherited lack of a hepatic conjugating enzyme (glucuronyl transferase).

Oestrogens impair bilirubin uptake and aggravate the jaundice in patients with this condition, as does fasting.

Transketolase deficiency

It has been found that some individuals inherit an abnormal form of transketolase with reduced avidity for its cofactor, thiamine pyrophosphate, inheritance being autosomal recessive. If dietary thiamine intake is reduced because of chronic alcoholism, the activity of transketolase becomes compromised. It is postulated that this explains why only some alcoholics develop Wernicke–Korsakov syndrome, whereas others with similar degrees of malnutrition are unaffected.

Polygenic influences on drug action

The above are examples of *discontinuous* variations in drug response, usually due to the effects of variations in a single allele. The response to most drugs in a population displays continuous variation and is the result of multiple genetic and environmental factors. Twin studies have been used to investigate the role of genetic influences acting in this type of distribution. There is much greater similarity between identical twins than between fraternal twins with regard to disposition of many drugs, including ethanol, phenytoin, halothane and nortriptyline (Figure 14.6). Family studies have confirmed this type of inheritance despite

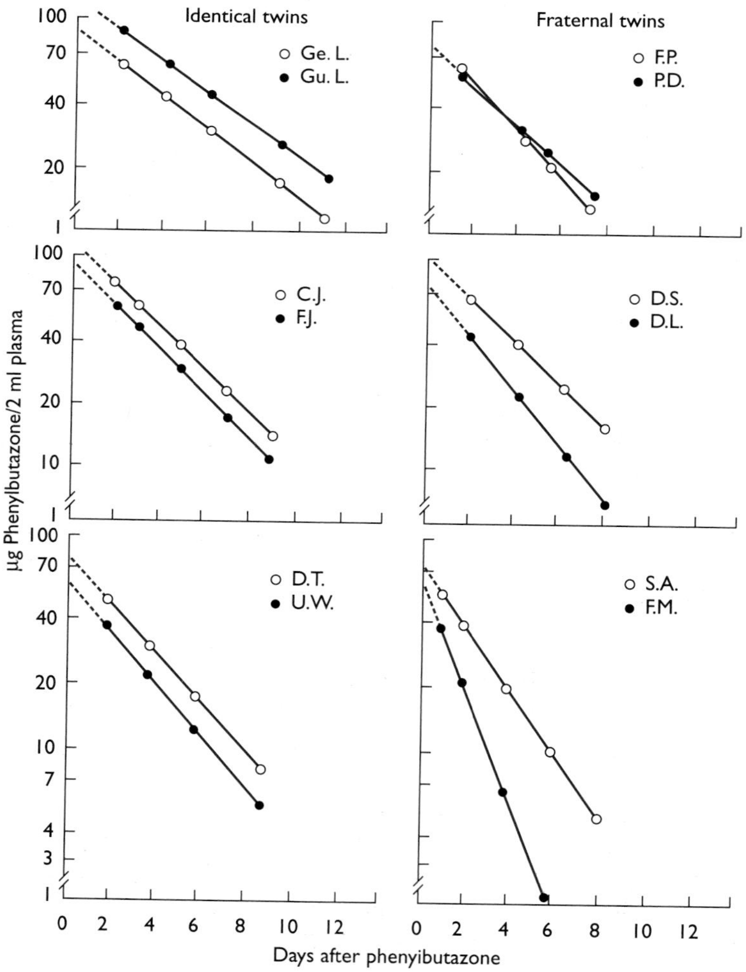

Figure 14.6 Decline in plasma phenylbutazone concentrations following a single dose of 6 mg/kg to three sets of identical twins and three sets of fraternal twins. (Reproduced from Vesell ES and Page JG 1968: *Science* **159**, 1479. Copyright 1968, American Association for the Advancement of Science.)

complications arising from differences in drug disposition according to age, sex, disease and exposure to chemicals in the environment. Thus, like blood pressure and height, which are also under polygenic control, the patterns of metabolism of these drugs in offspring tend to lie between those of the parents.

Estimates of heritability ($H = 1$ implying complete hereditary control and $H = 0$ implying no hereditary control) for antipyrine and ethanol metabolism have been put as high as 0.98 and 0.99, respectively, for identical twins and 0.47 and 0.38, respectively, for fraternal twins. Large inter-individual differences in the rates of elimination of these drugs are apparently remarkably free from environmental influences, at least under the environmental conditions in which these studies were conducted.

Drugs whose metabolism is mainly influenced by variations in a single gene may also show additional variation due to superimposed polygenic effects. Isoniazid is an example, where there is continuous variation within each of the two populations of rapid and slow acetylators (see Figure 14.1).

Key points

- Genetic differences contribute substantially to individual variation in responses to drugs.
- Mendelian traits that influence drug metabolism include:
  (a) acetylator status – balanced polymorphism that affects metabolism of several drugs, including isoniazid, hydralazine and dapsone;
  (b) deficient debrisoquine hydroxylation – a balanced polymorphism of a cytochrome P_{450} isoenzyme which hydroxylates several therapeutic drugs, including metoprolol and nortriptylene;
  (c) pseudocholinesterase deficiency – this leads to prolonged apnoea after suxamethonium, which is normally inactivated by this plasma enzyme.
- Several inherited diseases predispose to drug toxicity:
  (a) glucose-6-phosphate dehydrogenase deficiency predisposes to haemolysis following many drugs, including primaquine;
  (b) malignant hyperthermia is a Mendelian dominant affecting the ryanodine receptor in striated muscle, leading to potentially fatal attacks of hyperthermia and muscle spasm after treatment with suxamethonium and/or inhalational anaesthetics;
  (c) acute porphyrias, which are particularly triggered by enzyme-inducing agents as well as by other drugs.
- Polygenic influences are common and important determinants of drug response. This is currently being studied by genotyping populations with the aim of identifying markers that will identify optimum treatment for individuals (especially by avoiding idiosyncratic adverse effects).

Case history

A 52-year-old man underwent treatment for severe depression. Antidepressant drugs proved ineffective and he was admitted for a course of electroconvulsive therapy (ECT). He had previously been well and had never had an anaesthetic. There was no family history of problems with anaesthesia, and his parents were unrelated. He was given intravenous anaesthetic (thiopentone) and suxamethonium, and woke 4 h later in the intensive-care unit on a ventilator. Subsequent investigation demonstrated that he had a severe form of pseudocholinesterase deficiency.

Comment

This rare disorder is inherited as a Mendelian recessive, so the lack of family history is unsurprising. A relatively short-acting competitive neuromuscular blocker (such as mivacurium or rocuronium) could be used to provide muscle relaxation during ECT for this patient.

FURTHER READING

Cambien F, Poirier O, Lecerf L *et al.* 1992: Deletion polymorphism in the gene for angiotensin converting enzyme is a potent risk factor for myocardial infarction. *Nature* **359**, 641–4.

Grahame-Smith 1999: How will knowledge of the human genome affect drug therapy. *British Journal of Clinical Pharmacology* **47**, 7–10.

Kalow W. 1989: Race and therapeutic drug response. *New England Journal of Medicine* **320**, 588–90.

Price-Evans DA. 1993: *Genetic factors in drug therapy, clinical and molecular pharmacogenetics*. Cambridge: Cambridge University Press.

Zhou HH, Koshakji RP, Silberstein DJ, Wilkinson GR, Wood AJ. 1989: Altered sensitivity to and clearance of propranolol in men of Chinese descent as compared with American whites. *New England Journal of Medicine* **320**, 565–70. (Chinese have greater sensitivity to propranolol than whites, despite metabolizing propranolol more rapidly.)

CHAPTER FIFTEEN

INTRODUCTION *of* NEW DRUGS *and* CLINICAL TRIALS

- History
- UK regulatory system
- The process of drug development
- Preclinical studies
- Clinical trials
- Clinical drug development
- Generic drugs
- Ethics committees
- Globalization

HISTORY

Many years before Christ, man discovered, presumably by trial and error, that certain plant extracts influence the course of disease. Primitive tribes used extracts containing active drugs such as opium, ephedrine, cascara, cocaine, ipecacuanha and digitalis. These were probably often combined with strong psychosomatic therapies, and the fact that potentially beneficial agents survived the era of magic and superstition says a great deal about the powers of observation of those early 'researchers'.

Many useless and sometimes deleterious treatments also persisted through the centuries, but the desperate situation of the sick and their faith in medicine delayed recognition of the harmful effects of drugs. Any deterioration following drug administration was usually attributed to disease progression rather than to adverse drug effects. There were notable exceptions to this faith in medicine, and some physicians had a short life expectancy as a consequence!

During the present century there has been an almost exponential growth in the number of drugs introduced into medicine. The 1932 *British Pharmacopoeia* lists only 213 medicinal products. By 1990, this had increased to almost 3500. Many advances can be attributed to the necessities of war. However, properly controlled clinical trials, which are the cornerstone of new drug development and for which the well-organized vaccine trials of the Medical Research Council (MRC) must take much credit, only became widespread after World War Two. Some conditions did not require clinical trials (e.g. the early use of penicillin in conditions with a predictable natural history and high fatality rate). (Florey is credited with the remark that 'if you make a *real* discovery, you don't need to call in the statisticians'.) Ethical considerations relating to the use of a 'non-treatment' group in early trials were sometimes rendered irrelevant by logistic factors such as the lack of availability of drugs.

It was not until the 1960s that the appalling potential of drug-induced disease was realized world-wide. **Thalidomide** was first marketed in West Germany in 1956 as a sedative/hypnotic as well as a treatment for morning sickness. The drug was successfully launched in various countries, including Britain in 1958, and was generally accepted as a safe and effective compound with little hangover effect, and indeed its advertising slogan was 'the safe hypnotic'. However, in 1961 it became clear that its use in early pregnancy was causally related to a rare congenital abnormality, phocomelia, in which the long bones fail to develop. At least 600 such babies were born in England, and more than 10 000 afflicted babies were born world-wide. The thalidomide tragedy stunned the medical profession, the pharmaceutical industry and the general public. In 1963, the Minister of Health of the UK established a Committee on Safety of Drugs, since it was clear that some control over the introduction and marketing of drugs was necessary. These attempts at regulation culminated in the Medicines Act 1968.

UK REGULATORY SYSTEM

The Medicines Act 1968 provides for the licensing of all medicinal products, and controls their sale, supply and advertising. The Health and Agriculture Ministers are the 'licensing authority'. The Medicines Control Agency (MCA) performs the administrative and secretarial function. The Medicines Commission is an advisory body to the licensing authority and is distinct from the Committee on Safety of Medicines (CSM), which is an independent group of clinicians, clinical pharmacologists, toxicologists, pathologists and others who advise the licensing authority, on the safety, quality and efficacy of medicinal products as well as the investigation and monitoring of adverse reactions once a drug has been licensed. The CSM advises the MCA on the granting of clinical trial certificates (CTCs) or exemptions (CTXs) for trials concerning unlicensed drugs for 'new' indications. Eventually a product licence will be granted to the manufacturer if the CSM is satisfied with the quality, safety and efficacy of the drug. Cost is not a consideration for the CSM, nor is effectiveness in relation to other licensed products, but *risk–benefit* is considered. The granting of a product licence normally occurs approximately 10 years after the original patent is filed. The licence will state for what indications the drug may be marketed.

The UK is also subject to the European Union (EU) Pharmaceutical Directives, and the regulatory system has evolved to harmonize national and EU regulations. Medicines (unless derived from biotechnology) may be licensed directly by the MCA for use in the UK. In Europe, the EMEA is responsible for co-ordinating the assessment of medicines under a centralized procedure which enables approval to be granted for all EU member states.

THE PROCESS OF DRUG DEVELOPMENT

Drug development is a highly regulated process which should be performed under internationally recognized codes of practice, namely Good Manufacturing Practice (GMP), Good Laboratory Practice (GLP) and Good Clinical Practice (GCP). Good Clinical Practice is an international ethical and scientific quality standard for designing, conducting, recording and reporting trials that involve the participation of human subjects. Compliance with this standard provides public assurance that the rights, safety and well-being of trial subjects are protected, consistent with principles that have their origin in the Declaration of Helsinki, and that the clinical trial data are credible. The objective of the International Conference on Harmonization (ICH) GCP Guidelines is to provide a unified standard for the European Union (EU), Japan and the USA, to facilitate the mutual acceptance of clinical data by the regulatory authorities in these jurisdictions. The stages of drug development are outlined in Figure 15.1.

DRUG DISCOVERY, DESIGN AND SYNTHESIS

Whilst random screening and serendipity remain important in the discovery of new drugs, new knowledge of the role of receptors, enzymes, ion channels and carrier molecules in both normal physiological processes and disease now permits a more focused approach to drug design. Using advances in combinatorial chemistry, biotechnology and computer-aided drug design (see Chapter 16), new drugs can now be identified rationally rather than exclusively by the old methods of chance and grind.

PRECLINICAL STUDIES

New chemical entities are tested in animals to investigate their pharmacology, toxicology, pharmacokinetics and potential efficacy in order to select drugs of potential value in humans.

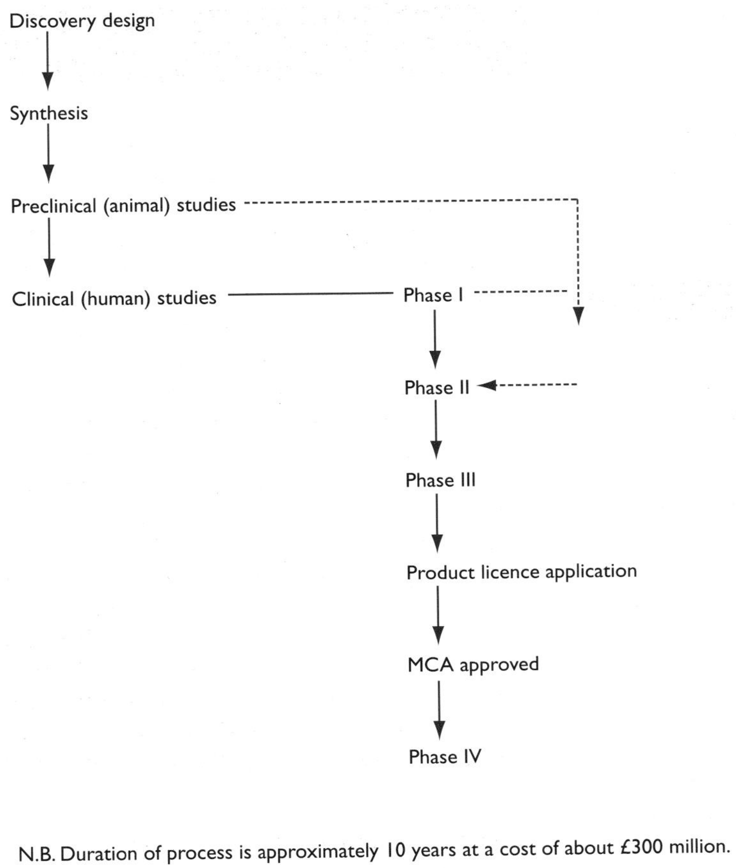

Figure 15.1: Stages of drug development.

These studies are summarized in Table 15.1. Although there is considerable controversy concerning the value of some studies performed in animals, human drug development has an excellent safety record, and there is understandable reluctance on the part of the regulatory authorities to reduce requirements. At present the European guidelines require that the effects of the drug should be assessed in two mammalian species (one non-rodent) after 2 weeks of dosing before a single dose is administered to a human. In addition, a batch of mutagenicity tests should have been completed and assessed. Additional and longer duration studies are conducted before product licence approval. The timing, specific tests and duration of studies may relate to the proposed human usage in both the clinical trials and eventual indications.

Table 15.1: Preclinical studies

Pharmacology*
Acute toxicity*
Chronic toxicity
Mutagenicity*/genotoxicity*
Carcinogenicity
Reproductive testing

*Minimum requirements before a single dose can be administered to a human in the EU guidelines.

Clinical trials

Physicians read clinical papers, review articles and pharmaceutical advertisements describing clinical trial results. Despite peer review, the incompetent or unscrupulous author can conceal deficiencies in design and possibly publish misleading data. The major medical journals are well refereed, although supplements to many medical journals are less rigorously reviewed for scientific value. An understanding of the essential elements of clinical trial design enables a more informed interpretation of published data.

Assessment of a new treatment by clinical impression is not adequate. Diseases may resolve or relapse spontaneously, coincidental factors may confound any interpretation, and the power of placebo and enthusiastic investigators are a major influence on subjective response. In order to minimize these factors and eliminate bias, any new treatment should be rigorously assessed by carefully designed, controlled clinical trials.

Objectives

The first step in clinical trial design is to determine the questions to be addressed. Primary and achievable objectives must be defined. The question may be straightforward. For example, does treatment A prolong survival in comparison with treatment B following diagnosis of small-cell carcinoma of the lung? Survival is a clear and objective end-point. Less easily measured end-points such as quality of life must also be assessed as objectively as possible. Prespecified subgroups of patients may be identified and differences in response determined. For example, treatment A may be found to be most effective in those patients with limited disease at diagnosis, whereas treatment B may be most effective in those with widespread disease at diagnosis. Any physician conducting a clinical trial must not forget that the ultimate objective of all studies is to benefit patients. The patients' welfare must be of paramount importance.

Randomization

Patients who agree to enter such a study must be randomized so that there is an equal likelihood of receiving treatment A or B. If treatment is not truly randomized, then bias will occur. For example, the investigator might consider treatment B to be less well tolerated and thus decide to treat particularly frail patients with treatment A. Multicentre studies are often necessary in order to recruit adequate numbers of patients, and it is essential to ensure that the treatments are fairly compared. If treatment A is confined to one centre/hospital and treatment B to another, many factors may affect the outcome of the study due to differences between the centres, such as interval between diagnosis and treatment, individual differences in determining entry criteria, facilities for treatment of complications, differing attitude to pain control, ease of transport, etc.

Inclusion and exclusion criteria

For any study, inclusion and exclusion criteria must be defined. It is essential to maximize safety and minimize confounding factors, whilst also ensuring that the criteria are not so strict that the findings will be applicable only to an unrepresentative subset of the patient population encountered in usual practice. The definition of a healthy elderly subject is problematic. Over the age of 65 years it is 'normal' (in the sense that it is common) to have a reduced creatinine clearance, to be on some concomitant medication and to have a history of allergy. If these are exclusion criteria, a trial will address a 'superfit' elderly population and not a normal population.

Double-blind design

A 'double-blind' design is often desirable to eliminate psychological factors such as enthusiasm for the 'new' remedy. This is not always possible. For example, if in the comparison of treatment A and treatment B described above, treatment A consists of regular intravenous infusions whilst treatment B consists of oral medication, the 'blind' is broken. As 'survival' duration is 'hard' objective data, this should not be influenced markedly, whereas softer end-points such as state of well-being are more easily confounded. In trials where these are especially important, it may be appropriate to use more elaborate strategies to permit blinding, such as the use of a 'double dummy' where there is a placebo for both dosage forms. In this case patients are randomized to active tablets plus placebo infusion or to active infusion plus placebo tablets.

Withdrawals

The number of patients who are withdrawn from each treatment and the reason for withdrawal (subjective, objective or logistic) must be taken into account. For example, if in an antihypertensive study comparing two treatments administered for 3 months only the data from those who completed 3 months of therapy with treatment X or Y are analysed, this may suggest that both treatments were equally effective. However, if 50% of the patients on treatment X withdrew after 1 week because of lack of efficacy, that conclusion is erroneous. Again, if patients are withdrawn after randomization but before dosing, this can lead to unrecognized bias if more patients in one group die before treatment is started than in the other group, leading to one group containing a higher proportion of fitter 'survivers'. Conversely, if patients are withdrawn after randomization but before dosing, adverse events cannot be attributed to the drug. Hence both an 'intention-to-treat' analysis and a 'treatment-received' analysis should be presented.

Placebo

If a placebo control is ethical and practical, this simplifies interpretation of trial data and enables efficacy to be determined more easily (and with much smaller numbers of subjects) than if an effective active comparator is current standard treatment (and hence ethically essential). It is well recognized that placebo treatment can have marked effects (e.g. lowering blood pressure). This is partly due to patient familiarization with study procedures, whose effect can be minimized by a placebo 'run-in' phase.

Trial design

There is no one perfect design for comparing treatments. Studies should be prospective, randomized, double-blind and placebo controlled whenever possible. Parallel-group studies are those in which patients are randomized to receive different treatments. Although tempting, the use of historical data as a control is often misleading and should only be employed in exceptional circumstances. Usually one of the treatments is the standard, established treatment of choice, i.e. the control, whilst the other is an alternative – often a new treatment which is a potential advance. In chronic stable diseases, a crossover design in which each subject acts as his or her own control can be employed. Intra-individual variability in response is usually much less than inter-individual variability. The treatment sequence must be evenly balanced to avoid order effects, and there must be adequate 'washout' to prevent a carry-over effect from the first treatment. This design is theoretically more 'economical' in subject numbers, but is often not applicable in practice.

Statistics

Research papers often quote P values as a measure of whether or not an observed difference is 'significant'. Conventionally, the null hypothesis is often rejected if $P < 0.05$ (i.e. a difference of the magnitude observed would be expected to occur by chance in less than 1 in 20 trials). This is of limited value, as a clinically important difference may be missed if the sample size is too small (type II error). To place reliance on a negative result, the statistical power of the study should be at least $P = 0.8$ and preferably $P = 0.9$ (i.e. a true difference of the magnitude prespecified would be missed in 20% or 10% of such trials, respectively). It is possible to calculate the number of patients required to establish a given difference between treatments at a specified level of statistical confidence. For a continuous variable, one needs an estimate of the mean and standard deviation which one would expect in the control group. This is usually available from historical data, but a pilot study may be necessary. The degree of uncertainty surrounding observed differences should be reported as confidence intervals (usually 95% confidence intervals). Such intervals will diminish as the sample size is increased. Confidence intervals reflect the effects of sampling variability on the precision of a procedure, and it is important to quote them when a 'non-significant' result is obtained, and when comparing different estimates of effectiveness (e.g. drug A in one trial may have performed twice as well as placebo, whereas drug B in another trial may have performed only 1.5 times as well as placebo; whether drug A is probably superior to drug B will be apparent from inspection of the two sets of confidence intervals).

The conventional threshold for a statistically significant result is usually $P < 0.05$, i.e. there is a 1:20 risk of a false-positive result (type I error).

If many parameters are analysed, some apparently 'significant' differences will be identified by chance. For example, if 100 parameters are analysed in a comparison of two treatments, one would expect to see a 'significant' difference in five of those parameters. One must also consider the clinical importance of any statistically significant result. For example, a drug may cause a statistically significant decrease in blood pressure in a study, but if it is only 0.2 mmHg it is not of any clinical relevance.

It is important to discuss the design and sample size of any clinical trial with a statistician at the planning phase. However, statistics cannot completely answer the question of when a randomized controlled trial should be stopped, and such trials may occasionally be unethical if one treatment is vastly superior to the other. Clearly it is neither ethically nor economically reasonable to continue with a trial once the result has clearly favoured one alternative. One trial design which permits timely and efficient termination of a comparison is the sequential design. In this design, patients are paired so that the alternative treatments are represented in each pair. For each pair a judgement based on agreed criteria is made as to the superiority of one of the treatments. This judgement is termed a *preference*. Pairs for which no preference for any one treatment can be made do not enter the analysis. The results of each preference are plotted on a chart such as that shown in Figure 15.2. The shape of boundaries in the chart is drawn up using statistical criteria. When the line of preference crosses the upper or lower boundaries of the chart the trial is terminated, since at this point a clear difference at a previously decided level of statistical significance has been demonstrated. Pairing of successive entrants to a trial automatically removes variation due to gradual trends in response occurring throughout the trial (e.g. changes in natural history of the disease, altered standards of assessment of response). The use of sequential trials may rapidly obtain an answer to a problem, but on the other hand if there is actually no difference, or only a small difference, between treatments the sequential trial requires more patients than non-sequential trials to establish this.

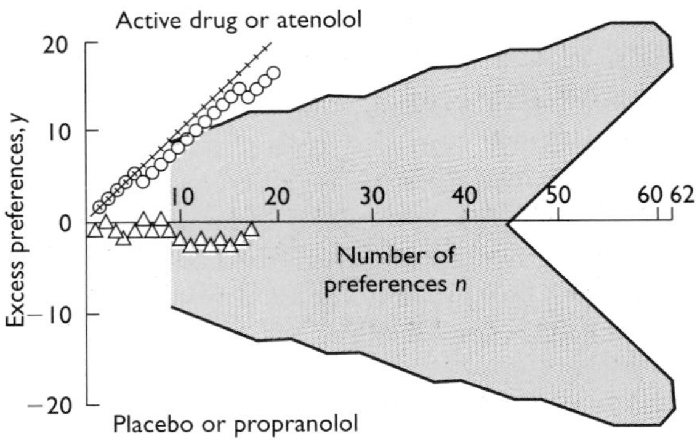

Figure 15.2: Sequential analysis of a trial of the effects of atenolol (×) and propranolol (○) vs. placebo in hyperthyroid patients using objective assessment of effects including heart rate. Both drugs are significantly better than placebo ($P = 0.05$) but a comparison of atenolol and propranolol (△) fails to distinguish between them with regard to efficacy. (Reproduced from McDevitt DG, Nelson JK. 1978: *British Journal of Clinical Pharmacology* **6**, 233.)

Sequential trials are not always suitable, and whether a trial should be stopped by breaking the double-blind if the organizers suspect that a proportion of the patients are responding well (or badly) to a new drug constitutes a dilemma. Independent data monitoring committees may be set up to address this concern.

Clinical drug development

For the majority of new drugs, the development process in humans – following a satisfactory preclinical safety evaluation – proceeds through four distinct phases. These are summarized below.

Phase I

The initial studies of drugs in humans usually involve healthy male volunteers unless toxicity is predictable (e.g. cytotoxic agents, murine monoclonal antibodies). The first dose to be administered to humans is usually 1/50–1/100 of a dose that produced no adverse effect in the most sensitive animal species tested. Subjective adverse events, clinical signs, haematology, biochemistry, urinalysis and eletrocardiography assess tolerance. Depending on the preclinical data, further evaluations may be appropriate (e.g. if toxicology data flagged a concern over cataract formation, detailed ophthalomoscopic examination should be part of the protocol). The studies are placebo controlled to reduce the influence of environment and normal variability. If the dose is well tolerated, a higher dose will be administered either to a different subject in a parallel design, or to the same group in an incremented crossover design.

This process is repeated until some predefined end-point such as a particular plasma concentration, a pharmacodynamic effect or maximum tolerated dose is reached. Data from the single-dose study will determine appropriate doses and dose intervals for subsequent multiple-dose studies. If the drug is administered by mouth, a food interaction study should be conducted before multiple-dose studies.

The multiple-dose study provides further opportunity for pharmacodynamic assessments, which may demonstrate a desired pharmacological effect and are often crucial for the selection of doses for phase II. Having established the dose range that is well tolerated by healthy subjects, and in some cases identified doses that produce the desired pharmacological effect, the phase II studies are initiated.

Key points

Phase I studies

- Not currently regulated in the UK unless patients are involved; local research ethics committee (LREC) approval is required.
- Initial exposure of humans to investigational drug.
- Assessment of tolerance, pharmacokinetics and pharmacodynamics in healthy subjects.
- Usually healthy male volunteers.
- Usually single site.
- 12–60 subjects per protocol.
- 40–100 subjects in total.

Key points

Phase II studies

- Require MCA and REC (usually local LREC) approval.
- Initial assessment of tolerance in 'target' population.
- Initial assessment of efficacy.
- Identification of doses for phase III studies.
- Well controlled with a narrowly defined patient population.
- Single or multicentre.
- 50–500 patients in total.
- Usually double-blind, randomized and controlled.

Phase II

If the drug completes the phase I programme satisfactorily and appears promising, the pharmaceutical, pharmacological, toxicological and phase I human study reports are submitted to the MCA in order to obtain a CTX to conduct therapeutic studies in patients.

Phase II studies are usually conducted in a small number of patients by specialists in the appropriate area to explore efficacy, tolerance and the dose–response relationship. If it is ethical and practicable, a double-blind design is used employing either a placebo control or a standard reference drug therapy as control. These are the first studies in the target population, and it is possible that drug effects, including tolerance and pharmacokinetics, may be different to those observed in the healthy subjects. If the exploratory phase II studies are promising, larger phase III studies are instigated.

Phase III

Phase III is the phase of large-scale formal clinical trials in which the efficacy and safety of the new drug is established. Patient groups who respond more or less well may be identified, patient exposure (both numbers and duration of therapy) is increased, and less common (type B, see Chapter 12) adverse reactions may be identified. During this period the manufacturers will be setting up

Key points

Phase III studies

- Require MCA and REC (usually multicentre, MREC) approval.
- Confirmation of effective doses.
- Expanded tolerance profile.
- Collection of data on a more varied patient population with indication.
- Data on overall benefit/risk.
- Can be placebo or more usually active controls.
- Multicentre.
- Commonly 1000–3000 patients in total.
- Usually double-blind.

plant for large-scale manufacture and undertaking further pharmaceutical studies on drug formulation, bioavailability and stability. The medical advisers to the company, in association with their pharmacological, pharmaceutical and legal colleagues, will begin to collate the large amount of data necessary to make formal application to the Licensing Authority via the CSM for a product licence. The size of the submission documents may extend to several hundredweights of paper! Marketing approval may be general or granted subject to certain limitations which may include restriction to hospital practice only, restriction in indications for use, or a requirement to monitor some particular action or organ function in a specified number of patients. All prescribing doctors are provided with a factual data sheet (summary of product characteristics, SPC) giving information on each new medicine, and the contents of this must be agreed with the CSM. It must provide all of the information necessary to make a proper decision as to whether the drug is indicated (i.e. it is not an advertisement), and it must detail the known hazards of the drug. Doctors are also reminded (by means of an inverted triangle symbol beside its entry in the *British National Formulary*) that this is a recently introduced drug, and that any suspected adverse reaction should be reported to the CSM.

Phase IV

Phase IV studies are prospective trials performed after marketing approval (the granting of a Product License). They may be studies to investigate new formulations, dosage requirements, drug interactions or patient groups, and may also help in the detection of previously unrecognized adverse events (see Chapter 12).

Key points

Phase IV Studies

- Performed after marketing approval and related to the approved indications.
- Exposure of drug to a wider population.
- Different formulations, dosages, duration of treatment, drug interactions and other drug comparisons are studied.
- Detection and definition of previously unknown or inadequately quantified adverse events and related risk factors.

Postmarketing surveillance

The CSM closely monitors newly licensed drugs for adverse events through the yellow card reporting system (see Chapter 12).

Generic drugs

Once the patent life of a drug has expired, anyone may manufacture and sell their version of that drug. The generic drug producer does not have to perform any of the research and development process other than to demonstrate that their version of the drug is 'bioequivalent' to the standard formulation. The convention accepted for such 'bioequivalence' is generous, and the issue is the subject of current debate by biostatisticians. In practice, the essential point is that clinically untoward consequences should not ensue if one preparation is substituted for the other.

Ethics committees

All protocols for clinical trials must be reviewed and approved by a properly constituted independent ethics committee. In the UK, any clinical trials that are conducted on NHS premises or involve NHS patients recruited by virtue of their past or present treatment by the NHS must involve consultation with a local research ethics committee (LREC) which follows the guidelines of the Department of Health. Multicentre studies (defined as studies involving five or more centres) require the approval of a Multicentre Research Ethics Committee (MREC), whose decision is notified to the appropriate LRECs. The objectives of the ethics committee are as follows:

1. to protect the subjects of research;
2. to preserve the rights of research subjects;
3. to provide public reassurance.

Key issues for ethical review include the importance of the research question, the scientific validity of the approach (for instance, it is unethical to enter subjects into a research protocol that is inadequately powered to answer the question that it poses), informed consent and indemnity of subjects.

GLOBALIZATION

In order to facilitate world-wide drug development and encourage good standards of practice, a series of international conferences on harmonization of requirements for registration of pharmaceuticals for human use have been conducted. The ICH conferences are leading to a globally accepted system of drug development, hopefully without stifling research with excessive bureaucracy, and without any lowering of standards. The goal is to facilitate the early introduction of valuable new therapies while at the same time maximizing patient protection.

Case history

Rather than a clinical case history, consider a chapter in the history of drug regulation which is instructive in illustrating the value of toxicity testing. Triparanol is a drug that lowers the concentration of cholesterol in plasma. It was marketed in the USA in 1959. In 1962, the Food and Drug Administration (FDA) received a tip-off and undertook an unannounced inspection. This revealed that toxicology data demonstrating cataract formation in rats and dogs had been falsified. Triparanol was withdrawn, but some of the patients who had been taking it for a year or longer also developed cataracts.

FURTHER READING

Collier J (ed.). 1996: *Drug and Therapeutics Bulletin; from trial outcomes to clinical practice*. London: Which? Ltd.

Griffin JP, O'Grady J, Wells FO (eds). 1998: *Textbook of pharmaceutical medicine*, 3rd edn. Belfast: Queen's University of Belfast.

Kirkness B (ed.). 1997: *The Association of British Pharmaceutical Industry. Pharma facts and figures*. London: White Crescent Press.

CHAPTER SIXTEEN

BIOTECHNOLOGY *and* GENE THERAPY

The term biotechnology encompasses not only the advances in our knowledge of cell and molecular biology since the discovery of DNA, but also the application of these advances to aid the diagnosis and treatment of disease. Recent progress in modern molecular genetics, cell biology and the human genome project has assisted the discovery of the mechanisms and potential therapies of disease. The identification of a gene sequence that has a particular function (e.g. production of a protein) and our ability to splice that human gene sequence into a bacterial or yeast chromosome, and to extract from those organisms large quantities of natural human and other proteins, has presented a whole array of new opportunities in medicine. The Centre for Medicines Research, when conducting a survey of the pharmaceutical industry, recently defined the product of biotechnology as 'a naturally occurring or modified protein, DNA or RNA product, produced by expression in cell lines (bacterial, yeast, mammal, insect, vertebrate or transgenic animals) ... for therapeutic, prophylactic or diagnostic use in humans'. In 1982 the first pharmaceutical product, namely human recombinant insulin, was marketed. Since then more than 50 medicines derived via biotechnology have been licensed for use in patients, whilst literally hundreds of biotechnology products are currently undergoing clinical trials. Once they have been discovered, some biotechnology products are manufactured by chemical synthesis rather than by biological processes. Examples of biotechnology products which are licensed or undergoing clinical trials are listed in Table 16.1. In parallel with these advances, the human genome project will be able to assist in establishing the associations between specific genes and specific diseases. Detailed medical histories and genetic information will be collected and collated from large samples of the population. This will identify not only who is at risk of a potential disease and may thus benefit from prophylactic therapy, but also who may be at risk of particular side-effects of certain drugs. It is not just the physical presence but, more importantly, the expression of a gene that is relevant. Often there is a complex interaction between many genes, the environment and experience that gives rise to disease. Despite these limitations, the human genome project linked with the products of biotechnology, including gene therapy, offers

Table 16.1: Examples of biotechnology products which are licensed or undergoing clinical trials

Calcitonin gene-related peptide
Luteinizing hormone-releasing factor
Granulocyte-colony-stimulating factor
Interferons
Interleukins
Human insulin
Growth hormone
Hirudin
Haemoglobin
Factors VIII and IX
Epoetin
Monoclonal antibodies for various cancers
Monoclonal antibodies against autoimmune mediators
Hepatitis vaccines
Anti-thrombin III

unprecedented opportunities for the treatment of disease.

Most biotechnologically produced proteins are not orally bioavailable, due to the efficiency of the human digestive system, and thus the majority of them cannot be administered by the oral route. However, the ability to use bacteria to produce legion numbers of modifications of proteins may aid the identification of orally bioavailable peptides.

Using biotechnology it is possible to produce human proteins from transgenic animals and bacteria to treat those diseases which are caused by the absence or impaired function of particular proteins. Before the cloning of genes and the subsequent synthesis of these human proteins in large quantities, the only source of these proteins, often in limited amounts, consisted of human tissues or body fluids, with the inherent problems of hypersensitivity and viral infections (e.g. hepatitis B and C and HIV). An example in which protein replacement is life-saving is the treatment of Gaucher's disease, a lysosomal storage disease which is caused by an inborn error of metabolism inherited as an autosomal recessive which results in a deficiency of glucocerebrosidase, which in turn results in the accumulation of glucosylcerimide in the lysosomes of the reticulo-endoethelial system, particularly the liver, bone marrow and spleen, which may result in hepatosplenomegaly, anaemia and pathological fractures. Originally a modified form of the protein, namely alglucerase, had to be extracted from human placental tissue. The deficient enzyme is now produced by recombinant technology and is effective in these patients.

The production of recombinant factor VIII for the treatment of haemophilia should minimize the risk of blood-borne viral infection such as hepatitis B and C and HIV which occurred with tragic consequences when factor VIII had been obtained from human donors. Likewise, the use of human growth hormone obtained from human pituitary glands was associated with Creutzfeldt-Jakob's disease, whereas recombinant growth hormone will now eliminate this risk.

Not only can recombinant technology be used to provide deficient proteins, but it can also be used to produce modifications of human molecules to advantage. The human insulin analogue, insulin lispro, has been produced using recombinant technology so that the order of just two amino acids is reversed in one chain of the insulin molecule, resulting in a shorter duration of action than soluble insulin. This is more convenient for some patients, and in certain circumstances will reduce the risk of hypoglycaemia.

In addition to producing recombinant human hormones (e.g. insulin) and biotechnology-derived proteins (e.g. hirudin, the anticoagulant protein of the leech), recombinant monoclonal antibodies for treating human diseases have been produced in animal species. Not surprisingly, the original murine antibodies induced antibody responses in humans which in turn caused disease or at the very least produced neutralizing antibodies, rendering the monoclonal antibodies ineffective. Immunoglobulins have been gradually humanized to reduce the risk of an immune response on repeated treatments.

Monoclonal antibodies have been produced that are of potential value in the treatment of various cancers, cardiovascular disease, septic shock and AIDS. In cancer therapy, monoclonal antibodies can be developed against a tumour-associated antigen. Most of them facilitate the body's immune system in destroying the cancer cells or reduce the blood supply to the tumour. Abciximab is a monoclonal antibody which very effectively inhibits platelet aggregation and thrombus formation. It is used in specialist centres as an adjunct to heparin and aspirin for the prevention of ischaemic complications in high-risk patients undergoing percutaneous transluminal coronary angioplasty. It is a murine monoclonal antibody, and can only be used in an individual patient once.

Recombinant techniques have also been of value in the development of vaccines, thereby avoiding the use of intact virus. Suspensions of hepatitis B surface antigen prepared from yeast cells by recombinant DNA techniques are already being widely used to prevent hepatitis B infection in high-risk groups in the UK.

An example of the use of genetic information to determine drug response is the recognition of the gene sequences responsible for the encoding of the cytochrome P_{450} enzymes. The CYP2D6 gene encodes a cytochrome P_{450} enzyme involved in the metabolism of nearly 25% of the most commonly prescribed drugs. Approximately 8% of the

Caucasian population lack CYP2D6 activity and exhibit relatively inefficient metabolism of dibrisoquine, thioridazine, amitriptylene, codeine and metoprolol. This can result in higher plasma concentrations than predicted with the standard dose, and possible drug toxicity. There are over 30 isoenzymes of cytochrome P_{450} recognized in humans, with different albeit often overlapping patterns of substrate preference. In the future, discerning the genetic blueprint of an individual may allow more appropriate dose selection. As more and more individuals are genotyped, it is hoped that those who are predisposed to severe idiosyncratic drug toxicity may be identified and subsequently avoid exposure to that particular drug. The term *pharmacogenomics* is used to describe the study of genetic differences that affect both therapeutics and adverse responses to a drug.

The increasing potential to exploit the advances in genetics and biotechnology raises the possibility of prevention by gene therapy both of some relatively common diseases which are currently reliant on symptomatic drug therapy, and of genetic disorders for which there is currently no satisfactory treatment, let alone a cure. Prevalence figures for some genetic disorders which result from a defect in a single gene are shown in Figure 16.1.

Gene therapy may be defined as the deliberate insertion of genes into human cells for therapeutic purposes to benefit the individual. Potentially gene therapy may involve the deliberate modification of the genetic material of either somatic or germ-line cells. Germ-line genotherapy by the introduction of a normal gene and/or deletion of the abnormal gene in germ cells (sperm, egg or zygote) has the potential to correct the genetic defect in many devastating inherited diseases and to be subsequently transmitted in Mendelian fashion from one generation to the next. The prevalence figures for inherited diseases in which a single gene is the major factor are listed in Figure 16.1. However, germ-line gene therapy is prohibited at present because of the unknown possible consequences and hazards, not only to the individual but also to future generations. Thus currently gene therapy only involves the introduction of genes into human somatic cells. At the beginning of 1997 more than 200 gene therapy protocols had been approved and more than 2100 patients had received gene therapy. Whereas the original gene therapy research was mainly directed at single-gene disorders, most of the research currently in progress is on malignant disease. Gene therapy trials in cancer usually involve destruction of tumour cells by the induction of an immune response against those cells, or by the introduction of 'suicide genes' into tumour cells.

Table 16.2: Prevalence of some genetic disorders which result from a defect in a single gene

Disorder	Estimated prevalence
Familial hypercholesterolaemia	1 in 500
Polycystic kidney disease	1 in 1250
Cystic fibrosis	1 in 2000
Huntington's chorea	1 in 2500
Hereditary spherocytosis	1 in 5000
Duchenne muscular dystrophy	1 in 7000
Haemophilia	1 in 10 000
Phenylketonuria	1 in 12 000

Cystic fibrosis (CF) is the most common life-shortening autosomal-recessive disease in Caucasians. It is caused by a mutation in the cystic fibrosis transmembrane conductants regulator (CFTR) gene. Over 600 different CF mutations have been recognized, although one mutation is present on over 70% of CF chromosomes. Phase I studies using both adenoviral and liposomal vectors to deliver copies of the normal CFTR gene to the airway epithelium are currently in progress. The results available to date suggest that gene transfer is feasible, but that it is only transient in duration and benefit.

A dramatic example of the potential benefit of gene therapy has been seen in the treatment of severe combined immunodeficiency secondary to adenosine deaminase deficiency by reinfusing genetically corrected autologous T-cells into affected children. One child has made a full and sustained recovery and is now able to lead a normal life mixing with the normal population, rather than being confined to a sterile isolation unit. Another success in gene therapy has occurred with recipients of allogenic bone-marrow transplants with recurrent malignancies. T-cells from the original bone-marrow donor can mediate regression of the malignancy, but can then potentially damage normal host tissues. The suicide gene was introduced into the donor T-cells, rendering them susceptible to ganciclovir before they were infused into the patients, so that they could be eliminated after the tumours had regressed and so avoid future damage to normal tissues.

A major problem in gene therapy is introducing the gene into human cells. In some applications, 'gene-gun' injection of plasma DNA may be sufficient. Minute metal particles coated with DNA are 'shot' into tissues using electrostatic force or gas pressure. Some DNA is trapped and expressed by a minority of cells, and this may be sufficient to induce an immune response.

The vectors most commonly used to introduce the therapeutic DNA into somatic cells are either viral (e.g. adenovirus vectors and retroviral vectors) or synthetic vectors (e.g. incorporating the DNA into liposomes which are then photocytosed by the host cells).

Not only is the load and poor expression of the transgene an obstacle, but also the most commonly used current vector systems raise concerns about viral infection (adenoviral vectors), integration into the genome (retroviral vectors) and tumour development. As the effects of inserting a gene are uncertain, there is concern that the genetic construct may not only directly produce abnormal function, possibly by causing expression of dormant bystander genes, but may also cause insertional mutagenesis.

Despite these inherent problems of gene therapy and the ethical concerns of how the information from the unravelling of the human genome and the genotyping of individuals will be used, the development of gene therapy has dramatic potential – not only for the replacement of defective genes in disabling diseases such as cystic fibrosis, Duchenne muscular dystrophy and Frederick's ataxia, but also for the treatment of malignant disease, and for prevention of cardiovascular disease and any other diseases for which there is a genetic predisposition.

FURTHER READING

Richards B. 1996: Biotechnology: principles, potential and pitfalls. *Pharmaceutical Medicine* **8**, 145–51.

Russell S. 1997: Gene therapy *British Medical Journal*; **315**, 1289–92.

See also articles on gene therapy by Caulfield and Cafferkey, Galas and Nevin in the *International Journal of Pharmaceutical Medicine* **12** (published in 1998).

PART II

THE NERVOUS SYSTEM

CHAPTER SEVENTEEN

HYPNOTICS *and* ANXIOLYTICS

- Introduction
- Hypnotics and sleep difficulties
- Anxiolytics

INTRODUCTION

Hypnotics induce sleep and anxiolytics reduce anxiety. There is considerable overlap between them. Thus drugs that induce sleep also reduce anxiety, and most anxiolytic drugs are sedative and will assist sleep when given at night. Neither hypnotics nor anxiolytics are suitable for the *long-term* management of insomnia or anxiety, due to their rapid induction of tolerance and dependence.

HYPNOTICS AND SLEEP DIFFICULTIES

Insomnia is common. Although no general optimal sleep duration can be defined, sleep requirements decline in old age. The average adult requires 7–8 h, but some function well on as little as 4 h while others perceive more than 9 h to be necessary. Dissatisfaction with sleep reportedly occurs in 35% of adults, and is most frequent in women aged over 65 years. Insomnia may include complaints such as difficulty in falling or staying asleep, and waking unrefreshed. Hypnotics are widely prescribed despite their ineffectiveness in chronic insomnia. Persistent insomnia is a risk factor or precursor of mood disorders, and may be associated with an increased incidence of daytime sleepiness predisposing to road traffic accidents, social and work-related problems. Insomnia lasting only a few days is commonly the result of acute stress, acute medical illness or jet lag. Insomnia lasting longer than 3 weeks is termed 'chronic' and requires careful evaluation.

SLEEP

Although we spend about one-third of our lives asleep, the function of sleep is not known. Two theories have been proposed concerning somatic and cerebral biochemical recuperation and neurophysiological functions such as consolidation of memory and sorting of sensory data.

Sleep consists of two alternating states, namely rapid eye movement (REM) sleep and non-REM sleep. During REM sleep dreaming occurs. This is accompanied by maintenance of synaptic connections and increased cerebral blood flow. Non-REM sleep includes sleep of different depths, and in the deepest form the electroencephalogram (EEG) shows a slow wave pattern, growth hormone is secreted and protein synthesis occurs.

Drugs produce states that superficially resemble physiological sleep but lack the normal mixture of REM and non-REM phases. Hypnotics usually suppress REM sleep, and when discontinued, there is an excess of REM (rebound) which is associated with troubled dreams punctuated by repeated wakenings. During this withdrawal state, falling from wakefulness to non-REM sleep is also inhibited by feelings of tension and anxiety. The result is that both patient and doctor are tempted to restart medication to suppress the withdrawal phenomena.

Management of insomnia

It is important to exclude causes of insomnia that require treating in their own right. These include the following:

1 pain (e.g. due to arthritis or dyspepsia);
2 dyspnoea (e.g. as a result of left ventricular failure, bronchospasm or cough);
3 frequency of micturition;
4 full bladder and/or loaded colon in the elderly;
5 drugs (see Table 17.1);
6 depression;
7 anxiety.

Much chronic insomnia is due to dependence on hypnotic drugs. In addition, external factors such as noise, snoring partner and an uncomfortable bed may be relevant.

Some individuals need very little sleep. Shortened sleep time is common in the elderly, and patients with dementia often have a very disturbed sleep rhythm.

1 Hypnotics should be considered if insomnia is severe and causing intolerable distress. They should be used for short periods (2–4 weeks at most) and, if possible, taken intermittently. On withdrawal the dose and frequency of use should be tailed off gradually.

Table 17.1: Drugs that may cause sleep disturbances

Caffeine
Nicotine
Alcohol withdrawal
Benzodiazepine withdrawal
Amphetamines
Certain antidepressants (e.g. imipramine)
Ecstasy
Drugs that can cause nightmares (e.g. cimetidine, corticosteroids, digoxin and propranolol)

2 **Benzodiazepines** are currently the hypnotics of choice, but may fail in the elderly, and alternatives such as **chlormethiazole** can be helpful.
3 Prescribing more than one hypnotic at a time is not recommended.
4 Drugs of other types may be needed when insomnia complicates psychiatric illness. Sleep disturbances accompanying depressive illness usually respond to sedative antidepressives such as **amitriptyline**. Antipsychotics such as **chlorpromazine** or **thioridazine** may help to settle patients suffering from dementia who have nocturnal restlessness.
5 Hypnotics should not be routinely given to hospital patients or in any other situation.
6 Whenever possible, non-pharmacological methods such as relaxation techniques, meditation, cognitive therapy, controlled breathing or mantras should be used. Some people experience sleepiness after a warm bath and/or sexual activity. A milk-based drink before bed can promote sleep but may cause weight gain. Caffeine-containing beverages should be avoided, and daytime sleeping should be discouraged. Increased daytime exercise improves sleep at night.
7 Alcohol is not recommended because it causes rebound restlessness and sleep disturbance after the initial sedation has worn off. Tolerance and dependence develop rapidly. It also causes dehydration (*gueule de bois*) and other unpleasant manifestations of hangover.

Drugs used to treat sleep disturbances

Benzodiazepines

These drugs share the same properties and are anxiolytic, anticonvulsant muscle relaxants that induce sleepiness. It is likely that some relative specificity occurs in individual drugs. For example, **clonazepam** is more anticonvulsant than other members of the group at equi-sedating doses.

Use

Indications for benzodiazepine treatment include the following:

1 panic attacks and some other forms of acute agitation;

2 intravenous benzodiazepines (e.g. **diazepam** and **midazolam**) are powerfully anxiolytic and at appropriate doses cause anterograde amnesia. These properties are useful for procedures such as endoscopy, electrocardioversion and operations under local anaesthesia;
3 relief of spasticity in neurological disease and reduction of muscle spasm due to pain;
4 intravenous benzodiazepines are rapidly effective in terminating some drug-induced abnormal movements such as acute dystonia caused by **metoclopramide;**
5 long-term treatment of some forms of epilepsy and the emergency treatment of status epilepticus;
6 tetanus;
7 short-term management of insomnia.

Note: The benzodiazepines are not suitable for the long-term treatment of anxiety or for chronic insomnia.

Long-acting benzodiazepines that are used as hypnotics include **nitrazepam**, **flunitrazepam** and **flurazepam**. **Loprazolam**, **lormetazepam** and **temazepam** act for a shorter time and therefore cause less hangover and accumulation. Members of the group that are classified as anxiolytics (e.g. diazepam) are as effective as hypnotics as these drugs.

MECHANISM OF ACTION

Benzodiazepines act by binding the γ-aminobutyric acid ($GABA_A$) receptor–chloride channel complex, and facilitate the opening of the channel in the presence of GABA. This increases hyperpolarization-induced neuronal inhibition.

ADVERSE EFFECTS

These mainly involve the nervous system, but other forms of toxicity may be encountered.

With regard to the *central nervous system*, adverse effects include:

1 sedation – feelings of fatigue, sleepiness and mental slowing down are usually dose dependent. Memory disturbances are common;
2 other consequences of CNS depression – ataxia, dysarthria, motor inco-ordination, diplopia, blurred vision, weakness, vertigo, increased risk of motor vehicle and other accidents, confusion, apathy;
3 states resembling Korsakoff's psychosis and alcoholic intoxication are sometimes produced. Occasionally these drugs precipitate outbreaks of rage and violence, presumably due to the release of anxiety-repressed hostility;
4 less common and more unpredictable effects include:
   - stimulation instead of sedation, similar to paradoxical excitement in children given barbiturates;
   - antisocial behaviour, which is probably a consequence of alcohol-like intoxication;
   - hypnagogic hallucinations during the induction of sleep. Nitrazepam can cause nightmares that often involve stressful incidents in the patient's past;
   - diazepam has occasionally been associated with depression and suicide;
   - patients with organic brain disease may respond adversely to large doses of diazepam and develop tremulousness, crying episodes, impaired concentration, nocturnal confusion and agitation;
   - diazepam inhibits stage 4 (slow-wave) sleep and suppresses attacks of night terrors (which arise during this phase of sleep). However, attacks may be displaced to the waking hours.

Allergic reactions are uncommon. **Chlordiazepoxide** has produced urticaria, angioedema and maculopapular eruptions. Light-sensitivity dermatitis, fixed drug eruptions, non-thrombocytopenic purpura and swelling of the tongue have been described with benzodiazepine treatment. Acute anaphylaxis has also been reported.

With regard to *other toxic effects*, there is no convincing evidence that these drugs are toxic to haematopoietic tissues, liver or fetus.

The adverse effects of *intravenous diazepam* include the following.

1 Cardiovascular and respiratory depression are uncommon. Patients particularly prone to develop hypotension or apnoea are those with serious underlying disease such as respiratory failure in chronic lung disease, and those who have been previously given other central depressant drugs.
2 Local pain is commonly experienced on repeated intravenous injections of diazepam, which can cause phlebitis. The incidence of this complication is reduced by flushing the vein

with 150–250 mL isotonic saline. Intra-arterial benzodiazepine can cause arterial spasm and gangrene.

An emulsion of diazepam in intralipid is less irritating to vein and perivenous tissues if leaking occurs. It is routinely used in the elderly and children. Rectal diazepam is also available.

DRUG DEPENDENCE AND WITHDRAWAL SYNDROME

Benzodiazepine dependence is usually caused by large doses taken for prolonged periods, but withdrawal states have also arisen after limited drug exposure. The full withdrawal picture may develop over 3 weeks with the longer-duration benzodiazepines. Short-acting benzodiazepines may produce withdrawal symptoms within a few hours. Withdrawal syndrome includes a cluster of features unusual in anxiety states, although frank anxiety and panic attacks commonly develop as well. Perceptual distortions (e.g. feelings of being surrounded by cotton wool), visual and auditory hallucinations, paranoia, feelings of unreality, depersonalization, paraesthesiae, perspiration, headaches and other pains, blurring of vision, dyspepsia and influenza-like symptoms are all characteristic. Depression and agoraphobia are also common. The syndrome may persist for many weeks. Withdrawal from benzodiazepines in patients who have become dependent should be gradual. If this proves difficult, then an equivalent dose of a long-acting benzodiazepine should be given as a single night-time dose instead of shorter-acting drugs. The dose should then be reduced in small fortnightly steps. Psychological support is usually needed. Beta-blockers or antidepressants should only be used if other measures fail.

PHARMACOKINETICS

Benzodiazepines are pharmacodynamically similar to one another, and the differences between them are usually due to their differing pharmacokinetics. Relationships between clinical effects and plasma concentrations of the benzodiazepines are imprecise, although in general terms the higher the plasma level, the greater the effect. Tolerance is a major contributory factor to the inter-individual variability in the pharmacokinetic– pharmacodynamic relationship. Routine measurement of plasma benzodiazepine concentrations is not useful as no clear therapeutic range has been established.

Benzodiazepines are well absorbed orally. Absorption of most benzodiazepines from intramuscular injections is less rapid and produces lower peak plasma levels than following oral administration. The unreliability of the intramuscular route is important when sedation of unco-operative patients is required (e.g. in alcohol withdrawal or acute anxiety). However, lorazepam is reliably and rapidly absorbed following intramuscular injection. Rectal diazepam is an alternative when the oral route is inappropriate.

Diazepam or midazolam are injected intravenously before procedures such as endoscopy. Early short-lived high peak blood levels are accompanied by amnesia. During the next 30–60 min there is a rapid α-phase decline and then a slower (β-phase) decline follows (diazepam half-life ($t_{\frac{1}{2}}$) = 20–50 h; midazolam $t_{\frac{1}{2}}$ = 2 h). The active desmethyl metabolite of diazepam has a $t_{\frac{1}{2}}$ of 36–200 h, but the α-hydroxy metabolite of midazolam has a $t_{\frac{1}{2}}$ of only 1–1.5 h.

Sometimes at 6 h there is a rise in blood concentration and reappearance of sedation, due to reabsorption of drug excreted in the bile (enterohepatic recirculation).

Benzodiazepines are highly protein bound in plasma (e.g. at therapeutic concentrations diazepam is 95% bound).

With the exception of chlorazepate, the major site of metabolism of benzodiazepines is the liver. There is an interrelated pattern of benzodiazepine metabolites, many of which are pharmacologically active and are used therapeutically. Desmethyldiazepam occupies a central position. This substance has a very long $t_{\frac{1}{2}}$ and at steady-state its concentration may exceed that of the parent substance. This explains the common hangover effects of continued administration of diazepam, for example. Temazepam, which does not form this metabolite and is largely excreted unchanged as glucuronide, has a shorter $t_{\frac{1}{2}}$ and causes less prolonged sedation. To increase this advantage, it is administered as a polyethylene glycol solution in capsules to speed absorption so that elimination of the total dose administered commences within a short time of administration (Figure 17.1). Unfortunately, this preparation is

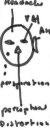

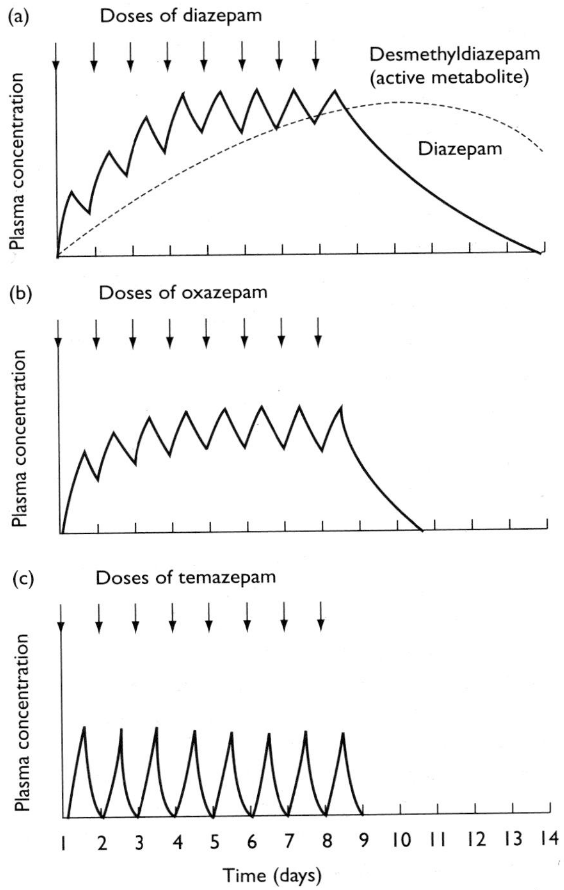

Figure 17.1: Schematic diagram of plasma concentrations following daily dosage of three benzodiazepines. Note in (a) the accumulation of both diazepam and its active metabolite, and in (b) and (c) the absence of accumulation and active metabolites for oxazepam and temazepam.

commonly used by drug abusers. It is now a controlled drug under the Misuse of Drugs Act (see Appendix) and is no longer available on NHS prescription.

Because of the long $t_{\frac{1}{2}}$ of most of these drugs, a single daily dose is sufficient to produce adequate steady-state levels. Benzodiazepines are only weak microsomal enzyme inducers, and are safe to administer with oral anticoagulants (in contrast to barbiturates). Age influences diazepam elimination, and the elderly have longer (up to 60%) half-lives for diazepam than the young. This means that with chronic dosing there is a greater delay in achieving steady state, with a consequent increased risk of failure to recognize adverse effects such as memory impairment as being drug related. The apparent volume of distribution of diazepam (which is lipid soluble) is also increased in old age because of the higher proportion of body fat in the elderly. Since clearance is directly proportional to volume of distribution and inversely proportional to $t_{\frac{1}{2}}$, diazepam clearance is unchanged as the altered $t_{\frac{1}{2}}$ and distribution volume offset one another. **Oxazepam** elimination does not require demethylation and is unaffected by ageing.

Clearance of many benzodiazepines is reduced in patients with cirrhosis of the liver, but clearance of oxazepam is unaffected, and the latter drug is therefore preferred for these patients.

DRUG INTERACTIONS

Pharmacodynamic interactions of benzodiazepines with other centrally acting drugs are common, whereas clinically significant pharmacokinetic interactions are not. Such pharmacodynamic interactions can lead to:

1 *acute potentiation* of the sedative effects of alcohol, histamine (H_1) antagonists, nabilone (a synthetic cannabinoid used as an anti-emetic for nausea and vomiting caused by cytotoxic drugs and unresponsive to conventional anti-emetics) and other hypnotics;
2 *chronic effects* – although benzodiazepines are highly protein bound, clinically significant interactions due to displacement of other protein-bound drugs (e.g. oral anticoagulants) are not observed.

Pharmacokinetic interactions include:

- cimetidine inhibition of the metabolism of benzodiazepines;
- omeprazole inhibition of the metabolism of diazepam;
- carbamazepine and phenytoin acceleration of the metabolism of clonazepam;
- erythromycin inhibition of the metabolism of midazolam.

Key points

Use of benzodiazepines for insomnia and anxiety

- Insomnia and anxiety are common. Most patients do not require drug therapy.
- Committee on Safety of Medicines (CSM) advice is as follows.

  (a) Benzodiazepines are indicated for the short-term relief (2–4 weeks only) of anxiety that is severe, disabling or subjecting the individual to unacceptable levels of distress, occurring alone or in association with insomnia or short-term psychosomatic, organic or psychotic illness.

  (b) The use of benzodiazepines to treat short-term 'mild' anxiety is inappropriate and unsuitable.

  (c) Benzodiazepines should be used to treat insomnia only when it is severe, disabling or subjecting the individual to extreme distress.

Flumazenil

Flumazenil is a benzodiazepine antagonist. It can be used to assist diagnosis in the management of multiple drug overdose, and to reverse benzodiazepine sedation. It is short acting, so sedation may return. Flumazemil can cause nausea, flushing, anxiety and fits.

Chlormethiazole

USES

Chlormethiazole has the following uses.

1 It is useful as a hypnotic in the elderly because its short action reduces the risk of severe hangover, ataxia and confusion the next day.
2 It is effective in acute withdrawal syndrome in alcoholics, but its use should be carefully supervised and treatment limited to a maximum of 9 days.
3 It can be given intravenously to terminate status epilepticus.
4 It can be used as a sedative during surgery under local anaesthesia.

MECHANISM OF ACTION

Although the structure of chlormethiazole shares some features with the thiamine molecule, there is no evidence that its actions have any relevance to this, and its mechanism remains unknown.

ADVERSE EFFECTS

1 Chlormethiazole readily causes dependence and should be used as a hypnotic only for short periods.
2 Nasal, pharyngeal and conjunctival discomfort and headache are frequently experienced during induction.
3 Gastric irritation is common.
4 High doses cause cardiovascular and respiratory depression. Especially during intravenous therapy the patient must be kept under close observation and the dose adjusted if necessary. Prolonged infusions result in drug accumulation which can lead to fatal respiratory depression.
5 Confusion and paradoxical excitement are uncommon.
6 Intravenous administration can cause thrombophlebitis. Intra-arterial infusion must be avoided because arterial spasm can lead to loss of a limb.
7 Despite the short half-life of the drug, drowsiness may be experienced on the following day and driving skills can be impaired.

CONTRAINDICATIONS

These include the following:

- pulmonary insufficiency;
- hepatocellular failure;
- alcohol dependence if alcohol is still being consumed;
- breast-feeding.

PHARMACOKINETICS

Absorption following oral administration is rapid, peak plasma levels being attained at 60 min. The $t_{\frac{1}{2}}$ is 50 min. Sedation and sleep usually occur 30–60 min after taking the drug orally. When given orally, chlormethiazole undergoes extensive first-pass metabolism (85%) which may be dose dependent and results in low bioavailability by this route. In cirrhosis, the oral bioavailability is increased about tenfold, although elimination of the drug is only slightly retarded. This results from decreased first-pass metabolism by the damaged liver. Chlormethiazole should therefore be given in reduced oral dosage to patients with cirrhosis of the liver.

DRUG INTERACTIONS

These include the following:

- potentiation of the actions of alcohol and other CNS depressants;
- cimetidine impairs the metabolism of chlormethiazole and so increases its action.

Promethazine

This H_1 antihistamine is sometimes used as a hypnotic, particularly for children. It is available without prescription for hypnotic purposes.

USES

Promethazine is of value in children if itching or allergy is causing sleep disturbance. Otherwise there is nothing to recommend promethazine as a hypnotic.

MECHANISM OF ACTION

Histamine mediates arousal and wakefulness by acting on receptors in the ventral posterior hypothalamus. Antihistamines produce sedation by inhibition of activity in long caudal tracts arising in this part of the hypothalamus.

ADVERSE EFFECTS

These include the following:

1. antimuscarinic actions – dry mouth, constipation, reduced sweating, hesitancy of micturition, aggravation of glaucoma, hallucinations, confusion in the elderly, excitement;
2. convulsions, involuntary movements;
3. nightmares;
4. hangover, bad temper;
5. respiratory and cardiovascular depression, abnormal cardiac rhythms.
6. dependence and tolerance.

CONTRAINDICATIONS

- Because of the antimuscarinic actions, promethazine should not be used in patients with glaucoma, prostatic syndrome or fever.
- Individuals with focal cerebral lesions are more likely to have fits with this drug.
- Liver failure is an absolute contraindication.

PHARMACOKINETICS

Promethazine is well absorbed from the gastrointestinal tract, but is subject to extensive first-pass metabolism. It is highly bound to plasma proteins, but freely passes the placental barrier and can cause sedation in the neonate when given to the mother during labour.

DRUG INTERACTIONS

These include the following:

- alcohol and other sedatives – enhanced sedation;
- antidepressants – tricyclics increase antimuscarinic and sedative effects.

Zopiclone and zolpidem

USES

Zopiclone and **zolpidem** are non-benzodiazepine hypnotics which enhance GABA activity and are used in the short-term management of insomnia.

MECHANISM OF ACTION

Zopiclone binds to the GABA–chloride channel complex, probably at the benzodiazepine-binding site. Although zopiclone has no structural similarity to the benzodiazepines, it appears to act in the same way by prolonging GABA-induced opening of the chloride channel.

ADVERSE EFFECTS

These are similar to those of the benzodiazepines, but there are some differences, including the following:

1. bitter, metallic taste (zopiclone);
2. anorexia, nausea, vomiting;
3. persistent drowsiness, ataxia, lack of co-ordination and confusion and depression the following day;
4. soon after the first dose, psychological toxic effects may develop – auditory and visual hallucinations, amnesia, aggression, and other behavioural disturbances (including agitation).

CONTRAINDICATIONS

These include previous psychiatric illness or history of drug abuse.

PHARMACOKINETICS

Peak blood levels occurs 1.5 h after oral administration, but this is delayed in patients with cirrhosis of the liver. The terminal $t_{\frac{1}{2}}$ is 3.5–6.5 h, although this may be prolonged to over 8 h in cirrhotic patients. Zopiclone enters breast milk, in which levels are about 50% of those in the plasma.

DRUG INTERACTIONS

These include potentiation of alcohol, benzodiazepines and other central depressants.

Chloral and derivatives

USES

Chloral was formerly often used in paediatric practice. There is no evidence that chloral derivatives have any advantages over benzodiazepines, and they are more likely to cause rashes and gastric irritation.

MECHANISM OF ACTION

Chloral has a 'type II' hypnotic action (like alcohol and volatile anaesthetics). Thus it enters hydrophobic regions of neuronal membranes and causes reversible swelling and disruption of crystalline structure. This inhibits the rapid opening of the sodium channel in neurones.

ADVERSE EFFECTS

These include the following:

1 gastric irritation (triclofos and dichloralphenazone are less irritating than chloral hydrate);
2 rashes;
3 headache, hangover;
4 ketonuria, disturbance of other urinary tests;
5 paradoxical excitement; delirium;
6 tolerance and dependence;
7 renal damage on prolonged use;
8 excreted in milk.

CONTRAINDICATIONS

These include the following:

- chronic obstructive lung disease;
- fever;
- heart failure;
- gastritis and peptic ulcer;
- renal failure (contraindicated if the glomerular filtration rate is less than 50 mL/min).

PHARMACOKINETICS

Chloral is well absorbed from the gastrointestinal tract and partly metabolized to trichlorethanol (active $t_{\frac{1}{2}}$ is 7–11 h) and trichloracetic acid (inactive).

DRUG INTERACTIONS

- Chloral enhances sedation due to alcohol and other CNS depressants. It may transitorily enhance the anticoagulant effects of warfarin.
- Dichloralphenazone (but not chloral) can interact with drugs such as warfarin by inducing cytochrome P_{450}.

SPECIAL PROBLEMS AND SPECIAL GROUPS

Jet lag

Jet lag consists of fatigue, sleep disturbances, headache and difficulty in concentrating. It is due to mismatching of the body clock (circadian dysrhythmia) against a new time environment with its own time cues (Zeitgebers). Resetting the internal clock is hastened by conforming to the new time regime. Thus one should rest in a dark room at night, even if not tired, and eat, work and socialize during the day. Sufferers should not allow themselves to sleep during the day. Taking hypnotics at night can make things worse if sleepiness is experienced the next day. However, short-acting benzodiazepines may sometimes be effective if taken before going to bed for two or three nights.

Melatonin may help sleep patterns, and improves daytime well being if taken in the evening. It is not yet generally available.

Night work

Night work causes more serious sleep difficulties than jet lag because hypnotics cannot be used for long periods. Moreover, drug-induced sleep during the day precludes family and other non-work activities. A better strategy is to allow the subject to have a short non-drug-induced sleep during the night shift. This will improve the subject's work efficiency towards the end of the night, and will also reduce his or her sleep needs during the day.

Children

The use of hypnotics in children is not recommended, except in unusual situations (e.g. on the night before an anticipated unpleasant procedure in hospital). Hypnotics are sometimes used for night terrors. Children are prone to experience paradoxical excitement with these drugs.

Elderly

Hypnotics increase the risk of falls and nocturnal confusion. Even short-acting drugs can lead to ataxia and hangover the next morning.

ANXIOLYTICS

Anxiety is fear, and is usually a normal reaction. Pathological anxiety is fear that is sufficiently severe as to be disabling. Such a reaction may be a response to a threatening situation (e.g. having to make a speech) or to a non-threatening event (e.g. leaving one's front door and going into the street). Episodes of paroxysmal severe anxiety associated with severe automonic symptoms (e.g. chest pain, dyspnoea and palpitations) are termed panic attacks and often accompany a generalized anxiety disorder.

GENERAL PRINCIPLES AND MANAGEMENT

1 Distinguish anxiety as a functional disturbance from a manifestation of organic brain disease, or general illness (e.g. rheumatoid arthritis and tuberculosis).
2 Assess the severity of any accompanying depression.
3 Most patients are best treated without drugs, and with cognitive therapy, relaxation techniques and simple psychotherapy instead.
4 Some patients are improved by taking regular aerobic exercise.
5 In the few selected severely anxious patients who are given anxiolytic drugs, these are only administered for a short period (up to 2–4 weeks) because of the risk of dependence.
6 Desensitization can be useful when severe anxiety develops in well-recognized situations (e.g. agoraphobia, arachnophobia, etc.). Anxiolytic drugs are sometimes given intermittently and with a flexible-dose scheme in such situations.
7 Benzodiazepines are the anxiolytics normally used in situations **5** and **6** above. Buspirone is as effective as and less hypnotic than the benzodiazepines.
8 Beta-blockers are sometimes useful in patients with prominent symptoms such as palpitations or tremor. They do not improve muscular tension.
9 Tricyclic antidepressants may be effective in severe anxiety and in preventing recurrent panic attacks.
10 Monoamine oxidase inhibitors (used only by specialists) can be useful for treating anxiety with depression, phobic anxiety, recurrent panic attacks and obsessive-compulsive disorders.
11 Individual panic attacks are usually terminated by benzodiazepines, which may have to be supplemented with phenothiazines such as chlorpromazine. Such antipsychotic drugs are not used for long-term treatment of anxiety because of the risk of Parkinsonism and tardive dyskinesias.
12 If hyperventilation reproduces the symptomatology and is considered to be the principal 'trigger', advice on controlled breathing exercises can be curative.

Buspirone

This drug belongs to a group of azaspirodecanediones which are relatively anxiolytic and do not have marked hypnotic, anticonvulsant or muscle relaxant properties.

USE

Buspirone is used in anxiety states, but prolonged treatment is avoided, as the risks of tolerance and dependence have not yet been fully evaluated. The response may be delayed for up to 2 weeks. Buspirone does not prevent or alleviate benzodiazepine withdrawal symptoms.

MECHANISM OF ACTION

The anxiolytic action of buspirone is probably related to partial agonistic effects in $5HT_{1A}$ receptors.

ADVERSE EFFECTS

These include the following:

1 nausea, dizziness, headache, nervousness and dysphoria. Drowsiness is uncommon;

Case history

A 67-year-old widow attends the Accident and Emergency Department complaining of left-sided chest pain, palpitations, breathlessness and dizziness. Relevant past medical history includes generalized anxiety disorder following the death of her husband 3 years earlier. She had been prescribed lorazepam, but had stopped it 3 weeks earlier because she had read in a magazine that it was addictive. When her anxiety symptoms returned she attended her GP, who prescribed buspirone, which she had started the day before admission.

Examination revealed no abnormality other than a regular tachycardia of 110 beats/min, dilated pupils and sweating hands. Routine investigations, including ECG and chest X-ray, were unremarkable.

Question 1

Assuming a panic attack is the diagnosis, what is a potential precipitant?

Question 2

Give two potential reasons for the tachycardia.

Answer 1

Benzodiazepine withdrawal.

Answer 2

1 Buspirone (note that buspirone, although anxiolytic, is not helpful in benzodiazpine withdrawal and may also cause tachycardia).

2 Anxiety.

3 Benzodiazepine withdrawal.

2 rarely, palpitations due to tachycardia. Chest pain;

3 sweating, dry mouth;

4 confusion and fatigue are uncommon. Driving performance may be impaired.

CONTRAINDICATIONS

These include the following:

- pregnancy, and during lactation;
- severe hepatic or renal failure;
- epilepsy.

DRUG INTERACTIONS

Potentiation of the actions of alcohol and other central depressants has not been documented, but it is prudent to avoid taking alcohol with buspirone.

FURTHER READING

Ashton CH. 1997: Management of insomnia. *Prescriber's Journal* **37**, 1–10.

Kupfer DJ, Reynolds CF. 1997: Management of insomina. *New England Journal of Medicine* **336**, 341–5.

Waterhouse J, Reilly T, Atkinson J. 1997: Jet lag. *Lancet* **350**, 1611–16.

CHAPTER EIGHTEEN

SCHIZOPHRENIA *and* BEHAVIOURAL EMERGENCIES

- Schizophrenia
- Behavioural emergencies

SCHIZOPHRENIA

INTRODUCTION

Schizophrenia is a devastating disease that affects approximately 1% of the population. The onset is usually in adolescence or young adulthood, and the disease is usually characterized by recurrent acute episodes which may develop into chronic disease. The introduction of antipsychotic drugs such as **chlorpromazine** revolutionized the treatment of schizophrenia so that the majority of patients, once the acute symptoms are relieved, can now be cared for in the community. Previously they would commonly be sentenced to a lifetime in institutional care.

Drugs that are effective in acute schizophrenia generally share many of the properties of chlorpromazine, the first member of the group to be used in western countries. These include central antidopaminergic actions on the extrapyramidal and mesolimbic systems and on the chemoreceptor trigger zone, antimuscarinic and α-adrenoceptor-blocking properties. The older terms 'major tranquillizer' and 'neuroleptic' can be misleading or uninformative. At present the label 'antipsychotic' seems to be most useful.

PATHOPHYSIOLOGY

The aetiology of schizophrenia, for which there is a genetic predisposition, is unknown. There is heterogeneity in clinical features, course of disease and response to therapy. It has been postulated that the disease is due to an interaction of an abnormal (biochemical/anatomical) mesolimbic system with life experience that triggers schizophrenia. The concept of an underlying neurochemical disorder is advanced by the dopamine theory of schizophrenia, summarized in Box 18.1. The majority of antipsychotics block dopamine receptors (D_1 and D_2) in the forebrain. 5-Hydroxytryptamine is also germane to the neurochemical theory of schizophrenia, as indicated in Box 18.2.

About 30% of patients with schizophrenia respond inadequately to the chlorpromazine type of D_2 antagonists. A high proportion of such refractory patients respond to **clozapine**, another type of antipsychotic drug which is an exception to the rule that antipsychotic potency is related to potency as a D_2 receptor antagonist. Clozapine has only weak D_2-blocking activity, but acts on other receptors, especially muscarinic, 5-hydroxytryptamine receptors ($5HT_2$) and D_1, and displays an especially high affinity for D_4 receptors. It is thus possible that antipsychotic activity could be due to anti-5HT or non-D_2

Box 18.1: Dopamine theory of schizophrenia

- There is excess dopamine activity in the mesolimbic system.
- Antipsychotic potency is often proportional to D_2-blocking potency
- Amphetamine (which increases dopamine release) can produce acute psychosis that is indistinguishable from acute schizophrenia (positive symptoms).
- D_2 agonists (bromocriptine and apomorphine) aggravate schizophrenia in schizophrenic patients.
- There is an increase in D_2 and D_4 receptors on PET in schizophrenic patients.
- L-dopa can cause hallucinations and acute psychotic reactions and paranoia, but does not cause all the features of these conditions.
- There is no definite increase in brain dopamine *in vivo* and post-mortem.

Box 18.2: 5-Hydroxytryptamine and Schizophrenia

- LSD acts on 5-HT receptors, causing hallucinations and dramatic psychological effects which may mimic some features of schizophrenia.
- 5-HT has a modulatory effect on dopamine pathways.
- Many effective antipsychotic drugs have dopamine *and* 5-HT_2 receptor-blocking properties.

dopamine antagonism in such patients. The D_4 receptor is localized to cortical regions, and may be the key receptor to be overexpressed in schizophrenia. Regional dopamine differences may be involved, such as low mesocortical activity with high mesolimbic activity.

General principles of management

Acute treatment

The main principles are as follows:

- prompt in-hospital management – delay worsens the prognosis;
- first-line treatment – **haloperidol** or chlorpromazine. In the near future it is likely that the preferred first-line treatment will be an 'atypical antipsychotic' (e.g. **risperidone** or **olanzapine**). At present there is no parental preparation of an atypical antipsychotic licensed in the UK;
- chlorpromazine may be preferred if sedation is advantageous (e.g. in very agitated patients);
- if the patient is very disturbed/aggressive, add benzodiazepine (e.g. IM **lorazepam**);
- antimuscarinic drugs (e.g. **orphenadrine** or **procyclidine** should be used if acute dystonia or Parkinsonian symptoms develop;
- psychosocial support/treatment;
- behaviour usually improves quickly, but hallucinations, delusions and affective disturbance may take weeks or months to improve;
- once first-rank symptoms have been relieved by drugs, the patient can usually return home and resume work on low-dose antipsychotic treatment.

Maintenance treatment

- Only 10–15% of patients remain in permanent remission after stopping drug therapy following a first schizophrenic episode.
- The decision to attempt drug withdrawal relates to the individual patient, their views, drug tolerance, social support, relatives and carers.
- Withdrawal of drug treatment requires attentive surveillance. Inappropriate withdrawal may lead to severe relapse.
- Most patients require lifelong drug therapy, so correct diagnosis is essential. All antipsychotic drugs have adverse effects. The newer 'atypical antipsychotic' drugs tend to be better tolerated and may improve neurological performance. Continuing psychosocial support is critical.
- Patient compliance is a major problem.
- An intramuscular depot preparation (e.g. **flupenthixol** IM) (Box 18.3) at its lowest effective dose is often used long term. This improves compliance. Antimuscarinic drugs (e.g. orphenadrine) are required to suppress Parkinsonian symptoms in approximately 30% of patients, but are only used if Parkinsonian symptoms develop. Tardive dyskinesia may be aggravated by antimuscarinic drugs.

Box 18.3: Intramuscular depot treatment

- Esters of the active drug are formulated in oil.
- There is slow absorption into the systemic circulation.
- It takes several months to reach steady state.
- After an acute episode, reduce the oral dose gradually, and overlap with depot treatment.
- Give a test dose in case the patient is allergic to the oil vehicle or very sensitive to extra pyramidal effects.
- Rotate the injection site.
- *Flupenthixol*, for example, is given once every 2–4 weeks.
- This form of treatment overcomes compliance problems.
- It also overcomes variations in first-pass metabolism.

DRUGS USED IN TREATMENT

Conventional antipsychotic drugs

The principal action of the conventional antipsychotic drugs (see Table 18.1), such as chlorpromazine (a phenothiazine) and haloperidol (a butyrophenone), is antagonism of D_2 receptors in the forebrain. The effect on D_1 receptors is variable. Blockade of the D_2 receptors induces extrapyramidal effects. Repeated adminstration causes an increase in D_2-receptor sensitivity due to an increase in abundance of these receptors. This appears to underlie the tardive dyskinesias that are caused by prolonged use of the conventional antipsychotic drugs.

The choice of drug is largely determined by the demands of the clinical situation, in particular the degree of sedation needed and the patient's susceptibility to extrapyramidal toxicity and hypotension.

USES

These include the following:

1 schizophrenia – antipsychotic drugs are more effective against first-rank (positive) symptoms (hallucinations, thought disorder, delusions, feelings of external control) than against negative symptoms (apathy and withdrawal). Piperazine phenothiazines are especially suitable for patients with circumscribed paranoid delusional states (e.g. monosymptomatic delusions);
2 other excited psychotic states, including mania and delirium;
3 anti-emetic and antihiccough;
4 premedication and in neuroleptanalgesia techniques in surgery;
5 terminal illness, including potentiating desired actions of opioids while reducing nausea and vomiting;
6 severe agitation and panic;
7 aggressive and violent behaviour;
8 movement and mental disorders in Huntington's disease.

Table 18.1: Conventional antipsychotic drugs

	Side-chain	Sedation	Extrapyramidal symptoms	Hypotension
Phenothiazines				
Chlorpromazine	Aliphatic	++	++	++
Fluphenazine*	Piperazine	+	+++	+
Thioridazine	Piperidine	++	+	++
Butyrophenones				
Haloperidol		–	+++	+
Thioxanthines				
Fluphenthixol*		+	++	+

*Depot preparation available.
All increase serum prolactin levels
Note: Pimozide α prolonged QT and cardiac arrhythmias.

ADVERSE EFFECTS

1 Akathisia is the most common movement disturbance caused by antipsychotics, and is an important cause of poor compliance. The spectrum of the disturbance includes agitation, insomnia and restlessness. The latter resembles the spontaneous condition of restless legs (Ekbom's syndrome) with aching at rest and the irresistible urge to move. The accompanying emotional changes include anxiety and feelings of inner tension. Acute akathisia starts soon after starting or increasing the dose of antipsychotics, even within 1 or 2 h. It can persist despite dose reduction, and sometimes persists after drug withdrawal. Such tardive akathisia may be difficult to distinguish from tardive dyskinesias. The two can coexist.

2 The tardive dyskinesias are several neurological disorders that produce persistent, repetitive, dystonic athetoid or choreiform movements of voluntary muscles. Usually the face and mouth are involved, causing repetitive sucking, chewing and lip smacking. The tongue may be injured. The movements are usually mild, but they can be severe and incapacitating. This effect follows months or years of antipsychotic treatment, and typically becomes more severe on stopping the drug .

3 The most common adverse effects are dose-dependent extensions of pharmacological actions:

- anticholinergic – dry mouth, nasal stuffiness, constipation, urinary retention, blurred vision;
- postural hypotension due to peripheral α-adrenergic blockade, which is rarely severe unless antipsychotics are used in conjunction with other vasoactive drugs (e.g. antihypertensives, anaesthetics). Gradual build-up of dose improves tolerability;
- sedation (which may be desirable in agitated patients), drowsiness and confusion. Tolerance usually develops after several weeks on a maintenance dose, but can be overcome by an increased dose. Emotional flattening is common, but it may be difficult to distinguish this feature from schizophrenia. Depression may develop, particularly following treatment of hypomania, and is again difficult to distinguish confidently from the natural history of the disease. Acute confusion is uncommon.

4 Abnormal involuntary movements occur, including tremor, seizures, Parkinsonism, dystonia and dyskinesia. All but the last of these are reversible. Acute dystonias can appear within 1 week of beginning the drug, but the other reactions can be delayed for months. There appears to be no relationship between the dose and their appearance. Their pathogenesis probably results from blockade of dopamine receptors, although tardive dyskinesias (described above) may involve actual structural change.

5 Jaundice occurs in 2–4% of patients taking chlorpromazine, usually during the second to fourth weeks of treatment. It is due to intrahepatic cholestasis, and is a hypersensitivity phenomenon associated with eosinophilia. Substitution of another phenothiazine may not reactivate the jaundice.

6 Ocular disorders observed during chronic administration include corneal and lens opacities and pigmentary retinopathy. This may be associated with cutaneous light sensitivity. Recent studies implicate the hydroxylated metabolites of chlorpromazine as the culprit in these ocular disorders.

7 Another type of hypersensitivity reaction involves the skin. About 5% of patients develop urticarial, maculopapular or petechial rashes. These disappear on withdrawal of the drug, and may not recur if the drug is reinstated. Contact dermatitis and light sensitivity are common complications. Abnormal melanin pigmentation may develop in the skin.

8 Chlorpromazine consistently raises serum cholesterol levels. Glucose tolerance may be impaired.

9 Blood dyscrasias are uncommon but may be lethal, particularly leukopenia and thrombocytopenia. These usually develop in the early days or weeks of treatment. The estimated incidence of agranulocytosis is approximately 1 in 10 000 patients receiving chlorpromazine.

10 Sudden cardiac arrhythmia and arrest occurs with phenothiazines in the absence of gross structural damage, although mitochondrial abnormalities have been noted in heart muscle. T-wave abnormalities and increased

frequency of ventricular premature beats are noted on the ECG.

11 Malignant neuroleptic syndrome is another rare and potentially fatal complication of neuroleptics. Its clinical features are rigidity, hyperpyrexia, stupor or coma, and autonomic disorders. It responds to treatment with **dantrolene** (an intracellular Ca^{2+} antagonist).

12 Seizures can be precipitated, particularly in alcoholics. Pre-existing epilepsy may be aggravated.

13 There may be impaired temperature control, with hypothermia in cold weather and hyperthermia in hot weather.

The Boston Collaborative Survey indicated that adverse reactions are most common in patients receiving high doses, and that they usually occur soon after starting treatment. The most common serious reactions were fits, coma, severe hypotension, leukopenia, thrombocytopenia and cardiac arrest.

CONTRAINDICATIONS

These include the following:

- coma due to cerebral depressants, bone-marrow depression, phaeochromocytoma, epilepsy, chronic respiratory disease, hepatic impairment or Parkinson's disease;
- *caution is needed in the elderly, especially in hot or cold weather*;
- pregnancy, lactation;
- alcoholism.

PHARMACOKINETICS

The pharmacokinetics of antipsychotic drugs have been little studied. They have multiple metabolites, and their large apparent volumes of distribution (V_d) (e.g. for chlorpromazine V_d = 22 L/kg) result in low plasma concentrations, presenting technical difficulties in estimation. Most is known about chlorpromazine. When given orally it is incompletely absorbed, with a bioavailability of about 30%. This is further decreased by the presence of food or by simultaneous administration of anticholinergic drugs and some antacids. Animal studies suggest that there is considerable degradation of chlorpromazine in the gut before it enters the portal circulation (a prehepatic first-pass effect). Peak plasma levels are reached in 2–3 h and the $t_{\frac{1}{2}}$ varies between 2 and 24 h in different individuals. Plasma steady-state concentrations are reached in around 1 week, and have been reported to range from 10 to 1200 ng/mL in psychotic patients. Changes of dose more often than every 5 days are therefore inadvisable, and daily dosing is adequate in most patients. A single night-time dose will increase compliance, and the sedative effects of the drug are maximal when they are most needed. Absorption is unreliable after intramuscular injection, possibly due to local precipitation of drug.

Chlorpromazine is an unstable molecule that rapidly forms an inactive sulphoxide on exposure to light. It has 168 potential metabolites, 70 of which have been identified in humans. Some of them are active. Metabolism is primarily by hepatic microsomes, although the brain, kidneys, lungs and gut also play a role. Chlorpromazine is 90–95% bound in plasma, mainly to albumin, and is concentrated in some tissues (e.g. the brain concentration is four to five times that in the plasma). Following a single dose, a clear relationship has been established between peak plasma concentration and effects such as sedation, pulse rate, pupil size, salivary secretion and orthostatic hypotension, although the threshold for response varies from one patient to another. With chronic administration, the plasma chlorpromazine concentration may fall while the antipsychotic effect becomes manifest.

DRUG INTERACTIONS

These include the following:

- alcohol and other CNS depressants – enhanced sedation;
- hypotensive drugs and anaesthetics – enhanced hypotension;
- increased risk of cardiac arrhythmias with drugs that prolong the QT interval (e.g. amiodarone, sotalol);
- tricyclic antidepressants – higher blood concentrations and increased antimuscarinic actions;
- anticonvulsants – reduced efficacy;
- domperidone and metoclopramide – increased extrapyramidal effects and akathisia;
- antagonism of anti-Parkinsonian dopamine agonists (e.g. L-dopa) (these are in any case contraindicated in schizophrenia).

check WBC every week for 18/12 months

Case history

A 50-year-old woman whose schizophrenia is treated with oral haloperidol is admitted to the Accident and Emergency Department with a high fever, fluctuating level of consciousness, muscular rigidity, pallor, tachycardia, labile blood pressure and urinary incontinence.

Question 1

What is the likely diagnosis?

Question 2

How should this patient be managed?

Answer 1

Neuroleptic malignant syndrome.

Answer 2

1 Stop the haloperidol.
2 Supportive therapy.
3 Bromocriptine (value uncertain).
4 Dantrolene (value uncertain).

ATYPICAL ANTIPSYCHOTIC DRUGS

The term 'atypical antipsychotic' is used very imprecisely. These drugs are less likely to cause extrapyramidal side-effects than conventional antipsychotics, but weight gain can be a problem. They are more expensive than conventional antipsychotic drugs. There is need for a parenteral atypical antipsychotic.

Clozapine

MECHANISM OF ACTION

Clozapine blocks D_4, 5–HT_2, D_1 > D_2 and α-receptors.

USE

1 Clozapine is at least as effective as other antipsychotics in schizophrenia, and furthermore it is effective in up to 60% of patients who have not responded to other drugs.
2 Unlike D_2 antagonists, clozapine is effective against negative as well as positive symptoms.
3 Because of the relatively high incidence of agranulocytosis, the use of clozapine is reserved for those patients who are resistant to or intolerant of other antipsychotic treatments.

ADVERSE EFFECTS

1 Neutropenia or agranulocytosis develops in up to 3% of patients taking clozapine for 1 year (compared to 0.01–0.1% with other antipsychotics). Because of this, only psychiatrists should prescribe clozapine, and blood monitoring is mandatory, including a pretreatment full blood picture.
2 Clozapine is virtually free from extrapyramidal effects.
3 Other adverse effects include fits (3-4% of patients), drowsiness, salivation, dizziness, constipation, nausea, vomiting, weight gain, transient hypertension, severe postural hypotension (predominantly first-dose effect; initial therapy should be in hospital).

DRUG INTERACTIONS

Lithium increases the adverse effects of clozapine on the central nervous system.

Risperidone

Risperidone blocks 5-HT_2 receptors in particular, but also D_2 receptors. The drug shows improved tolerance over the conventional antipsychotic drugs. Extrapyramidal symptoms in particular are rare, but the dose needs careful titration in order to maximize benefits and reduce adverse effects. Risperidone is effective against negative and positive symptoms.

Olanzapine

Olanzapine is a recently introduced broad-spectrum antagonist of D_1, D_2, D_4, 5-HT_2 and muscarinic receptors. This drug also shows improved tolerability compared to conventional antipsychotic drugs, and in particular the extrapyramidal disorders are rare. It is effective against negative and positive symptoms.

Sulpiride

Sulpiride is chemically different to other antipsychotics, and shows some selectivity in activity in schizophrenia with relatively little extrapyramidal toxicity. In high doses, sulpiride controls florid positive schizophrenic symptoms. Lower doses have an alerting effect on apathetic and withdrawn schizophrenics. Sulpiride toxicity is similar to that of phenothiazines, with the exception of a lack of jaundice or skin reactions.

Key points

Pharmacological treatment

- Receptor blockade:
  $5HT_2$.
- Although there may be a rapid behavioural benefit, a delay (usually of the order of weeks) in reduction of many symptoms implies secondary effects (e.g. receptor up-/down-regulation.)
- Conventional antipsychotics (e.g. chlorpromazine, haloperidol, thioridazine), act predominantly by D_2 blockade.
- Atypical antipsychotics (e.g. clozapine, risperidone, olanzapine) are less likely to cause extrapyramidal side effects.

Key points

Adverse effects of antipsychotic drugs

- Extrapyramidal motor disturbances, related to dopamine blockade.
- Endocrine distributions (e.g. gynaecomastia), related to prolactin release secondary to dopamine blockade.
- Autonomic effects, dry mouth, blurred vision, constipation due to antimuscarinic action and postural hypotension due to α-blockade.
- Cardiac arrhythmias, which may be related to prolonged QT e.g. sertindole (an atypical antipsychotic), pimozide.
- Sedation.
- Impaired temperature homeostasis.
- Weight gain.
- Idiosyncratic reactions;
  jaundice (e.g. chlorpromazine);
  leucopenia and agranulocytosis (e.g. clozapine);
  skin reactions;
  neuroleptic malignant syndrome.

BEHAVIOURAL EMERGENCIES

MANIA

Acute attacks are managed with antipsychotics, but the long-term prophylactic treatment of choice is **lithium**. The control of hypomanic and manic episodes with chlorpromazine is often dramatic.

ACUTE PSYCHOTIC EPISODES

Patients with organic disorders may experience fluctuating confusion, hallucinations and transient paranoid delusions. Violent incidents sometimes complicate schizophrenic illness.

Management

Antipsychotics and benzodiazepines, either separately or together, are most often used in the treatment of patients with violent and disturbed behaviour. **Paraldehyde** is an effective and safe parenteral drug, but can cause painful lesions unless given by deep intramuscular injection.

Haloperidol can rapidly terminate violent behaviour, but hypotension, although uncommon, can be severe, particularly in patients who are already critically ill. Doses should be reduced in the elderly.

Chlorpromazine by intramuscular injection is no longer recommended because of the formation of painful and irritating crystalline deposits in the tissues. It also causes hypotension.

Case history

A 60-year-old man with schizophrenia who has been treated for 30 years with chlorpromazine develops involuntary (choreo-athetoid) movements of the face and tongue.

Question 1

What drug-induced movement disorder has developed?

Question 2

Will an anticholinergic drug improve the symptoms?

Question 3

Name three other drug-induced movement disorders associated with antipsychotic drugs.

Answer 1

Tardive dyskinesia.

Answer 2

No. Anticholinergic drugs may unmask or worsen tardive dyskinesia.

Answer 3

1 Akathisia.
2 Acute dystonias.
3 Chronic dystonias.
4 Pseudo-Parkinsonism.

When treating violent patients, large doses of antipsychotics are needed. Consequently, extrapyramidal toxicity, in particular acute dystonias, develops in up to one-third of patients. Prophylactic anti-Parkinsonian drugs such as procyclidine may be given, especially in patients who are particularly prone to movement disorders.

The combination of lorazepam and haloperidol has been successful in treating otherwise resistant delirious behaviour.

Oral medication, especially in liquid form, is the preferred mode of administration, but rectal, intramuscular or intravenous routes may have to be used. **Droperidol** acts equally rapidly whether given intramuscularly or intravenously.

Antipsychotics such as chlorpromazine should not be given in alcohol withdrawal states, in alcoholics or in those dependent on benzodiazepines because of the risk of causing fits.

Further reading

Kane JM. 1996: Drug therapy: schizophrenia. *New England Journal of Medicine* **334**, (1) 34–41.

Livingston MG. 1996: Management of schizophrenia, *Prescriber's Journal* **36**, 206–15.

McGrath J., Emmerson WB. 1999: Treatment of Schizophrenia. *British Journal of Medicine* **319**, 1045–8.

CHAPTER NINETEEN

MOOD DISORDERS

- Depressive illnesses and antidepressants
- Lithium and tryptophan
- Special groups

DEPRESSIVE ILLNESSES AND ANTIDEPRESSANTS

Many forms of depression respond well to drugs. However, one of the difficulties in finding out which types of illness improve with drug treatment is that psychiatrists often move the diagnostic goalposts. Hence the definitions of subtypes of depression in the *Diagnostic and Statistical Manual of Mental Disorders* (American Psychiatric Association, Washington, DC) differ in the versions published in 1952, 1968, 1980, 1987 and 1992.

From a biochemical viewpoint there are probably different types of depression (which do not correspond predictably to clinical variants) depending on which neurotransmitter is involved, and these may respond differently to different drugs.

PATHOPHYSIOLOGY

The monoamine theory of mood is mainly based on evidence from the actions of drugs.

1 Reserpine, which depletes neuronal stores of noradrenaline (NA) and 5-hydroxytryptamine (5HT) and α-methyltyrosine, which inhibits NA synthesis, cause depression.
2 Tricyclic drugs of the amitriptyline type (which raise the synaptic concentration of NA and 5HT) are antidepressant.
3 Monoamine oxidase inhibitors (which increase total brain NA and 5HT) are antidepressant.

On the basis of these actions it was suggested that depression could be due to a cerebral deficiency of monoamines. One difficulty with this theory is that amphetamine and cocaine, which act like tricyclic drugs in raising the synaptic NA content, are not antidepressive, although they do alter mood. Even worse, the tricyclic antidepressants block amine reuptake from synapses within 1 or 2 h of administration, but take from 10 days to 4 weeks to alleviate depression. Such a long time-course suggests a resetting of postsynaptic or presynaptic receptor sensitivity. For example, inhibiting presynpatic receptors could down-regulate reducing feedback inhibition and lead to increased release of monoamine transmitters. There is evidence that long-term antidepressant treatment does down-regulate monoamine receptors (including presynaptic α-adrenoceptors). 5-Hydroxytryptamine ($5HT_2$) receptors are also down-regulated by these drugs. Moreover, it is likely that the brain stem râphé systems have a built-in inertia which slows down mood changes. The pontine and medullary râphé nuclei are the main CNS sites of $5HT_{1A}$ receptors.

Dysregulation of the hypothalamo–pituitary–adrenal axis is a common biological marker of depression. This is demonstrated by a relative failure of a standard dose of dexamethasone to suppress endogenous cortisol secretion. Cushing's disease, stroke, chronic alcoholism and stress can also disrupt the hypothlamo–pituitary axis and may all precipitate depression. However, underactivity of the hypothalamo–pituitary axis is associated with post-traumatic stress disorder. Part of the activity of traditional antidepressants may be mediated by monoamine activity in the hippocampus, which has a direct effect on the hypothalamo–pituitary axis. The therapeutic potential of antiglucocorticoid drugs is currently under investigation.

At present there is considerable interest in the potential of substance P (a peptide neurotransmitter) antagonists in depression. It has been postulated that substance P may be a final common pathway for the action of various classes of antidepressant.

General principles of management

1. Depression is common but it is underdiagnosed. It can be recognized during routine consultations, but additional time may be needed. Genetic and social factors are often relevant.
2. Patients should talk about their depression symptoms, but need encouragement to do so because of feelings of shame, admission of failure and fear that the doctor will not understand (or has no time).
3. Drug treatment is not usually appropriate at the mild end of the severity range. Listening and simple psychotherapy may be helpful. The possibility of altering social factors should be examined. Regular aerobic exercise may improve mild depression.
4. Drugs are used in more severe depression, especially if it has melancholic ('endogenous') features. Even if depression is related to interpersonal difficulties or other life stresses (including physical illness), antidepressant drugs may be useful. Drugs used in the initial treatment of depression include the older tricyclics (e.g. **amitriptyline** and **imipramine**), related drugs (e.g. **lofepramine**), selective serotonin reuptake inhibitors (SSRIs, e.g. **fluoxetine**), and serotonin and noradrenaline reuptake inhibitors (SNRIs, e.g. **venlafaxine**). Although clinical experience is most extensive with the tricyclic antidepressants, the side-effect profile of the SSRIs is usually less troublesome, and these drugs are safer in overdose. Therefore many psychiatrists and general practitioners use SSRIs rather than tricyclics as first-line treatment for depression. SSRIs are more expensive than tricyclic antidepressants. The relative side-effects of the different antidepressant drugs are summarized in Table 19.1.
5. Antidepressant drugs should be given as part of a combined therapeutic programme. The aims and strategy of the various measures must be agreed with the patient, and the toxic effects of the drugs discussed before treatment is started. The fact that there will be a delay of 10 days to 3 weeks before improvement starts should also be stressed.
6. After successful treatment of the acute episode, drug treatment is usually continued for at least 4–6 months to avoid relapse. The initial effective dose is maintained during this time unless toxic effects necessitate a reduction in dose. The drug is withdrawn gradually to avoid insomnia, panic and other withdrawal symptoms.
7. In refractory depression, other drug treatment or electroconvulsive therapy (ECT) are considered. Alternative drug strategies include (a) adding lithium to a tricyclic to give a lithium blood level of 0.6–0.8 mmol/L, (b) monoamine oxidase inhibitors (MAOIs), usually prescribed only by psychiatrists, (c) MAOI plus a tricyclic – but only in expert psychiatric hands or (d) small doses of **flupenthixol** (for short-term treatment only).
8. Prophylaxis with lithium or a low-dose tricyclic is considered in recurrent illness (e.g. in unipolar or bipolar affective disorders). Patients and their families should be warned about the possibility of relapse and advised what to do if it occurs. Cognitive therapy has a protective effect against relapse.
9. Electroconvulsive therapy (ECT) is considered when a delay before the drug acts in a major depressive episode cannot be tolerated or is hazardous.
10. Chronic mood depression (dysthymia) responds less well to drugs. Major depression

Table 19.1: Relative antidepressant side-effects

Drug	Anti-cholinergic effects	Cardiac effects	Nausea	Sedation	Overdose	Pro-convulsant	Tyramine interaction
Tricyclics and related antidepressants							
Amitriptyline	+++	+++	+	+++	++	++	–
Clomipramine	+++	++	+	++	+	++	–
Dothiepin	++	++	–	+++	+++	++	–
Imipramine	++	++	+	+	++	++	–
Lofepramine	++	+	+	+	–	–	–
Trazodone	+	+	++	++	+	–	–
Selective serotonin reuptake inhibitors							
Citalopram	–	–	++	–	+	–	–
Fluoxetine	–	–	++	–	–	?	–
Paroxetine	–	–	++	–	–	?	–
Sertraline	–	–	++	–	–	?	–
Monoamine oxidase inhibitors							
Phenelzine	+	+	++	–	+	–	+++
Moclobemide	+	–	+	–	–	?	+
Others							
Venlafaxine	–	++	++	+	?	+	–
Nefazodone	–	–	++	+	?	?	–

–, little or nothing reported; +, mild; ++, moderate; +++, high; ?, insufficient information available.

can be superimposed on dysthymia (double depression) and successful treatment of the major depression, may leave residual dysthymia.

11 Melancholic depression (which used to be called endogenous depression) usually responds well to tricyclics, SSRIs and SNRI's if there was a stable personality before the illness.

12 Atypical depression is used to describe depressed patients without melancholic features who respond positively to favourable life events, but are chronically oversensitive to rejection. These patients do not usually respond well to drugs. There may be a marginally better response to MAOIs than to tricyclics.

13 Major depression with psychotic features (e.g. delusions) requires specialist treatment. Antidepressants and antipsychotics may be needed in combination. Such patients may respond to ECT.

14 Psychiatric referral is advised if there is no response to treatment – partly because there could be a more severe underlying psychiatric illness or drug/alcohol abuse. Other important reasons for referral to a specialist centre include suicide potential, violent behaviour, self-neglect or other forms of self-harm.

15 Monoamine-oxidase inhibitors (e.g. **phenelzine** are used much less frequently than tricyclics and SSRIs because of their dangerous drug and dietary interactions. **Moclobemide**, a reversible and selective monoamine oxidase inhibitor, is less likely to potentiate such interactions.

Selective 5-hydroxytryptamine (serotonin) reuptake inhibitors (SSRIs)

These drugs are safer in overdose than the tricyclic group. Selective serotonin reuptake inhibitors do not stimulate appetite and have much fewer antimuscarinic side-effects than the tricyclics and other catecholamine-uptake inhibitors. They are also well tolerated in the elderly. Examples include fluoxetine, **fluvoxamine**, **paroxetine**, **sertraline** and **citalopram**.

USES

These include the following:

1 in depression (they have similar efficacy to tricyclics, but are much more expensive);
2 in chronic anxiety, and as prophylaxis for panic attacks;
3 obsessive-compulsive states;
4 bulimia nervosa;
5 seasonal affective disorder, especially if accompanied by carbohydrate craving and weight gain;
6 possibly effective as prophylactic agents in recurrent depression.

MECHANISM OF ACTION

Selective serotonin reuptake inhibitors block neuronal uptake of 5HT and do not primarily influence other neurotransmitter systems.

5-Hydroxytryptamine pathways influence mood and behaviour and regulate appetite, sleep, aggression and anxiety levels. Selective serotonin reuptake inhibitors augment 5HT activity in depression without unwanted effects on histamine, cholinergic and noradrenergic pathways.

ADVERSE EFFECTS

1 The most common adverse reactions to SSRIs are nausea, dyspepsia, diarrhoea, dry mouth, headache, insomnia and dizziness. Sweating, erectile dysfunction and delayed orgasm are well-recognized associations. These tend to become less severe after 1–2 months of treatment.
2 Selective serotonin reuptake inhibitors have less anticholinergic and cardiotoxic actions than tricyclic drugs.
3 Epilepsy can be precipitated.
4 Selective serotonin reuptake inhibitors are usually non-sedating, but may cause insomnia and do not usually cause orthostatic hypotension.
5 Fluoxetine has been associated with a rare fatal systemic vasculitis, of which rash may be the first clinical sign. It has also been said to cause violent and suicidal thoughts, but such thoughts are more likely to be due to the underlying psychiatric illness for which the drug is being used.
6 Delayed ejaculation affects a substantial minority of men treated with SSRIs.

CONTRAINDICATIONS

These include the following:

- hepatic and renal failure;
- epilepsy;
- manic phase.

PHARMACOKINETICS

Selective serotonin reuptake inhibitors have similar pharmacokinetic profiles, but differ in their half-lives. The elimination half-lives of fluvoxamine, paroxetine and sertraline range from 15 to 30 h, while fluoxetine has a half-life of approximately 2 days and its active metabolite, norfluoxetine, has a half-life of approximately 7 days.

DRUG INTERACTIONS

- Combinations of SSRI with lithium, **tryptophan** or MAOIs may enhance efficacy, but are currently contraindicated because they increase the severity of 5HT-related toxicity. In the worst reactions, the life-threatening 5HT syndrome develops. This consists of hyperthermia, restlessness, tremor, myoclonus, hyperreflexia, coma and fits. After using MAOIs it is recommended that 2 weeks should elapse before starting SSRIs. Avoid fluoxetine for at least 5 weeks before using MAOI.
- The action of **warfarin** is probably enhanced by fluoxetine and paroxetine.
- There is antagonism of anticonvulsants.
- Fluoxetine raises blood concentrations of haloperidol.

RELATED ANTIDEPRESSANTS

Nefazadone A modest inhibitor of serotonin and noradrenaline uptake, but an effective $5\text{-}HT_{2A}$ receptor antagonist, associated with less sexual, gastrointestinal and sleep disturbance than SSRIs.

Venlafaxine A potent serotonin and noradrenaline uptake inhibitor that appears to be as effective as tricyclic antidepressants, but without anticholinergic effects. It may have a more rapid onset of therapeutic action than other antidepressants, but this has yet to be confirmed. It is associated with more cardiac toxicity than the SSRIs.

Tricyclics and related antidepressants

USES

These include the following:

1. depressive illnesses, especially major depressive episodes and melancholic depression;
2. atypical oral and facial pain;
3. prophylaxis of panic attacks;
4. phobic anxiety;
5. obsessive–compulsive disorders;
6. imipramine has some efficacy in nocturnal enuresis.

Although these drugs share many properties, their profiles vary in some respects, and this may alter their use in different patients. The more sedative drugs include amitriptyline, **dothiepin** and **doxepin**. These are more appropriate for agitated or anxious patients than for withdrawn or apathetic patients, for whom **imipramine** or **nortriptyline**, which are less sedative, are preferred. **Protriptyline** is usually stimulant.

Imipramine and amitriptyline (tertiary amines) have more powerful anticholinergic and cardiac toxic effects than secondary amines (e.g. nortriptyline).

MECHANISM OF ACTION

The tricyclics block uptake 1 of monoamines into cerebral (and other) neurones. Thus the concentration of amines in the synaptic cleft rises. Imipramine causes equally powerful inhibition of NA and 5HT uptake, whereas amitriptyline has a more powerful effect on 5HT. Nortriptyline acts mainly on NA uptake. In general the tertiary amines have a more powerful action on 5HT uptake than do secondary amines.

Inhibition of uptake 1 is established long before depression is alleviated, so the two events are not directly related. A slow adaptive decrease in presynaptic amine receptor (e.g. α_2) sensitivity may be the physiological basis for clinical benefit, by enhancing amine release from the prejunctional neurone.

ADVERSE EFFECTS

Autonomic (anticholinergic) Dry mouth, constipation (rarely paralytic ileus, gastroparesis), tachycardia, paralysis of accommodation, aggravation of narrow-angle glaucoma, retention of urine, dry skin due to loss of sweating, and (due to α-blockade) postural hypotension.

Central nervous system Fine tremor and sedation, but also (paradoxically) sometimes insomnia, decreased rapid eye movement (REM) sleep, twitching, convulsions, dysarthria, paraesthesia, ataxia. Uncommonly, confusion, mania, schizophrenic excitement. Anticholinergic and sedating actions are more pronounced with tertiary amine drugs than with secondary amines.

Increased appetite and weight gain, particularly with the sedative tricyclics, are common. On withdrawal of the drug, there may be gastrointestinal symptoms such as nausea and vomiting, headache, giddiness, shivering and insomnia. Sometimes anxiety, agitation and restlessness follow sudden withdrawal..

Cardiovascular Postural hypotension. Rarely, sudden death due to a cardiac arrhythmia. In overdose a range of tachyarrhythmias and intracardiac blocks may be produced.

Allergic and idiosyncratic reactions These include bone-marrow suppression and jaundice (both rare). Hyponatraemia, possibly due to inappropriate ADH release, more common in the elderly.

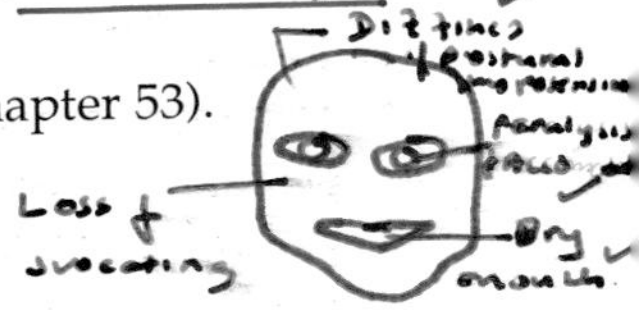

Dangerous in overdose (see Chapter 53).

CONTRAINDICATIONS

These include the following:

- epilepsy;
- recent myocardial infarction, heart block;
- mania;
- porphyria.

PHARMACOKINETICS

Tricyclic antidepressants, being lipid soluble, are readily absorbed from the gastrointestinal tract. Tricyclics may delay their own absorption and that of other drugs, due to their anticholinergic effect in decreasing gastric emptying rate and intestinal peristalsis.

Protein binding of these drugs is high (e.g. 85% for imipramine). This and their large apparent volume of distribution (V_d) (e.g. imipramine, 28–61 L/kg body weight) make dialysis inappropriate in overdose. These drugs are therefore present in free form in plasma only at very low concentrations after distribution. Tricyclics are extensively metabolized, and there is considerable presystemic hepatic metabolism (e.g. 53% for imipramine). Demethylation of the side-chain commonly occurs, and thus imipramine is metabolized to desipramine and amitriptyline is similarly converted into nortriptyline. These monomethyl derivatives are pharmacologically active. Ring hydroxylation, which abolishes activity, also occurs before conjugation and excretion of polar metabolites in urine.

There is a wide scatter (5- to 30-fold) in plasma steady-state levels between individuals on the same dose. Thus patients receiving imipramine at a dose of 3.5 mg/kg/day have steady-state plasma concentrations of 95–1020 ng/mL, and nortriptyline given at a dose of 100 mg at night produces steady-state concentrations in the range 120–681 ng/mL. There is much less inter-individual variation between monozygotic twins. Hepatic enzyme induction is also important, and lower plasma steady-state levels of tricyclic antidepressants are present in patients who smoke (nicotine and polycyclic hydrocarbons are inducing agents), drink alcohol or take barbiturates.

Only 70% of depressed patients respond adequately to tricyclic antidepressants. One of the factors involved may be the wide variation in individual plasma concentrations of these drugs that is obtained with a given dose. However, the relationship between plasma concentration and response is not well defined. A multicentre collaborative study organized by the World Health Organization failed to demonstrate any relationship whatsoever between plasma amitriptyline concentration and clinical effect.

Related non-tricyclic antidepressant drugs

This is a mixed group which includes 1-, 2- and 4-ring structured drugs with broadly similar properties. Specific characteristics of the group are summarized below.

Maproptiline – sedative, with less antimuscarinic effects, but rashes are more common and fits are a significant risk.

Mianserin – blocks central α_2 receptors. It is sedative, with much fewer anticholinergic effects, but can cause postural hypotension and blood dyscrasias, particularly in the elderly. Full blood count must be monitored.

Lofepramine – less sedative, and with less cardiac toxicity, but occasionally hepatotoxic.

Mirtazapine – increases noradrenergic and serotonergic neurotransmission via central α_2 adrenoreceptors. The increased release of serotonin stimulates 5-HT_1 receptors whilst the 5-HT_2 and 5-HT_3 receptors are blocked. H_1 receptors are also blocked. This combination of actions appear to be associated with antidepressant activity, anxiolytic and sedative effects. Reported adverse effects include increased appetite, weight gain, drowsiness, dry mouth and (rarely) blood dyscrasias.

DRUG INTERACTIONS

These include the following:

- antagonism of anti-epileptics;
- potentiation of sedation with alcohol and other central depressants;
- antihypertensives and diuretics increase orthostatic hypotension;
- hypertension and cardiac arrhythmias with adrenaline, noradrenaline and ephedrine.

Monoamine oxidase inhibitors (MAOIs)

These drugs were little used for many years because of their toxicity, and particularly poten-

Case history

A 75-year-old woman with endogenous depression is treated with amitriptyline. After 3 weeks she appears to be responding, but then seems to become increasingly drowsy and confused. She is brought to the Accident and Emergency Department following a series of convulsions.

Question

What is the likely cause of her drowsiness, confusion and convulsions?

Answer

Hyponatraemia.

tially lethal food and drug interactions causing hypertensive crises. Non-selective MAOIs should only be prescribed by specialists who are experienced in their use. They can be effective in some forms of refractory depression and anxiety states, for which they are generally reserved. The introduction of **moclobemide**, a reversible selective MAO-A inhibitor, may lead to more widespread use of this therapeutic class.

Tranylcypromine is the most hazardous MAOI because of its stimulant activity. The non-selective MAOIs of choice are **phenelzine** and **isocarboxazid**.

USES

These include the following:

1 monoamine oxidase inhibitors can be used alone or (with close psychiatric supervision) with a tricyclic antidepressant, in depression which has not responded to tricyclic antidepressants;
2 in phobic anxiety and depression with anxiety;
3 in patients with anxiety who have agoraphobia, panic attacks or multiple somatic symptoms;
4 hypochondria and hysterical symptoms may respond well;
5 for atypical depression with biological features such as hypersomnia, lethargy and hyperphagia.

MECHANISM OF ACTION

Phenelzine, isocarboxazid and tranylcypromine irreversibly inhibit both A and B forms of monoamine oxidase, whereas moclobemide reversibly inhibits the A form. Inhibition of the A form decreases deamination of NA and (to a lesser extent) 5HT. The antidepressant effect is presumably related in some way to the increase in vesicular neuronal stores of NA and 5HT. However, the extent of improvement of patients on MAO varies considerably and may be slow, some patients requiring treatment for 6–8 weeks before showing any response. Clinical efficacy of MAOI does not correspond to their efficacy in MAO inhibition. The stores of adrenaline and NA in the adrenal medulla and NA in peripheral sympathetic nerves also increase. This is part of the basis of the hypertensive crisis, due to massive release of these amines when indirectly acting sympathomimetic drugs are given concurrently.

Selective inhibitors of MAO-B preferentially decrease deamination of dopamine. This occurs with theraputic doses of selegiline (see Chapter 20). Higher doses inhibit both A and B types of MAO and have antidepressant activity.

ADVERSE EFFECTS

1 Common effects include orthostatic hypotension, weight gain, sexual dysfunction, headache and aggravation of migraine, insomnia, anticholinergic actions and oedema.
2 Rare and potentially fatal effects include hypertensive crisis and 5HT syndrome (see interactions), psychotic reactions, hepatocellular necrosis, peripheral neuropathy and convulsions.
3 Stopping a MAOI is more likely to produce a withdrawal syndrome than is the case with tricyclics. The syndrome includes agitation, restlessness, panic attacks and insomnia.

CONTRAINDICATIONS

These include the following:

- liver failure;
- cerebrovascular disease;
- phaeochromocytoma;
- porphyria;
- epilepsy.

PHARMACOKINETICS

Monoamine oxidase inhibitors are generally lipophilic and are well absorbed from the gut. They freely penetrate cell membranes and the blood–brain barrier. The hydrazine MAOIs produce irreversible inhibition of monoamine oxidase, whereas the inhibition produced by the non-hydrazines is reversible. Thus with many of the MAOIs, even after cessation of treatment when the drug can no longer be detected in the body, the effects of treatment persist and dangerous toxicity may arise until new enzyme is synthesized, a process that requires several weeks.

Hydrazine MAOIs are partly metabolized by acetylation, and slow acetylators more frequently experience toxicity. Differences in therapeutic responsiveness can be detected between acetylator phenotypes. Blood-concentration studies relating to clinical effect are not available, but would not be expected to correlate usefully with response in the case of irreversible enzyme inhibitors. In one trial, depressed patients treated with phenelzine and demonstrating an 80% inhibition of platelet monoamine oxidase were more likely to benefit than those with less enzyme inhibition. The relationship between peripheral and central inhibition of monoamine oxidase is unclear.

It has been suggested that response to MAOI is genetically determined, and that efficacy could be predicted in a patient if the response of a first-degree relative to the same drug were known. This possible pharmacogenetic variation could reflect biochemical factors, but more evidence is required before it can be accepted.

DRUG INTERACTIONS

Many important interactions occur with MAOI. A treatment card for patients should be carried at all times, which describes precautions and lists some of the foods to be avoided. The interactions are as follows:

- hypertensive and hyperthermic reactions sufficient to cause fatal subarachnoid haemorrhage, particularly with tranylcypromine. Such serious reactions are precipitated by amines, including indirectly acting sympathomimetic agents such as tyramine (in cheese), dopamine (in broad bean pods and formed from levodopa), amines formed from any fermentation process (e.g. in yoghurt, beer, wine), **phenylephrine** (including that administered as nosedrops and in cold remedies), **ephedrine**, **amphetamine** (all can give hypertensive reactions), other amines, **pethidine** (excitement, hyperthermia), **levodopa** (hypertension), and tricyclic, tetracyclic and bicyclic antidepressants (excitement, hyperpyrexia). **Buspirone** should not be used with MAOIs. Hypertensive crisis may be treated with α-adrenoceptor blockade analogous to medical treatment of patients with phaeochromocytoma (see Chapter 39). Interactions of this type are much less likely to occur with moclobemide, as its MAO inhibition is reversible, competitive and selective for MAO-A. MAO-B is free to deaminate biogenic amines. Although experience with moclobemide is limited, its side-effect profile is similar to that of placebo, and it appears to be relatively safe in overdose;
- failure to metabolize drugs that are normally oxidized, including opioids, benzodiazepines, alcohol (reactions with alcoholic drinks occur mainly because of their tyramine content). These drugs will have an exaggerated and prolonged effect;
- enhanced effects of oral hypoglycaemic agents, anaesthetics, suxamethonium, caffeine and anticholinergics (including benzhexol and similar anti-Parkinsonian drugs);
- antagonism of anti-epileptics;
- enhanced hypotension with antihypertensives;
- central nervous system (CNS) excitation and hypertension with oxypertine (an antipsychotic) and tetrabenazine (used for chorea);
- increased CNS toxicity with sumatriptan.

Key points

Drug treatment of depression

- Initial drug treatment is usually with SSRIs, tricyclic antidepressants or related drugs.
- The choice is usually related to the side-effect profile of relevance to the particular patient.
- Tricyclic antidepressants are more dangerous in overdose.
- Tricyclic antidepressants commonly cause antimuscarinic and cardiac effects.
- Tricyclic antidepressants tend to increase appetite and weight, whereas SSRIs more commonly reduce appetite and weight.
- SSRIs are associated with nausea and sleep disturbance.
- There is a variable delay (10 days–4 weeks) before therapeutic benefit is obtained.

Key points

Antidepressant contraindications

- Tricyclic antidepressants – recent myocardial infarction, arrhythmias, manic phase, severe liver disease.
- SSRIs – manic phase.
- Monamine oxidase inhibitors – acute confused state, phaeochromocytoma.
- Caution is needed – cardiac disease, epilepsy, pregnancy and breast-feeding, elderly, hepatic and renal impairment, thyroid disease, narrow-angle glaucoma, urinary retention, prostatism, porphyria, psychoses, electroconvulsive therapy (ECT), anaesthesia.

Key points

CSM advice on hyponatraemia

Hyponatraemia (usually in the elderly and possibly due to inappropriate ADH secretion) has been associated with all types of antidepressants. Consider hyponatraemia in patients who develop drowsiness, confusion or convulsions while taking antidepressants.

Case history

A 45-year-old man with agoraphobia, anxiety and depression associated with hypochondriacal features is treated with phenelzine. He has no history of hypertension. He is seen in the Accident and Emergency Department because of a throbbing headache and palpitations. On examination he is hypertensive 260/120 mmHg with a heart rate of 40 beats/min. He is noted to have nasal congestion.

Question 1

What is the likely diagnosis?

Question 2

What is the most appropriate treatment?

Answer 1

Hypertensive crisis, possibly secondary to taking a cold cure containing an indirectly acting sympathomimetic.

Answer 2

Phentolamine, a short-acting alpha-blocker, may be given by intravenous injection, with repeat doses titrated against response.

LITHIUM AND TRYPTOPHAN

Lithium

Although lithium is widely used in affective disorders, it has a low toxic to therapeutic ratio, and serum concentration monitoring is essential. Serum is used rather than plasma because of possible problems due to lithium heparin, which is often used as an anticoagulant. Plasma lithium levels fluctuate between doses, and serum concentrations should be measured at a standard time, preferably 12 h after the previous dose. This measurement is made frequently until steady state is attained, and is then made every 3 months, unless some intercurrent event occurs that could cause toxicity (e.g. desalination or diuretic therapy).

USE

Lithium is effective in acute mania, but its action is slow (1–2 weeks), so antipsychotic drugs such as haloperidol are preferred in this situation (see Chapter 18). Its main use is in prophylaxis in unipolar and bipolar affective illness (therapeutic serum levels 0.4–1 mmol/L). Lithium is also used on its own or with another antidepressant in refractory depression to terminate a depressive episode or to prevent recurrences and aggressive or self-mutilating behaviour.

Patients should avoid major dietary changes that alter sodium intake, and maintain an adequate water intake.

Different lithium preparations have different bioavailabilities, so the form should not be changed.

MECHANISM OF ACTION

Lithium increases 5HT actions in the CNS. It acts as a $5HT_{1A}$ agonist, and is also a $5HT_2$ antagonist. This may be the basis for its antidepressant activity and may explain why it increases the CNS toxicity of selective 5HT uptake inhibitors.

The basic biochemical activity of lithium is not known. It has actions on two second messengers.

1 Hormone stimulation of adenyl cyclase is inhibited, so that hormone-stimulated cyclic adenosine monophosphate (cAMP) production is reduced. This probably underlies some of the adverse effects of lithium, such as goitre and nephrogenic diabetes insipidus, since thyroid-stimulating hormone (TSH) and antidiuretic hormone activate adenyl cyclase in thyroid and collecting duct cells, respectively. The relevance of this to its therapeutic effect is uncertain.

2 Lithium at a concentration of 1 mmol/L inhibits hydrolysis of myoinositol phosphate in the brain, so lithium may reduce the cellular content of phosphatidyl inositides, thereby altering the sensitivity of neurones to neurotransmitters that work on receptors linked to phospholipase C (including muscarinic and α-receptors).

From these actions it is clear that lithium can modify a wide range of neurotransmitter effects, but its efficacy both in mania and in depression indicates a subtlety of action that is currently unexplained, but may be related to activation of the brain stem râphé nuclei.

ADVERSE EFFECTS

1. When monitored regularly lithium is reasonably safe in the medium term. However, adverse effects occur even in the therapeutic range – in particular, tremor, weight gain, oedema, polyuria, nausea and loose bowels.
2. Above the therapeutic range tremor coarsens, diarrhoea becomes more severe and ataxia and dysarthria appear. Higher levels cause gross ataxia, coma, fits, cardiac arrhythmias and death. Serum lithium concentrations greater than 1.5 mmol/L may be dangerous and if greater than 2 mmol/L, are usually associated with serious toxicity.
3. Goitre, hypothyroidism and exacerbation of psoriasis are less common.
4. Renal tubular damage has been described in association with prolonged use.

CONTRAINDICATIONS

These include the following:

- renal disease;
- cardiac disease;
- sodium-losing states (e.g. Addison's disease, diarrhoea, vomiting);
- myasthenia gravis;
- during surgical operations;
- avoid when possible during pregnancy and breast-feeding.

PHARMACOKINETICS

Lithium is readily absorbed after oral administration, and injectable preparations are not available. Peak plasma concentrations occur 3–5 h after dosing. The $t_{\frac{1}{2}}$ varies with age because of the progressive decline in glomerular filtration rate, being 18–20 h in young adults and up to 36 h in healthy elderly people. Sustained-release preparations are available, but in view of the long $t_{\frac{1}{2}}$ they are not kinetically justified. The evidence that they produce more even plasma levels is not established. They are erratically absorbed in the upper gut and can cause lower intestinal upset. The long absorption $t_{\frac{1}{2}}$ also means that it takes several days to reach steady state, and the first samples for plasma level monitoring should be taken after about 1 week unless loading doses are given. Lithium elimination is almost entirely renal. Like sodium, lithium does not bind to plasma protein, and it readily passes into the glomerular filtrate; 70–80% is reabsorbed in the proximal tubules but, unlike sodium, there is no distal tubular reabsorption and its elimination is not *directly* altered by diuretics acting on the distal tubule. However, states such as sodium deficiency and sodium diuresis increase lithium retention (and cause toxicity) by stimulating proximal tubular sodium and lithium reabsorption. An important implication of the renal handling of lithium is that neither loop diuretics, thiazides nor potassium-sparing diuretics can enhance lithium loss in a toxic patient, but all of them do enhance its toxicity. Dialysis reduces elevated plasma lithium concentration effectively.

DRUG INTERACTIONS

- Lithium concentration in the plasma is increased by diuretics and non-steroidal anti-inflammatory drugs.
- Lithium toxicity is increased by concomitant administration of haloperidol, serotonin uptake inhibitors, calcium antagonists (e.g. diltiazem) and anticonvulsants (phenytoin and carbamazepine) without a change in plasma concentration.
- Lithium increases the incidence of extrapyramidal effects of antipsychotics.

L-TRYPTOPHAN

Tryptophan is the amino acid precursor of 5HT. On its own or with other antidepressants or lithium it sometimes benefits refractory forms of depression. However, L-tryptophan has been withdrawn from general use because of its association with an eosinophilic myalgic syndrome characterized by intense and incapacitating fatigue, myalgia and eosinophilia. Arthralgia, fever, cough, dyspnoea and rash may also develop over several weeks. A few patients develop myocarditis.

L-Tryptophan remains available on a named patient basis, for those whom no other treatment has helped.

Special groups

The elderly

Depression is common in the elderly, in whom it tends to be chronic and has a high rate of recurrence. Treatment with drugs is made more difficult because of slow metabolism and sensitivity to anticholinergic effects. Lower doses are therefore needed than in younger patients.

Lack of response may indicate true refractoriness of the depression, or sadness due to social isolation or bereavement. The possibility of underlying disease such as hypothyroidism (the incidence of which increases with age) should be considered.

Lofepramine and SSRIs cause fewer problems in patients with prostatism or glaucoma than do the tricyclic antidepressants because they have less antimuscarinic action. Dizziness and falls due to orthostatic hypotension are less common with nortriptyline than with imipramine. Mianserin has fewer anticholinergic effects, but blood dyscrasias occur in about 1 in 4000 patients and postural hypotension can be severe.

Epilepsy

No currently used antidepressive is entirely safe in epilepsy, but SSRIs are less likely to cause fits than the amitriptyline group, mianserin or maprotiline.

Suicide

Successful suicide is a less likely outcome with overdoses of mianserin, trazodone and SSRIs than with maprotiline and members of the amitriptyline group.

Seasonal affective disorder

Seasonal affective disorder may respond well to SSRIs, as well as to summer sky fluorescent tube lighting.

Further reading

Anon 1996: Three new antidepressants. *Drug and Therapeutics Bulletin* **34**, 65–8.

Leonard B. 1997: Drug treatment of depression. In *Fundamentals of psychopharmacology*, 2nd edn. 118–42.

CHAPTER TWENTY

MOVEMENT DISORDERS *and* DEGENERATIVE CNS DISEASE

- Parkinson's syndrome and its treatment
- Spasticity
- Chorea
- Dyskinesias
- Treatment of other movement disorders
- Myasthenia gravis
- Alzheimer's disease

PARKINSON'S SYNDROME AND ITS TREATMENT

PATHOPHYSIOLOGY

James Parkinson first described the tremor, rigidity and bradykinesia/akinesia that characterize the syndrome that now bears his name in his *Essay on the Shaking Palsy* in 1817. Most cases of Parkinson's disease are caused by idiopathic degeneration of the nigrostriatal pathway. Atherosclerotic, toxic (related to antipsychotic–neuroleptic treatment, manganese or carbon monoxide poisoning) and postencephalitic cases also occur. Treatment of parkinsonism caused by antipsychotic drugs differs from treatment of the idiopathic disease, but other aetiologies are treated similarly to the idiopathic disease. Parkinsonian symptoms manifest after loss of 80% or more of the nerve cells in the substantia nigra (zona compacta). The nigrostriatal projection consists of very fine nerve fibres travelling from the zona compacta of the substantia nigra to the corpus striatum. This pathway is dopaminergic and inhibitory, and the motor projections to the putamen are more affected than either those to the cognitive areas (caudate nucleus and the nucleus accumbens) or those to the limbic and hypolimbic regions (Figure 20.1). Other fibres terminating in the corpus striatum include excitatory cholinergic nerves and noradrenergic and serotoninergic fibres, and these are also affected, but to varying extents, and the overall effect is a complex imbalance between inhibitory and excitatory influences.

Parkinsonism arises because of deficient neural transmission at the postsynaptic D_2 receptors, but it appears that stimulation of both D_1 and D_2 is required for optimal response. D_1 receptors activate adenylyl cyclase, which increases intracellular cyclic adenosine monophosphate (cAMP). The antagonistic effects of dopamine and acetylcholine within the striatum have suggested that parkinsonism results from an imbalance between these neurotransmitters (Figure 20.2). The therapeutic basis for treating parkinsonism is to increase dopaminergic activity or to reduce the effects of acetylcholine. Ideally, treatment of parkinsonism should start with removal of the cause. However, in most patients with chronic progressive parkinsonism this is unknown. Exposure to toxic agents has been considered. 1-Methyl-4-phenyl-1,2,5,6-tetrahydropyridine (MPTP) has been used illicitly on the West Coast of the USA as a 'designer drug'. It causes severe parkinsonism, and led to the development of animal models of the disease. MPTP is converted, in neuronal mitochondria, by the enzyme monoamine oxidase-B (MAO-B) to a toxic free-radical metabolite (MPP^+), which is specifically toxic to dopamine-producing cells. This led to the proposal of one hypothesis that

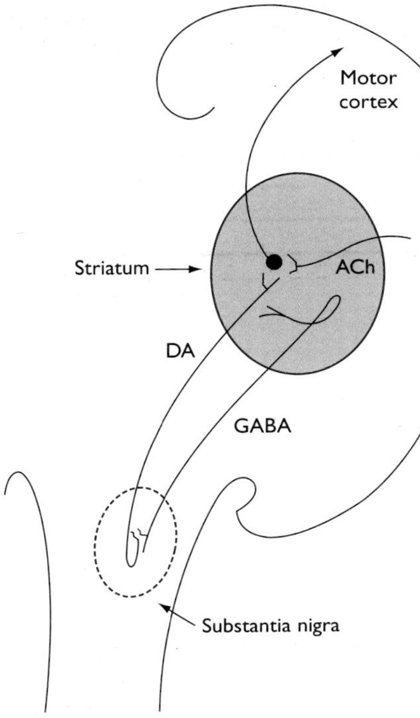

Figure 20.1: Representation of relationships between cholinergic (ACh), dopaminergic (DA) and GABA-producing neurones in the basal ganglia.

idiopathic Parkinson's disease may be due to chronically increased free-radical damage to the cells of the substantia nigra. Evidence supporting this view includes the following: mitochondrial glutathione activity (a free-radical scavenger) is low; superoxide dismutase activity is high; monoamine oxidase activity is high; and there is reduced activity of mitochondrial site 1 (NAD-DH) complex in the substantia nigra (this complex is inhibited by MPP^+). Free-radical scavengers prevent or retard the progression of MPTP-induced extrapyramidal disease in primate models, and this offers a potential clinical use of anti-oxidants/free-radical scavengers in an attempt to reduce the rate of disease progression. So far, clinical studies using adjunctive anti-oxidants have been disappointing.

The free-radical hypothesis has raised the worrying possibility that treatment with levodopa (see below) could accelerate disease progression by increasing free-radical formation as the drug is metabolized in the remaining nigro-striatal nerve fibres. This is consistent with the clinical impression of some neurologists, but in the absence of randomized clinical trials it is difficult to tell whether clinical deterioration is due to the natural history of the disease or is being accelerated by the therapeutic agent. Such trials, comparing early treatment with levodopa with dopamine agonists (see below), are currently in progress.

PRINCIPLES OF TREATMENT IN PARKINSONISM

Idiopathic Parkinson's disease is a progressive disorder, and is treated with drugs that relieve symptoms and if possible reduce the rate of progression of the disease. In the mildest cases treatment may be postponed early on. At present there is no optimal, well-defined, single-drug therapy, and thus generally a multi-drug regimen is the preferred treatment. A levodopa/decarboxylase inhibitor combination is standard therapy in patients with definite disability. The dose is titrated to produce optimal results. Occasionally, **amantidine** or anticholinergics may be useful as monotherapy in early disease, especially in younger patients where tremor is the dominant symptom. The occurrence of motor fluctuations (on–off phenomena) heralds a more drastic phase of the illness. Initially, such fluctuations may be controlled by giving more frequent doses of levodopa (or a sustained-release preparation). The

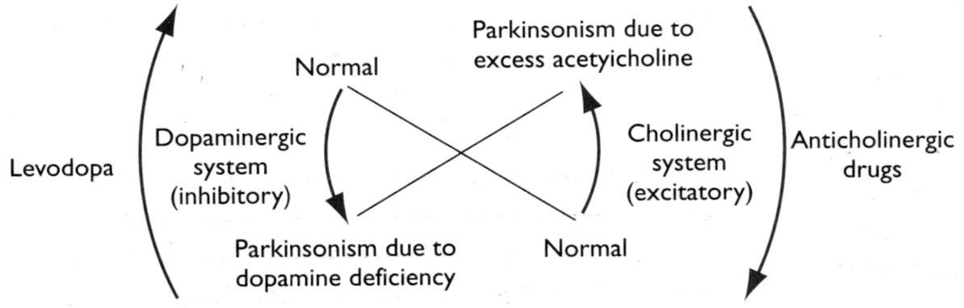

Figure 20.2: Antagonistic actions of the dopaminergic and cholinergic systems in the pathogenisis of Parkinsonian symptoms.

addition of either a dopamine receptor agonist (e.g. **bromocriptine** or one of the newer non-ergot derivatives, such as **ropinirole**) or one of the recently available calechol-O-methyl transferase (COMT) inhibitors (**entacapone**, **tolcapone**) to the drug regimen may improve mobility. In addition, this usually allows dose reduction of the L-dopa while improving 'end-of-dose' effects as well as improving motor fluctuations. If on-off phenomena are refractory, the dopamine agonist **apomorphine** will reverse most 'off' periods after 15 mins, but its use is complex (see below). Preliminary evidence from the DATATOP study suggested that **selegiline** (an MAO-B inhibitor) improved parkinsonian symptoms and retarded disease progression. Subsequent studies have been ambiguous, with a (disputed) suggestion the the drug may cause *reduced* survival. Selegiline probably still has a role in combined therapy for patients who are already on it and who have improved; otherwise we do not recommend it, pending the availability of new data. Physiotherapy and psychological support are helpful. The experimental approach of implantation of fetal adrenal cells into the substantia nigra of severely affected parkinsonian patients (perhaps with low-dose immunosuppression) offers an exciting potential therapy, the efficacy of which awaits further research. The potential of stereotactic unilateral pallidotomy, and of fetal neuronal transplantation, for severe refractory cases of Parkinson's disease is being re-evaluated.

Drugs that cause parkinsonism, notably the older, less specific dopaminergic antagonist antipsychotic drugs (e.g. chlorpromazine, haloperidol) (see Chapter 18) are withdrawn if possible, or substituted by the newer 'clozapine-like' antipsychotics (e.g. risperidone or olanzapine), since these have a lower incidence of extrapyramidal side-effects. Antimuscarinic drugs (e.g. **benzhexol**) are useful if changing the drug/reducing the dose is not therapeutically acceptable, whereas drugs that increase dopaminergic transmission are contraindicated because of their effect on psychotic symptoms.

Key points

Parkinson's disease

- Clinical diagnosis is based on the triad of tremor, rigidity and bradykinesia.
- Parkinsonism is caused by the degeneration of dopaminergic pathways in basal ganglia leading to imbalance between cholinergic (stimulatory) and dopaminergic (inhibitory) transmission.
- It is induced/exacerbated by centrally acting dopamine antagonists (e.g. haloperidol), but less so by clozapine, risperidone or olanzapine.

ANTI-PARKINSONIAN DRUGS

Drugs affecting the dopaminergic system

Dopaminergic activity can be enhanced by the following:

1 administration of levodopa with a peripheral dopa decarboxylase inhibitor;
2 increasing release of endogenous dopamine;
3 stimulation of dopamine receptors;
4 inhibition of catechol-O-methyl transferase (COMT);
5 inhibition of monoamine oxidase type B (MAO-B).

Levodopa and dopa decarboxylase inhibitors

USE

Levodopa (unlike dopamine) can enter nerve terminals in the basal ganglia where it undergoes decarboxylation to form dopamine, partially correcting the nigrostriatal deficiency and improving rigidity and bradykinesia. Levodopa is used in combination with a peripheral (extracerebral) dopa decarboxylase inhibitor (e.g. carbidopa or benserazide). This allows a four- to fivefold reduction in levodopa dose, and the incidence of vomiting and arrhythmias is reduced. However, central adverse effects (e.g. hallucinations) are predictably as common as when large doses of levodopa are given without a dopa decarboxylase inhibitor.

Combined preparations (**co-careldopa** or **co-beneldopa**) are available and appropriate for idiopathic Parkinson's disease. (Levodopa is contraindicated in schizophrenia and must not be used for parkinsonism caused by antipsychotic drugs, as explained above.) Combined preparations are given three times daily starting at a low dose, increased initially after 2 weeks and then reviewed at intervals of 6–8 weeks. Without dopa decarboxylase inhibitors, 95% of levodopa is metabolized outside the brain. In their presence, plasma levodopa concentrations rise (Figure 20.3), excretion of dopamine and its metabolites falls, and the availability of levodopa within the brain for conversion to dopamine increases. The two available inhibitors are similar.

ADVERSE EFFECTS

These include the following:

1 nausea and vomiting;
2 postural hypotension – this usually resolves after a few weeks, but excessive hypotension may result if antihypertensive treatment is given concurrently;
3 involuntary movements (dystonic reactions) – these include akathisia (abnormal restlessness and inability to keep still), chorea and jerking of the limbs (myoclonus). Involuntary movements may become worse as treatment is continued, and may necessitate drug withdrawal;
4 psychological disturbance, including vivid dreams, agitation, paranoia, confusion and hallucinations;
5 cardiac arrhythmias;

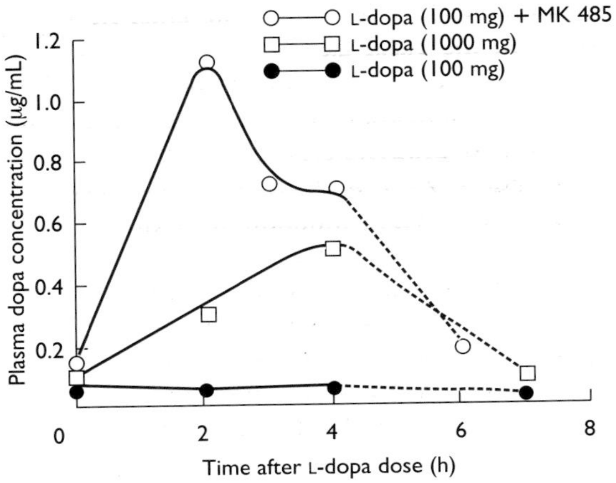

Figure 20.3: Increased plasma dopa concentrations following combination with a peripheral dopa decarboxylase inhibitor in one patient. (Reproduced from Dunner DL *et al.* 1971: *Clinical Pharmacology and Therapeutics* **12**, 213.)

6 endocrine effects of levodopa, including stimulation of growth hormone and suppression of prolactin.

PHARMACOKINETICS

Levodopa is absorbed from the proximal small intestine and is metabolized both by decarboxylases in the intestinal wall and by the gut flora. Oral absorption is therefore somewhat variable. Absorption is improved by coadministration of decarboxylase inhibitors. The elimination $t_{\frac{1}{2}}$ following intravenous infusion is short (30–60 min) and is only moderately prolonged (by about 30%) by dopa-decarboxylase blockade. Following oral administration of 15 mg/kg levodopa, peak plasma concentrations occur at 1–2 h. A further increase in $t_{\frac{1}{2}}$ and AUC may be achieved by combining levodopa with a COMT inhibitor (e.g. tolcapone, see below).

DRUG INTERACTIONS

Monoamine oxidase inhibitors can produce hypertensive reactions if given concurrently with levodopa. The hypotensive actions of other drugs are potentiated by levodopa.

Increased release of endogenous dopamine

Amantidine

USE

Amantidine seldom produces substantial clinical improvement, but approximately 60% of patients experience some benefit. The usual dose is 100 mg twice daily. Severe toxicity is rare.

MECHANISM OF ACTION

Endogenous dopamine release is stimulated by amantadine, which also inhibits reuptake of dopamine into nerve terminals.

ADVERSE EFFECTS

These include the following:

1 peripheral oedema;
2 gastrointestinal upsets and dry mouth;
3 livedo reticularis;
4 CNS toxicity – nightmares, insomnia, dizziness, hallucinations, convulsions;
5 leukopenia (uncommon).

PHARMACOKINETICS

The $t_{\frac{1}{2}}$ of amantidine varies from 10 to 30 h, so steady-state concentrations are reached after 4–7 days of treatment. About 95% is eliminated by the kidney, and it should not be used in patients with renal failure.

DOPAMINE RECEPTOR AGONISTS

Dopamine receptor agonists are used as adjuncts to levodopa–dopa decarboxylase inhibitor combinations in patients with severe motor fluctuations (on–off phenomena). A vexed question (see above) is whether early use of dopamine agonists in place of levodopa-based therapy could retard the progression of the neurodegenerative process, and this is currently being investigated. Dopamine agonists share many of their adverse effects, particularly nausea due to stimulation of dopamine receptors in the chemoreceptor trigger zone. This brain region is unusual in that it is accessible to drugs in the systemic circulation, so domperidone (a dopamine antagonist that does not cross the blood–brain barrier) is used to prevent this symptom without blocking dopamine receptors in the striatum, and hence worsening the movement disorder. Dopamine agonists are divided into those that are related to ergot, and those that are not. (See also Chapter 41 for use in pituitary disorders, and Chapter 40 for use in suppression of lactation).

Ergot derivatives – bromocriptine, lysuride and pergolide

Bromocriptine

USES

There is great individual variation in the efficacy of **bromocriptine**. It is seldom more effective than levodopa, and has more marked adverse effects. Its plasma $t_{\frac{1}{2}}$ is 6–8 h, i.e. longer than that of levodopa, which may be of relevance in patients with severe motor fluctuations. The initial dose is 1–2.5 mg at night, increased to a total of 10–40 mg in three divided doses.

Lysuride

USE

Lysuride is used in similar situations to bromocriptine. The starting dose of lysuride is 200 μg with food at bedtime, increasing to a maximum of 5 mg daily in four divided doses. It stimulates D_2 receptors, and is an agonist at 5-hydroxytryptamine receptors ($5HT_1$ and $5HT_2$).

ADVERSE EFFECTS

These are primarily due to its D_2 agonist activity, and include the following:

1 gastrointestinal – nausea and vomiting, constipation or diarrhoea;
2 central nervous system – headache, drowsiness, confusion;
3 Orthostatic hypotension (particularly in the elderly);
4 Cardiac arrhythmias – bradycardia.

PHARMACOKINETICS

Following oral administration, absorption is complete, but variable first-pass metabolism with extensive hepatic clearance explains the bioavailability of 10–25%. The elimination $t_{\frac{1}{2}}$ is approximately 8 h.

Pergolide

This drug is very similar to lysuride in its use, mechanism of action (in addition it stimulates D_1 receptors) and toxicity. **Pergolide** is licensed for use in combination with levodopa, allowing a reduction in levodopa dose. The initial pergolide dose is 50 μg at bedtime, increasing to 2–5 mg daily in divided doses. It undergoes hepatic metabolism with a long elimination half-life (15–42 h).

Non-ergot derivatives – ropinirole

USE

Ropinirole is started at a dose of 0.25 mg tds and increased gradually up to a maximum of 24 mg/day. The usual dose range is 3–9 mg/day. It may permit a reduction in the dose of levodopa of approximately 20%.

MECHANISM OF ACTION

Ropinirole is an agonist at the D_2 receptor, and also stimulates the other D_2-like receptors, D_3 and D_4.

ADVERSE EFFECTS

These include the following:

1. somnolence; sleep 'episodes'
2. nausea;
3. orthostatic hypotension, syncope;
4. nightmares, hallucinations.

PHARMACOKINETICS

Ropinirole is well absorbed after oral ingestion, and is metabolized in the liver to inactive metabolites mainly by cytochrome $P_{450\ 1A2}$. The elimination $t_{\frac{1}{2}}$ is approximately 6 h.

DRUG INTERACTIONS

Ciprofloxacin inhibits cytochrome $P_{450\ 1A2}$ and reduces clearance of ropinirole.

Apomorphine

Apomorphine is a powerful dopamine agonist at both D_1 and D_2 receptors, and is used in patients with refractory motor oscillations (on–off phenomena). It is difficult to use, necessitating specialist input. The problems stem from its pharmacokinetics and from side-effects of severe nausea and vomiting (it was used as part of 'aversive conditioning therapy' in less enlightened times, in order to 'cure' people of behaviour patterns such as homosexuality, which was classified as a psychiatric diagnosis until relatively recently). The gastrointestinal side-effects can be controlled with domperidone. Apomorphine is started in hospital after pretreatment with domperidone for at least 3 days, and withholding other anti-Parkinsonian treatment at night to provoke an 'off' attack. Initially 0.5 mg is given subcutaneously into the lower abdomen or outer thigh every 2 h when an 'off' state is reached. The dose is increased, and when the individual dose requirement has been established, with reintroduction of other drugs if necessary, administration is sometimes changed from intermittent dosing to subcutaneous infusion via a syringe pump, with patient-activated extra boluses if needed. Apomorphine is extensively hepatically metabolized, and is given parenterally. The mean plasma $t_{\frac{1}{2}}$ is only 30 min.

CATECHOL-O-METHYL TRANSFERASE (COMT) INHIBITORS

Tolcapone

USE

Tolcapone has recently been removed from the therapeutic armamentarium due to hepatic toxicity. It is used for adjunctive therapy in patients who are already taking L-dopa/dopa decarboxylase inhibitor combinations with unsatisfactory control (e.g. end-of-dose deterioration). These agents improve symptoms with less on–off fluctuations, as well as reducing the levodopa dose requirement by 20–30%. Adverse effects arising from increased availability of L-dopa centrally can be minimized by decreasing the dose of levodopa combination treatment prospectively. The role in treatment of COMT inhibitors has yet to be defined fully.

MECHANISM OF ACTION

Tolcapone is a reversible competitive inhibitor of COMT, thereby reducing metabolism of L-dopa and increasing its availability within nigrostriatal nerve fibres. It is relatively specific for central (CNS) COMT, with little effect on the peripheral COMT, thus causing increased brain concentrations of L-dopa, while producing less of an increase in plasma concentration.

ADVERSE EFFECTS

These include the following:

1. nausea;
2. CNS – hallucinations and dyskinesias;
3. orthostatic hypotension, syncope;
4. hepatitis.

PHARMACOKINETICS

Tolcapone is rapidly absorbed, and is cleared by hepatic metabolism. At recommended doses it produces approximately 80–90% inhibition of central COMT.

DRUG INTERACTIONS

Apomorphine is metabolized by O-methylation, so interaction with entapone is to be anticipated. Entapone should not be administered with MAOIs, as blockade of both pathways of monoamine metabolism simultaneously has the potential to enhance the effects of endogenous and exogenous amines and other drugs in an unpredictable manner.

MONOAMINE OXIDASE INHIBITORS – TYPE B

SELEGILINE

USE

Initial small controlled studies in Parkinson's disease reported that disease progression was slowed in patients treated with selegiline alone, delaying the need to start levodopa. Larger-scale studies have refuted this conclusion. Selegiline may be used in conjunction with levodopa, allows a dose reduction of approximately 30%, and prolongs the duration of action of levodopa. It is given as a single oral dose of 10 mg in the morning, or as two divided doses of 5 mg at breakfast and lunchtime.

MECHANISM OF ACTION

There are two forms of monoamine oxidase (MAO), namely type A (substrates include 5–hydroxytryptamine and tyramine) and type B (substrates include phenylethylamine, benzylamine and tyramine). Pargyline (an antidepressant monoamine oxidase inhibitor) inhibits both MAO-A and MAO-B. Selegiline selectively and irreversibly inhibits only MAO-B, which is mainly localized in neuroglia. MAO-A metabolizes adrenaline, noradrenaline and 5-hydroxytryptamine, while the physiological role of MAO-B is unclear. Both isoenzymes metabolize dopamine. Inhibition of MAO-B could raise brain dopamine levels without affecting other major transmitter amines. Because selegiline selectively inhibits MAO-B, it is much less likely to produce a hypertensive reaction with cheese or other sources of tyramine than non-selective MAOIs such as pargyline, iproniazid and phenelzine.

ADVERSE EFFECTS

Selegiline is generally well tolerated, but side-effects include the following:

1 agitation and involuntary movements;
2 confusion, insomnia and hallucinations;
3 nausea.

PHARMACOKINETICS

Oral selegiline is well absorbed (100%), but is extensively metabolized by the liver, first to an active metabolite, desmethylselegiline (which also inhibits MAO-B) and then to amphetamine and metamphetamine. Its plasma $t_{\frac{1}{2}}$ is long (with a mean value of 39 h).

DRUG INTERACTIONS

Hypertension occurs at very high doses (60 mg/day: six times the therapeutic dose), MAO-B selectivity is lost and pressor responses to tyramine are potentiated. Hypertensive reactions to tyramine-containing products (e.g. cheese or yeast extract) have been described, but are rare. Amantadine and centrally active antimuscarinic agents potentiate the anti-parkinsonian effects of selegiline.

DRUGS AFFECTING THE CHOLINERGIC SYSTEM

Muscarinic receptor antagonists

USE

Muscarinic antagonists (e.g. benzhexol, **benztropine**) are effective in the treatment of parkinsonian tremor and – to a lesser extent – rigidity, but produce only a slight improvement in bradykinesia. They are usually given in divided doses, which are increased every 2–5 days until optimum benefit is achieved or until toxic effects occur. Their main use is in patients with parkinsonism caused by antipsychotic agents that cannot be withdrawn.

MECHANISM OF ACTION

Non-selective muscarinic receptor antagonism is believed to restore, in part, the balance between dopaminergic/cholinergic pathways in the striatum.

> **Key points**
>
> Treatment of Parkinson's disease
>
> - A combination of levodopa and a dopa-decarboxylase inhibitor (carbidopa or benserazide) is standard first-line therapy.
> - Dopamine agonists (e.g. ergot derivatives – bromocriptine; non-ergot derivatives – ropinirole) and COMT inhibitors (entapone) are helpful as adjuvant drugs for patients with loss of effect at the end of the dose interval, and to reduce 'on–off' motor fluctuations.
> - The benefit of early treatment with an MAO-B inhibitor, selegiline, to retard disease progression is unproven, and it may even increase mortality.
> - Polypharmacy is almost inevitable in patients with longstanding disease.
> - Ultimately, disease progression requires increasing drug doses with a regrettable but inevitable increased incidence of side-effects, especially involuntary movements and psychosis.
> - Anticholinergic drugs reduce tremor but dose-limiting CNS side-effects are common, especially in the elderly. These drugs are first-line treatment for parkinsonism caused by indicated (essential) antipsychotic drugs.

ADVERSE EFFECTS

These include the following:

1. antimuscarinic side-effects – dry mouth, blurred vision, constipation;
2. precipitation of glaucoma or urinary retention – they are therefore contraindicated in some forms of glaucoma, and in men with prostatic hypertrophy;
3. confusion, excitement or psychosis, especially in the elderly.

PHARMACOKINETICS

Table 20.1 lists some drugs of this type that are in common use, together with their major pharmacokinetic properties.

SPASTICITY

Spasticity is the increase in muscle tone which accompanies a decrease in voluntary muscle power due to damage to the corticomotor neurone pathways in the brain or spinal cord. It can be painful as well as disabling, and is an important problem in patients with upper motor neurone lesions (e.g. following neck injuries to the cord, following stroke, in some patients with multiple sclerosis, and in congenital or perinatal spasticity). Treatment is seldom very effective, but physiotherapy or limited surgical release procedures have some place. Drugs that reduce spasticity include diazepam, baclofen and dantrolene, but they have considerable limitations.

Diazepam (see Chapter 17) facilitates γ-aminobutyric acid (GABA) action. Although spasticity and flexor spasms may be diminished, sedating doses are often needed to produce this effect.

Baclofen also reduces spasticity and flexor spasms by stimulating the peripheral spinal GABA receptors (GABA-B). Effective doses are 5–20 mg 8-hourly. Larger doses may cause fits. Less sedation is produced than by equi-effective doses of diazepam (15–50 mg daily), but baclofen

Table 20.1: Common muscarinic receptor antagonists, dosing and pharmacokinetics

Drug	Route of administration	Half-life	Metabolism and excretion	Dose (mg)	Special features
Benzhexol	Oral	3–7 h	Hepatic	1–4 mg tds Maximum 15 mg/day	
Orphenadrine	Oral	13.7–16.1 h	Hepatic-active metabolite	150–400 mg dose twice a day	Central stimulation
Procyclidine	Oral	12.6 h	Hepatic	2.5 mg tds Maximum 60 mg	

can produce vertigo, nausea and hypotension. There is specialist interest in chronic administration of low doses of baclofen intrathecally via implanted intrathecal cannulae in selected patients in order to maximize efficacy without causing side-effects.

Dantrolene

USE

Dantrolene is generally less useful for symptoms of spasticity than baclofen because muscle power is reduced as spasticity is relieved. It is used intravenously to treat malignant hyperthermia and the neuroleptic malignant syndrome, for both of which it is uniquely effective (see Chapter 23).

MECHANISM OF ACTION

Dantrolene acts directly on striated muscle and inhibits excitation–contraction coupling by inhibiting the release of calcium ions from the sarcoplasmic reticulum by blocking calcium channels (known as ryanodine receptors) in the sarcoplasmic reticulum.

ADVERSE EFFECTS

These include the following:

1 drowsiness, vertigo, malaise, weakness and fatigue;
2 diarrhoea;
3 increased serum potassium levels.

DRUG INTERACTIONS

If used in conjunction with voltage-operated calcium-channel blockers (e.g. verapamil) intravenous dantrolene may cause severe myocardial depression.

CHOREA

The γ-aminobutyric acid content in the basal ganglia is reduced in patients with Huntington's disease. Dopamine receptor antagonists (e.g. haloperidol) or **tetrabenazine** suppress the choreiform movements in these patients, but dopamine antagonists are best avoided, as they themselves may induce dyskinesias. Tetrabenazine is therefore preferred. It depletes neuronal terminals of dopamine and serotonin, and is given in doses of 25 mg twice daily, increasing to 50 mg three or four times a day. It can cause severe dose-related depression. Diazepam may be a useful alternative, but there is no effective treatment for the dementia and other manifestations of Huntington's disease.

DYSKINESIAS

Antipsychotic drugs can produce any kind of dyskinesia, including drug-induced parkinsonism, acute dystonic reactions and chronic tardive dyskinesias.

1 Drug-induced parkinsonism is due to a reduction in dopamine effects in the striatum. Antipsychotic drugs vary in their propensity to produce parkinsonism because of their varying antimuscarinic activities (high antimuscarinic activity reducing parkinsonian activity). The newer clozapine-like antipsychotics (risperidone, olanzapine) produce less extrapyramidal side-effects than the older neuroleptics.
2 Acute dystonic reactions can be induced by several antipsychotic drugs (the incidence is approximately 2–10%), or by metoclopramide. Drug-induced dystonic reactions are caused by an increase in transmitter turnover. This normally occurs in younger patients, and develops rapidly, usually within 48 h of the start of treatment. Akathisia (a state of intense restlessness) may precede torticollis, facial grimacing, dysarthria, laboured breathing and involuntary movements. Accompanying these may be scoliosis, lordosis, opisthotonus and dystonic gait. The signs can be abolished by an intravenous injection of 2 mg benztropine, or 5–10 mg procyclidine or 10 mg diazepam.
3 Tardive dyskinesias consist of orofacial chewing and sucking movements, often accompanied by distal limb chorea and dystonia of the trunk. About 15% of patients treated with neuroleptics for over 2 years develop this complication. If treatment is continued, the syndrome persists, but stopping the neuroleptics results in a slow improvement in only 40% of patients, and sometimes the dyskinesia worsens. Tardive dyskinesia is thought to result from the

development of 'denervation hypersensitivity' in dopaminergic postsynaptic receptors of the nigrostriatal pathway following chronic receptor blockade by neuroleptics. It is therefore due to a relative excess of dopaminergic effects. This accounts for its exacerbation by drug discontinuation, because of the reduction in receptor blockade, and allows more dopamine to stimulate the sensitized receptors. Administration of increased doses of dopamine antagonists paradoxically initially improves tardive dyskinesia. Use of these drugs in this way can lead to escalating doses, with more and more drug being required to suppress the dyskinesia.

Treatment of other movement disorders

Tics and idiopathic dystonias

Botulinum toxin A

Botulinum toxin A is one of seven distinct neurotoxins produced by *Clostridium botulinum*, and it is a glycoprotein. It is available for clinical use as *Clostridium botulinum* toxin A-haemagglutinin complex, and is used by neurologists to treat hemifacial spasm, blepharospasm, cervical dystonia (torticollis), jaw-closing oromandibular dystonia and adductor laryngeal dysphonia. Botulinum toxin A is given by local injection into affected muscles, the injection site being best localized by electromyography. Recently it has also proved successful in the treatment of achalasia. Injection of botulinum toxin A into a muscle weakens it by irreversibly blocking the release of acetylcholine at the neuromuscular junction. Muscles injected with botulinum toxin A atrophy and become weak over a period of 2–20 days and recover over 2–4 months as new axon terminals sprout and restore transmission. Repeated injections can then be given. Most patients continue to respond to repeated injections over a period of 5–10 years. Long-term side-effects have not yet been noted, but the best long-term treatment plan is not established. Symptoms are seldom abolished, and adjuvant conventional therapy should be given. Adverse effects due to toxin spread causing weakness of nearby muscles and local autonomic dysfunction can occur. In the neck this may cause dysphagia and aspiration into the lungs. Electromyography has detected evidence of systemic spread of the toxin, but generalized weakness does not occur with standard doses. Occasionally, a flu-like reaction with brachial neuritis has been reported, suggesting an acute immune response to the toxin. Neutralizing antibodies to botulinum toxin A cause loss of efficacy in up to 10% of patients. **Botulinum toxin F** does not cross-react with neutralizing antibodies to botulinum toxin A, and is effective in patients with torticollis who have botulinum toxin A-neutralizing antibodies.

Amyotrophic lateral sclerosis (MND)

Riluzole 50 mg orally twice a day is used to extend life or time to mechanical ventilation in patients with motor neurone disease (MND). It acts by blocking Na characters and inhibits pre-synaptic release of glutamate aspartate as well as improving NMDA receptor events. It is metabolized by receptor cytochrome $P_{450\,1A2}$ + glucuronidation with a $t_{\frac{1}{2}}$ of 12 h. Major side effects are gastro-intestinal aspects, nephritis and neutropenia.

Myasthenia gravis

Pathophysiology

Myasthenia gravis is a syndrome of increased fatiguability and weakness of striated muscle, and it results from an autoimmune process with antibodies to nicotinic acetylcholine receptors. These interact with postsynaptic nicotinic cholinoreceptors at the neuromuscular junction. (Such antibodies may be passively transferred via purified immunoglobulin or across the placenta to produce a myasthenic neonate.) Antibodies vary from one patient to another, and are often directed against receptor-protein domains distinct from the acetylcholine-binding site. They none the less interfere with neuromuscular transmission by reducing available receptors, by increasing receptor turnover by activating complement and/or cross-linking adjacent receptors. Endplate potentials are reduced in amplitude, and in some fibres may be below the threshold for initiating a muscle action potential, thus reducing the force of contraction of the muscle. The precise stimulus for the production of the antireceptor antibodies is not known, although since antigens in the thymus cross-react with acetylcholine receptors, it is possible that these are responsible for autosensitization in some cases.

Diagnosis is aided by the use of **edrophonium**, a short-acting inhibitor of acetylcholinesterase, which produces a transient increase in muscle power in patients with myasthenia gravis. The initial drug therapy of myasthenia consists of oral anticholinesterase drugs, usually neostigmine, 15 mg, administered 8-hourly. If the disease is non-responsive or progressive, then thymectomy or immunosuppressant therapy with glucocorticosteroids and azathioprine are needed. Thymectomy is beneficial in patients with associated thymoma and in patients with generalized disease who can withstand the operation. It reduces the number of circulating T-lymphocytes that are capable of assisting B-lymphocytes to produce antibody, and a fall in antibody titre occurs after thymectomy, albeit slowly. Corticosteroids and immunosuppressive drugs also reduce circulating T-cells. Plasmapheresis is useful in emergencies, and reduces the amount of antibody present, producing a striking short-term clinical improvement in a few patients.

ANTICHOLINESTERASE DRUGS

The defect in neuromuscular transmission may be redressed by cholinesterase inhibitors that inhibit synaptic acetylcholine breakdown and increase the concentration of transmitter available to stimulate the nictonic receptor at the motor end plate.

NEOSTIGMINE

Neostigmine is initially given orally in doses of 15 mg 8-hourly, but usually requires more frequent administration (up to 2-hourly) because of its short duration of action (2–6 h). It is rapidly inactivated in the gut, so the corresponding parenteral dose (1–2 mg) is much smaller. Cholinesterase inhibitors enhance both muscarinic and nicotinic cholinergic effects. The former results in increased bronchial secretions, abdominal colic, diarrhoea, miosis, nausea, hypersalivation and lachrymation. Excessive muscarinic effects may be blocked by giving atropine or propantheline, but this increases the risk of overdosage and consequent cholinergic crisis.

PYRIDOSTIGMINE

Pyridostigmine has a more prolonged action than neostigmine, and it is seldom necessary to give it more frequently than 4-hourly. The initial dose is 60 mg 8-hourly (equivalent to 15 mg neostigmine), although individual requirements vary, and some patients may need up to 2000 mg in a day.

Adjuvant drug therapy

Remissions of myasthenic symptoms are produced by oral administration of prednisolone. Increased weakness may occur at the beginning of treatment, which must therefore be instituted in hospital. This effect has been minimized by the use of alternate-day therapy, starting with 20 mg prednisolone with a gradual increase of the dose to 100 mg on alternate days. With such high doses the usual acute side-effects of corticosteroids (see Chapter 39) should be anticipated. The dose is reduced by 5 mg each month for as long as improvement is maintained. Azathioprine, 2.5 mg/kg (see Chapter 49), has been used either on its own or combined with glucocorticosteroids for its 'corticosteroid-sparing' effect.

MYASTHENIC AND CHOLINERGIC CRISIS

Severe weakness leading to paralysis may result from either a deficiency (myasthenic crisis) or an excess (cholinergic crisis) of acetylcholine at the neuromuscular junction. Clinically the distinction may be difficult, but it is assisted by the edrophonium ('Tensilon') test.

Edrophonium

Edrophonium (Tensilon), a short-acting cholinesterase inhibitor, is given intravenously as a 10-

mg bolus, and is very useful in diagnosis and for differentiating a myasthenic crisis from a cholinergic one. It transiently improves a myasthenic crisis and aggravates a cholinergic crisis. Because of its short duration of action, any deterioration of a cholinergic crisis is unlikely to have serious consequences, although facilities for artificial ventilation must be available. In this setting it is important that the strength of essential (respiratory or bulbar) muscles be monitored using simple respiratory spirometric mesaurements (FEV_1 and FVC) during the test, rather than the strength of non-essential (limb or ocular) muscles.

Myasthenic crises may develop as a spontaneous deterioration in the natural history of the disease, or as a result of infection or surgery, or be exacerbated due to concomitant drug therapy with the following agents:

1 aminoglycosides (e.g. gentamicin, tobramycin, streptomycin);
2 other antibiotics, including erythromycin and polymyxin;
3 myasthenics demonstrate increased sensitivity to non-depolarizing neuromuscular-blocking drugs;
4 anti-arrhythmic drugs, which reduce the excitability of the muscle membrane, and quinidine (quinine), lignocaine, procainamide and propranolol, which may increase weakness;
5 benzodiazepines, due to their respiratory depressant effects and inhibition of muscle tone.

Key points

Myasthenia gravis

- Auto-antibodies to nicotinic acetylcholine receptors lead to increased receptor degradation and neuromuscular blockade.
- Treatment is with an oral anticholinesterase (e.g. neostigmine or physostigmine). Over- or under-treatment both lead to increased weakness ('cholinergic' and 'myasthenic' crises, respectively).
- Cholinergic and myasthenic crises are differentiated by administering a short-acting anticholinesterase, edrophonium IV. This test transiently improves a myasthenic crisis while transiently worsening a cholinergic crisis, allowing the appropriate dose adjustment to be made safely.
- Immunotherapy with azathioprine and/or corticosteroids or thymectomy may be needed in severe cases.
- Weakness is exacerbated by aminoglycosides or erythromycin, and patients are exquisitely sensitive to non-depolarizing neuromuscular blocking drugs (e.g. vecuronium).

TREATMENT

MYASTHENIC CRISIS

Myasthenic crisis is treated with neostigmine, 0.5 mg given intramuscularly, repeated every 20 min with frequent edrophonium tests. Mechanical ventilation may be needed.

CHOLINERGIC CRISIS

Treatment of myasthenia with anticholinesterases can be usefully monitored clinically by observation of the pupil (a diameter of 2 mm or less in normal lighting suggests overdose). Overdosage produces a cholinergic crisis, and further drug should be withheld.

ALZHEIMER'S DISEASE

Alzheimer's disease (AD) is the commonest cause of dementia in the Western world. Its incidence increases with age, and its prevalence in North America and Europe has been estimated to be 3–11% of the population over 65 years of age. In the USA this currently represents about 4 million patients and, because of the ageing of this population, epidemiologists have predicted that there will be 14 million sufferers by the year 2040. The symptoms of Alzheimer's disease are progressive memory impairment associated with a decline in language, visuospatial function, calculation and judgement. Ultimately this leads to major behavioural and functional disability. Only recently have anticholinesterases (e.g. **donepezil**) become available for treating the primary disorder. Other drug therapy, such as oestrogens, non-steroidal anti-inflammatory drugs (NSAIDs) and vitamin E, has not been conclusively shown to be of benefit. Depression is commonly associated with Alzheimer's disease and can be treated with a selective serotonin reuptake inhibitor (SSRI) e.g.

sertraline). Antipsychotic drugs and benzodiazepines are sometimes indicated in such patients for symptoms of psychosis or agitation.

Pathophysiology

Degeneration of cholinergic neurones has been implicated in the pathogenesis of Alzheimer's disease. Neurochemically, low levels of acetylcholine are related to damage in the ascending cholinergic tracts of the nucleus basalis of Meynert to the cerebal cortex. Other neurotransmitter systems have been shown to be affected in the brains of Alzheimer's sufferers, but the cholinergic system is most consistently affected and remains the primary target for therapeutic attack. The brains of patients with Alzheimer's disease show a reduction in acetylcholinesterase, the enzyme in the brain that is primarily responsible for the hydrolysis of acetylcholine. This loss is mainly due to the depletion of cholinesterase-positive neurones within the cerebral cortex and basal forebrain.

These findings led to pharmacological attempts to augment the cholinergic system by means of cholinesterase inhibitors (e.g. **physostigmine** and **tacrine**). These have short half-lives, and tacrine has significant hepatotoxicity. A search for a longer-acting and less toxic agent resulted in donepezil, which has not been linked to hepatotoxicity to date.

Key points

Alzheimer's disease

- The prevalence of Alzheimer's disease is increasing in ageing populations.
- Currently, the only specific therapeutic target is reduced cholinergic transmission.
- Placebo-controlled studies in patients with mild or moderate Alzheimer's disease of donepezil (a central cholinesterase inhibitor) showed that scores of cognitive function were greater at 3–6 months in patients treated with the active drug. The clinical importance of this difference is uncertain.
- The therapeutic benefits of donepezil appear to be modest and have not yet been demonstrated to be sustained. This drug does not appear to affect underlying disease progression or mortality.

Donepezil

USE

Donepezil, given at a dose of 5 or 10 mg once daily, maintained neuropsychiatric scores and assessments of behaviour in patients with mild or moderate disease compared to placebo (for which scores continued to fall compared to baseline) over 3–6 months. There are no data relating to functional improvement, mortality or duration of survival, and the clinical impact of the effect is uncertain. The drug is administered as a single daily dose starting at 5 mg/day, taken at bedtime. The dose should only be increased to 10 mg/day after 4–6 weeks on the lower dose.

Case history

A 21-year-old woman was treated with an anti-emetic because of nausea and vomiting secondary to viral labyrinthitis. She received an initial intramuscular dose of 10 mg of metoclopromide and then continued on oral metoclopramide 10 mg tds, which relieved her nausea and vomiting. Two days later she was brought into the local casualty department because her husband thought she was having an epileptic fit. Her arms and feet were twitching, her eyes were deviated to the left, and her neck was twisted, but she opened her mouth and tried to answer your questions. Muscle tone in the limbs was increased.

Question

What is the diagnosis here, and what is the most appropriate and diagnostic acute drug treatment?

Answer

Her posture, dystonia and head and ocular problems all point to a major dystonia with oculogyric crisis, almost certainly caused by metoclopramide. This side-effect is more common in young women on high doses (a similar syndrome can occur with neuroleptics such as prochlorperazine, used to treat nausea). It is probably due to excessive dopamine blockade centrally in a sensitive patient. It usually resolves within several hours of discontinuing the offending drug, and in mild cases this is all that may be needed. In more severe cases, the drug of choice is intravenous benztropine (2 mg) or procyclidine (5–10 mg) anticholinergic agents, and further doses may be required, given orally. An alternative, equi-effective but less satisfactory therapy because it is not diagnostic is intravenous diazepam (5–10 mg).

MECHANISM OF ACTION

Donepezil is a centrally acting, non-competitive, reversible inhibitor of acetyl cholinesterase. Preclinical data suggest that it has a high degree of selectivity for acetylcholinesterase in the CNS and little effect on the peripheral enzyme.

ADVERSE EFFECTS

These include the following:

1. effects of cholinergic excess – nausea, vomiting and diarrhoea;
2. insomnia.

PHARMACOKINETICS

Donepezil is rapidly absorbed from the gastrointestinal tract, reaching peak plasma concentrations at 3–4 h. It is highly bound to plasma proteins. The drug is cleared from the body both by hepatic metabolism and via renal excretion. The major drug-metabolizing enzymes are cytochrome $P_{450\ IID6}$ and cytochrome $P_{450\ 3A4}$. Donepezil and its active metabolites are excreted in the urine and faeces. The elimination $t_{\frac{1}{2}}$ is long (approximately 70 h).

DRUG INTERACTIONS

Theoretically, donepezil might interact with a number of other drugs that are metabolized by cytochrome P_{450}, but at present there is no clinical evidence of an interaction with theophylline, warfarin or cimetidine. Ketoconazole and quinidine inhibit the metabolism of donepezil *in vitro*, but the clinical implication (if any) of this is unknown.

FURTHER READING

Abrahams KR. 1998: Selegiline or the problem of early termination of clinical trials. *British Medical Journal* **316**, 1182–3.

National Prescribing Centre. 1996: Therapy of Parkinson's disease. *MeRec Bulletin* **7**, 41–4.

Nutt JG. 1998: Catechol-O-methyltransferase inhibitors in the treatment of Parkinson's disease. *Lancet* **351**, 1221–2.

Small GW, Rabins PV, Barry PP *et al.* 1997: Diagnosis and treatment of Alzheimer's disease and related disorders. Consensus statement of the American Association for Geriatric Psychiatry, the Alzheimer's Association and the American Geriatric Society. *Journal of the American Medical Association* **278**, 1363–71.

CHAPTER TWENTY-ONE

ANTICONVULSANTS

- Introduction
- Mechanisms of action of anticonvulsants
- General principles of treatment of epilepsy
- Drug interactions with anticonvulsants
- Anticonvulsants and pregnancy
- Anticonvulsant osteomalacia
- Status epilepticus
- Withdrawal of anticonvulsant drugs
- Febrile convulsions

INTRODUCTION

Epilepsy is characterized by recurrent seizures. An epileptic seizure is a paroxysmal discharge of cerebral neurones associated with a clinical event apparent to an observer (e.g. a tonic clonic seizure), or as an abnormal sensation perceived by the patient (e.g. a distortion of consciousness in temporal lobe epilepsy, which may not be apparent to an observer but which is perceived by the patient as flashing lights, macropsia, micropsia, etc.).

A 'funny turn', black-out or apparent seizure may be secondary to many events, including hypoglycaemia, a vasovagal episode, cardiac arrhythmias, drug withdrawal, migraine and transient ischaemic attacks. Precise differentiation is essential not only to avoid the damaging social and practical stigma associated with epilepsy, but also to ensure appropriate medical treatment. Febrile seizures are a distinct problem and are discussed at the end of this chapter.

Key points

- Epilepsy affects 0.5% of the population.
- It is characterized by recurrent seizures.

MECHANISMS OF ACTION OF ANTICONVULSANTS

The pathophysiology of epilepsy and the mode of action of anti-epileptic drugs are poorly understood. These agents are not all sedative, but selectively block repetitive discharges at concentrations below those that block normal impulse conduction. Carbamazepine and phenytoin prolong the inactivated state of the sodium channel, and reduce the likelihood of repetitive action potentials. Consequently, normal cerebral activity, which is associated with relatively low action-potential frequencies, is unaffected, whilst epileptic discharges are suppressed.

α-Aminobutyric acid (GABA) acts as an inhibitory neurotransmitter by opening receptor-operated chloride channels that lead to hyperpolarization and suppression of epileptic discharges. In addition to the receptor site for GABA, the GABA receptor–channel complex includes benzodiazepine and barbiturate recognition sites which can potentiate GABA anti-epileptic activity. Vigabatrin (γ-vinyl-γ-aminobutyric acid) irreversibly inhibits GABA transaminase, the enzyme that inactivates GABA. The resulting increase in synaptic GABA probably explains its anti-epileptic activity.

Glutamate is an excitatory neurotransmitter. A glutamate receptor, the N-methyl-D-aspartate

Key points

Mechanisms of action of anticonvulsants

- They are poorly understood
- They cause blockade of repetitive discharges at a concentration that does not block normal impulse conduction
- This may be achieved via enhancement of GABA action or inhibition of sodium channel function.

(NMDA) receptor, is important in the genesis and propagation of high-frequency discharges. Lamotrigine inhibits glutamate release and has anticonvulsant activity.

GENERAL PRINCIPLES OF TREATMENT OF EPILEPSY

Before treatment is prescribed, the following questions should be asked.

1 Are the fits truly epileptic and not due to some other disorder (e.g. syncope, cardiac arrhythmia)?
2 Is the epilepsy caused by a condition that requires treatment in its own right (e.g. brain tumour, brain abscess, alcohol withdrawal)?
3 Are there remediable or reversible factors that aggravate the epilepsy or precipitate individual attacks?
4 Is there a clinically important risk if the patient is left untreated?
5 What type of epilepsy is present?

The ideal anticonvulsant would completely suppress all clinical and electroencephalographic evidence of the patient's epilepsy, while at the same time producing no immediate or delayed side-effects. This ideal does not exist (in the UK at least 16 anticonvulsant preparations are available), and the choice of drug depends on the balance between efficacy and toxicity and the type of epilepsy being treated. Table 21.1 summarizes the commonest forms of seizure and their drug treatment.

Control should initially be attempted using a single drug which is chosen on the basis of the type of epilepsy. The dose is increased until either the seizures cease or the blood drug concentration (see Chapter 8) is in the toxic range and/or signs of toxicity appear. It should be emphasized that some patients have epilepsy which is controlled at drug blood concentrations below the usual therapeutic range, and others do not manifest toxicity above the therapeutic range. Thus estimation of drug plasma concentration is to be regarded as a guide but not an absolute arbiter. The availability of plasma concentration monitoring of anticonvulsant drugs has allowed the more efficient use of individual drugs, and is a crude guide to compliance. In a study of phenytoin monotherapy for tonic clonic and partial seizures, only 10% of new patients required the addition of a second drug,

Table 21.1: Choice of drug in various forms of seizure

Form of seizure	First choice	Other drugs
Partial with or without secondary generalized tonic clonic seizures	Carbamazepine Valproate Phenytoin	Vigabatrin Lamotrigine Phenobarbitone/primidone Clobazam/clonazepam Topiramate Tiagabine
Primary generalized seizures (tonic clonic)	Valproate	Phenytoin Lamotrigine Clobazam/clonazepam Phenobarbitone/primidone Topiramate
Absence/myclonic	Valproate Lamotrigine	Ethosuximide Clobazam/clonazepam

> **Key points**
>
> Choice of anticonvulsant
>
> - Use a single drug based on type of epilepsy.
> - Generally increase the dose every 2 weeks until either the seizures cease or signs of toxicity appear and/or the plasma drug concentration is in the toxic range.
> - If unsatisfactory, substitute another drug.
> - Probably less than 10% of epileptic patients benefit from two or more concurrent anticonvulsants.

whereas over 50% would have done so if concentrations had not been measured. If a drug proves to be ineffective, it should not be withdrawn suddenly, as this may provoke status epilepticus. Another drug should be introduced in increasing dosage while the first is gradually withdrawn.

Few studies have investigated combined drug therapy, although empirically this is sometimes necessary. In most but not all cases, effects are additive. Combinations of three or more drugs probably do more harm than good by increasing the likelihood of adverse drug reaction without improving seizure control. Many anticonvulsant drugs are enzyme inducers, so pharmacokinetic reactions are common (e.g. carbamazepine reduces plasma concentrations of phenytoin).

INDIVIDUAL ANTI-EPILEPTIC DRUGS

Phenytoin

USE

Phenytoin is one of the drugs of choice in the treatment of tonic clonic and partial seizures, including complex partial seizures. For adults the usual dose is approximately 300 mg/day given as a single dose, but individualization is essential. Plasma concentration is measured after 2 weeks. According to clinical response and plasma concentration, adjustments should be small (e.g. 50 mg at a time) and no more frequent than every 4–6 weeks. Phenytoin illustrates the usefulness of therapeutic drug monitoring (see Chapter 8), but not all patients require a plasma phenytoin concentration within the therapeutic range of 10–20 mg/L for optimum control of their seizures. In status epilepticus, phenytoin may be given by intravenous infusion diluted in sodium chloride together with continuous ECG monitoring.

ADVERSE EFFECTS

These include the following:

- effects on nervous system – high concentrations produce a cerebellar syndrome (ataxia, nystagmus, intention tremor, dysarthria), involuntary movements and sedation. Seizures may paradoxically increase with phenytoin intoxication. High concentrations cause psychological disturbances;
- 'allergic' effects – rashes, drug fever and hepatitis may occur. Predisposition to these associated severe but rare effects (and also to lymphadenopathy, see below) is probably genetically predetermined by an abnormality in phenytoin metabolism. Oddly, but importantly, such patients can show cross-sensitivity to carbamazepine;
- skin and collagen changes – coarse facial features, gum hypertrophy, acne and hirsutism may appear;
- haematological effects – macrocytic anaemia which responds to folate is common; rarely there is aplastic anaemia, or lymphadenopathy ('pseudolymphoma', which rarely progresses to true lymphoma);
- effects on fetus – (these are difficult to distinguish from effects of epilepsy). There is increased perinatal mortality, raised frequency of cleft palate, hare lip, microcephaly and congenital heart disease;
- effects on heart – too rapid IV injection causes arrhythmia.

PHARMACOKINETICS

Intestinal absorption is variable. There is wide variation in the handling of phenytoin, and in patients taking the same dose there is 50 fold variation in steady-state plasma concentrations. The following factors contribute to the variation:

1. age – phenytoin clearance increases with age, and this is correlated with lower protein binding and plasma albumin levels in the elderly. Young children metabolize phenytoin faster than adults;
2. body weight – this influences volume of distribution (0.6 L/kg);

3 gender – this makes a small contribution, steady-state levels being lower in females;
4 metabolism – this is under polygenic control and varies widely between patients, accounting for most of the inter-individual variation in steady-state plasma concentration.

Phenytoin is extensively metabolized by the liver, and less than 5% is excreted unchanged. The enzyme responsible for elimination becomes saturated at concentrations within the therapeutic range, and phenytoin exhibits dose-dependent kinetics which, because of its low therapeutic index, makes clinical use of phenytoin difficult. Successive equal dose increments result in a disproportionate increase in plasma concentration (see Figure 21.1) as drug metabolism approaches saturation. The clinical implications are as follows.

1 Dosage increments should be 50 mg or less once the plasma concentration is within the therapeutic range.
2 Fluctuations above and below the therapeutic range occur relatively easily due to changes in the amount of drug absorbed, or as a result of forgetting to take a tablet. This behaviour also magnifies bioavailability differences, and on one occasion clinical intoxication resulted from alteration of the excipient in phenytoin capsules from calcium sulphate to lactose (see Chapter 4).
3 Drug interactions are common, as administration of a second drug (e.g. isoniazid, which inhibits phenytoin metabolism, or carbamazepine, which enhances it) results in clinically important effects on steady-state plasma concentrations.

The saturation kinetics of phenytoin make it invalid to calculate $t_{\frac{1}{2}}$, as the rate of elimination depends on the plasma level and enzyme saturation. The time to reach a plateau plasma concentration is longer than is predicted from the $t_{\frac{1}{2}}$ of a single dose of the drug. Hence, if necessary (e.g. in patients with status epilepticus), a loading dose (800–1000 mg) is used. Eight-hourly dosing is unnecessary, and a single daily dosage is effective and aids compliance.

Phenytoin is extremely insoluble and crystallizes out in intramuscular injection sites, so this route should never be used. For the rapid attainment of therapeutic plasma concentrations, intravenous injection is needed. To improve solubility, the parenteral preparation has a pH of 10 and precipitation of the free acid occurs if the injection is added to intravenous infusion fluids. The high pH is irritant to veins and tissues. Phenytoin should not be given at rates of > 50 mg/min, because at higher rates of administration cardiovascular collapse, respiratory arrest and seizures may occur. Electrocardiographic monitoring with measurement of blood pressure every minute during

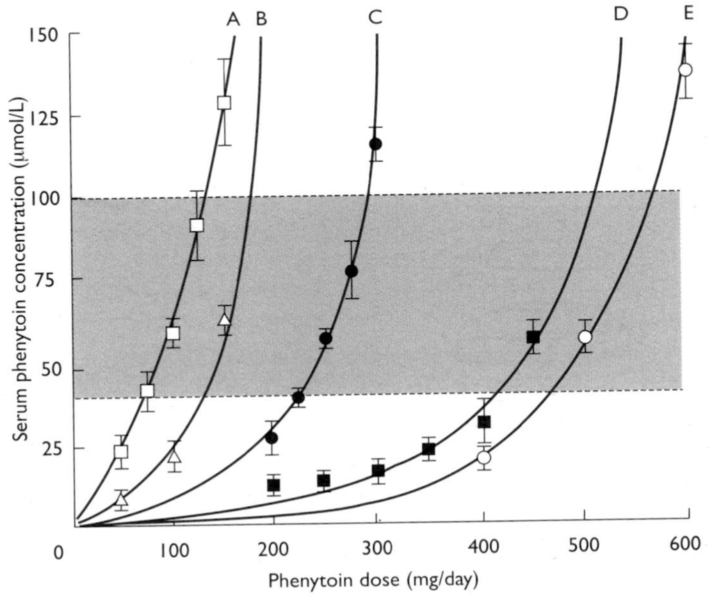

Figure 21.1: Relationship between daily dose of phenytoin and resulting steady-state serum level in five patients on several different doses of the drug. The curves were fitted by computer assuming Michaelis–Menten kinetics. (Reproduced with permission from Richens A, and Dunlop A. 1975: *Lancet* **ii**, 247.) © The Lancet Ltd.

administration is essential. If blood pressure falls, administration is temporarily stopped until the blood pressure has risen to a satisfactory level.

At therapeutic concentrations, 90% of phenytoin is bound to albumin and to two α-globulins which also bind thyroxine. In uraemia, displacement of phenytoin from plasma protein binding results in lower total plasma concentration and a lower therapeutic range. If this is not appreciated and the dose is increased, toxicity will result.

> **Key points**
>
> Phenytoin pharmacokinetics
>
> - There is enormous inter-individual variation, so individualize the dose.
> - Absorption is variable.
> - There is reduced protein binding in uraemia, pregnancy and displacement by valproate.
> - Saturable hepatic metabolism is under polygenic control.
> - The $t_{\frac{1}{2}}$ is 7–60 h (dose dependent).
> - Many use an oral loading dose when initiating therapy.
> - Once daily dosing is used in chronic therapy.
> - Metabolism is induced by concurrent carbamazepine and inhibited by cimetidine.

Sodium valproate also increases the ratio of free to total phenytoin by this mechanism.

Other important interactions occur via alterations in the hepatic metabolism of phenytoin. The drugs that impair or induce metabolism are summarized in Table 21.2.

Phenytoin elimination is impaired in liver disease. Chronic renal disease may result in unusually low levels because of hypoalbuminaemia in patients with nephrotic syndrome, or displacement of protein-bound phenytoin by accumulated endogenous metabolites in patients with renal failure.

Phenobarbitone

Phenobarbitone is an effective drug for tonic and partial seizures, but is sedative in adults and causes behavioural disturbances and hyperkinesia in children. It may be tried as a second-line drug for atypical absence, atonic and tonic seizures. Rebound seizures may occur on withdrawal. Monitoring plasma concentrations is less useful than with phenytoin because tolerance occurs, and the relationship between plasma concentrations and therapeutic and adverse effects is less predictable than is the case with phenytoin.

Table 21.2: Metabolic interactions of anticonvulsants

Enzyme-inducing effect of anti-epilepetic drugs		**Drugs that inhibit the metabolism of anticonvulsants**	
Anti-epileptic drug	**Drugs whose metabolism is enhanced**	**Inhibitor**	**Anticonvulsant**
Carbamazepine	Warfarin	Amiodarone	Phenytoin
Phenobarbitone	Oral contraceptives	Fluoxetine	Phenytoin, carbamazepine
Phenytoin	Theophylline	Diltiazem, nifedipine	Phenytoin
Primidone	Cyclosporin	Chloramphenicol	Phenytoin
	Some tricyclic antidepressants	Disulfiram	Phenytoin
	Doxycycline	Erythromycin and clarithromycin	Carbamazepine
	Corticosteroids		
	Anticonvulsants	Cimetidine	Phenytoin
		Isoniazid	Carbamazepine, ethosuximide, phenytoin
		Metronidazole	Phenytoin
		Miconazole, fluconazole	Phenytoin
		Valproate	Lamotrigine

Other adverse effects include rashes, anaphylaxis, folate deficiency, aplastic anaemia and congenital abnormalities.

Carbamazepine

USE

Carbamazepine is structurally related to the tricyclic antidepressants. It is the drug of choice for simple and complex partial seizures and for tonic-clonic seizures secondary to a focal discharge seizure, and it is effective in trigeminal neuralgia and in the prophylaxis of mood swings in manic-depressive illness (see Chapter 19). A dose of 100–200 mg is given twice daily followed by a slow increase in dose until seizures are controlled. At higher doses, the daily dose may have to be divided into a three or four times daily regime to reduce side-effects. A dose of 1200 mg daily is sometimes required. Assays of serum concentration are a useful guide to compliance, rapid metabolism, or drug failure if seizures continue. The therapeutic range is 4–12 mg/L.

PHARMACOKINETICS

Carbamazepine is slowly but well absorbed following oral administration. The plasma levels fluctuate widely during absorption. Plasma $t_{\frac{1}{2}}$ after a single dose is 25–60 h, but on chronic dosing this decreases to 10 h, possibly due to enzyme induction. A controlled-release preparation reduces the peak plasma concentration and fluctuations in carbamazepine concentration during treatment. It is indicated in patients whose adverse effects (dizziness, diplopia and drowsiness) correlate with peak drug concentrations, and in patients who have difficulty in complying with three or more doses per day.

At therapeutic concentrations, carbamazepine is 75% bound to plasma protein, and it is feasible to use salivary carbamazepine concentrations (which reflect unbound drug in the plasma) as an alternative to blood analysis.

ADVERSE EFFECTS

Adverse effects are common but seldom severe. They are particularly troublesome early in treatment. Sedation, ataxia, giddiness, nystagmus, diplopia, blurred vision and slurred speech occur in 50% of patients with plasma levels over 8.5 mg/L. Other effects include rash and (much more rarely) blood dyscrasia, cholestatic jaundice, renal impairment and lymphadenopathy. Carbamazepine can cause hyponatraemia and water intoxication due to an antidiuretic action. It is contraindicated in patients with atrioventricular (AV) conduction abnormalities and a history of bone-marrow depression or porphyria. Its use in pregnancy has been associated with fetal neural-tube defects and hypospadias.

DRUG INTERACTIONS

Carbamazepine should not be combined with monoamine oxidase inhibitors. It is a potent enzyme inducer and, in particular, it accelerates the metabolism of warfarin, theophylline and the oral contraceptive.

Benzodiazepines

See Chapter 17.

USE

Benzodiazepines (e.g. diazepam, clobazepam and clonazepam) have anticonvulsant properties in addition to their anxiolytic and other actions. Unfortunately, on prolonged usage, tolerance of their anti-epileptic properties tends to develop. Clonazepam was introduced specifically as an anticonvulsant. Its chief uses are as maintenance therapy and in status epilepticus, in which diazepam or clonazepam given intravenously is the treatment of choice. Clonazepam has a wide spectrum of activity, having a place in the management of the motor seizures of childhood, particularly absences and infantile spasms. It is also useful in complex partial seizures and myoclonic epilepsy in patients who are not adequately controlled by phenytoin or carbamazepine. Oral treatment is usually started with a single dose at night. The dose is gradually titrated upwards until control is achieved or adverse effects become unacceptable. Despite their long half-lives, the drugs appear to be better tolerated at higher doses if given in divided doses.

Clonazepam is given in divided doses of 4–8 mg/day in adults. The intravenous dose is 0.5–2 mg. Intravenous diazepam is indicated in status epilepticus. Rectal diazepam is a useful alternative in children.

ADVERSE EFFECTS

Adverse effects are frequent, and about 50% of patients experience lethargy, somnolence and dizziness with clonazepam. This is minimized by starting with a low dose and then gradually increasing it. In many cases sedation disappears on chronic treatment. More serious effects are muscular inco-ordination, ataxia, dysphoria, hypotonia and muscle relaxation, increased salivary secretion and hyperactivity with aggressive behaviour.

PHARMACOKINETICS

Clonazepam is well absorbed orally and the $t_{\frac{1}{2}}$ is about 30 h. Neither therapeutic nor adverse effects appear to be closely related to plasma concentrations. Control of most types of epilepsy occurs within the range 30–60 ng/mL. Clonazepam is extensively metabolized to inactive metabolites.

Sodium valproate

USE

Sodium valproate (dipropylacetate) is effective against several forms of epilepsy, including tonic clonic, absence, partial seizures and myoclonic epilepsy. Dosage starts at 600 mg daily in divided (8-hourly) doses after meals, and is increased every 3 days by 200 mg/day until control is achieved. This is generally in the range 1000–2000 mg/day, but may be up to 2500 mg/day. The onset of effect is slow and may take several days.

ADVERSE EFFECTS

Adverse effects most commonly involve the alimentary system. Toxic effects include the following:

1. nausea, vomiting and abdominal pain (these effects may be reduced by enteric-coated tablets);
2. enhancement of sedatives (including alcohol);
3. thrombocytopenia (usually associated with high dosage). Platelet count should be checked before surgery and if any abnormal bruising occurs;
4. temporary hair loss;
5. a false-positive ketone test in urine, which may cause confusion in the management of diabetes, has been reported;
6. teratogenic effects (neural-tube defects and hypospadias) have been reported;
7. rarely, hepatic necrosis has developed, particularly in children taking high doses and suffering from congenital metabolic disorders;
8. acute pancreatitis is another rare complication.

PHARMACOKINETICS

Valproate is well absorbed when given orally (95–100% bioavailability). Like other fatty acids, it is highly bound (approximately 90%) to plasma protein, showing a twofold inter-individual variation in the amount of free drug. Like phenytoin, there is reduced binding in uraemia and the unbound drug a strong good correlation with serum creatinine levels. The plasma $t_{\frac{1}{2}}$ is 7–10 h. Possibly the presence of active metabolites explains the relatively slow onset and long time-course of action. The brain to plasma ratio is low (0.3) and a large dose (1–2 g/day) is necessary. There is substantial inter-individual variation in the handling of the drug. Plasma valproate concentrations do not correlate closely with efficacy.

Key points

Sodium valproate

Pharmacokinetics

- Well absorbed.
- Interindividual variation in metabolism.
- Relatively short $t_{\frac{1}{2}}$ <10 h therefore adjust dose every 3 days.

Use

- Effective in all forms of epilepsy.

Adverse effects

- Nausea, vomiting, abdominal pain.
- Enhancement of sedatives.
- Thrombocytopaenia.
- Hair loss.
- Teratogen – neural tube defects.
- Rarely hepatic necrosis.

Chlormethiazole

Chlormethiazole (see Chapter 17) is a powerful anticonvulsant which can be given intravenously in the treatment of status epilepticus. When given orally it has a short half-life (1 h) and is therefore not convenient for use in the day-to-day treatment of epilepsy. It can cause respiratory depression and, if given by intravenous infusion, careful monitoring of respiratory function is mandatory. In addition, if the infusion is prolonged accumulation may occur.

Vigabatrin

USE

Vigabatrin, a structural analogue of GABA, increases the brain concentration of GABA (an inhibitory neurotransmitter) through irreversible inhibition of GABA transaminase. It is reserved for the treatment of epilepsy that is unsatisfactorily controlled by more established drugs. Lower doses should be used in the elderly and in those with impaired renal function. Vigabatrin should be avoided in those with a psychiatric history.

ADVERSE EFFECTS

1 The commonest reported adverse event (in up to 30% of patients) is drowsiness.
2 Fatigue, irritability, dizziness, confusion and weight gain have all been reported.
3 Behavioural side-effects (e.g. ill temper) may occur.
4 Psychotic reactions, including hallucinations and paranoia, may occur.
5 Nystagmus, ataxia, tremor, paraesthaesia, retinal disorders, visual-field defects and photophobia have been reported. Regular testing of visual fields is recommended. The patient should be warned to report any visual symptoms and an urgent opthalmological opinion should be sought if visual-field loss is suspected.

PHARMACOKINETICS

Absorption is not influenced by food, and peak plasma concentrations occur within 2 h of an oral dose. In contrast to most other anticonvulsants, vigabatrin is not metabolized in the liver but is excreted unchanged via the kidney and has a plasma half-life of about 5 h. Its efficacy does not correlate with the plasma concentration, and its duration of action is prolonged due to irreversible binding to GABA transaminase.

Lamotrigine

Lamotrigine prolongs the inactivated state of the sodium channel, thereby inhibiting transmitter release, particularly glutamate. It is indicated as monotherapy and adjunctive treatment of partial seizures, generalized tonic clonic seizures that are not satisfactorily controlled with other drugs, and seizures associated with Lennox–Gastaut syndrome. It is contraindicated in hepatic and renal impairment. Lamotrigine is generally well tolerated. Side-effects include rashes (rarely angioedema, Steven–Johnson syndrome and toxic epidermal necrolysis), flu-like symptoms, visual disturbances, dizziness, drowsiness, gastrointestinal disturbances and aggression. The patient must be counselled to seek urgent medical advice if rash or influenza symptoms associated with hypersensitivity develop.

Gabapentin

Gabapentin has been licensed as an 'add-on' therapy in the treatment of partial seizures. It is a GABA analogue, but its mechanism of action is thought to occur at calcium channels. Initial studies suggest that it is generally well tolerated, with somnolence being the most frequently reported side effect. It is well absorbed after oral administration, and is eliminated by renal excretion; the average half-life is 5–7 h. It does not interfere with the metabolism or protein binding of other anticonvulsants.

Topiramate

Topiramate blocks sodium channels, attenuates neuronal excitation and enhances GABA–mediated inhibition. It is licensed for adjunctive therapy of partial seizures, with or without secondary generalization. It may also be of value for seizures associated with Lennox–Gastaut syndrome and primarily generalized tonic-clonic seizures. Topiramate is an inducer of cytochrome P_{450}, and its own metabolism is induced by carbamazepine and phenytoin. Adverse effects include poor concentration and memory, impaired speech, mood disorders, ataxia, somnolence, anorexia and weight loss.

Tiagabine

Tiagabine inhibits the neuronal and glial uptake of GABA. Tiagabine has recently been licensed as adjunctive therapy in the UK for partial seizures with or without secondary generalization. Reported adverse events include dizziness, asthenia, nervousness, tremor, depression and diarrhoea. It has a $t_{\frac{1}{2}}$ of approximately 7 h, which may be halved by concurrent administration of carbomazepine and phenytoin.

Ethosuximide

USE

Ethosuximide is one of a group of succinimide drugs and is the drug of choice in absence seizures. It is continued into adolescence and then gradually withdrawn over several months. If a drug for tonic clonic seizures is being given concurrently, this is continued for a further 3 years. The daily dose is usually in the range 0.5–2 g by mouth. It may also be used in myoclonic seizures and in atypical absences.

ADVERSE EFFECTS

Apart from dizziness, nausea and epigastric discomfort, side-effects are rare, and there are few doubts about its safety. Tonic clonic and absence seizures may coexist in the same child, and a drug such as phenytoin may need to be added, as ethosuximide is not effective against tonic clonic seizures.

PHARMACOKINETICS

Ethosuximide is well absorbed following oral administration. Its plasma $t_{\frac{1}{2}}$ is 70 h in adults, but only 30 h in children. Thus ethosuximide need be given only once daily, and steady-state values are reached within 7 days.

Plasma concentration estimations are not usually required, but effective concentrations lie in the range 40–120 mg/L; the average dose which will achieve this is 20 mg/kg/day. In practice, 500 mg are given as the initial dose, and this is increased by 250 mg every week until attacks are prevented. Extensive hepatic metabolism produces two major metabolites which are inactive. No significant plasma protein binding occurs, and the cerebrospinal fluid (CSF) drug concentration is similar to that in plasma.

Drug interactions with anticonvulsants

Clinically important interactions with other drugs occur with several anti-epileptics. The therapeutic ratio of anti-epileptics is often small, and changes in plasma concentrations can seriously affect both efficacy and toxicity. In addition, anti-epileptics are prescribed over long periods, so there is a considerable likelihood that sooner or later they will be combined with another drug.

Several mechanisms are involved:

1. enzyme induction, so the hepatic metabolism of the anti-epileptic is enhanced, plasma concentration lowered and efficacy reduced;
2. enzyme inhibition, so the metabolism of the anti-epileptic is impaired with the development of higher blood concentrations and toxicity;
3. displacement of the anti-epileptic from plasma binding sites.

In addition to this, several anti-epileptics (e.g. phenytoin, phenobarbitone, carbamazepine) are themselves powerful enzyme inducers and may alter the metabolism of other drugs. Table 21.2 lists the effects of some drugs on the metabolism of widely used anti-epileptics, and the effects of anti-epileptics on the metabolism of other drugs.

Anti-epileptics and the oral contraceptive

Phenytoin, phenobarbitone, toprimate and carbamazepine induce the metabolism of oestrogen and can lead to unwanted pregnancies. Patients taking anti-epileptics and wishing to take an oral contraceptive should use one containing at least 50 μg oestrogen.

Anticonvulsants and pregnancy

The benefit of treatment outweighs the risk to the fetus. The risk of teratogenicity is greater if more than one drug is used (see Chapter 9).

Anticonvulsant osteomalacia

Enzyme induction reduces serum 25-hydroxycholecalciferol. Subclinical or symptomatic rickets or osteomalacia can develop due to deficient vitamin D. However, clinically significant anticonvulsant osteomalacia is exceedingly rare. The deficit is increased by the poor diet and lack of sunlight which is the lot of many institutionalized epileptics. Associated hypocalcaemia rarely causes fits. Good diet should be encouraged in epileptics, and a vitamin D supplement prescribed if necessary.

Status epilepticus

Status epilepticus is a medical emergency with a mortality of about 10%, with neurological and psychiatric sequelae possible in the survivors. Rapid suppression of seizure activity is essential, and can usually be achieved with intravenous benzodiazepines (e.g. diazepam, formulated as an emulsion, 10 mg IV). The rectal route is useful in children and if venous access is difficult (see Chapter 10). Alternative benzodiazepines include clonazepam and lorazepam, the latter having a longer duration of action. False teeth should be removed, an airway established and oxygen administered as soon as possible. The dose of diazepam is repeated if fitting continues. Transient respiratory depression and hypotension may occur. Relapse may be prevented with intravenous phenytoin and/or early recommencement of regular anticonvulsants. Identification of any precipitating factors, such as hypoglycaemia, alcohol, drug overdose, low anticonvulsant plasma concentrations and non-compliance, may influence the immediate and subsequent management. If intravenous benzodiazepines and phenytoin fail to control the fits, removal to an intensive-care unit and assistance from an anaesthetist are essential. Intravenous chlormethiazole, phenobarbitone or thiopentone are commonly used in this situation. EEG or cerebral function monitoring are mandatory if general anaesthesia is used. Where facilities for resuscitation are poor, paraldehyde administered rectally or, less commonly, by deep intramuscular injection is valuable, as it causes little respiratory depression.

Key points

Status epilepticus

If fits are > 5 min in duration or there is incomplete recovery from fits of shorter duration, suppress seizure activity *as soon as possible*.

- Remove false teeth, establish an airway, and give oxygen at a high flow rate. Assess the patient, verify the diagnosis and place them in the lateral semi-prone position.
- Give *IV diazepam* (diazemuls) as a 10-mg bolus.
- Give diazepam 10 mg over 12 min (rectal diazepam and rectal paraldehyde are alternatives if immediate IV access is not possible).
- The above procedure may be repeated once if fits continue.
- Take blood for anticonvulsant, alcohol and sugar analysis, as well as calcium, electrolytes and urea (if there is doubt about the diagnosis, test for prolactin).
- If glucose levels are low, give 50% dextrose. If alcohol is a problem, give IV vitamins B and C.
- If fits continue, give *IV phenytoin* by infusion, and monitor ECG.
- If fits continue, give a *chlormethiazole* infusion – intensive-care unit (ITU), consult anaesthetist, paralyse if necessary, ventilate, give thiopentone, monitor cerebral function, check pentobarbitone levels.

Withdrawal of anticonvulsant drugs

All anticonvulsants are associated with adverse effects. It has been estimated that up to 70% of patients eventually enter a prolonged remission and do not require medication. However, it is difficult to know whether a prolonged seizure-free interval is due to efficacy of the anti-epileptic drug treatment or to true remission. Individuals with a history of adult-onset epilepsy of long duration which has been difficult to control, partial seizures and/or underlying cerebral disorder have a less favourable prognosis. Drug withdrawal itself may precipitate seizures, and the possible medical and social consequences of recurrent seizures (e.g. loss of driving licence; see Table 21.3) must be carefully discussed with the patient. If drugs are to be withdrawn, the dose should be reduced gradually (e.g. over 6 months) with strict instructions to the patient to report any seizure activity. Patients should not drive during withdrawal or for 6 months afterwards.

Table 21.3: Driving and epilepsy

- Patients with epilepsy may drive a motor vehicle (but not an HGV* or public service vehicle) provided that they have been seizure free for 1 year or have established a 3-year period of seizures whilst asleep
- Patients affected by drowsiness should not drive or operate machinery
- Patients should not drive during withdrawal of anticonvulsants or for 6 months afterwards

*An HGV licence can be held by a person who has been seizure free and off all anticonvulsant medication for 10 years or longer.

FEBRILE CONVULSIONS

Febrile seizures are the most common seizures of childhood. A febrile convulsion is defined as a convulsion that occurs in a child aged between 3 months and 5 years with a fever but without any other evident cause, such as an intracranial infection or previous non-febrile convulsions. Approximately 3% of children have at least one febrile convulsion, of whom about one-third will have one or more recurrences and 3% will develop epilepsy in later life.

Despite the usually insignificant medical consequences, a febrile convulsion is a terrifying experience to parents. Most children are admitted to hospital following their first febrile convulsion. If prolonged, the convulsion can be terminated with either rectal or intravenous diazepam. If the child is under 18 months old, pyogenic meningitis should be excluded. It is usual to reduce fever by giving paracetamol, removal of clothing, tepid sponging and fanning. Fever is usually due to viral infection, but if a bacterial cause is found this should be treated.

Uncomplicated febrile seizures have an excellent prognosis, so the parents can be confidently reassured. They should be advised how to reduce the fever and how to deal with a subsequent fit, should it occur. Although phenobarbitone and sodium valproate have been used as long-term regular prophylaxis in children to reduce the occurrence of febrile convulsions, there is no evidence that this reduces the likelihood of developing epilepsy in later life, and their benefits are outweighed by the sedation and behavioural disturbances caused by phenobarbitone, and the small risk of hepatic necrosis associated with sodium valproate. Rectal diazepam may be administered by parents as prophylaxis during a febrile illness, or to stop a prolonged convulsion.

Case history

A 24-year-old woman whose secondary generalized tonic clonic seizures have been well controlled with carbamazepine for the previous 4 years develops confusion, somnolence, ataxia, vertigo and nausea. Her concurrent medication includes the oral contraceptive – Loestrin 20 (which contains norethisterone 1 mg and ethinoloestradiol 20 mg) – and erythromycin, which was started 1 week earlier for sinusitis. She has no history of drug allergy.

Question 1

What is the likely cause of her symptoms?

Question 2

Is the oral contraceptive preparation appropriate?

Answer 1

Erythromycin inhibits the metabolism of carbamazepine, and the symptoms described are attributable to a raised plasma concentration of carbamazepine.

Answer 2

This patient is not adequately protected against conception with the low-dose oestrogen pill, since carbamazepine induces the metabolism of oestrogen.

FURTHER READING

Stephen LJ, Brodie MJ. 1998: New drug treatments for epilepsy. *Prescriber's Journal* **38**, 98–106.

1996: Stopping status epilepticus. *Drugs and Therapeutics Bulletin* **34**.

CHAPTER TWENTY-TWO

MIGRAINE

- Pathophysiology
- Drugs used for the acute migraine attack
- Drugs used for migraine prophylaxis

PATHOPHYSIOLOGY

Migraine is common and prostrating, yet its pathophysiology remains poorly understood. The aura is associated with intracranial vasoconstriction and localized cerebral ischaemia, as demonstrated by angiographic and isotopic blood-flow studies. Shortly after this, the extracranial vessels dilate and pulsate in association with local tenderness and the classical unilateral headache, although it is unclear whether this or a neuronal abnormality ('spreading cortical depression') is the cause of the symptoms.

5-Hydroxytryptamine (5HT, serotonin) is strongly implicated, but this longstanding hypothesis remains unproven. 5HT is a potent vasoconstrictor of extracranial vessels in humans, and also has vasodilator actions in some vascular beds. Excretion of 5-HIAA (the main urinary metabolite of 5HT) is increased following a migraine attack, and blood 5HT (reflecting platelet 5HT content) is reduced, suggesting that platelet activation and 5HT release may occur during an attack. This could contribute to vasoconstriction during the aura and either summate with or oppose the effects of kinins, prostaglandins and histamine to cause pain in the affected arteries. The initial stimulus for platelet 5HT release is unknown. One hypothesis is that migraineurs have inherently unstable cerebral vasculature prone to excessive contraction and dilatation when stimulated by factors that in normal subjects produce only minor effects (see Figure 22.1).

Ingestion by a migraine sufferer of vasoactive amines in food may cause inappropriate responses of intra- and extracranial vessels. Several other idiosyncratic precipitating factors are recognized anecdotally, although in some cases, (e.g. precipitation by chocolate) they are not easily demonstrated scientifically. These include physical trauma, local pain from sinuses, cervical spondylosis, sleep (too much or too little), ingestion of tyramine-containing foods such as cheese, alcoholic beverages (especially brandy), allergy (e.g. to wheat, eggs or fish), stress, hormonal changes, (e.g. during the menstrual cycle and pregnancy, and at menarche or menopause), fasting and hypoglycaemia.

Some of the most effective prophylactic drugs against migraine inhibit 5HT reuptake by platelets and other cells. Several of these have additional antihistamine and anti-5HT activity. Assessment of drug efficacy in migraine is bedevilled by variability in the frequency and severity of attacks both within an individual and between different sufferers. Drugs are divided into those administered for the acute attack and those used for prophylaxis.

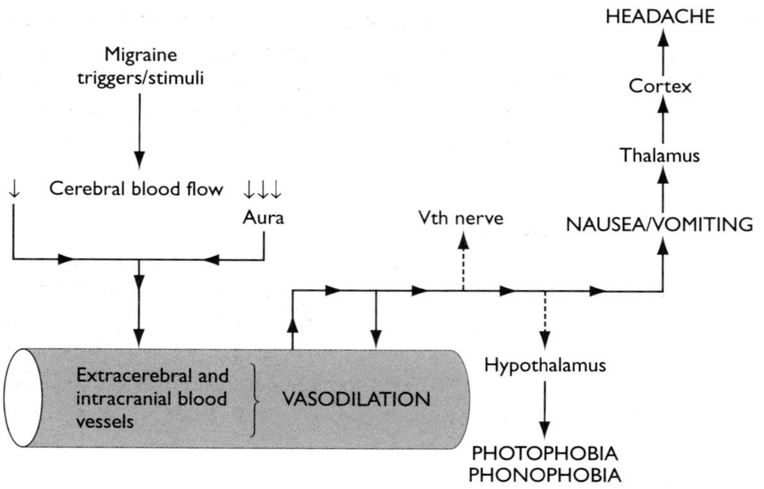

Figure 22.1: Pathophysiology of migraine.

Drugs used for the acute migraine attack

In the majority of patients with migraine, the combination of a mild analgesic with an anti-emetic and, if possible, a period of rest aborts the acute attack. Until recently, the small proportion of migraine sufferers in whom this treatment was inadequate were given ergotamine taken orally, by suppository or by inhaler. The therapeutic armamentarium has been extended with the introduction of 5-HT_{1D} agonists (e.g. sumatriptan). These are expensive, but they are less toxic than ergotamine and play an important role in relieving migraine which is resistant to simple therapy.

Simple analgesics

Aspirin, 900 mg, or **paracetamol**, 1 g, are useful in treatment of the headache. They are inexpensive, and are effective in up to 75% of patients. During a migraine attack, gastric stasis occurs and this impairs drug absorption. If necessary, soluble aspirin should be used with metoclopramide (as an anti-emetic and to enhance gastric emptying). Combination preparations of metoclopramide, 5 mg, and aspirin, 325 mg (or with paracetamol, 500 mg) are available. They should be avoided if possible in adolescents and women in their twenties because of the risk of spasmodic torticollis and dystonia (see Chapter 20).

Anti-emetics for migraine

Metoclopramide, a dopamine and weak $5HT_4$ antagonist, or **domperidone**, a dopamine antagonist that does not penetrate the blood–brain barrier, are appropriate choices. Sedative anti-emetics (e.g. antihistamines, phenothiazines) should generally be avoided.

$5HT_{1D}$ agonists (sumatriptan, naratriptan and zolmitriptan)

Sumatriptan

Use

Sumatriptan (6 mg) is injected subcutaneously or given by mouth (100 mg) and now available as a nasal spray (20 mg). It has largely replaced ergotamine. Prepacked dosage vials are available for self-injection, and the maximum recommended dose is 12 mg/24 h, a second injection being administered no sooner than 1 h after the first. The maximum recommended dose (PO) is 300 mg/24 h. It can be taken at any time during a migraine attack, but is most effective if taken early. It is used to treat acute migraine or cluster headache, and relieves symptoms in 65–85% of attacks. Because of its short half-life, the headache recurs after a single dose in about one-third of attacks.

Mechanism of action

Sumatriptan is a selective agonist of $5HT_{1D}$ receptors which are found predominantly in the cranial circulation, and causes dose-dependent carotid vasoconstriction. There is less marked vasoconstriction in other vascular beds, notably the coronary and pulmonary vasculature, and a significant but transient increase in blood pressure.

ADVERSE EFFECTS

These include the following:

1 transient pain at the injection site;
2 flushing, dizziness and weakness;
3 paraesthesiae;
4 pressure or tightness in any part of the body, especially the chest. Chest pain is particularly worrying as it is possible that it could be due to coronary artery vasoconstriction, although there is no conclusive evidence to support this view;
5 nausea and vomiting after oral administration.

PHARMACOKINETICS

Sumatriptan is rapidly absorbed after both oral and subcutaneous administration, with a T_{max} of 45 and 15 min, respectively. The drug is approximately 100% bioavailable after subcutaneous injection, compared to 14% bioavailability after oral administration; food does not affect oral absorption. Sumatriptan undergoes substantial presystemic hepatic metabolism to an inactive indoleacetic-acid metabolite. About 8% is metabolized and 20% is excreted unchanged via the kidney. The $t_{\frac{1}{2}}$ is 2 h, protein binding is low and, because of its lipid solubility, it has a large volume of distribution.

CONTRAINDICATIONS AND DRUG INTERACTIONS

Sumatriptan should not be used in patients with ischaemic heart disease or Prinzmetal's angina, or severe systemic hypertension. Sumatriptan should not be combined with ergotamine, MAOIs, lithium or selective serotonin reuptake inhibitors (SSRIs).

The properties of other new $5HT_{1D}$ agonists are summarized in Table 22.1.

DRUGS USED FOR MIGRAINE PROPHYLAXIS

Migraine prophylaxis is not justified unless the attack frequency is more than once per month. Due to the relapsing/remitting natural history of migraine, prophylactic therapy should be given for 4–6 months and then withdrawn with monitoring of the frequency of attacks. Several drugs that are quite widely used for migraine

Table 22.1: New $5HT_{1D}$ agonists

Drug	Recommended oral dose	Pharmacokinetic properties	Adverse effects	Drug interactions	Other comments
Naratriptan	2.5 mg as soon as possible after onset, and repeat dose in 4 h if migraine recurs. Maximum of 5 mg per 24 h	$t_{\frac{1}{2}}$ = 6 h. Cleared by renal excretion and hepatic cytochrome P_{450} metabolism. Onset of action may be slower than Sumatriptan	Drowsiness, hypertension, bradycardia, chest pain, visual disturbances	Contraindicated with other serotonergic agents (e.g. ergotamine, SSRIs, etc.)	Not to be used in patients >65 yrs or with coronary artery disease or PVD
Rizatriptan*	5–10 mg po	$t_{\frac{1}{2}}$ = 2 h. Hepatic cytochrome P_{450} MAO metabolism	Somnolence dizziness/ fatigue	As above + MAOIs	As above
Zolmitriptan	2.5 mg orally for acute attack (Range = 2.5–5.0 mg)	$t_{\frac{1}{2}}$ = 3 h. Rapid onset. Hepatic metabolism to active metabolite	Nausea, dizziness, dry mouth, chest pain	As above + MAOIs	As above

*Formulation also available for sublingual use

prophylaxis are not licensed for this indication; folklore abounds and scientific evidence is scarce.

Pizotifen

USE

Pizotifen is licensed, and is an appropriate first choice for migraine prophylaxis. It is related to the tricyclic antidepressants. The initial dose is 0.5 mg (given at night as it causes drowsiness), and this can be increased up to 3 mg if necessary.

MECHANISM OF ACTION

Pizotifen is a $5HT_2$ antagonist. It also has mild antimuscarinic and antihistaminic activity.

ADVERSE EFFECTS

These include the following:

1 drowsiness;
2 appetite stimulation and weight gain;
3 dizziness;
4 muscle pain.

PHARMACOKINETICS

Pizotifen is well absorbed (80%) and undergoes extensive hepatic metabolism. Only 1% of a dose is excreted unchanged in the urine, and its $t_{\frac{1}{2}}$ is 26 h.

DRUG INTERACTIONS

Pizotifen should not be used with monoamine oxidase inhibitors, and potentiates the drowsiness and sedation of sedatives, tranquillizers and antidepressants.

Propranolol and other beta-adrenoceptor antagonists

β-Adrenoreceptor antagonists have prophylactic efficacy compared to placebo in migraine. Their mechanism in this regard is uncertain, but they may act by opposing dilatation of extracranial vessels. **Atenolol** or **metoprolol** are effective and easy to use (see Chapters 27 and 28). β-Adrenoreceptor antagonists potentiate the peripheral vasoconstriction caused by ergotamine *and these drugs should not be given concurrently*.

Methysergide

USE

***Methysergide** should only be used under specialist hospital supervision because of its severe toxicity*. It is highly effective as prophylaxis (up to 80% of patients) in a dose of 1–2 mg two or three times daily with meals. Initially 1 mg is given at night and the dose is slowly increased up to 2 mg 8-hourly. After 6 months it is stopped for at least 1 month. *It is only indicated in patients who, despite other attempts at control, experience such severe and frequent migraine as to interfere substantially with their work or social activities*. The smallest dose that suppresses about 75% of the headaches is used.

MECHANISM OF ACTION

Methysergide has powerful $5HT_2$-blocking activity with partial agonist activity at $5HT_1$ receptors and also some anti-inflammatory and vasoconstrictor effects.

ADVERSE EFFECTS

These include the following:

> **Key points**
>
> Migraine and its drug treatment
>
> - The clinical features of classical migraine consist of aura followed by unilateral and then generalized throbbing headache, photophobia and visual disturbances (e.g. fortification spectra) with nausea and vomiting.
> - The pathophysiology of migraine is poorly understood. 5HT in particular, but also norepinephrine, prostaglandins and kinins, have all been implicated. Initial cranial vasoconstriction gives way to vasodilatation, and spreading neuronal depression occurs.
> - Attacks may be precipitated by relaxation after stress, tyramine, caffeine or alcohol. Avoiding these and other precipitants is worthwhile for individuals with a clear history.
> - Up to 70% of acute attacks are aborted with simple analgesics (e.g. paracetamol/aspirin), together with an anti-emetic (e.g. metoclopramide/domperidone) if necessary.
> - Unresponsive and disabling attacks merit more specific therapy with $5HT_{1D}$ agonists (e.g. sumatriptan).
> - Prophylaxis is not indicated unless the patient suffers more than one attack per month. The preferred drugs are pizotifen or β-adrenoceptor antagonists. Ca^{2+} antagonists, tricyclic antidepressants and (in exceptional cases only) methysergide may also be effective.

Case history

A 29-year-old woman has suffered from migraine for many years. Her attacks are normally ameliorated by oral cafergot tablets (containing ergotamine and caffeine) which she takes up to two at a time. One evening she develops a particularly severe headache and goes to lie down in a darkened room. She takes 2 cafergot tablets. Two hours later there has been no relief of her headache, and she takes some metoclopramide 20 mg and 2 further cafergot tablets, followed about 1 h later by another 2 cafergot tablets as her headache is unremitting. Approximately 30 min later her headache starts to improve, but she feels nauseated and notices that her fingers are turning white (despite being indoors) and are numb. She is seen in the local casualty department where her headache has now disappeared, but the second and fifth fingers on her left hand are now blue, and she has lost sensation in the other fingers of that hand.

Question

What is the problem and how would you treat her?

Answer

The problem is that the patient has inadvertently ingested an overdose of cafergot (ergotamine tartrate 1 mg and caffeine 100 mg). No more than 4 cafergot tablets should be taken during any 24-h period (a maximum of 8 tablets per week). The major toxicity of ergotamine is related to its potent α-agonist activity, which causes severe vasoconstriction and potentially leads to digital and limb ischaemia. Cardiac and cerebral ischaemia may also be precipitated or exacerbated. Treatment consists of keeping the limb warm but not hot, together with a vasodilator – either an alpha-blocker to antagonize the α_1 effects of ergotamine, or another potent vasodilator such as a calcium-channel antagonist or nitroglycerin. Blood pressure must be monitored, carefully as must blood flow to the affected limb/digits. The dose of the vasodilating agents should be titrated, preferably in an intensive-care unit.

1 gastrointestinal disturbances – nausea, vomiting, diarrhoea and abdominal pain;
2 neurological disturbances – mild euphoria, dissociation, experiences of unreality, hyperaesthesia;
3 weight gain and oedema;
4 reversible vasoconstriction – angina, intermittent claudication, abdominal angina;
5 fibrosis in the peritoneum and thorax – retroperitoneal fibrosis is not clearly dose related but is related, to prolonged use. Symptoms may be minimal, and progression to end-stage renal failure may occur insidiously.

Calcium-channel blockers

Flunarizine, 10 mg daily, is effective. Verapamil, 40 mg three times a day, is sometimes used as prophylaxis against cluster headaches.

Tricyclic antidepressants and other agents

Tricyclic antidepressants (see Chapter 19) prevent attacks in some patients independent of mood. The probable mechanism is via 5HT and noradrenaline reuptake blockade. Amitriptyline in low dose (e.g. 10–25 mg at night) may be adequate. Sodium valproate, 300 mg twice daily (see Chapter 21), is also used.

Further reading

Diener HC, May A. 1997: New aspects of migraine pathophysiology: lessons learnt from positron emission tomography. *Current Opinion in Neurology* **9**, 199–201.

Saper JR. 1997: Diagnosis and symptomatic treatment of migraine. *Headache* **37** (**Supplement 1**), S1–S14.

Welch KM. 1993: Drug therapy of migraine. *New England Journal of Medicine* **329**, 1976–83.

CHAPTER TWENTY-THREE

ANAESTHETICS *and* MUSCLE RELAXANTS

- General anaesthetics
- Inhalational anaesthetics
- Intravenous anaesthetics
- Supplementary drugs
- Sedation in the intensive-care unit
- Premedication for anaesthesia
- Muscle relaxants
- Malignant hyperthermia
- Local anaesthetics

GENERAL ANAESTHETICS

The modern practice of anaesthesia most commonly involves the administration of an intravenous anaesthetic agent to induce rapid loss of consciousness, amnesia and inhibition of autonomic and sensory reflexes. Anaesthesia is maintained conventionally by the continuous administration of an inhalational anaesthetic agent, and cessation of administration results in rapid recovery. An opioid is often administered for analgesia, and in many cases a muscle relaxant is given in order to produce skeletal paralysis. A combination of drugs is normally used, as any one agent cannot produce all of the desired effects, and in this way the side-effects of each agent can be minimized. The concept of 'balanced anaesthesia' describes general anaesthesia as a balance between relaxation, hypnosis and analgesia.

General anaesthetics are usually considered in two groups:

1 inhalational anaesthetics;
2 intravenous anaesthetics.

INHALATIONAL ANAESTHETICS

PHARMACOKINETICS

Uptake and distribution

A few inhalational general anaesthetics are gases (e.g. **nitrous oxide**). However, most are volatile liquids which are administered as vapours from calibrated vaporizers (e.g. **isoflurane**). The anaesthetic vapours are carried to the patient in a mixture of nitrous oxide and oxygen or oxygen-enriched air. The concentration of an individual gas in a mixture of gases is proportional to its partial pressure or tension. It is the partial pressure of an anaesthetic agent in the brain that determines the onset of anaesthesia, and this equates with the alveolar partial pressure of that agent. The rate of induction and recovery from anaesthesia depends on a number of factors that determine the rate of transfer of anaesthetic agent from alveoli to arterial blood and from arterial blood to brain. The rate at which a given anaesthetic concentration is reached in the brain depends on the following factors:

1 anaesthetic concentration in the inspired air – increases in the inspired anaesthetic concentration will increase the rate of induction of anaesthesia by increasing the rate of transfer into the blood;

2 relative solubility in blood – the blood:gas solubility coefficient defines the relative affinity of an anaesthetic for blood compared to air. Anaesthetic agents that are not very soluble in blood have a low blood:gas solubility coefficient, and the alveolar concentration during inhalation will rise rapidly as little drug is taken up into the circulation. Agents with low blood solubility rapidly produce high arterial tensions and therefore large concentration gradients between the blood and brain. This leads to rapid induction and, on discontinuing administration, rapid recovery. Agents with a relatively high blood solubility are associated with less rapid induction and more prolonged recovery.
3 pulmonary blood flow – an increase in cardiac output results in an increase in pulmonary blood flow and more agent is removed from the alveoli, thereby slowing the rate of increase in arterial tension and making induction longer, particularly in those agents with moderate to high blood solubility. A fall in pulmonary blood flow, as occurs in shock, hastens induction.
4 pulmonary ventilation – changes in minute ventilation have little influence on induction with insoluble agents, as the alveolar concentration is always high. However, soluble agents show significant increases in alveolar tension with increased minute ventilation;
5 arteriovenous concentration gradient – the amount of anaesthetic in venous blood returning to the lungs is dependent on the rate and extent of tissue uptake. The greater the difference in tension between venous and arterial blood, the more slowly equilibrium will be achieved.

Pharmacodynamics

Mechanism of action

The molecular mechanism of action of anaesthetics is still not clearly understood. All general anaesthetics depress spontaneous and evoked activity of neurones, especially synaptic transmission in the central nervous system. They cause hyperpolarization of neurones by activating potassium and chloride channels, and this leads to an increase in action potential threshold and decreased firing. Progressive depression of ascending pathways in the reticular activating system produces complete but reversible loss of consciousness. The probable principal site of action is a hydrophobic site on specific neuronal membrane protein channels, rather than bulk perturbations in the neuronal lipid plasma membrane. Support for the theory that anaesthetics have a non-specific action on the structure of the membrane lipid matrix includes the observation that the anaesthetic potency of drugs is strongly correlated with their lipid solubility. Moreover, high atmospheric pressures (applied experimentally in animal experiments) can lead to reversal of anaesthesia, presumably as a result of reversing physical changes in cell membranes.

The relative potencies of different anaesthetics can be expressed in terms of their minimum alveolar concentration (MAC) expressed as a percentage of alveolar gas mixture at atmospheric pressure. The MAC of an anaesthetic is defined as the minimum alveolar concentration that prevents reflex response to a standard noxious stimulus in 50% of the population. MAC represents one point on the dose–response curve, but the curve for anaesthetic agents is steep, and 95% of patients will not respond to a surgical stimulus at 1.2 times MAC. Nitrous oxide has an MAC of 105% (MAC of 52.5% at 2 atmospheres, calculated using volunteers in a hyperbaric chamber) and is a weak anaesthetic agent, whereas **halothane** is a potent anaesthetic with an MAC of 0.75%. If nitrous oxide is used with halothane, it will have an additive effect on the MAC of halothane, 60% nitrous oxide reducing the MAC of halothane by 60%. The MAC of an anaesthetic is also reduced by concomitant use of opioids in the elderly, and is increased in neonates.

Commonly used inhalational anaesthetic agents include halothane, **isoflurane**, **enflurane**, **sevoflurane**, **desflurane** and nitrous oxide:

Halothane

USE

Halothane is a halogenated hydrocarbon and a potent inhalational anaesthetic. It is a clear, colourless liquid with a pleasant sweet smell. It is decomposed by light, so is stored in amber-coloured bottles. It is non-inflammable. Halothane is administered via a calibrated vaporizer; 2–4%

vapour is required for induction of anaesthesia, which is smooth as the vapour is non-irritant and 0.5–2% is required for maintenance. It is a poor analgesic, but with nitrous oxide and oxygen it is effective and convenient. It is inexpensive and widely used world-wide, although in the UK it has been replaced by isoflurane in many centres as the standard inhalational agent of first choice. Although apparently simple to use, its therapeutic index is relatively low and overdose is easily produced. Warning signs of overdose are bradycardia, hypotension and tachypnoea. Halothane produces moderate muscular relaxation, but this is rarely sufficient for major abdominal surgery. As with other volatile anaesthetics, the actions of most non-depolarizing muscle relaxants are augmented.

ADVERSE EFFECTS

1 Effects on the cardiovascular system include the following:
   - increased myocardial excitability leads to ventricular arrhythmias. Predisposing factors include hypercapnia, hypoxaemia, increase in circulatory catecholamines, atropine and sensory stimulation during light anaesthesia. Adrenaline infiltration should be avoided;
   - bradycardia mediated by the vagus;
   - halothane depresses cardiac muscle fibres and blood pressure usually falls during halothane anaesthesia, which is augmented by any bradycardia;
   - cerebral blood flow is increased, which contraindicates its use where reduction of intracranial pressure is desired (e.g. head injury, intracranial tumours).

2 Effects on respiratory system – respiratory depression commonly occurs, resulting in decreased alveolar ventilation due to a reduction in tidal volume, although the rate of breathing increases.

3 Effects on liver – there are two types of hepatic dysfunction following halothane anaesthesia. A mild subclinical hepatitis due to the reaction of halothane with hepatic macromolecules can occur, and its effects are transient. However, there is a very rare incidence of massive hepatic necrosis due to halothane. This is due to formation of a hapten–protein complex and has a mortality of 30–70%. Patients most at risk are middle-aged, obese women who have previously (within the last 28 days) had halothane anaesthesia. Halothane anaesthesia is contraindicated in those who have had jaundice or unexplained pyrexia following halothane anaesthesia, and repeat exposure is not advised within 3 months.

4 Effects on the uterus – halothane can cause uterine atony and postpartum haemorrhage.

PHARMACOKINETICS

Because of the relatively low blood:gas solubility, induction of anaesthesia is rapid but slower than the newer agents. Excretion is predominantly by exhalation, but approximately 20% is metabolized by the liver. Metabolites can be detected in the urine for up to 3 weeks following anaesthesia.

Isoflurane

USE AND ADVERSE EFFECTS

Isoflurane is an isomer of enflurane. It has a pungent smell and the vapour is irritant, making gas induction difficult. Compared to halothane and enflurane, it has less myocardial depressant effect and reduces systemic vascular resistance through vasodilation. It is popular in hypotensive anaesthesia and cardiac patients, although there is the theoretical concern of a 'coronary steal' effect in patients with ischaemic heart disease. Cerebral blood flow is little affected, and uterine tone is well preserved. Isoflurane has muscle-relaxant properties and potentiates other muscle relaxants. Isoflurane depresses respiration and is rarely associated with hepatotoxicity in individuals sensitized to halogenated anaesthetics. Isoflurane has replaced halothane as the inhalational anaesthetic of first choice for many indications in the UK.

PHARMACOKINETICS

Only desflurane and sevoflurane are less soluble volatile anaesthetics than isoflurane, and therefore it has a more rapid onset and recovery than halothane or enflurane. The rate of induction is limited by the pungency of the vapour. Because of its low solubility, isoflurane is even less metabolized than enflurane (0.17%), so fluoride accumulation is rare, and is only seen after prolonged administration (e.g. when used for sedation in intensive care).

Enflurane

USE

Enflurane is a halogenated ether and a volatile anaesthetic agent. It is less potent than halothane. Enflurane is non-irritant and does not increase airway secretions, but inhalational induction is not as smooth as with halothane. Enflurane causes muscle relaxation and potentiation of non-depolarizing muscle relaxants to a greater extent than halothane.

ADVERSE EFFECTS

1. Effects on cardiovascular system – enflurane depresses myocardial contractility more than halothane and causes a tachycardia, but sensitizes the myocardium to catecholamines less than halothane.
2. Effects on respiratory system – in common with other volatile agents, enflurane causes respiratory depression.
3. Effects on central nervous system – high concentrations (> 3%) can produce spike and wave activity in the electroencephalogram (EEG), particularly in children. Enflurane should be avoided in epileptic patients.
4. Effects on uterus – uterine tone is reduced, increasing the risk of postpartum haemorrhage.
5. Effects on kidney – transient loss of renal concentrating ability leading to polyuria has been reported following prolonged enflurane anaesthesia.
6. Effects on liver – lower risk if there is hypertoxicity compared to halothane in patients sensitized to halogenated anaesthetics.

PHARMACOKINETICS

Because of its low blood:gas solubility, enflurane has a rapid onset and recovery. Approximately 2.5% of enflurane is metabolized. This process releases free fluoride and may potentially lead to nephrotoxicity in susceptible patients.

Sevoflurane

This inhalational agent is relatively new to the UK but has been widely used in Japan. It has a sweet smell, a blood:gas solubility coefficient of 0.6 and an MAC of 2%. It has cardiovascular stability and has gained popularity for rapid and smooth gaseous induction in children, with rapid recovery. Its theoretical disadvantages are that it is 3% metabolized producing fluoride similar to enflurane. It may also react with soda lime.

Desflurane

This is also a relatively new inhalational anaesthetic agent, and is similar in structure to isoflurane. It has an MAC of 6% and a boiling point of 23.5°C, so it requires a special heated vaporizer. It has a blood:gas coefficient of 0.42, and therefore induction and recovery are faster than with any other volatile agents, allowing rapid alteration of depth of anaesthesia. It is cardiovascularly stable. It cannot be used for inhalational induction because it is irritant to the respiratory tract and has a pungent odour.

Nitrous oxide

USE

Nitrous oxide is a sweet-smelling, non-irritant gas which is compressed and stored in pressurized cylinders. It is analgesic but only a weak anaesthetic. It is commonly used in the maintenance of general anaesthetic in concentrations of 50–70% in oxygen in combination with other inhalational or intravenous agents. It can reduce the MAC value of the volatile agent by up to 65%.

A 50:50 mixture of nitrous oxide and oxygen is available as Entonox®, which is useful as a rapid recovery demand analgesic in labour, for emergency paramedics, and to cover certain painful procedures such as changing surgical dressings and removal of drainage tubes.

ADVERSE EFFECTS

1. When nitrous oxide anaesthesia is terminated, nitrous oxide diffuses out of the blood into the alveoli faster than nitrogen is taken up. This dilutes the concentration of gases in the alveoli, including oxygen, and causes hypoxia. This effect is known as diffusion hypoxia, and it is countered by the administration of 100% oxygen for 10 min.
2. Nitrous oxide in the blood equilibrates with closed gas-containing spaces inside the body, and if the amount of nitrous oxide entering a space is greater than the amount of nitrogen leaving, the volume of the space will increase. Thus pressure can increase in the gut, lungs,

middle ear and sinuses. Ear complications and tension pneumothorax may occur.

3 Prolonged use may result in megaloblastic anaemia due to interference with vitamin B_{12}, and agranulocytosis.

4 Nitrous oxide is a direct myocardial depressant, but this effect is countered by indirectly mediated sympathoadrenal stimulation.

PHARMACOKINETICS

Nitrous oxide is eliminated unchanged from the body, mostly via the lungs. Despite its high solubility in fat, most is eliminated within minutes of ceasing administration.

OCCUPATIONAL HAZARDS OF INHALATIONAL ANAESTHETICS

There is evidence to suggest that prolonged exposure to inhalational agents is hazardous to anaesthetists and other theatre personnel. Some studies have reported an increased incidence of spontaneous abortion and low-birth-weight infants among female operating-department staff. Although much of the evidence is controversial, scavenging of expired or excessive anaesthetic gases is standard practice.

Key points

Inhaled anaesthetics

Volatile liquid anaesthetics administered via calibrated vaporizers using carrier gas (air, oxygen or nitrous oxygen mixture):

- halothane;
- isoflurane;
- sevoflurane;
- enflurane;
- desflurane.

Gaseous anaesthetic

- nitrous oxide

Key points

Volatile liquid anaesthetics

- All cause dose-dependent cardiorepiratory depression.
- Halothane is convenient, inexpensive and widely used, but due to association with severe hepatotoxicity it is being superseded by isoflurane (which is also associated with less cardiac depression) in the UK.

Key points

Committee on Safety of Medicines (CSM) advice (halothane hepatoxicity)

Recommendations prior to use of halothane

1 A careful anaesthetic history should be taken to determine previous exposure and previous reactions to halothane.

2 Repeated exposure to halothane within a period of at least 3 months should be avoided unless there are overriding clinical circumstances.

3 A history of unexplained jaundice or pyrexia in a patient following exposure to halothane is an absolute contraindication to its future use in that patient.

INTRAVENOUS ANAESTHETICS

UPTAKE AND DISTRIBUTION

There is a rapid increase in plasma concentration after administration of a bolus dose of an intravenous anaesthetic agent; this is followed by a slower decline. Anaesthetic action depends on the production of sufficient brain concentration of anaesthetic. The drug has to diffuse across the blood–brain barrier from arterial blood, and this depends on a number of factors, including protein binding of the agent, blood flow to the brain, degree of ionization and lipid solubility of the drug, and the rate and volume of injection. Redistribution from blood to viscera is the main factor influencing recovery from anaesthesia following a single bolus dose of an intravenous anaesthetic. Drug diffuses from the brain along the concentration gradient into the blood. Metabolism is generally hepatic, and elimination may take many hours.

Sodium thiopentone

USE AND PHARMACOKINETICS

Sodium thiopentone is a potent general anaesthetic induction agent with a narrow therapeutic index which is devoid of analgesic properties. Recovery of consciousness occurs within 5–10 min after an intravenous bolus injection over 15. The solution for injection has a pH of 10.8 and is extremely irritant. The plasma $t_{\frac{1}{2}\beta}$ of the drug is 6 h, but the rapid course of action is explained by its high lipid solubility coupled with the rich cerebral blood flow which ensures rapid penetration into the brain. The short-lived anaesthesia results from the rapid fall (α phase) of the blood concentration, which occurs due to the distribution of drug into the tissues when the drug is transferred rapidly out of the brain to maintain equilibrium (see Figure 23.1). The main early transfer is into the muscle. In the hypovolaemia and vasoconstriction occurring in shock, this transfer is reduced and sustained high concentrations develop in the brain and heart, producing prolonged depression of these organs.

Relatively little of the drug enters fat initially because of its poor blood supply, but 30 min after injection the thiopentone concentration continues to rise in this tissue. Such absorption by fat is responsible for the termination of anaesthesia from 0.5–2 h after injection if sufficient thiopentane has been given to achieve equilibrium between the anaesthetic concentration in the brain and the concentration in the blood. Following administration of even larger doses, sustained blood levels result in prolonged anaesthesia due to saturation of tissue stores and slow metabolism. The latter only occurs at 10–15% per hour. The depth of anaesthesia depends not only on the plasma concentration but also on the duration of exposure of the brain to the drug.

Thiopentone is 75% bound to plasma proteins, and thus only about 25% of the total plasma drug concentration is in equilibrium with the extravascular fluids. Hypocapnia and the associated rise in pH increase the proportion of unbound drug, and this prolongs the anaesthetic action. Sulphonamides, aspirin and naproxen may also have the same effect. Thiopentone binding is also reduced in uraemia and hepatic failure, and this may in part explain the sensitivity of such patients to the drug.

Metabolism occurs in the liver, muscles and kidneys. The metabolites are excreted via the kidneys. Reduced doses are used in the presence of impaired liver or renal function. Thiopentone has anticonvulsant properties and may be used in refractory status epileptics (see Chapter 21).

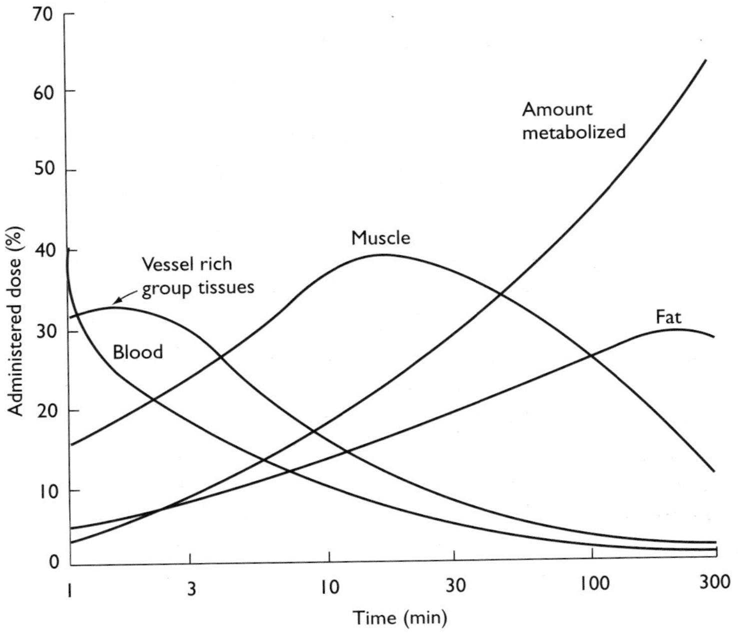

Figure 23.1: Tissue distribution of thiopentone following intravenous injection.

ADVERSE EFFECTS

1 Central nervous system – many central functions are depressed, including respiratory and cardiovascular centres. The sympathetic system is depressed to a greater extent than the parasympathetic system, and this can result in bradycardia. Thiopentone is not analgesic, and at sub-anaesthetic doses it reduces the pain threshold. Cerebral blood flow, metabolism and intracranial pressure are reduced (this is turned to advantage when thiopentone is used in neuroanaesthesia).
2 Cardiovascular system – cardiac depression and therefore cardiac output are reduced. There is dilatation of peripheral capacitance vessels with a fall in blood pressure. Severe hypotension can occur if the drug is administered in excessive dose or too rapidly, especially in hypovolaemic patients in whom cardiac arrest may occur.
3 Respiratory system – there is centrally mediated respiratory depression and a short period of apnoea is common. There is an increased tendency to laryngeal spasm if anaesthesia is light and there is increased bronchial tone.
4 Miscellaneous adverse effects – allergic reactions can manifest as urticaria or anaphylactic shock due to histamine release. Local tissue necrosis and peripheral nerve injury can occur due to accidental extravascular administration. Accidental injection into an artery causes severe burning pain due to severe arterial constriction, and can lead to ischaemia and gangrene, so must be avoided. Post-operative restlessness and nausea are common.
5 Thiopentane should be avoided or the dose reduced in patients with hypovolaemia, uraemia, hepatic disease, asthma and cardiac disease. In patients with porphyria, thiopentone (like other barbiturates) can precipitate paralysis and cardiovascular collapse.

Propofol

USES

Propofol has superseded thiopentone as an intravenous induction agent in many centres, owing to its short duration of action, anti-emetic effect and the rapid clear-headed recovery. It is formulated as a white emulsion in soya-bean oil and egg phosphatide. It is rapidly metabolized in the liver and extrahepatic sites, and has no active metabolites. Its uses include the following:

1 intravenous induction – a dose of 2–2.5 mg/kg will provide generally smooth induction of anaesthesia within 20–40 s lasting for approximately 5 min, making it especially useful for short procedures. Propofol is considered to be the drug of choice for insertion of a laryngeal mask, because of suppression of laryngeal reflexes. The lack of hangover effect makes it a popular anaesthetic agent for day surgery, although delayed convulsions have been reported.
2 maintenance of anaesthesia – propofol administered as an infusion in doses of 6–12 mg/kg/h can provide total intravenous anaesthesia (TIVA). It is often used in conjunction with oxygen or oxygen-enriched air, opioids and muscle relaxants. Although recovery is slower than that following a single dose, accumulation does not occur. It allows the use of a high concentration of oxygen in compromised patients. It is particularly useful in middle-ear surgery (where nitrous oxide is best avoided) and in patients with raised intracranial pressure (in whom volatile anaesthetics should be avoided).
3 Sedation – doses of 2–3 mg/kg/h can be used in cases where sedation is required (e.g. in intensive care, during investigative procedures or regional anaesthesia). Long-term sedation in intensive care using propofol can lead to a substantial extra calorie load (in the form of lipid), which should be accounted for if the patient is receiving parenteral nutrition.

ADVERSE EFFECTS

1 Cardiovascular system – propofol produces a greater degree of arterial hypotension than thiopentone, which is mainly due to vasodilation, although there is some myocardial depression. It should be administered particularly slowly and cautiously in patients with hypovolaemia or cardiovascular compromise. It can also cause bradycardia.
2 Respiratory system – apnoea following injection may require assisted ventilation. If opioids are also administered, as with other agents the respiratory depression is more marked.
3 Pain on injection – this is common, and the inci-

dence is reduced if a larger vein is used or lignocaine, 10 mg, is mixed with propofol.

Ketamine

USE AND PHARMACOKINETICS

Ketamine is chemically related to **phencyclidine**, and produces dissociative anaesthesia, amnesia and profound analgesia. It is a relatively safe anaesthetic and this relates to the fact that, unlike other intravenous anaesthetics, it is a respiratory and cardiac stimulant. A patent airway is maintained and it is a bronchodilator. Ketamine may also be administered by intramuscular injection, and this has proved useful when venous cannulation is difficult. Because of its ease of administration and safety, its use is widespread in countries where there are few skilled anaesthetists. It has been used for management of mass casualties or for anaesthesia of trapped patients to carry out amputations, etc.

The plasma $t_{\frac{1}{2}}$ of ketamine is 2.5–4 h. It is 5–10 times more lipid soluble than thiopentone, and rapidly passes the blood–brain barrier. An intravenous dose of 2 mg/kg produces anaesthesia within 30–60 s, which lasts for 10–15 min. An intramuscular dose of 10 mg/kg is effective within 3–4 min, and has a duration of action of 15–25 min. Unconsciousness is probably terminated by redistribution of drug from the brain to other tissues. This occurs more slowly than with thiopentone. Metabolism occurs in the liver and some of its metabolites have pharmacological activity, which may be responsible for post-anaesthetic hallucinations.

ADVERSE EFFECTS

1 Ketamine causes hallucinatory experiences of a vivid and unpleasant nature in approximately 15% of patients during recovery, often accompanied by delirium. Nightmares can occur over many months, but are thought to be uncommon in children and the elderly. The incidence of these effects can be reduced by the concomitant administration of benzodiazepines.
2 Intracranial pressure is increased by ketamine, and it is contraindicated in patients with raised intracranial pressure.
3 Blood pressure is raised by 25–30 mmHg and pulse rate by 10–15 beats/min, so ketamine should not be used in patients with hypertension, heart failure or ischaemic heart disease.
4 Salivation and muscle tone are increased.
5 Recovery is relatively slow.

Other agents

Sodium methohexitone is an intravenous anaesthetic agent, which has a more rapid recovery than thiopentone, but causes excitatory phenomena

Key points

- Intravenous anaesthetics may cause apnoea and hypotension.
- Adequate resuscitation facilities must be available.

Key points

Intravenous induction agents

All have a rapid onset of action, with propofol gradually replacing thiopentone in the UK as the usual agent of choice.

- Propofol – rapid recovery, pain on injection, bradycardia which may be avoided by use of an antimuscarinic agent, rarely anaphylaxic and causing convulsions.
- Thiopentone – smooth induction but narrow therapeutic index, cardiorespiratory depression, awakening usually rapid due to redistribution, but metabolism slow and sedative effects prolonged, very irritant injection.
- Methohexitone – barbiturate similar to thiopentone, less smooth induction, less irritant, may cause hiccup, tremor and involuntary movements.
- Etomidate – rapid recovery and less hypotensive effect than propofol and thiopentone, but painful on injection. Extraneous muscle movements and repeated doses cause adrenocortical suppression.
- Ketamine – good analgesic, increases cardiac output and muscle tone, due to unpleasant psychological effects (e.g. nightmares and hallucinations) it is restricted to high-risk patients. Useful in children (in whom CNS effects are less problematic), particularly when repeated doses may be required, and in mass disasters (relatively wide therapeutic index, may be used intramuscularly, slow recovery, safer than other agents in less experienced hands).

and pain on induction. It is commonly used during electroconvulsive therapy.

Etomidate is an intravenous anaesthetic with a rapid onset and duration of action of 2–3 min. It is thought to cause less cardiovascular depression than thiopentone in healthy patients. Its use has declined because it causes pain on injection, nausea and vomiting, and excitatory phenomena including extranenous muscle movements. Etomidate can also suppress synthesis of cortisol (see below).

SUPPLEMENTARY DRUGS

BENZODIAZEPINES

See Chapters 17 and 21.

USE

Midazolam is a water-soluble benzodiazepine which is a popular intravenous sedative. It has a more rapid onset of action than diazepam and a shorter duration of action, with a plasma half-life of 1.5–2.5 h. It is more potent than diazepam, and an initial dose should not exceed 2.5 mg and further doses should be titrated to effect. Midazolam causes amnesia, which is useful for procedures such as endoscopy or dentistry. It should not be used in repeated doses, as accumulation occurs. The use of benzodiazepines for induction of anaesthesia is usually confined to the slow induction of poor-risk patients. The prior administration of a small dose of midazolam decreases the dose of intravenous anaesthetic required for induction. Large doses can cause cardiovascular and respiratory depression. Repeated doses of midazolam accumulate and recovery is prolonged.

Diazepam has been used for induction, but large doses are required, onset is slow and full recovery is prolonged. Despite good amnesia and less cardiorespiratory depression than with the other short-acting intravenous agents, it is not popular for induction. It is mainly used for premedication (10 mg orally), sedation (5–15 mg by slow intravenous injection) and as an anticonvulsant (10–20 mg intravenously). Using a preparation made up as an emulsion in soya-bean oil has substantially reduced the incidence of thrombophlebitis with intravenous diazepam.

OPIOIDS

Opioids (see Chapter 24) in high doses have been used to induce and maintain anaesthesia in poor-risk patients undergoing major surgery. Opioids such as fentanyl provide cardiac stability and a reduction in the stress response to anaesthesia and surgery. The onset is slow and the duration of action prolonged to the extent that ventilatory support is required after the operation. A small dose of volatile anaesthetic, benzodiazepine or propofol infusion needs to be administered in order to avoid awareness even with large doses of opioids. High-dose opioids can also cause marked chest wall rigidity, which interferes with mechanical ventilation. This can be abolished by the use of muscle relaxants.

Fentanyl

Fentanyl is a synthetic opioid and is the most commonly employed analgesic supplement during anaesthesia. It is very lipid soluble, and has an onset time of 1–2 min. It is exceptionally potent, having approximately 100 times the analgesic activity of morphine. Fentanyl is rapidly and extensively metabolized, the $t_{\frac{1}{2}}$ being 2–4 h, but the short duration of action (the peak effect lasts only 20–30 min) is probably due to redistribution of drug from brain to tissues. Particular care should therefore be taken after multiple injections due to accumulation of the drug because of saturation of tissue stores. Depression of ventilation can occur for several minutes. Fentanyl and the other potent opioids must not be used in situations where ventilation cannot be controlled. Fentanyl has little cardiovascular effect, but bradycardia may occur.

Neuroleptanalgesia is produced by a combination of a butyrophenone (**droperidol**) and an opioid (fentanyl). This is a state of inactivity and reduced response to external stimuli, which can be useful in complex diagnostic procedures, although it is rarely used.

Alfentanil

This is a highly lipid-soluble derivative of fentanyl that acts in one arm-brain circulation time. It has a short duration of action of 5–10 min, and is often used as an infusion, but causes marked respiratory depression for some minutes.

Remifentanil

This is a new (μ-agonist with a rapid onset and short duration. It has an ester linkage, making it susceptible to rapid hydrolysis by a number of non-specific esterases in blood and tissues. It is administered as an infusion and does not accumulate even after a 3-h infusion. Its $t_{\frac{1}{2}}$ is 5–7 min. It is a useful adjunct to anaesthetics, particularly in patients with renal or hepatic impairment.

α_2-Adrenoceptor agonists

Clonidine has analgesic, anxiolytic and sedative properties. It reduces the dose of inhalational and intravenous anaesthetics. The reduction of MAC of anaesthetics is more marked with the more specific α_2-adrenoceptor agonist dexmetomidine, but this is not currently available in the UK. Adverse effects include hypotension and bradycardia.

Sedation in the intensive-care unit

Patients in the intensive-care unit frequently require sedative/analgesic drugs in order to facilitate controlled ventilation, to provide sedation and analgesia during painful procedures, to allay anxiety and psychological stress, and to manage confusional states. The choice of agent(s) used is tailored to meet the needs of the individual patient, and must be frequently reviewed. Most sedative and analgesic drugs are given by continuous intravenous infusion both for convenience of administration and for control. Opioids are often used to provide analgesia. They also suppress the cough reflex and are respiratory depressants, which is useful in ventilated patients. **Morphine** and fentanyl have been used for long-term sedation. **Alfentanil** has a short half-life and is given by infusion. Opioids are often combined with benzodiazepines (e.g. midazolam). Monitoring the level of sedation is particularly important in cases where long-acting opioids or benzodiazepines are being used whose action may be prolonged due to accumulation of drug and active metabolites. **Propofol** is increasingly used where short-term sedation or regular assessment is required, because its lack of accumulation results in rapid recovery. It is not recommended in children. **Etomidate** was used for intensive care sedation before it was shown to increase mortality by adrenocortical suppression. Inhalational agents such as isoflurane have also been successfully used to provide sedation. Occasionally muscle relaxants are indicated in critically ill patients to facilitate ventilation. **Atracurium** is then the drug of choice, and sedation must be adequate to avoid awareness.

Premedication for anaesthesia

Premedication was originally introduced to facilitate induction of anaesthesia with agents such as chloroform and ether that are irritant and produce copious amounts of secretions. Modern induction methods are simple and not unpleasant, and the chief aim of premedication is now to allay anxiety in the patient awaiting surgery. Oral **temazepam** is often the only premedication used before routine surgery. Adequate premedication leads to the administration of smaller doses of anaesthetic than would otherwise have been required, thereby resulting in fewer side-effects and improved recovery. Intravenous midazolam, which causes anxiolysis and amnesia, are often used. Opioids such as **morphine**, phenothiazines and muscarinic receptor antagonists (e.g. **hyoscine**) are also used. Gastric prokinetic agents, anti-emetics and H_2-receptor antagonists are used to enhance gastric emptying, decrease the incidence of nausea and vomiting, and reduce gastric acidity and volume in certain situations.

Muscle relaxants

Muscle relaxants are neuromuscular blocking drugs which cause reversible muscle paralysis. They are grouped as follows:

1 non-depolarizing agents (competitive blockers), such as **vecuronium** and **atracurium**, which bind reversibly to the postsynaptic nicotinic acetylcholine receptors on the motor end-plate, competing with acetylcholine and thereby preventing end-plate depolarization and blocking neuromuscular transmission;
2 depolarizing agents, such as **suxamethonium**, which bind acetylcholine receptors at the neuromuscular junction, but act as agonists. There is an initial depolarization and muscle contraction known as fasciculation. As this effect persists, the motor end-plate is prevented from responding normally to acetylcholine.

All muscle relaxants are highly charged molecules and do not readily pass through plasma membranes into cells. They are usually administered intravenously and are distributed throughout the body by blood flow and diffusion. Changes in muscle blood flow or cardiac output can thus alter the speed of onset of neuromuscular blockade. At the end of a procedure, the concentration of relaxant at the end-plate decreases as the drug diffuses down a concentration gradient into the plasma. At this point, the effect of non-depolarizing drugs can be reversed by the injection of an anticholinesterase such as **neostigmine**, which increases the amount of acetylcholine at the end-plate by preventing its breakdown by acetylcholinesterase. **Atropine** or **glycopyrrolate** is administered before neostigmine, to prevent the parasympathetic effects of acetylcholine by blocking muscarinic receptors.

In the presence of respiratory acidosis, myasthenic syndromes, concurrent administration of β-receptor blockers, aminoglycosides, frusemide and some tetracyclines, prolongation of neuromuscular blockade occurs. Volatile anaesthetics intensify and prolong the action of non-depolarizing muscle relaxants. The muscle relaxants have poor penetration of the placental barrier, and normal doses do not affect the fetus or cross the blood–brain barrier.

Key points

Muscle relaxants in anaesthesia

- Neuromuscular blocking drugs:
  - non-depolarizing (e.g. atracurium);
  - depolarizing (e.g. suxamethonium).
- Used to:
  - facilitate tracheal intubation;
  - relax muscles of the abdomen and diaphragm during surgery.
- Following administration, respiration must be assisted or controlled until the effects have subsided.

Non-depolarizing agents

Pancuronium bromide

Pancuronium has a peak effect at 3–4 min following an intubating dose, and duration of action of 60–90 min. It is partly metabolized by the liver, but 60% is eliminated unchanged by the kidneys, so patients with reduced renal or hepatic function show reduced elimination and prolonged neuromuscular blockade. Pancuronium has a direct vagolytic effect as well as sympathomimetic effects, which can cause tachycardia and slight hypertension. This may prove useful when it is used in cardiovascularly compromised patients. **Pipecuronium bromide** has similar actions to pancuronium, but with marked cardiovascular stability. It is only available in the USA.

Vecuronium

A full intubating dose of **vecuronium** has an onset of action within 3 min, which is slightly faster than pancuronium but slower than atracurium. The duration of action is approximately 30 min, and can usually be reversed successfully by anticholinesterases after only 15–20 min. It has minimal effect on heart rate and blood pressure, and does not generally release histamine. Vecuronium undergoes hepatic de-acetylation, and the kidneys excrete 30% of the drug.

Rocuronium bromide

This is the most recent steroid muscle relaxant to be introduced into clinical practice. Good intubating conditions are achieved within 60–90 s. **Rocuronium bromide** has the most rapid onset of any non-depolarizing muscle relaxant, and is only slightly slower than suxamethonium. The drug is similar to vecuronium, except that the duration of action is 30–45 min.

Atracurium besylate

USE

Atracurium is a non-depolarizing muscle relaxant with a rapid onset time of 2.0–2.5 min, although it is not as rapid as suxamethonium, with a duration of 20–25 min. The intubating dose is 0.5 mg/kg. Histamine release may cause flushing of the face and chest, local wheal and flare at the site of injection and, more rarely, bronchospasm and hypotension. Atracurium is cardiovascularly stable and does not accumulate. Therefore continuous infusion is popular in intensive care to facilitate intermittent positive pressure ventilation (IPPV). During long surgical cases it can provide stable and readily reversible muscle relaxation. It is unique in that it is inactivated spontaneously at body temperature and pH by Hofman elimination, a chemical process that requires neither hepatic metabolism nor renal excretion. This makes it the agent of choice for use in patients with significant hepatic and renal impairment. **Cisatracurium**, a sterioisomer of atracurium, is the most recently introduced neuromucular blocker. It is four times more potent than its parent compound and has a slightly longer duration of action. It has the advantage of causing less histamine release.

Mivacurium chloride

USE

Mivacurium has an onset time and propensity for histamine release similar to those of atracurium. Because it is metabolized by plasma cholinesterase, reversal with an anticholinesterase may not always be necessary, and recovery occurs within 20 min. It is useful for short procedures requiring muscle relaxation (e.g. oesophagoscopy) and avoids the side-effects of suxamethonium.

Key points

Non-depolarizing muscle relaxants

- Compete with acetylcholine at the neuromuscular junction.
- Action is reversed by anticholinesterases (e.g. neostigmaine) (*note that atropine or glycopyrrolate is required to prevent dangerous bradycardia and hypersalivation*).
- May cause histamine release.
- Allergic cross-reactivity has been reported.
- Prolonged effect in myasthenia gravis and hypothermia.
- Examples include atracurium, vecuronium and pancuronium (longer duration of action).

DEPOLARIZING AGENTS

Suxamethonium

USE

Suxamethonium (known as succinylcholine in the USA) is the dicholine ester of succinic acid and thus structurally resembles two molecules of acetylcholine linked together. Solutions of suxamethonium are unstable at room temperature and must be stored at 4°C. A single adult dose of 1 mg/kg administered intravenously produces rapid paralysis within 1 min with good tracheal intubating conditions. Therefore suxamethonium is particularly useful when it is important to intubate the trachea rapidly, as in patients at risk of aspiration of gastric contents and patients who may be difficult to intubate for anatomical reasons. Suxamethonium is also used to obtain short-duration muscle relaxation as needed during bronchoscopy, orthopaedic manipulation and electroconvulsive therapy. The drug is metabolized rapidly by plasma cholinesterase, and recovery begins within 3 min and is complete within 15 min. The use of an anticholinesterase such as neostigamine is contraindicated because it inhibits plasma cholinesterase.

ADVERSE REACTIONS

1 In about 1 in 2800 of the population a genetically determined abnormal plasma pseudocholinesterase is present which has poor metabolic activity (see Chapter 14). Suxamethonium undergoes slow hydrolysis by non-

specific esterases in these patients, producing prolonged apnoea, sometimes lasting for several hours. Acquired deficiency of cholinesterase may be caused by renal disease, liver disease, carcinomatosis, starvation, pregnancy and anticholinesterases. However, even very low blood cholinesterase levels acquired due to these causes only prolong suxamethonium apnoea by several minutes.

2 Muscle fasciculations are often produced several seconds after injection of suxamethonium, and are associated with muscular pains after anaesthesia. They occur in particular in patients who are muscular and those who are ambulatory soon after surgery.
3 Rarely, suxamethonium can trigger malignant hyperthermia (see below).
4 Owing to its muscarinic action, repeated doses of suxamethonium without prior administration of atropine or glycopyrrolate can cause bradycardia or asystole.
5 Suxamethonium may cause an increase in intragastric pressure; regurgitation of stomach contents is unlikely to occur with a normal lower oesophageal sphincter. It can also increase intra-ocular pressure, and its use may be contraindicated in glaucoma and open eye injuries.
6 Suxamethonium can increase the plasma potassium concentration, due to potassium released from muscle during fasciculation. This release is increased if the muscle cells are damaged, and for this reason suxamethonium is contraindicated in patients with neuropathies, myopathies or severe burns.
7 Anaphylactic reactions are rare, but do occur, especially after repeated exposure.

Key points

Depolarizing muscle relaxant – suxamethonium

- Most rapid onset of action.
- Action not reversed by anticholinesterases.
- Paralysis usually preceded by painful muscle fasciculations. Therefore it should be given immediately after induction. May result in myalgia after surgery.
- Premedication with atropine reduces bradycardia and hypersalivation.
- Prolonged paralysis in patients with low plasma cholinesterase (genetically determined).
- Contraindicated in patients with neuropathies, myopathies, or severe burns, due to risk of hyperkalaemia.

MALIGNANT HYPERTHERMIA

This is a rare autosomal-dominant inherited complication of anaesthesia. If untreated, the mortality is 80%. All of the *volatile anaesthetic agents and suxamethonium* have been implicated in its causation. It consists of a rapid increase in body temperature of 2°C per hour accompanied by tachycardia, increased carbon dioxide production and generalized muscle rigidity. Severe acidosis, hypoxia, hypercarbia and hyperkalaemia can lead to serious arrhythmias.

TREATMENT

Treatment includes the following measures.

1 Discontinue the anaesthetic and administer 100% oxygen via a vapour-free breathing system.
2 Administer **dantrolene sodium** intravenously. This inhibits excitation–contraction coupling in striated muscle by interfering with intracellular calcium mobilization, thus relieving muscle spasm. Intravenous boluses of 1 mg/kg are given as required at 5 to 10-min intervals to a maximum of 10 mg/kg.
3 Correct acidosis and treat serious arrhythmias promptly.
4 Administer of 50% glucose and insulin to correct hyperkalaemia.
5 Employ cooling measures such as tepid sponging, ice packs and cold fluids.

LOCAL ANAESTHETICS

INTRODUCTION

Local and regional techniques can be used alone to provide anaesthesia for many surgical procedures. They also offer the advantage of good-quality post-operative analgesia, especially when using continuous epidural infusions. A local anaesthetic may well be considered the method of choice for patients with severe cardiorespiratory disease, as the risks of general anaesthesia and systemic narcotic analgesics are avoided. Local anaesthetic techniques have also proved useful in combination with general anaesthesia. Local anaesthetics are substances that reversibly block impulse transmission in peripheral nerves. They have the same general structure of an aromatic group joined by an intermediate chain to an amine. The intermediate chain may be either an amide bond (e.g. lignocaine, bupivacaine, and prilocaine) or an ester (e.g. cocaine, amethocaine). Local anaesthetics are injected in their ionized water-soluble form, and in tissues a proportion of the drug dissociates to lipid-soluble unionized free base. The free base is able to cross neuronal lipid membrane, where reionization takes place. The reionized portion then enters and blocks sodium channels. As sodium ions cannot enter the cell, no nerve action potential is generated or propagated. Esters are rapidly metabolized by plasma cholinesterase, and amides are metabolized by liver amidases, the tissue concentration decreasing below that in the nerves and drug diffusing out, restoring the normal function of nerves. Local anaesthetics depress small unmyelinated fibres first and larger myelinated fibres last. The order of loss of function is therefore as follows:

1 pain;
2 temperature;
3 touch;
4 motor function.

Systemic toxicity

Inadvertent intravascular injection is the most common cause of systemic toxicity. Therefore careful aspiration is vital before injection. Toxicity may result from absolute overdose, so recommended safe doses should not be exceeded. Early signs are circumoral numbness and tingling, which may be followed by drowsiness, anxiety and tinnitus. In severe cases there is loss of consciousness, and there may be convulsions with subsequent coma, apnoea and cardiovascular collapse. The addition of a vasoconstrictor such as adrenaline to a local anaesthetic solution slows the rate of absorption, prolongs duration and reduces toxicity. The concentration of adrenaline should not be greater than 1:200 000. Preparations containing adrenaline are *contraindicated* for injection close to end-arteries ('ring' blocks of the digits and penis) because of the risk of vasospasm and consequent ischaemia.

Lignocaine

Lignocaine is the most widely used local anaesthetic in the UK (its use as an anti-arrhythmic drug is discussed in Chapter 31). It has a quick onset and medium duration of action, potency and toxicity. It is available as an injectable hydrochloride salt in 0.5–2.0% solution. Lignocaine is also available as 2–4% gel or aerosol preparations for topical use. Lignocaine may be used in all forms of local anaesthesia, although its most frequent use is for local infiltration or applied topically as a gel or drops to mucous membranes. Lignocaine does not affect vascular smooth muscle, but is available in combination with adrenaline, which causes vasoconstriction and hence prolongs its duration of action from 1 to 2 h. Toxicity (see Chapter 31) is uncommon after lignocaine is used as a local anaesthetic, but cardiovascular and central nervous complications can occur. The recommended maximum safe dose for local administration is 3 mg/kg without adrenaline and 6 mg/kg with adrenaline. Absorption following topical application can be rapid (e.g. from the larynx, bronchi or urethra), and levels in the plasma may be reached similar to those after intravenous injection. Systemic allergy is uncommon.

Prilocaine

Prilocaine is similar to lignocaine, but its clearance is more rapid, so it is less toxic. It is most useful when a large total amount of local anaesthetic is needed or a high plasma concentration is likely, (e.g. injection into vascular areas such as the perineum) or for use in intravenous regional anaesthesia (e.g. Biers' block). Prilocaine is available as 0.5–2.0% injectable solution and, for topical analgesia, as a 4% solution. EMLA is a eutectic mixture of local anaesthetic and is a combination of equal amounts of crystalline 2.5% prilocaine and 2.5 % lignocaine in the form of a cream. If applied topically for 30–60 mins and covered with an occlusive dressing it provides reliable anaesthesia for venepuncture or skin grafting. In dental procedures prilocaine is often used with the peptide vasoconstrictor **felypressin**. Excessive doses can lead to systemic toxicity, dependent on plasma concentration, and the maximum safe dose is approximately 600 mg.

Prilocaine is metabolized by amidases in the liver, kidney and lungs. The rapid production of oxidation products may rarely give rise to methaemoglobinaemia. This is of clinical importance only if there is severe anaemia or circulatory failure, and the treatment is methylene blue (1 mg/kg).

Bupivacaine

Bupivacaine is a long-acting amide local anaesthetic commonly used for epidural and spinal anaesthesia. Bupivacaine hydrochloride is available as a 0.25–0.75% solution. Although it has a slower onset of action, peripheral nerve and plexus blockade with 0.5% bupivacaine can have a duration of action of 5–12 h. Epidural blockade is much shorter, at about 2 h, but is still longer than for lignocaine. The relatively short duration of epidural block is related to the high vascularity of the epidural space and consequent rapid uptake of anaesthetic into the bloodstream. Bupivacaine is the agent of choice for continuous epidural blockade in obstetrics, as the rise in maternal (and therefore fetal) plasma concentration occurs less rapidly than with lignocaine. Increasing the concentration of bupivacaine increases the motor nerve block; dilute solutions of 0.1% bupivacaine combined with an opioid such as fentanyl have been used to provide satisfactory epidural analgesia without motor block. Bupivacaine has a mild vasodilator action that makes the addition of adrenaline less effective than with lignocaine. Therefore the maximum recommended dose is 2 mg/kg with or without adrenaline. Although the acute central nervous system toxicity of bupivacaine is similar to that of lignocaine, it is thought to be more toxic to the myocardium. The first sign of toxicity can be cardiac arrest from ventricular fibrillation, which is often resistant to defibrillation.

Ropivicaine

This new local anaesthetic is the propyl homologue of bupivacaine, and is the only local anaesthetic that occurs in a single enantiomeric form. It is marginally less potent than bupivacaine, with a slightly shorter duration of action. Its advantages are that it produces less motor block and cardiac toxicity.

Cocaine

The use of cocaine (see also Chapter 53) as a local anaesthetic is restricted to topical application in ear, nose and throat (ENT) procedures because of its adverse effects. Acute intoxication can occur, consisting of restlessness, anxiety, confusion, tachycardia, angina, cardiovascular collapse, convulsions, coma and death. In the central nervous system, initial stimulation gives rise to excitement and raised blood pressure followed by vomiting. This may be followed by fits and CNS depression. Cocaine is an ester, so has a tendency to cause allergic reactions, and it is also a drug of addiction. It causes vasoconstriction, so the addition of adrenaline is not recommended. The safe dose for surface analgesia is 1.5 mg/kg, with a maximum total of 100 mg.

Benzocaine

Benzocaine is a topical anaesthetic which is comparatively non-irritant and has low toxicity. Compound benzocaine lozenges (containing 10 mg benzocaine) are used to alleviate the pain of local oral lesions such as aphthous ulcers, lacerations and carcinoma of the mouth.

Amethocaine

The use of this drug in the UK is restricted to topical application, especially in ophthalmic surgery. The 4% gel has also proved useful for anaesthetiz-

Key points

Toxicity of local anaesthetics

- Inadvertent intravenous injection may lead to convulsions and cardiovascular collapse.
- Initial symptoms of overdose (excess local dose resulting in high plasma concentrations and systemic toxicity) may include light-headedness, sedation, circumoral paraesthesia and twitching.
- The total dose of lignocaine should not exceed 200 mg (or 500 mg if given in solutions containing adrenaline).

Case history

An 18-year-old girl who had recently commenced the oral contraceptive was admitted with abdominal pain and proceeded to have a laparotomy. Anaesthesia was induced using thiopentone and suxamethonium, and was maintained with isoflurane. A normal appendix was removed. Post-operatively the patient's abdominal pain worsened, and was not significantly improved with a morphine injection. A nurse reported that the patient's urine appeared dark in colour and her blood pressure was high.

Question

What is the likely post-operative diagnosis, and what may have precipitated this?

Answer

Acute intermittent porphyria in association with:

- oral contraceptive pill;
- thiopentone.

Opiates such as morphine and pethidine are thought to be safe in porphyria. (Ectopic pregnancies should always be considered in sexually active female patients with abdominal pain..)

ing the skin for venepuncture. However, amethocaine is popular in the USA (where it is known as tetracaine) for use in spinal anaesthesia because of its potency and long duration of action.

Chloroprocaine

This local anaesthetic agent is claimed to have the most rapid onset of all, and has low toxicity. Although not available in the UK, it is widely used in North America.

Further reading

Aitkenhead AR, Jones RM. 1995: *Clinical anaesthesia.* Edinburgh: Churchill Livingstone.

McKinnon RP, Wildsmith JAW, 1995: Histaminoid reactions to anaesthesia. *British Journal of Anaesthesia* **74**, 217–28.

Wiklund RA, Rosenbaum SH 1997: Anaesthesiology. *New England Journal of Medicine* **337**, 1132–41.

CHAPTER TWENTY-FOUR

ANALGESICS *and the* CONTROL *of* PAIN

- Introduction
- Mechanism of pain
- Potential sites of action of analgesics
- Analgesics in terminal disease
- Management of post-operative pain
- Drugs used to treat mild or moderate pain
- Drugs for severe pain
- Opioid antagonists

INTRODUCTION

Pain is a common symptom and is important because it both signals 'disease' (in the broadest sense) and aids diagnosis. However, by definition it is a wretched sensation, and its relief is one of the most important duties of a doctor. Fortunately, pain relief was one of the earliest triumphs of pharmacology, although less happily physicians and nurses have only recently started to use the drugs that are available adequately and rationally.

MECHANISM OF PAIN

Pain is usually triggered by a potentially harmful peripheral stimulus. The perception of such stimuli is termed nociception, and is not quite the same as the subjective experience of pain, which contains a strong central and emotional component. Consequently, the intensity of pain is often poorly correlated with the intensity of the nociceptive stimulus, and many clinical states associated with pain are due to a derangement of the central processing of afferent information such that a stimulus that is innocuous is perceived as painful. *Trigeminal neuralgia* is an extreme example where a minimal mechanical stimulus to the face can trigger excruciating pain. *Post-operative* pain provides a striking demonstration of the importance of higher functions in the perception of pain. When patients are provided with devices that enable them to control their own analgesia (see below), they report superior pain relief but use less analgesic medication than when this is administered by nursing staff.

The afferent nerve fibres involved in nociception consist of slowly conducting unmyelinated C-fibres that are activated by stimuli of various kinds (mechanical, thermal and chemical) and fine myelinated (Aδ) fibres that conduct more rapidly but respond to similar stimuli. These afferents synapse in the dorsal horn of grey matter in the spinal cord in laminae I, V and II (the substantia gelatinosa). The cells in laminae I and V cross over and project to the contralateral thalamus, whereas cells in the substantia gelatinosa have short projections to laminae I and V and function as a 'gate', inhibiting transmission of impulses from the primary afferent fibres. The gate provided by the substantia gelatinosa can also be activated centrally by descending pathways. There is a similar gate mechanism in the thalamus. Descending inhibitory controls are very important, a key component being the small region of grey matter in the mid-brain known as the periaqueductal grey (PAG). Electrical stimulation of the PAG causes profound analgesia. The main pathway from this area runs to the nucleus raphe magnus in the medulla, and thence back to the dorsal horn of the cord connecting with the interneurones involved in nociception.

Stimulation of nociceptive endings in the periphery is predominantly chemically mediated. *Bradykinin, prostaglandins* and various neurotransmitters (e.g. 5-hydroxytryptamine, 5HT) and metabolites (e.g. lactate) or ions (e.g. K^+) released from damaged tissue have been implicated. **Capsaicin**, the active principle of red peppers, potently stimulates and then desensitizes nociceptors. The neurotransmitters of the primary nociceptor fibres include fast neurotransmitters – including glutamate and probably adenosine triphosphate (ATP) – and various neuropeptides – including substance P and calcitonin gene-related peptide (CGRP), whose function is uncertain. Neurotransmitters that are known to play a part in modulating the nociceptive pathway include opioid peptides (metenkephalin and β-endorphin) (which are present in the substantia gelatinosa, the PAG and the nucleus raphe magnus), 5HT (which is the transmitter of the axons running from the nucleus raphe magnus to the dorsal horn) and noradrenaline (which is the transmitter of inhibitory fibres running from the locus ceruleus to the dorsal horn).

Potential sites of action of analgesics

Drugs can inhibit pain by acting either peripherally or centrally as follows:

- at the site of injury by interfering with the chemical mediators involved in nociception (e.g. inhibition of prostaglandin synthesis by the non-steroidal anti-inflammatory drugs, NSAIDs);
- transmission in peripheral nerves, as with local anaesthetics;
- transmission in the dorsal horn and thalamus. This explains some of the actions of opioids and of **nefopam** and some of the antidepressants that inhibit axonal reuptake of 5HT and noradrenaline. It is also believed to account for the effect of vibromassage, transcutaneous electrical nerve stimulation (TENS) and perhaps acupuncture;
- pathways involved in the central appreciation of pain. This is an important mode of action of the opioids, and may also contribute to the analgesic action of antidepressants.

> **Key points**
>
> Mechanisms of pain and actions of analgesic drugs
>
> - Nociception and pain involve peripheral and central mechanisms; 'gating' mechanisms in the spinal cord and thalamus are key features.
> - Pain differs from nociception because of central mechanisms, including an emotional component.
> - Many mediators are implicated, including prostaglandins, various peptides that act on μ receptors (including endorphins), 5HT and noradrenaline.
> - Analgesics inhibit, mimic or potentiate natural mediators (e.g. aspirin inhibits prostaglandin biosynthesis, morphine acts on μ-receptors, and nefopam and tricyclic drugs block neuronal amine uptake).

Analgesics in terminal disease

The relief of pain in terminal disease, usually cancer, requires skilful use of analgesic drugs.

1. **Morphine** (or a congener) is the key treatment for severe pain.
2. It is important to use a large enough dose, if necessary given intravenously or intramuscularly, to relieve the pain completely. There is an extraordinarily wide range (about 1000-fold variation) in dose needed to suppress pain in different individuals, but very few patients need very high doses, and most need 200 mg/day or less of oral morphine.
3. Drug dependence is *not* a problem in this type of patient.
4. It is much easier to keep the patient free from pain than to relieve pain and its attendant anxiety when it has fully developed.
5. If possible, use oral medication, and once pain control is established (e.g. with frequent doses of morphine elixir by mouth) change to a slow-release morphine preparation. In addition to convenience, this produces a smoother control of pain, without peaks and troughs of analgesia.

6 Tolerance is *not* a problem in this setting, the dose being increased until pain relief is obtained.

A variety of analgesic drugs may be used depending on the severity of the pain and the preference of the patient. The World Health Organization (WHO) has endorsed a simple stepwise approach of moving from non-opioid to weak opioid to strong opioid. For mild pain, **paracetamol**, **aspirin** or **codeine** (a weak opioid) or a combined preparation (e.g. **cocodamol**) are usually satisfactory.

Bone pain is often most effectively relieved by local radiotherapy rather than by drugs, but non-steroidal anti-inflammatory drugs are useful in some patients in whom such pain is partly prostaglandin mediated, and they reduce opioid requirements in such patients. **Buprenorphine**, dissolved under the tongue, is useful for more severe pain and it has the advantage of a rather longer action than most powerful analgesics, but should not be combined with other opioids because it is a partial agonist (see below).

For short-term analgesia to cover dressings, etc., **dextromoramide** administered orally or by injection is effective for 2–3 h. For severe pain, morphine or **diamorphine** are the drugs of choice. Their use is described in the sections on these drugs below. Doses are adjusted so that the patient is kept pain-free. Rarely, because of vomiting or the severity of the pain, morphine has to be given by injection, but such nausea and vomiting often resolve after a few days. **Chlorpromazine** or **prochlorperazine** can be used to reduce nausea and vomiting, and may increase analgesia. Narcotic drugs are constipating and suppress appetite, which is often very poor. Despite hydration and as much fibre as can be tolerated in the form of fruit and vegetables, patients inevitably require a stimulant laxative such as **senna**, and/or glycerine suppositories. Spinal administration of opioids is not routinely available, but is sometimes useful for those few patients with opioid-responsive pain who experience intolerable systemic side-effects when morphine is given orally. Perhaps around 25% of patients with terminal cancer have some degree of endogenous depression. A trial of an antidepressant is worthwhile if this is suspected, starting with a low dose which is increased gradually.

Key points

Analgesics in terminal care

- Stepwise use of non-opioid (e.g. paracetomol)/weak opioid (e.g. codeine)/strong opioid (e.g. morphine) is rational when the patient presents with mild symptoms.
- In cases where severe pain is already established, parenteral morphine is often needed initially, followed by regular frequent doses of morphine elixir by mouth with additional ('top-up') doses prescribed as needed, followed by conversion to an effective dose of long-acting (slow-release) oral morphine, individualized to the patient's requirements.
- Chronic morphine necessitates adjunctive treatment with:
  - anti-emetic;
  - laxative.
- Additional measures that are often useful include:
  - radiotherapy (for painful metastases);
  - a cyclo-oxygenase inhibitor (especially with bone involvement);
  - an antidepressant.

MANAGEMENT OF POSTOPERATIVE PAIN

Unfortunately, post-operative pain has traditionally been managed by analgesics prescribed by the most inexperienced surgical staff and administered at the discretion of nursing staff. Recently, anaesthetists have become more involved in the management of post-operative pain, and pain teams have led to notable improvements. There are several general principles.

1 Surgery results in pain as the anaesthetic wears off. This causes fear in the patient, reinforcing anxieties about his or her illness and about the hospital environment, and thus making the pain worse. This vicious circle can be avoided by time spent pre-operatively explaining the procedure, and giving reassurance that pain is expected, will be transient and will be controlled.

2 Analgesics are always more effective in preventing the development of pain than in treating it when it has developed. Regular use

of mild analgesics can be highly effective. Non-steroidal anti-inflammatory drugs (e.g. **ketorolac**, which can be given parenterally) can have comparable efficacy to opioids when used in this way. They are particularly useful after orthopaedic surgery.

3 Parenteral administration is usually only necessary for a short time post-operatively, after which analgesics can be given orally. If suitable devices are available, the best way to give parenteral opioid analgesia is often by intravenous or subcutaneous infusion under control of the patient ('patient-controlled analgesia,' PCA). Opioids are effective in visceral pain, and are especially valuable after abdominal surgery. Some operations (e.g. cardiothoracic surgery) cause both visceral and somatic pain, and regular prescription of both an opioid and a non-opioid analgesic is appropriate. Once drugs can be taken by mouth, slow-release morphine, **meptazinol** or buprenorphine prescribed on a regular basis are effective. Breakthrough pain can be treated by additional oral or parenteral doses of morphine.

4 **Pethidine** does not cause bronchoconstriction, and is therefore more suitable for asthmatics than morphine, which causes bronchoconstriction via liberation of histamine. However, pethidene must still be used with great care in such patients because of its respiratory depressant action. Nefopam is useful when respiratory depression is a particular concern.

5 Anti-emetics (e.g. **metoclopramide**, prochlorperazine) should be routinely prescribed on an 'as-needed' basis. They are only required by a minority of patients, but should be available without delay when needed.

6 A nitrous oxide/oxygen mixture (50/50) can be self-administered and is useful during painful procedures such as dressing changes or physiotherapy, and in obstetrics. It should not be used for very prolonged periods (e.g. in intensive-care units), as it can cause vitamin B_{12} deficiency in this setting.

Key points

Analgesia and post-operative pain

- Pre-operative explanation minimizes analgesic requirements.
- Prevention of post-operative pain is initiated during anaesthesia (e.g. local anaesthetics, parenteral cyclo-oxygenase inhibitor).
- Patient-controlled analgesia using morphine is safe and effective.
- The switch to oral analgesia should be made as soon as possible.
- Anti-emetics should be written up on the 'as needed' part of the prescription chart, to avoid delay if they are required.

DRUGS USED TO TREAT MILD OR MODERATE PAIN

Paracetamol

USES

Paracetamol is an antipyretic and mild analgesic with few, if any anti-inflammatory properties and no antiplatelet action. It has no irritant effect on the gastric mucosa and can be used in in individuals who are intolerant of aspirin. It is useful in paediatrics since, unlike aspirin, it has not been associated with Reye's syndrome and can be formulated as a stable suspension. The usual adult dose is 0.5–1 g repeated at intervals of 4–6 h if needed.

MECHANISM OF ACTION

Paracetamol inhibits prostaglandin biosynthesis, but by a different mechanism to aspirin and the other NSAIDs. Prostaglandin biosynthesis requires the presence of peroxides as cofactors for the action of cyclo-oxygenase, and paracetamol reduces peroxide tone. This effectively prevents prostaglandin biosynthesis in tissues where the peroxide concentration is low (e.g. brain), but not where it is high (e.g. at sites of inflammation, especially in the presence of pus).

ADVERSE EFFECTS

Rashes and blood dyscrasias have been reported, but are rare. There is no evidence of nephrotoxicity following short-term therapeutic use. The most important toxic effect is hepatic necrosis leading to liver failure after overdose, but renal failure in the absence of liver failure has also been reported after overdose. There is no convincing evidence

Renal failure can occur without hepatic failure.

that paracetamol causes chronic liver disease when used regularly in therapeutic doses, earlier reports that it does so probably being attributable to concomitant alcohol abuse. Paracetamol is structurally closely related to phenacetin, raising the question of whether its long-term abuse causes analgesic nephropathy, an issue which is as yet unresolved. In any event, long-term use of large doses is to be discouraged.

PHARMACOKINETICS, METABOLISM AND INTERACTIONS

Absorption of paracetamol following oral administration is increased by concomitant administration of metoclopramide, and there is a significant relationship between gastric emptying and absorption. Paracetamol is rapidly metabolized in the liver and has a plasma ($t_{\frac{1}{2}}$) of 75–180 min. Sulphate and glucuronide conjugates are excreted in the urine accompanied by 1–4% unchanged drug. When paracetamol is taken in *overdose* (see Chapter 53) the capacity of the conjugating mechanisms is exceeded, the plasma $t_{\frac{1}{2}}$ of paracetamol is increased, and a reactive metabolite, N-acetyl benzoquinone imine (NABQI), is formed by a cytochrome P_{450}-dependent metabolic pathway. NABQI is extremely toxic and causes hepatocellular damage unless it is inactivated by conjugation with reduced glutathione. This is the reason for giving **acetylcysteine** to such patients (see Chapter 53), as this repletes the supply of reduced glutathione in the liver.

Aspirin

USE

Antiplatelet uses of aspirin are described in Chapters 28 and 29. As an *antipyretic* and *mild analgesic* it has similar efficacy to paracetamol. However, unlike paracetamol it has anti-inflammatory properties, especially when used in high doses (3.6 g daily or more), and is useful in disorders (including rheumatic fever) where there is an inflammatory component. The dose of aspirin varies, depending on the type of pain being treated. For minor pain the usual dose for an adult is 600 mg repeated 4- to 6-hourly if required, taken after food. Various preparations are available, including regular as well as buffered, soluble and enteric-coated forms. Enteric coating is intended to reduce local gastric irritation, but these preparations have variable bioavailability, and much of the gastric toxicity of aspirin is due to inhibition of prostaglandin biosynthesis (see below), rather than to direct gastric irritation. Consequently, slow-release preparations do not obviate the adverse effects of aspirin on the gastric mucosa, although symptoms from direct irritation may be less troublesome in some individuals. The same applies to **benorylate**, a prodrug ester of aspirin with paracetamol.

MECHANISM OF ACTION

Salicylates exert their major analgesic and anti-inflammatory effects by inhibition of prostaglandin biosynthesis. Their antipyretic effect is due to inhibition of the synthesis of prostaglandins E_2 and D_2 in the hypothalamus, which is the site of temperature regulation. Aspirin inhibits cyclo-oxygenase irreversibly by acetylating a serine residue in the active site. There are two isoforms of cyclo-oxygenase (COX-1 and COX-2). COX-1 is a constitutive enzyme which is present in platelets and other cells under basal conditions. COX-2 is an inducible form of the enzyme, which is produced in response to cytokine stimulation in areas of inflammation, and produces very large amounts of prostaglandins. Acetylation of serine in COX-1 prevents access of substrate (arachidonic acid) to the active site. By contrast, COX-2 can still metabolize arachidonic acid after it has reacted with aspirin, but the product is another fatty acid and not a prostaglandin. Salicylic acid (to which aspirin is metabolized) and other salicylates inhibit the enzyme reversibly, and less potently than does aspirin. In *overdose*, (see Chapter 53) salicylates increase respiration by a direct stimulant action on the respiratory centre, and they also uncouple oxidative phosphorylation, leading to inefficient cellular respiration, lactic acidosis and fever.

ADVERSE EFFECTS AND CONTRAINDICATIONS

These include the folowing:

1 *salicylism* – toxic doses of salicylates cause tinnitus, deafness, nausea, vomiting and occasionally abdominal pain and flushing;
2 regular use of aspirin frequently causes *dyspepsia*. Blood loss from the stomach can be life-threatening. With prolonged treatment, chronic low-grade gastrointestinal blood loss may be

sufficient to cause iron-deficiency anaemia. The mechanism of the gastrotoxicity of aspirin is inhibition of gastric prostaglandin (PGE_2) biosynthesis. PGE_2 is the main prostaglandin made by the human stomach, which it protects in several ways. It inhibits acid secretion, stimulates mucus secretion and increases the clearance of acid that has diffused into the submucosa by causing local vasodilatation. Aspirin and other NSAIDs damage the stomach by impairing these protective mechanisms, and perhaps also by damaging the mucosal barrier directly. Aspirin should not be given to patients with active peptic ulceration;

3 *Aspirin-sensitive asthma* (which occurs in approximately 2% of asthmatics; see Chapter 32) is associated with the presence of nasal polyps and similar reactions to other NSAIDs, tartrazine (a yellow food dye) and sometimes (but not always) paracetamol. The mechanism of this adverse effect is evidently linked to the pharmacological action of aspirin rather than to an allergic reaction to the drug. An individual who is aspirin sensitive is predictably sensitive to structurally unrelated NSAIDs that share its pharmacological effect on cyclo-oxygenase. It is probably related to an alteration in the proportions of cyclo-oxygenase products (prostaglandins) to lipoxygenase products (leukotrienes) in the lung (see Chapter 32).

4 *gout* – due to reduced uric acid excretion as a result of inhibition of tubular urate secretion (conversely, high doses of salicylates are uricosuric because of inhibition of tubular urate reabsorption, but this is not clinically useful);

5 hepatitis, especially in patients with systemic lupus erythematosus and other connective tissue disorders. This is dose dependent. The main changes are elevation of the serum enzymes. Histological change is minimal, and liver function tests revert to normal on stopping the drug;

6 Reye's syndrome, a rare disease of children, with high mortality, is characterized by hepatic failure and encephalopathy, often occurring in the setting of a viral illness. The cause of its epidemiological association with aspirin use is not known.

PHARMACOKINETICS

The gastrointestinal absorption of salicylates is rapid, with an apparent absorption $t_{\frac{1}{2}}$ of soluble aspirin of 5–15 min. Aspirin is subject to considerable presystemic metabolism to salicylate, so the plasma concentration of aspirin is much lower than that of salicylate following an oral dose (Figure 24.1). Some of the selectivity of aspirin for platelet cyclo-oxygenase is probably due to exposure of platelets to high concentrations of aspirin in portal blood, whereas tissues are exposed to the lower concentrations present in the systemic circulation. Salicylates are extensively bound (80–85%) to plasma albumin. Salicylate is metabolized in the liver by five main parallel pathways, two of which are saturable (Michaelis–Menten kinetics), and is also excreted unchanged in the urine by a first-order process. This is summarized in Figure 24.2. The formation of salicylurate is of interest since it is one of the relatively few drug metabolism processes that occur in mitochondria, and is easily saturable. Consequently, salicylate has dose-dependent (non-linear) kinetics at high therapeutic doses or after overdose. Urinary elim-

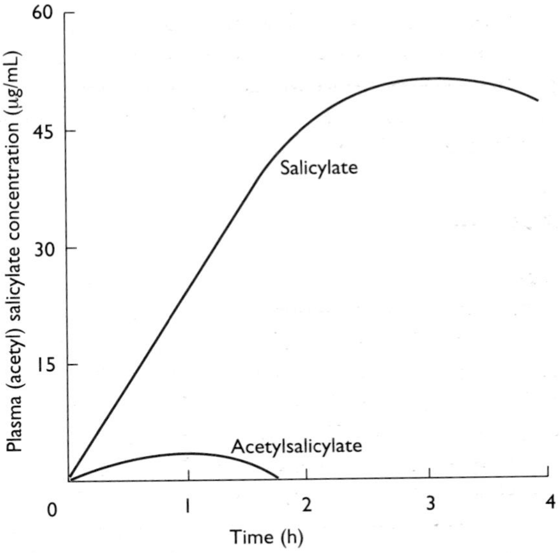

Figure 24.1: Plasma levels of salicylate and acetylsalicylate following 640 mg aspirin given orally, demonstrating rapid conversion of acetylsalicylate to salicylate.

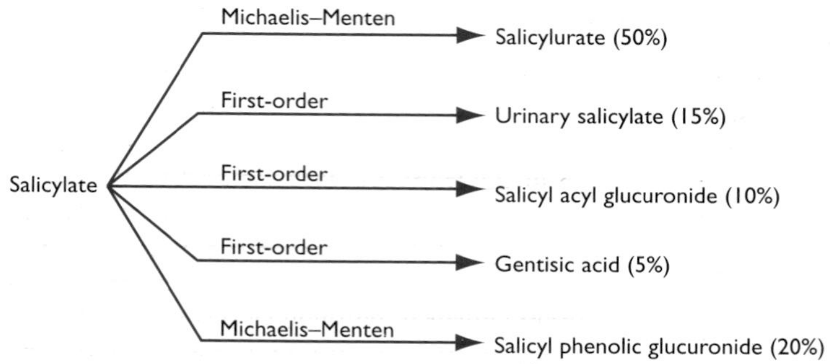

Figure 24.2: The main pathways of salicylate metabolism.

ination of salicylate is influenced by pH, being more rapid in alkaline urine, which favours the charged (polar) anionic form that is not reabsorbed, rather than the free acid (see Chapter 6). This property is utilized in the treatment of salicylate overdose by alkalinization of the urine by administration of sodium bicarbonate (see Chapter 53).

DRUG INTERACTIONS

Misoprostol, a prostaglandin E analogue, or acid suppressant drugs, may permit aspirin to be tolerated by individuals who would otherwise experience unacceptable dyspepsia. Salicylates potentiate gastric irritation by alcohol, and also potentiate the effects of some oral hypoglycaemic agents (see Chapter 36). They increase the risk of bleeding in patients receiving oral anticoagulants by their effects on platelets, their gastrotoxicity and, in overdose, by a hypoprothrombinaemic effect. Aspirin should not be given to neonates with hyperbilirubinaemia because of the risk of kernicterus as a result of displacement of bilirubin from its binding site on plasma albumin (see Chapter 13).

IBUPROFEN

Ibuprofen has a similar analgesic potency to paracetamol and, in addition, has useful anti-inflammatory activity, so it is an alternative to aspirin for painful conditions with an inflammatory component (e.g. sprains and minor soft tissue injury). It is also useful in dysmenorrhoea. It is a reversible cyclo-oxygenase inhibitor, but causes rather less gastric irritation than aspirin and other NSAIDs at normal doses, and is available over the counter in the UK. The usual dose is 400–800 mg three times a day after food. A suspension is available for use in children. It is not recommended in the more severe inflammatory disorders such as gout. It can cause other adverse reactions common to the NSAIDs, including reversible renal impairment in patients with cirrhosis, nephrotic syndrome or heart failure, and it reduces the efficacy of antihypertensive medication and of diuretics by a non-specific pharmacodynamic interaction.

Topical non-steroidal anti-inflammatory drugs

Several NSAIDs (incuding ibuprofen and **piroxicam**) are available as topical preparations. Systemic absorption does occur, but is modest. Their effectiveness in soft tissue injuries and other localized inflammatory conditions is modest. They occasionally cause local irritation of the skin, but adverse effects are otherwise uncommon.

Nefopam

USE

Nefopam is chemically and pharmacologically unrelated to other analgesics, being a cyclized analogue of orphenadrine. It is used for moderately severe pain, being intermediate in potency between aspirin and morphine. Unlike the NSAIDs, it does not injure the gastric mucosa. It is less of a respiratory depressant than the opioids, and does not cause dependence. It is used in postoperative or acute pain, and in the relief of cancer pain, and is particularly useful in patients in whom the levels of respiratory depression caused by opioids is unacceptable. It is more expensive than opioids or NSAIDs. The usual dose is in the range 30–90 mg by mouth three times a day, adjusted according to response. The usual intramuscular dose is 20 mg every 8 h.

MECHANISM OF ACTION

Nefopam is a potent inhibitor of uptake of 5HT, noradrenaline and dopamine by nerve terminals, and it potentiates descending 5HT and other aminergic pathways that operate the gate mechanism for pain described above. When given intravenously it has mild positive chronotropic and inotropic effects due to potentiation of endogenous catecholamines. It has activity in some animal models that suggests it may have antidepressant activity, in common with other 5HT reuptake inhibitors that are marketed for this indication (e.g. sertraline). In higher concentrations it has antimuscarinic activity, which accounts for some of its adverse effects.

ADVERSE EFFECTS AND CONTRAINDICATIONS

Nefopam has few severe (life-threatening) effects, although convulsions, cerebral oedema and fatality can result from massive overdose. It is contraindicated in patients with a history of epilepsy, and also in patients receiving monoamine oxidase inhibitors (see below). It should not be used in acute myocardial infarction, as it increases myocardial oxygen demand and may also be pro-arrhythmogenic. In contrast to the relative paucity of severe adverse effects, nefopam causes a high incidence of minor adverse effects, especially after parenteral use. These include sweating, nausea, headache, dry mouth, insomnia, dizziness and anorexia. Nefopam is contraindicated in glaucoma, and can cause urinary retention in men with prostatic hypertrophy. Neither tolerance nor drug dependence has been demonstrated.

PHARMACOKINETICS

Nefopam is rapidly absorbed (within 15–30 min) following oral administration. The plasma $t_{\frac{1}{2}}$ is 4–8 h. It is extensively metabolized by the liver to inactive compounds excreted in the urine. Presystemic metabolism is substantial.

Drug interactions

Nefopam can cause potentially fatal hypertension with monoamine oxidase inhibitors (MAOIs), and potentiates the arrhythmogenic effect of halothane.

Combined analgesic tablets

A large number of fixed combinations of analgesics are marketed, and a number of problems are associated with them. **Coproxamol** is a combination of **dextropropoxyphene** and paracetamol. Dextropropoxyphene is structurally similar to **methadone**, but it is a weaker analgesic. Its elimination $t_{\frac{1}{2}}$ is 12–24 h and the $t_{\frac{1}{2}}$ of its active metabolite norpropoxyphene is 24–48 h. Although the combination is very widely used, there is no clear evidence that it is superior to other mild

Key points

Drugs for mild pain

- The main drugs for mild pain are paracetamol, aspirin and ibuprofen.
- These work by inhibiting prostaglandin synthesis, and are available over the counter.
- Paracetamol:
  - is analgesic;
  - is antipyretic but not anti-inflammatory;
  - lacks gastric toxicity, and can be used safely in children;
  - does not cause bleeding;
  - is dangerous in overdose via a toxic metabolite (N-acetyl-β-benzoquinone imine, NABQI)
- Aspirin:
  - is anti-inflammatory as well as analgesic and antipyretic;
  - is uniquely useful for its antiplatelet effect (see Chapters 28 and 29);
  - is a common cause of indigestion, and severe gastrointestinal bleeding can occur;
  - is associated with Reye's syndrome in children;
  - is dangerous in overdose (salicylate toxicity).
- Ibuprofen:
  - is similar as an analgesic to aspirin, but is preferred by some patients (e.g. for dysmenorrhoea);
  - is not proven to have a clinically useful antiplatelet effect.
- Topical NASIDs (e.g. piroxicam gel):
  - have modest efficacy (at best);
  - have low toxicity.

analgesics given alone for acute pain. The disparity in half-lives of the two components is a disadvantage when single doses are used, but with repeated doses a higher steady-state blood concentration is obtained, which may account for its effect when taken regularly. Overdose can be fatal (due to respiratory depression or atrioventricular (AV) block), particularly if alcohol is taken in addition. Large doses of **naloxone** are required to displace dextropropoxyphene from opioid receptors, and treatment for paracetamol toxicity (see Chapter 53) will also be required. Both abuse and dependence occur.

DRUGS FOR SEVERE PAIN

OPIOIDS

Opium is derived from the dried milky juice exuded by incised seed capsules of a species of poppy, *Papaver somniferum*, that is grown in Turkey, India and South-East Asia. Homer refers to it in the *Odyssey* as 'nepenthes', a drug given to Odysseus and his followers 'to banish grief or trouble of the mind'. Sydenham introduced laudanum (tincture of opium) into English medicine in the seventeenth century and wrote that 'few would be willing to practise medicine without opium'. Osler referred to it as 'God's own medicine'. Opium had social as well as medical uses. Several literary figures were 'opium eaters', including Scott and Coleridge, as well as de Quincey. A number of notably discreditable events, including the opium wars and the mistreatment of Chinese labourers on the Panama Canal, ensued from the commercial, social, moral and political interests involved in its world-wide trade and use. Opium is a complex mixture of alkaloids, the principal components being morphine, **codeine** and **papaverine**. The main analgesic action of opium is due to morphine. Papaverine is a vasodilator without analgesic actions.

Until 1868, opium could be purchased without prescription from grocers' shops in the UK. During the last 100 years it has been realized that it is not without disadvantages, notably addiction and dependence. Much work has gone into synthesizing morphine analogues in the hope of producing a drug with the therapeutic actions of morphine but without its disadvantages. However, the analgesic actions of opioids are closely related to their potential for abuse, and the history of this field has not been encouraging. Morphine was introduced as a non-addictive alternative to opium, and this in turn was superseded by diamorphine, which was believed to be non-addicting! Synthetic drugs such as pethidine, **dextropropoxyphene** and **pentazocine** were originally incorrectly thought to lack potential for abuse.

Morphine is active when given by mouth, and a more rapid effect can be obtained if it is administered intramuscularly or intravenously, but the potential for abuse is also greatly increased. Some anaesthetists give opioids such as **fentanyl** by the epidural route, especially during obstetric surgery (e.g. Caesarean section).

OPIOID RECEPTORS

Stereospecific receptors with a high affinity for opioid analgesics are present in neuronal membranes. They are found in high concentrations in the PAG, the limbic system, the pulvina of the thalamus, the hypothalamus, medulla oblongata and the substantia gelatinosa of the spinal cord. Several endogenous peptides with analgesic properties are widely distributed throughout the nervous system. They can be divided into the following three groups:

1. encephalins (leu-encephalin and met-encephalin) are pentapeptides differing in only one amino acid;
2. dynorphins are extended forms of encephalins;
3. endorphins (e.g. β-endorphin).

These peptides are derived from larger precursors (pro-opiomelanocortin, pro-encephalin and prodynorphin) and may act as neurotransmitters or as longer-acting neurohormones.

There are three types of opioid receptor, namely μ, δ and κ. A fourth category, the σ-receptors, are now generally not classified as opioid receptors because they bind non-opioid psychotomimetic drugs such as phencyclidine and the only opioids that bind appreciably to them are the benzomorphans (e.g. pentazocine) that have psychotomimetic properties.

Blocking opioid receptors with naloxone has little effect in normal individuals, but in patients suffering from chronic pain it produces hyperalgesia. This suggests that a pre-existing stimulus is required to activate the pain-inhibiting function of the opioid system. Physical and emotional stress can produce analgesia which is reversed by naloxone. Electrical stimulation of areas of the brain that are rich in encephalins and opioid receptors elicits analgesia which is abolished by naloxone, implying that it is caused by liberation of endogenous opioids. Pain relief by acupuncture may also be mediated by encephalin release, because it is antagonized by naloxone.

Narcotic analgesics exert their effects by binding to opioid receptors. The resulting pattern of pharmacological activity depends on their affinity for the various receptors and whether they are full or partial agonists. The affinity of narcotic analgesics for μ-receptors parallels their analgesic potency. In addition to their involvement in brain function, the opioid peptides may well play a neuroendocrine role. Administration in humans suppresses the pituitary–gonadal and pituitary–adrenal axis and stimulates the release of prolactin, thyroid-stimulating hormone (TSH) and growth hormone. High concentrations of opioid peptides are present in sympathetic ganglia and the adrenal medulla. Their function at these sites has not been elucidated, but they may play an inhibitory role in the sympathetic system.

Following repeated administration of an exogenous opioid, the sensitivity of the receptors decreases, necessitating an increased dose to produce the same effect ('tolerance'). On withdrawal of the drug, endogenous opioids are not sufficient to stimulate the insensitive receptors, resulting in a withdrawal state characterized by autonomic disturbances, including pallor, sweating and piloerection ('cold turkey').

Morphine

USE

1 The most important use of morphine is for pain relief. The effective dose is highly variable. Previous analgesic requirements (if known) should be taken into account when selecting a dose.

2 Morphine may be given as an intravenous bolus if rapid relief is required (e.g. during myocardial infarction), and the usual dose is 5 mg.

3 Alternatively, morphine can be given continuously by an infusion pump (e.g. postoperatively), either intravenously or subcutaneously. This is very effective, and relatively small doses are required.

4 Morphine is effective orally, although larger doses are needed due to presystemic metabolism. Morphine is given by mouth initially regularly 4-hourly as an elixir, giving additional doses as needed between the regular doses as a 'top-up', the daily dose being reviewed and titrated. Once the dose requirement is established, sustained-release morphine (12-hourly) is substituted.

5 Spinal (epidural or intrathecal) administration of morphine is effective at much lower doses than when given by other routes, and causes fewer systemic side-effects. It is useful in those few patients with opioid-responsive pain who experience intolerable side-effects when morphine is administered by other routes.

6 Continuous subcutaneous infusions by pump are useful in the terminally ill. There is an advantage in using diamorphine rather than morphine for this purpose, since its greater solubility permits smaller volumes of more concentrated solution to be used.

7 Morphine is effective in the relief of acute left ventricular failure. How this is achieved is unknown, but it probably involves depression of pulmonary reflexes and dilatation of capacitance vessels (pulmonary vessels and great veins), thus reducing cardiac preload. The usual dose is 5–10 mg intravenously.

8 Morphine inhibits cough, but codeine is preferred for this indication. Cough suppression does not involve endorphin receptors, and this property of opiates is not stereospecific, so that D-isomers, such as dextromethorphan, are effective antitussives.

9 Morphine relieves diarrhoea, but codeine is preferred for this indication.

MECHANISM OF ACTION

Morphine relieves both the perception of pain and the emotional response to it, as a result of its action as a full agonist on μ-opioid receptors. It causes pupillary constriction by stimulating μ/δ-receptors in the Edinger–Westphal nucleus in the mid-brain. This action is not of therapeutic importance, but provides a useful diagnostic sign in narcotic overdosage or chronic abuse. Morphine dilates capacitance and resistance vessels by both neurally and locally mediated mechanisms. It also causes peripheral histamine release and thus vasodilatation and, in some patients, bronchoconstriction. Moreover, in some patients it causes bradycardia due to stimulation of the vagal centre in the medulla.

ADVERSE EFFECTS

Certain patients are particularly sensitive to the pharmacological actions of morphine. These include the very young, the elderly, and those with chronic lung disease, myxoedema, chronic liver disease and chronic renal failure. Overdose leads to coma. Morphine depresses the sensitivity of the respiratory centre to carbon dioxide, thus causing a progressively decreased respiratory rate. Patients with decreased respiratory reserve due to asthma, bronchitis, emphysema or hypoxaemia of any cause are more sensitive to the respiratory depressant effect of opioids. Bronchoconstriction occurs via histamine release, but is usually mild and clinically important only in asthmatics, in whom morphine is best avoided. Morphine causes vomiting in 10–15% of patients by stimulation of the chemoreceptor trigger zone. This action is mediated by dopamine receptors rather than opioid receptors, and can be antagonized by dopamine-receptor antagonists (e.g. chlorpromazine). Morphine increases smooth muscle tone throughout the gastrointestinal tract, which is combined with decreased peristalsis. The result is constipation with hard dry stool. The increase in muscle tone also involves the sphincter of Oddi, and morphine increases intrabiliary pressure for 2–3 h. Dependence (both physical and psychological) is particularly likely to occur if the drug is used for the pleasurable feeling it produces rather than in a therapeutic context. Patients with prostatic hypertrophy may suffer acute retention of urine, as morphine increases the tone in the sphincter of the bladder neck.

PHARMACOKINETICS

Like other organic bases, opioids are well absorbed and morphine can be given orally or by subcutaneous, intramuscular or intravenous injection. After intramuscular injection, the peak therapeutic effect is achieved within about 1 h and lasts for 3–4 h. Morphine is metabolized largely by combination with glucuronic acid, but also by N-dealkylation and oxidation, about 10% being excreted in the urine as morphine and 60–70% as the glucuronide. Metabolism occurs in the liver and gut wall, and the oral bioavailability of morphine is 16–64%. The dose–plasma relationship for morphine and its main metabolite is linear over a wide range of oral dosage. Morphine-6-glucuronide has analgesic properties, and may account for much of the analgesic action of morphine. Only low concentrations of this active metabolite appear in the blood after a single oral dose. With repeated dosing the concentration of morphine-6-glucuronide increases, correlating with the high efficacy of repeated-dose oral morphine. Morphine-6-glucuronide is eliminated in the urine, so patients with renal impairment may experience severe and prolonged respiratory depression. The birth of opiate-dependent babies born to addicted mothers demonstrates the ability of morphine to cross the placenta.

DRUG INTERACTIONS

- Morphine augments other central depressants, and should not be combined with MAOIs.
- Antagonists (e.g. naloxone) are used in overdose and sometimes (e.g. naltrexone) in managing addicts after withdrawal.

Diamorphine

USE

Diamorphine is diacetylmorphine. Its actions are similar to those of morphine, although it is more potent as an analgesic when given by injection (7.5 mg of morphine are equivalent to 5 mg of diamorphine). Diamorphine has a reputation for having a greater addictive potential than morphine, and is banned in the USA. The more rapid central effect of intravenous diamorphine than of morphine (the faster 'buzz'), due to rapid penetration of the blood–brain barrier, makes this plausible (see below). Diamorphine is used for the same purposes as morphine. It is more soluble than morphine, and this may be an advantage if large doses are being given by injection (e.g. as a continuous subcutaneous infusion).

ADVERSE EFFECTS

The adverse effects of diamorphine are same as those for morphine.

PHARMACOKINETICS

Diamorphine is hydrolysed (deacetylated) to form 6-acetylmorphine and morphine, the $t_{\frac{1}{2}}$ being about 3 min. Diamorphine enters the brain more rapidly than morphine, which accounts for its rapid effect.

Pethidine

USE

The actions of pethidine are similar to those of morphine. It causes similar respiratory depression, vomiting and gastrointestinal smooth muscle contraction to morphine, but does not constrict the pupil, release histamine or suppress cough. It produces little euphoria, but does cause dependence. Pethidine is widely used in obstetrics because it does not reduce the activity of the pregnant uterus. The usual dose is 25–100 mg parenterally or 50–150 mg orally.

PHARMACOKINETICS

Hepatic metabolism is the main route of elimination, with less than 50% being excreted unchanged in the urine. The major metabolites are an N-demethylated product, norpethidine, and a hydrolysis product, pethidinic acid, and its conjugates. Norpethidine has twice the convulsant activity of pethidine. The $t_{\frac{1}{2}}$ of pethidine is 3–4 h in healthy individuals, but this is increased in the elderly and in patients with cirrhosis or hepatitis. Pethidine crosses the placenta and causes respiratory depression of the neonate. This is exacerbated by the prolonged elimination $t_{\frac{1}{2}}$ in neonates of about 22 h (seven times longer than in healthy adults).

DRUG INTERACTIONS

- When pethidene and monoamine oxidase inhibitors are given together, a syndrome characterized by rigidity, hyperpyrexia, excitement, hypotension and coma has occurred. Its mechanism is unknown.
- Pethidine, like other opiates, delays gastric emptying, thus interfering with the absorption of co-administered drugs. Delayed gastric emptying is of particular concern in obstetrics, as gastric aspiration is a leading cause of maternal mortality.

Methadone

USE

Methadone has very similar actions to morphine, but is less sedating and longer acting. Its main use is by mouth to replace morphine or diamorphine when these drugs are being withdrawn in the treatment of drug dependence. A single oral dose of methadone given once daily under supervision is less damaging than leaving addicts to seek diamorphine illicitly. Many of the adverse effects of opioid abuse are related to parenteral administration, with its attendant risks of infection, (e.g. endocarditis, human immunodeficiency virus (HIV) or hepatitis). The objective is to reduce craving by occupying opioid receptors, simultaneously reducing the 'buzz' from any additional dose taken. The slower onset following oral administration reduces the reward and reinforcement of dependence. The relatively long half-life reduces the intensity of withdrawal and permits once-daily dosing under supervision.

PHARMACOKINETICS

After oral dosage, the peak blood concentration is achieved within about 4 h. Methadone is 40% protein bound to albumin. The metabolism of methadone is variable, particularly with repeated doses, and accumulation can occur with prolonged administration.

Codeine

USE

Codeine is the methyl ether of morphine, but has only about 10% of its analgesic potency. (**Dihydrocodeine** is similar, and is a commonly prescribed alternative.) Although codeine is converted to morphine, it produces little euphoria and has low addiction potential. As a result, it has been used for many years as an analgesic for moderate pain (15–60 mg given 4-hourly), as a cough suppressant (codeine linctus BPC contains 15 mg/5 mL) and for symptomatic relief of diarrhoea.

ADVERSE EFFECTS

Constipation and nausea are the most commonly encountered adverse effects.

PHARMACOKINETICS

Codeine has a plasma $t_{\frac{1}{2}}$ of 3.2 h, but free morphine also appears in plasma following codeine administration, and it has been suggested that codeine acts as a prodrug, producing a low but sustained concentration of morphine. Sufficient morphine may enter the brain to produce analgesia without causing a high risk of abuse. Some individuals are poor metabolizers of codeine and consequently produce little morphine and experience less, if any, analgesic effect.

Pentazocine

Pentazocine is a partial agonist on opioid receptors (especially κ-receptors, with additional actions on σ-receptors, which result in hallucinations and thought disturbance). It also increases pulmonary artery pressure. Its use is not recommended.

Buprenorphine

USE

Buprenorphine is a partial agonist. It is given sublingually in doses of 0.2–0.4 mg for chronic pain. In common with other partial agonists, buprenorphine occupies a much larger fraction of the receptors to produce its analgesic effect than does a full agonist. Consequently, it antagonizes full agonists and can precipitate pain and cause withdrawal symptoms in patients who are already receiving morphine. Much larger doses of naloxone are required to displace it from the receptors in the treatment of overdose than are needed to treat overdosage with a full agonist, for the same reason.

PHARMACOKINETICS

Like other opiates, buprenorphine is subject to considerable hepatic first-pass metabolism, but this is circumvented by sublingual administration. It is metabolized by dealkylation and glucuronidation before excretion predominantly in the bile. The duration of pain relief is a little longer than with morphine.

OPIOID ANTAGONISTS

Minor alterations in the chemical structure of opioids result in drugs that are competitive antagonists.

Naloxone

Naloxone is derived from oxymorphone. It is a pure competitive antagonist of opioid agonists at μ-receptors. It is given intravenously, the usual dose being 0.8–2.0 mg for the treatment of poisoning with full agonists (e.g. morphine), higher doses (up to 10 times the recommended dose, depending on clinical response) being required for overdosage with partial agonists (e.g. dextropropoxyphene, buprenorphine). Its effect is rapid, and if a satisfactory response has not been obtained within 3 min, the dose may be repeated. If the patient still does not respond, the diagnosis of opioid overdose should be reconsidered. The action of many opioids outlasts that of naloxone, which has a $t_{\frac{1}{2}}$ of 1 h, and a constant-rate infusion of naloxone (e.g. up to 5 mg/h) may be needed. Naloxone can also be used to reverse the effects of morphine post-operatively, or in the management of the apnoeic infant after birth when the mother has received an opioid during labour. Naloxone precipitates acute withdrawal symptoms in opiate-dependent patients.

Naltrexone

Naltrexone hydrochloride is an orally active opioid antagonist at μ- and other opioid receptors that is used in specialized clinics as adjunctive treatment to reduce the risk of relapse in former opioid addicts who have been detoxified. Such patients who are receiving naltrexone in addition to supportive therapy are less likely to resume illicit opiate use (detected by urine measurements) than those receiving placebo plus supportive therapy. However, the drop-out rate is high due to non-compliance. Naltrexone has weak agonist activity, but this is not clinically important, and withdrawal symptoms do not follow abrupt cessation of treatment. The usual dose is 25 mg increasing to 50 mg daily, and it should not be started until the addict has been opioid free for at least 7 days for short-acting drugs (e.g.

Key points

Opioids

- The main drug is morphine, which is a full agonist at μ-receptors.
- Effects of morphine include:
  - analgesia;
  - relief of left ventricular failure;
  - miosis (pupillary constriction);
  - suppression of cough ('antitussive' effect);
  - constipation;
  - nausea/vomiting;
  - liberation of histamine (pruritus, bronchospasm);
  - addiction;
  - tolerance;
  - withdrawal symptoms following chronic use.
- Diamorphine ('heroin'):
  - is metabolzed rapidly to morphine;
  - gains access to the CNS more rapidly than morphine (when given IV);
  - for this reason gives a rapid 'buzz';
  - may therefore have an even higher potential for abuse than morphine;
  - is more soluble than morphine.
- Codeine and dihydrocodeine are:
  - weak opioids;
  - slowly metabolized to morphine;
  - used in combination with paracetamol for moderate pain;
  - used for diarrhoea or as antitussives.
- Pethidine:
  - is a strong synthetic opioid;
  - does not inhibit uterine contraction;
  - is widely used in obstetrics;
  - can cause respiratory depression in neonates;
  - is less liable than morphine to cause bronchial constriction;
  - does not cause miosis;
  - has potential for abuse.
- Buprenorphine and dextropropoxyphene are partial agonists.
  1. Buprenorphine:
     - is used sublingually in severe chronic pain.
  2. Dextropropoxyphene:
     - is combined with paracetamol for moderately severe chronic pain;
     - this combination is not more effective than paracetamol alone for acute pain;
     - is dangerous in overdose.
- Opioid effects are antagonized competitively by naloxone:
  - very large doses are needed to reverse the effects of partial agonists.

Case history

A 55-year-old retired naval officer presents to Accident and Emergency with sudden onset of very severe back pain. A chest X-ray reveals a mass, and he is admitted at 9 a.m. for further investigation. On examination he is pale, sweaty and distressed. The Senior House Officer writes him up for morphine 10 mg subcutaneously, 4-hourly as needed, and the pain responds well to the first dose, following which the patient falls into a light sleep.

That evening his wife, scarcely able to contain her anger, approaches the consultant on the Firm's round to beg that her husband be given some more analgesic.

Comment

Communication is key in managing pain. There are often difficulties when, as in the present case, the diagnosis is probable but not confirmed, and when the patient is admitted to a general ward which may be short of nursing staff. The Senior House Officer was concerned not to cause respiratory depression, so did not write up regular analgesia, but unfortunately neither medical nor nursing staff realized that the patient had awoken with recurrent severe pain. He had not himself asked for additional analgesia (which was written up) because his personality traits would lead him to lie quietly and 'suffer in silence'. The good initial response suggests that his pain will respond well to regular oral morphine, and this indeed proved to be the case. A subsequent biopsy confirmed squamous-cell carcinoma, and a bone scan demonstrated multiple metastases, one of which had led to a crush fracture of a vertebral body visible on plain X-ray. A non-steroidal drug reduced his immediate requirement for morphine, and radiotherapy resolved his back pain completely and morphine was discontinued. He remained pain-free at home for the next 4 months, and was then found dead in bed by his wife. Autopsy was not performed. One of several possibilities is that he died from pulmonary embolism.

diamorphine or morphine), or 10 days for longer-acting drugs (e.g. methadone), because it can precipitate a severe and prolonged abstinence syndrome. Naltrexone has not been extensively studied in non-addicts, and most of the symptoms that have been attributed to it are those that arise from opioid withdrawal. In addition, one reversible case of idiopathic thrombocytopenic purpura and several cases of other rashes have been reported. Naltrexone has a number of neuroendocrine effects, including increased plasma concentrations of β-endorphin, cortisol and luteinizing hormone (LH). Indeed, it has been used experimentally to induce ovulation in women with amenorrhoea secondary to hypothalamic disease, although it is not licensed for such use in the UK. Evidence of reversible hepatocellular damage is inconclusive, but it is recommended that liver enzymes are determined before and at intervals during treatment. Naltrexone is completely absorbed following oral administration, but is rapidly and variably metabolized ($t_{\frac{1}{2}}$ = 1–10 h). The main metabolite is 6-β-naltrexol, which is much less potent than the parent drug but which may none the less have important biological activity by virtue of its slower elimination rate.

Further reading

Dahl JB, Kehlet H. 1993: The value of pre-emptive analgesia in the treatment of post-operative pain, *British Journal of Anaesthesia*, **70**, 434–9.

Fields HL. 1987: *Pain*. New York: McGraw-Hill.

Raineville P, Duncan GH, Price DD, Carrier B, Bushnell MC. 1997: Pain effect encoded in human anterior cingulate but not somatosensory cortex. *Science* **277**, 968–71.

Wall PD, Melzac R. (eds) 1994: *Textbook of pain*. Edinburgh: Churchill Livingstone.

PART III

THE MUSCULOSKELETAL SYSTEM

CHAPTER TWENTY-FIVE

ANTI-INFLAMMATORY DRUGS *and the* TREATMENT *of* ARTHRITIS

- Rheumatoid arthritis and other chronic inflammatory joint diseases
- Non-steroidal anti-inflammatory drugs (NSAIDs)
- Glucocorticoids
- Disease-modifying anti-rheumatic drugs (DMARDs)
- Hyperuricaemia and gout

RHEUMATOID ARTHRITIS AND OTHER CHRONIC INFLAMMATORY JOINT DISEASES

INTRODUCTION

The cause of rheumatoid arthritis is unknown, and current treatment involves the use of drugs that have been found empirically to influence some aspect of the disease. *Non-steroidal anti-inflammatory drugs* (NSAIDs) play a major part in controlling symptoms, but do not alter the underlying disease process. When the disease is resistant and progressive despite NSAIDs, one of the *disease-modifying anti-rheumatic drugs* (DMARDs) can be added to the therapeutic regime. The efficacy of these drugs is established, but their toxicities make close monitoring mandatory. However, patients should not be allowed to become permanently disabled without a trial of DMARDs being at least considered. The place of *glucocorticoids* in treatment has changed over the years. There is no doubt that they suppress the inflammatory process and produce rapid and dramatic relief. However, with prolonged use, side-effects become increasingly prominent and glucocorticoids are now only used systemically when other measures have failed, or sometimes in elderly patients in whom a rapid therapeutic response is required to prevent them becoming permanently bedridden.

NON-STEROIDAL ANTI-INFLAMMATORY DRUGS (NSAIDS)

Many NSAIDs are available for clinical use. They are chemically diverse (see Table 25.1), but all of them inhibit prostaglandin biosynthesis by inhibiting cyclo-oxygenase (COX). This is the basis of most of their therapeutic as well as their undesired actions. COX is a key enzyme in the synthesis of prostaglandins and thromboxanes (see also Chapters 24 and 28), and these COX products are important mediators of the erythema, oedema, pain and fever of inflammation. Inflammatory effects result both from direct actions of prostaglandins (on the microvasculature, on nociceptive afferents and on temperature-regulating centres in the hypothalamus) and, indirectly, by synergy with other inflammatory mediators including bradykinin, histamine, activated complement components (c5a) and platelet-activating factor. There are two isoforms of the enzyme, namely a constitutive form (COX-1) that is present in platelets, stomach and other tissues, and an inducible form (COX-2) that is expressed in inflamed tissues as a result of stimulation by cytokines. Current NSAIDs are relatively non-specific for the two isoforms. There is currently great interest in inhibitors specific for COX-2, the first of which have been licensed, which it is hoped will lack the adverse effects caused by inhibition of the constitutive enzyme. Some NSAIDs have additional actions, including inhibition of superoxide and hydroxyl anion radical production, and inhibition of leucocyte migration, but it is unclear to what extent these effects contribute to their anti-inflammatory actions in clinical use.

Use

NSAIDs are widely used in the treatment of rheumatoid and other inflammatory joint diseases, including ankylosing spondylitis, psoriatic arthropathy and gout, and for cases of osteoarthrosis with a marked inflammatory component. They are valuable for suppressing inflammation in these miserable and chronic conditions, but do not influence the course of the disease favourably in terms of progression to disability and deformity. Differences in anti-inflammatory activity between different NSAIDs are small, but there is considerable inter-patient variation in clinical response. About two-thirds of patients respond to any NSAID, but among the remaining third, individuals may respond to one drug after having failed to respond to another. Consequently, if no response is obtained after 3 weeks, a drug of a chemically distinct class should be substituted on an empirical basis. Some NSAIDs are also used as general-purpose analgesics for other types of pain both mild, (e.g. dysmenorrhoea, muscular sprains and other soft tissue injuries) and severe, (e.g. pain from metastatic deposits in bone). Parenteral NSAIDs (e.g. ketorolac) are used for post-operative analgesia, and topical preparations (e.g. of piroxicam) are sold over the counter for mild musculo-skeletal pain, as described in Chapter 24. Aspirin irreversibly inhibits COX-1, and has a unique role as an antiplatelet drug (see Chapter 28). It is not especially potent as an anti-inflammatory drug, and the doses required to achieve an adequate anti-inflammatory effect in rheumatoid arthritis and other inflammatory diseases are associated with considerable toxicity. More potent reversible NSAIDs are preferred for this indication. It has a place as a mild analgesic (see Chapter 24) and as an anti-inflammatory drug in treating rheumatic fever, but apart from this condition its use is avoided in children because of its assoiation with Reye's syndrome (see Chapter 24). Juvenile chronic arthritis is treated with

Table 25.1: Non-steroidal anti-inflammatory drugs (NSAIDs)

Chemical class	Examples	Comments
Salicylates	Aspirin	Indicated for rheumatic fever; not otherwise used in children because of risk of Reye's syndrome
Indoleacetic acids	Indomethacin Sulindac	Widely used potent drug Relatively 'renal sparing'
Propionic acids	Ibuprofen Naproxen	Mild in recommended dose; see Chapter 24
Anthranilic acids	Mefenamic acid	–
Phenylacetic acids	Diclofenac	–
Oxicams	Piroxicam	–
Pyrazolones	Phenylbutazone	Used in ankylosing spondylitis when other NSAIDs are unsatisfactory. Causes agranulocytosis

NSAIDs and DMARDs in most cases, but the pattern of disease with systemic onset (previously termed Still's disease) requires corticosteroids.

Adverse effects and interactions common to NSAIDs

Several adverse effects of NSAIDs are common to the group as a whole, and are the result of their main pharmacological action, namely inhibition of COX, although not all NSAIDs cause these effects to an equal extent when used at recommended doses. The main adverse effects of NSAIDs are on the following:

- gastrointestinal tract;
- kidneys (and hence indirectly on the cardiovascular system);
- airways;
- liver.

Prostaglandin E_2 is the main COX product in the stomach, which it protects in several ways. NSAIDs cause gastritis and peptic ulceration. Dyspepsia is common with all NSAIDs and haematemesis (the severity of which is exacerbated by inhibition of platelet function) is their most frequent life-threatening adverse effect. Ibuprofen (which is available over the counter in the UK) is less potent than other NSAIDs, and gastric toxicity associated with it is correspondingly less common at recommended doses.

The main prostaglandins produced in human kidneys are prostacyclin (PGI_2) and prostaglandin E_2. NSAIDs predictably cause functional renal impairment in patients with pre-existing glomerular disease (e.g. lupus nephritis), or with systemic diseases in which renal blood flow is dependent on the kidneys' ability to synthesize vasodilator prostaglandins. These include heart failure, salt and water depletion, cirrhosis and nephrotic syndrome. The elderly, with their reduced glomerular filtration rate and reduced capacity to eliminate NSAIDs, are especially at risk. Renal impairment manifests as a progressive increase in serum creatinine levels that is reversible within a few days if the NSAID is stopped promptly. All NSAIDs can cause this effect, but it is less common with aspirin (which is a weak inhibitor of renal cyclo-oxygenase) or low doses of **sulindac**. This is because sulindac is a prodrug that acts through an active sulphide metabolite; the kidney converts the sulphide back into the inactive sulphone. Sulindac is therefore relatively 'renal sparing' although, at higher doses, inhibition of renal prostaglandin biosynthesis and consequent renal impairment in susceptible patients do occur. For the same reason (inhibition of renal prostaglandin biosynthesis), *NSAIDs all interact non-specifically with antihypertensive medication*, rendering them less effective, and concurrent use of NSAIDs is a common cause of loss of control of blood pressure in treated hypertensive patients. Again, and for the same reasons, aspirin and sulindac are less likely to cause this interaction. PGE_2 and PGI_2 are natriuretic as well as vasodilators, and *NSAIDs consequently cause salt and water retention*, antagonize the effects of diuretics and exacerbate heart failure. (Some of their interaction with diuretics also reflects competition for the renal tubular weak acid secretory mechanism.) As well as reducing sodium excretion, NSAIDs reduce lithium ion clearance, and plasma concentrations of lithium should be closely monitored in patients on maintenance doses of lithium in whom treatment with an NSAID is initiated. NSAIDs also increase the plasma potassium ion concentration, especially in patients with diabetes who may have associated hyporeninaemic hypoaldosteronism, and in patients with renal impairment or who are receiving drugs that elevate the plasma potassium ion concentration (e.g. potassium supplements, potassium-sparing diuretics or converting-enzyme inhibitors).

In addition to their type A effects on the kidney due to inhibition of renal prostaglandins, NSAIDs can cause acute interstitial nephritis, which presents as nephrotic syndrome or renal impairment that slowly resolves on withdrawing the drug. This is an idiosyncratic effect, unique to a particular drug within one susceptible individual. NSAIDs have also been implicated in analgesic nephropathy (see Chapter 24), although this is controversial.

NSAIDs worsen bronchospasm in aspirin-sensitive asthmatics (who sometimes have a history of nasal polyps and urticaria, see Chapter 32). All NSAIDs cause wheezing in aspirin-sensitive individuals.

NSAIDs cause hepatitis in some patients. The mechanism is not understood, but the elderly are particularly susceptible. Different NSAIDs vary in how commonly they cause this problem. (Indeed, hepatotoxicity was one of the reasons for the withdrawal of one such drug, **benoxaprofen**, from the market.) Aspirin is a recognized cause of hepatitis, particularly in patients with systemic lupus erythematosus.

Indomethacin

USE

Indomethacin has a powerful anti-inflammatory action but only a weak analgesic action. It is used to treat rheumatoid arthritis and associated disorders, ankylosing spondylitis and gout. Adverse effects are rather common, so in chronic disorders it is best to start treatment with a single dose of 25 mg daily and increase this gradually to 25 mg three times daily. A further increase in dosage is unlikely to increase the effectiveness of the drug. In acute gout the initial dose is 50 mg orally repeated after 4 h and then 6-hourly for a few days. It can be given as a suppository (100 mg) at night to relieve morning stiffness in rheumatoid arthritis, and slow-release preparations are available.

ADVERSE EFFECTS

Indomethacin produces side-effects in at least 25% of patients. The most common adverse effects are headaches and occasionally other central nervous symptoms such as light-headedness, confusion or hallucination. Gastric intolerance is common, and renal and pulmonary toxicities occur as with other NSAIDs (see above).

PHARMACOKINETICS

Indomethacin is readily absorbed by mouth or from suppositories. It undergoes extensive hepatic metabolism, and both the parent compound and its metabolites take part in enterohepatic circulation. The mean $t_{\frac{1}{2}}$ is 7–10 h, but hepatic elimination is prolonged in patients with biliary obstruction. Both the parent drug and inactive metabolites are also excreted in the urine.

DRUG INTERACTIONS

Anticoagulants worsen haemorrhage should peptic ulceration or gastritis occur during treatment with indomethacin. The actions of antihypertensive drugs and diuretics are opposed by indomethacin. **Triamterene** (as commonly prescribed in the combination product, cotriamterzide – 'Dyazide™') in particular should be avoided, as its addition to maintenance doses of indomethacin resulted in reversible renal failure in two of four previously healthy volunteers.

Naproxen

USE

Naproxen is used in rheumatic and musculoskeletal diseases. It is also useful in dysmenorrhoea and in the prophylaxis and treatment of migraine. The usual dose is 250–500 mg twice daily.

MECHANISM OF ACTION

Naproxen is approximately 20 times as potent an inhibitor of COX as aspirin. An additional property of note is inhibition of leucocyte migration, with a potency similar to that of colchicine.

ADVERSE EFFECTS

Adverse effects (and adverse interactions) are generally mild, although naproxen does cause all of the adverse effects common to NSAIDs.

Key points

NSAIDs

- They inhibit cyclo-oxygenase (COX).
- Examples include indomethacin, naproxen and ibuprofen.
- Uses:
  short term – analgesia/anti-inflammatory;
  chronic – symptomatic relief in arthritis.
- Adverse effects:
  gastritis and other gastrointestinal inflammation/bleeding;
  reversible renal impairment (haemodynamic effect);
  interstitial nephritis (idiosyncratic);
  asthma in 'aspirin-sensitive' patients;
  hepatitis (idiosyncratic).
- Interactions:
  antihypertensive drugs (reduced effectiveness);
  diuretics (reduced effectiveness).
- COX-2-selective drugs are currently being developed. It is hoped that they will have reduced adverse effects.

Glucocorticoids

Glucocorticoids are discussed in Chapters 39 and 49. Despite their rapid and often profound effect on the inflammatory component of rheumatoid arthritis, they have such severe long-term effects if used systemically in pharmacological doses that their use is now highly circumscribed. **Prednisolone** is generally preferred for systemic use when a glucocorticoid is specifically indicated (e.g. for giant-cell arteritis, for which high-dose daily steroid treatment saves sight, in lower dose for polymyalgia rheumatica), for selected patients with systemic lupus erythematosus with ongoing inflammatory problems (especially in renal glomeruli or brain), active polyarteritis nodosa, myositis or dermatomyositis. A brief course of high-dose prednisolone is usually given to suppress the disease, followed if possible by dose reduction to a maintenance dose of 7.5 mg or less, given as a single dose first thing in the morning when endogenous glucocorticoids are at their peak. A marker of disease activity, such as the erythrocyte sedimentation rate (ESR) in patients with polymyalgia or giant-cell arteritis, is followed as a guide to dose reduction. An important use of glucocorticoids in rheumatoid arthritis and inflammatory osteoarthritis is by intra-articular injection to reduce pain and deformity in a joint. Glucocorticoids can be administered locally to soft tissues (avoiding direct injection into a tendon, as this can lead to rupture) to relieve peri-articular pain, and when injected into the subacromial bursa are more effective in the treatment of painful shoulder than is an oral NSAID. It is essential to rule out infection before injecting steroid into a joint, and meticulous aseptic technique is needed to avoid introducing infection. A suspension of a poorly soluble drug such as **triamcinolone** acetonide (a potent halogenated synthetic steroid also used topically to treat a variety of skin diseases) is used to give a long-lasting effect. The patient is warned to avoid excessive weight-bearing or over-use of the joint should the desired improvement materialize, since this predisposes to joint destruction. Multiple injections over a period of time also cause joint destruction and bone necrosis, and should be avoided. Steroid-induced myopathy is a particular problem with the fluorinated derivatives, and triamcinolone should therefore be avoided in patients with a history of steroid myopathy.

Disease-modifying anti-rheumatic drugs (DMARDs)

DMARDs are not analgesic and do not inhibit COX, but they do suppress the inflammatory process in rheumatoid arthritis and psoriatic arthritis. They are not effective in spondarthritis or other inflammatory joint disorders. Their mechanism of action is not well understood, but may involve inhibition of excessive cytokine liberation. They only have a part to play in the management of patients with *progressive* disease. Response is not invariable, and is usually maximal within 4–10 weeks. Unlike NSAIDs, DMARDs reduce the erythrocyte sedimentation rate (ESR), a non-specific index of inflammatory activity (historically, it was this effect that led to them being referred to as 'disease modifying'). It is difficult to prove that a drug influences the natural history of a relapsing/remitting and unpredictably progressing disease such as rheumatoid arthritis, but immunosuppressants retard the radiological progression of erosions. DMARDs are toxic necessitating careful patient monitoring, and are best used by physicians experienced in rheumatology. This is even more important when the possibility of using these drugs in combination with one another is contemplated. There is a tendency among rheumatologists to use them earlier than in the past (despite the lack of regulatory authority approval of some of the DMARDs for this indication), with close monitoring for toxicity, and the patient fully informed about toxic as well as desired effects. This is especially important since many of these drugs are licensed for quite different indications to arthritis. In terms of efficacy, **methotrexate**, **gold**, **D-penicillamine**, **azathioprine** and **sulphasalazine** are similar, and are all more potent than **hydroxychloroquine**. Methotrexate (see Chapter 47) is better tolerated than the other DMARDs, and is therefore usually the first choice. Sulphasalazine (see Chapter 33) is the second choice. Alternative DMARDs, and some of their adverse effects, are summarized in Table 25.2.

Table 25.2: Disease-modifying anti-rheumatic drugs (DMARDs)

Drug	Adverse effects	Comments
Immunosuppressants: azathioprine, methotrexate, cyclosporin	Blood dyscrasias, carcinogenesis, opportunistic infection, alopecia, nausea; methotrexate also causes mucositis and cirrhosis; cyclosporin also causes nephrotoxicity, hypertension and hyperkalaemia	Methotrexate is usual first-choice DMARD
Sulphasalazine	Blood dyscrasias, nausea, rashes, colours urine/tears orange	First introduced for arthritis, now used mainly in inflammatory bowel disease (see Chapter 23)
Gold salts	Rashes, nephrotic syndrome, blood dyscrasias, stomatitis, diarrhoea	Oral preparation (auranofin) more convenient, less toxic but less effective than intramuscular aurothiomalate
Penicillamine	Blood dyscrasias, proteinuria, urticaria	
Antimalarials: chloroquine, hydroxychloroquine	Retinopathy, nausea, diarrhoea, rashes, pigmentation of palate, bleaching of hair	See Chapter 46 (p. 537)

Gold salts

USE

Gold was originally introduced to treat tuberculosis. Although ineffective, it was found serendipitously to have anti-rheumatic properties, and it has been used to treat patients with rheumatoid arthritis since the 1920s. **Sodium aurothiomalate** is administered weekly by deep intramuscular injection as follows: week 1, 10 mg; week 2, 20 mg; week 3, 50 mg; and thereafter 50 mg weekly until a total of 1.0 g has been given followed by maintenance treatment of 50 mg monthly. A benefit is not anticipated until 300–600 mg have been administered. About 75% of patients improve, with a reduction in joint swelling, disappearance of rheumatoid nodules and a fall in ESR. Urine must be tested for protein and full blood count (with platelet count and differential white cell count) performed before each injection. **Auranofin** is an oral gold preparation with less toxicity but also less efficacy than aurothiomalate. The usual starting dose is 3 mg twice daily, changing to 6 mg as a single daily dose if the drug is tolerated. If the response is inadequate after 6 months, the dose is increased to 3 mg three times a day. If there is no response after a further 3 months, the drug is stopped. Monitoring of blood counts and urine is performed monthly.

MECHANISM OF ACTION

The precise mechanism of the therapeutic action of gold salts is unknown. Several effects could contribute to their efficacy in rheumatoid arthritis. Gold–albumin complexes are phagocytosed by macrophages and polymorphonuclear leucocytes and concentrated in their lysosomes, where gold inhibits lysosomal enzymes that have been implicated in causing damage to joints. Furthermore, gold binds to sulphydryl groups and inhibits sulphydryl–disulphide interchange in immunoglobulin and complement, which could influence the progression of autoimmune processes.

ADVERSE EFFECTS

The adverse effects of gold are often troublesome and sometimes dangerous. Some adverse effects occur in up to 50% of all treated patients, in half of whom they are severe.

1 Rashes are an indication to stop treatment, as they can progress to exfoliation.

2 Photosensitive eruptions, urticaria and erythematous reactions to gold are often preceded by itching.
3 Glomerular injury can be severe, resulting in nephrotic syndrome, so treatment must be withheld if more than a trace of proteinuria is present, and should not be resumed until the urine is protein free.
4 Blood dyscrasias can develop rapidly and consequently become established despite frequent routine blood counts.
5 Stomatitis can be troublesome, and suggests the possibility of neutropenia.
6 Diarrhoea is uncommon, but gold colitis can be life-threatening.

PHARMACOKINETICS

The plasma half-life of gold increases with repeated administration, and may range from 1 day to several weeks. Gold is bound to plasma proteins and is concentrated in inflamed areas. It is excreted in urine and a small amount is lost in the faeces. Total elimination from the body takes a long time, and gold continues to be excreted in the urine for up to 1 year after a course of treatment.

Pencillamine

USE

Penicillamine is a breakdown product of penicillin. It is effective in Wilson's disease and in cystinuria, and more recently has found a place in the management of rheumatoid arthritis. It is given orally between meals (ideally 1 h before food). The initial dose is 125 mg daily for 1 month, then 250 mg daily for a further month, increasing by 125–250 mg per month until a response is achieved. Clinical improvement is anticipated only after 6–12 weeks. When improvement is well established, the dose is gradually reduced (by 125–250 mg every 6 weeks) to the minimum effective maintenance dose. This is usually 500–750 mg daily, but doses as high as 1.5 g are sometimes used. The results are similar to those obtained with gold. Weekly blood and urine tests (including platelet and differential and absolute white-cell counts and urine protein) are performed initially, and then monthly during maintenance treatment. Treatment should be discontinued if there is no improvement within 1 year.

MECHANISM OF ACTION

Penicillamine acts by several mechanisms, including metal-ion chelation via its sulphydryl group, and dissociation of macroglobulins. It also inhibits the release of lysosomal enzymes in inflamed connective tissue.

ADVERSE EFFECTS

The commonest adverse effects of penicillamine are anorexia and weight loss. Other effects are more serious, and they are more common in patients with poor sulphoxidation.

1 Bone-marrow hypoplasia, thrombocytopenia and leukopenia occur and can be fatal. They are all indications to stop treatment.
2 Immune-complex glomerulonephritis is common and causes mild proteinuria in 30% of patients. The drug should be stopped until the condition resolves, and then treatment should be resumed at a lower dose. Heavy proteinuria, with or without oedema, is an indication to stop the drug permanently.
3 Other symptoms include hypersensitivity reactions with urticaria, nausea (minimized by taking the drug on an empty stomach), anorexia, taste loss (usually transient) and systemic lupus erythematosus-like and myasthenia gravis-like syndromes.

The toxicity of penicillamine is such that it should only be used by clinicians with experience of the drug and with meticulous patient monitoring.

CONTRAINDICATIONS

Penicillamine is contraindicated in patients with systemic lupus erythematosus, and should be used with caution, if at all, in individuals with renal or hepatic impairment.

PHARMACOKINETICS

Penicillamine is well absorbed from the gut in the fasting state. A number of hepatic metabolites are formed and rapidly excreted after acute dosing. Some of the active substance is tightly bound to plasma proteins and tissues, and is slowly excreted over several months during and after chronic dosing.

Key points

Disease-modifying anti-rheumatic drugs (DMARDs)

- Mechanisms are poorly understood; these drugs are often licensed for indications other than arthritis. Examples include:
  - methotrexate;
  - sulphasalazine;
  - gold;
  - D-pencillamine;
  - hydroxychloroquine.
- Uses – these drugs are used by rheumatologists to treat patients with progressive rheumatoid or psoriatic arthritis. A trial should be considered before a patient becomes disabled.
- All of these drugs can have severe adverse effects, and informed consent should be obtained before they are prescribed (especially those that are unlicensed for this indication).
- Their action is slow (of the order of weeks) in onset.
- In contrast to NSAIDs, these drugs:
  - reduce ESR;
  - retard progression of erosions on X-ray.
- Close monitoring for toxicity (blood counts, urinalysis and serum chemistry) is essential.

DRUG INTERACTIONS

The absorption of penicillamine is prevented by antacids, iron or zinc (which bind to its sulphydryl group). It should not be used with concurrent gold, chloroquine or immunosuppressive treatment, because of increased toxicity.

HYPERURICAEMIA AND GOUT

Uric acid is the end-product of purine (adenine and guanine) metabolism in humans, and gives rise to problems because of its limited solubility. Crystals of uric acid evoke a severe inflammatory response in patients with gout, cause chalky deposits (tophi) in cool extremities (e.g. pinna of the ear, toes), and cause renal stones and/or renal tubular obstruction. The final stages in the production of uric acid are shown in Figure 25.1. Two of these stages are dependent on xanthine oxidase. In most mammals, uricase converts uric acid into allantoin, which is rapidly eliminated by the

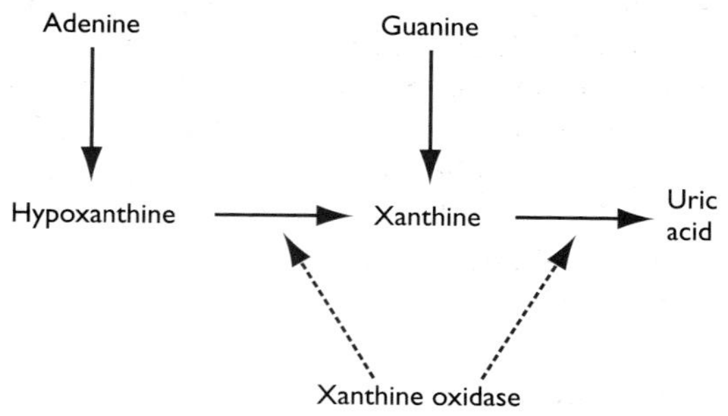

Figure 25.1: The final stages of the production of uric acid.

kidneys, but humans (as well as higher apes and Dalmatian dogs) lack uricase, so the less soluble uric acid must be excreted. Uric acid is filtered by the glomerulus, but 98% is reabsorbed in the proximal tubule with subsequent secretion into the distal tubule. It is more soluble in an alkaline urine (which favours the charged anionic urate, rather than free uric acid), and one factor in the development of uric acid stones is impairment of the ability to excrete alkaline urine. It is possible to lower the plasma uric acid concentration either by increasing renal excretion of uric acid or by inhibiting its synthesis.

Hyperuricaemia is almost always a result of relative impairment of urate clearance, often occurring in the setting of obesity and excessive alcohol consumption. Genetically determined defects of metabolism causing overproduction of uric acid are extremely rare. Increased breakdown of nuclear material occurs in leukaemia and similar disorders, particularly when treated by cytotoxic drugs, and is extremely important because it can lead to acute renal failure if measures are not taken to reduce urate formation and enhance its excretion in this setting (see below). Hyperuricaemia also occurs when excretion is decreased, as occurs in renal failure or when tubular excretion of uric acid is diminished by diuretics, pyrazinamide, or low doses of salicylate.

Acute gout

The acute attack is treated with anti-inflammatory analgesic agents (e.g. indomethacin, see above). Aspirin is contraindicated because of its effect on urate excetion. Colchicine (derived from the autumn crocus) is relatively specific in relieving the symptoms of acute gout, and is an alternative to an NSAID. It does not inhibit COX, so it lacks the side-effects of NSAIDs, but it commonly causes diarrhoea. *Pseudogout* is characterized by crystals of pyrophosphate rather than urate. It commonly affects the knee, and usually responds to joint aspiration, with intra-articular steroid injection if necessary.

Colchicine

USE

Colchicine is a useful alternative to NSAIDs in patients with gout in whom NSAIDs are contraindicated (e.g. patients with heart failure). Its efficacy is similar to that of indomethacin. It is also used in patients with familial Mediterranean fever and certain forms of Behçet's disease that are associated with excessive polymorphonuclear leucocyte migration into sites of tissue injury. Unlike several NSAIDs, it does not interact with warfarin. For acute attacks, it is given in doses of 0.5 mg orally up to four times a day. It can also be used prophylactically in doses of 0.5 mg two or three times daily. It is relatively contraindicated in the elderly and in those with renal or gastrointestinal disease.

MECHANISM OF ACTION

The primary action of colchicine is to bind to microtubular protein. This has two important results:

1 toxic concentrations cause arrest of cell division at metaphase (this phenomenon is exploited in making chromosome preparations *ex vivo*);
2 inhibition of leucocyte migration and hence reduced inflammation.

ADVERSE EFFECTS

1 The most important adverse effects are nausea, vomiting and diarrhoea, probably due to a direct effect on dividing cells in the intestinal mucosa. Some patients cannot tolerate the drug because of this.
2 Excessive doses cause gastrointestinal haemorrhage, rashes and renal failure.
3 Peripheral neuropathy (probably related to the role of microtubular proteins in axonal transport), alopecia and blood dyscrasias occur with prolonged use.

Alopecia
Blood dyscrasias

PHARMACOKINETICS

Colchicine is rapidly absorbed from the gastrointestinal tract. The mean $t_{\frac{1}{2}}$ is 30 min. The drug is partly metabolized, and a major portion is excreted via the bile and undergoes enterohepatic circulation, contributing to its gastrointestinal toxicity.

PROPHYLAXIS FOR RECURRENT GOUT

Allopurinol

USE

Allopurinol is used as long-term prophylaxis for patients with recurrent gout, especially those with severe tophaceous gout, urate renal stones, gout with renal failure and acute urate nephropathy, and to prevent this complication in patients about to undergo treatment of leukaemias and lymphomas with cytotoxic drugs. The plasma uric acid concentration should be kept below 0.42 mmol/L. The initial dose is 100 mg daily after food, increased gradually if necessary to a maximum of 600 mg daily. Allopurinol is of no use for the treatment of acute gout, and its use may provoke acute gout during the first few weeks of treatment. Concurrent indomethacin or colchicine is therefore given during the first month of treatment.

MECHANISM OF ACTION

Allopurinol is a xanthine oxidase inhibitor and decreases the production of uric acid. This reduces the concentration of uric acid in extracellular fluid, thereby preventing precipitation of crystals in joints or elsewhere. Uric acid is mobilized from tophaceous deposits which slowly disappear.

ADVERSE EFFECTS

The theoretical risk of forming xanthine stones has not proved to be a problem in ordinary clinical practice, although crystals of xanthine, hypoxanthine and oxypurinol (which appear to be harmless) are found in the muscles of allopurinol-treated patients. Mild dose-related rashes and more serious hypersensitivity reactions (including Stevens–Johnson syndrome) occur, especially in patients with renal failure, and are probably due to accumulation of metabolites. Malaise, nausea, vertigo, alopecia and hepatotoxicity are uncommon.

PHARMACOKINETICS

Allopurinol is well absorbed from the intestine. The mean plasma $t_{\frac{1}{2}}$ is about 3 h. Hepatic metabolism yields oxypurinol, which is itself a weak xanthine oxidase inhibitor.

DRUG INTERACTIONS

- Allopurinol decreases the rate of breakdown of 6-mercaptopurine (the active metabolite of azathioprine). If these drugs are used concomitantly with allopurinol (as in the treatment of leukaemia), their dose should be reduced.
- Metabolism of warfarin is inhibited, so when allopurinol is prescribed for patients receiving this anticoagulant, the international normalized ratio (INR) must be checked repeatedly during the first few days and weeks, with warfarin dose adjustment if necessary.

Uricosuric drugs

USE

These drugs (e.g. sulphinpyrazone, probenecid) have been largely rendered obsolete by allopurinol, but continue to be useful in the few patients who require prophylactic therapy and who have severe adverse reactions to allopurinol. Uricosuric drugs inhibit active transport of organic acids by renal tubules. Their main effect on the handling of uric acid by the kidney is to prevent the reabsorption of filtered uric acid by the proximal tubule, thus greatly increasing excretion. After 1 week the initial dose (250 mg daily for probenecid, 100 mg daily for sulphinpyrazone) is increased until a satisfactory plasma concentration of uric acid is

Key points

Gout

- Gout is caused by an inflammory reaction to precipitated crystals of uric acid.
- Always consider possible contributing factors, including drugs (especially diuretics) and alcohol.
- Treatment of acute attack:
  - NSAIDs (e.g. indomethacin);
  - colchicine (useful in cases where NSAIDs are contraindicated);
- Prophylaxis (for recurrent disease or tophaceous gout):
  - allopurinol (xanthine oxidase inhibitor) is only started well after the acute attack has resolved, and with NSAID cover to prevent a flare;
  - uricosuric drugs (e.g. sulphinpyrazone, which has additional NSAID and antiplatelet actions) are less effective than allopurinol. They are a useful alternative when allopurinol causes severe adverse effects (e.g. rashes). A high output of alkaline urine should be maintained to prevent crystalluria.

Case history

A 45-year-old publican presented to a locum GP with symptoms suggestive of acute gout in his big toe. There was a history of essential hypertension, and he had a similar but less severe attack 3 months previously which settled spontaneously. Following this serum urate levels were determined and found to be within the normal range. His toe was now inflamed and exquisitely tender. His blood pressure was 180/106 mmHg, but the examination was otherwise unremarkable. The locum was concerned that treatment with an NSAID might increase the patient's blood pressure, and that, since his uric acid level was recently found to be normal, he might not have gout. He therefore prescribed coproxamol for the pain and repeated the serum urate assay. The patient returns the following day unimproved, having spent a sleepless night, and you see him yourself for the first time. The examination is as described by your locum, and serum urate remains normal. What would you do?

Comment

Normal serum urate does not exclude gout. The patient requires treatment with an NSAID such as indomethacin. Review his medication (is he on a diuretic for his hypertension?) and enquire about his alcohol consumption. Blood pressure is commonly increased by acute pain. Despite his occupation, the patient is in fact teetotal, and he was receiving bendrofluazide for hypertension. This was discontinued, atenolol was substituted, and his blood pressure fell to 162/100 mmHg during treatment with indomethacin. A short period of poor antihypertensive control in this setting is not of great importance. After the pain had settled and indomethacin was stopped, the patient's blood pressure decreased further to 140/84 mmHg on atenolol. He did not have any recurrence of gout. (Only if recurrent gout was a problem would prophylactic treatment with allopurinol be worth considering.)

obtained. An acute attack of gout may be precipitated if treatment is started with a large dose. Concurrent treatment with an anti-inflammatory drug while initiating treatment with probenecid reduces this risk, but at the expense of increased risk of NSAID toxicity, since these drugs are also eliminated by the organic acid secretory mechanism (see Chapter 6). Sulphinpyrazone is a weak NSAID in its own right, and a flare of gout is less likely to occur when using it. Unlike other NSAIDs, there is also evidence that it has a clinically useful antiplatelet action. The patient should drink enough water to have a urine output of 2 L/day during the first month of treatment, and a sodium bicarbonate or potassium citrate mixture should be given to keep the urinary pH above 7.0. Other adverse effects include rashes and gastrointestinal upsets.

Further reading

De Broe ME, Elseviers MM. 1998: Analgesic nephropathy. *New England Journal of Medicine* **338**, 446–42.

Emmerson BT. 1996: The management of gout. *New England Journal of Medicine* **334**, 445–51.

O'Dell JR, Haire CE, Erikson N et al. 1996: Treatment of rheumatoid arthritis with methotrexate alone, sulfasalazine and hydroxychloroquine or a combination of all three medications. *New England Journal of Medicine* **334**, 1287–91.

Rongean JC, Kelly JP, Naldi L. 1995: Medication use and the risk of Stevens-Johnson syndrome or toxic epidermal necrolysis. *New England Journal of Medicine* **333**, 1600–7.

Vane JR, Bakhle YS, Botting RM. 1998: Cyclo-oxygenases 1 and 2. *Annual Review of Pharmacology and Toxicology* **38**, 97–120.

PART IV

THE CARDIOVASCULAR SYSTEM

CHAPTER TWENTY-SIX

PREVENTION *of* ATHEROMA: LOWERING PLASMA CHOLESTEROL *and* OTHER APPROACHES

- Introduction
- Pathophysiology
- Prevention of atheroma
- Screening/primary prevention
- Approach to therapy
- Drugs used to treat dyslipidaemia
- Treatment of dyslipidaemia at extremes of age and during pregnancy

INTRODUCTION

Atheroma is the commonest cause of ischaemic heart disease, stroke and peripheral vascular disease. Since these are the major causes of morbidity and mortality among adults in industrialized societies, its prevention is of great importance. An important practical distinction is made between preventive measures in healthy people (called 'primary prevention') and measures in people who have survived a stroke or a heart attack or who are symptomatic from angina or claudication (called 'secondary prevention'). The absolute risk per unit time is greatest in those with clinical evidence of established disease, so secondary prevention is especially worthwhile (and cost-effective), and is pursued more aggressively (e.g. with drug treatment) than primary prevention. Primary prevention inevitably involves larger populations who are at relatively low absolute risk per unit time, so interventions must be inexpensive and have a very low risk of adverse effects (e.g. advice regarding a healthy lifestyle).

A family history of myocardial infarction in a first-degree relative, especially at an early age, confers an increased risk of ischaemic heart disease, and *genetic factors* are important in the development of atheroma. Epidemiological observations, including the rapid change in incidence of coronary disease in Japanese migrants from Japan (low risk) through Hawaii (intermediate risk) to the west coast of the USA (high risk), and the recent substantial decline in coronary risk in the USA, indicate that *environmental factors* are also of paramount importance in the pathogenesis of atheroma. Such observations further suggest that if environmental risk factors are altered, this quite rapidly results in an altered incidence of disease.

PATHOPHYSIOLOGY

Atheromatous plaques are *focal* lesions of large and medium-sized arteries. They start as fatty streaks in the intima, and progress to proliferative fibro-fatty growths that protrude into the vascular lumen and limit blood flow. These plaques are rich in both extracellular and intracellular cholesterol. During their development they do not initially give rise to symptoms, but as they progress they may cause angina pectoris, intermittent claudication or other symptoms according to their anatomical location. They may rupture or ulcerate, in which event the subintima acts as a focus for thrombosis: platelet–fibrin thrombi propagate and can occlude the artery, causing myocardial infarction or stroke.

Epidemiological observations (e.g. the Framingham Study) have shown that there is a strong positive relationship between the concentration of circulating cholesterol, specifically of the low-density-lipoprotein (LDL) fraction, and the risk of atheroma. This relationship is non-linear and depends strongly on the presence or absence of other risk factors, including male sex, arterial hypertension, cigarette smoking, diabetes mellitus, positive family or personal history of premature ischaemic heart disease, and electrocardiographic or echocardiographic abnormalities (Figure 26.1).

Figure 26.2 shows an outline of the metabolic pathways involved in lipid transport. Approximately two-thirds of cholesterol circulating in the blood is synthesized in the liver. Hepatocytes synthesize cholesterol and bile acids from acetate, and secrete them in bile into the intestine, where they are involved in fat absorption. The rate-limiting enzyme in cholesterol biosynthesis is 3-hydroxyl 3-methylglutaryl coenzyme A reductase (HMG-CoA reductase). Fat is absorbed in the form of triglyceride-rich chylomicra. Free fatty acid is cleaved from triglyceride in these particles by lipoprotein lipase, an enzyme on the surface of endothelial cells. Free fatty acids are used as an energy source by striated muscle, or stored as fat in adipose tissue. Chylomicron remnants are taken up by hepatocytes to complete the exogenous cycle. The endogenous cycle consists of the secretion of triglyceride-rich (and hence very-low-density) lipoprotein particles (VLDL) by the liver into the blood, followed by removal of free fatty acid by lipoprotein lipase. This results in progressive enrichment of the particles with cholesterol, with an increase in their density through intermediate-density to low-density lipoprotein (LDL). It is circulating LDL that is especially atherogenic. Low-density-lipoprotein particles bind to receptors (LDL receptors) located in coated pits on the surface of hepatocytes, so the plasma concentration of LDL is determined by a balance between LDL synthesis and hepatic uptake. Low-density lipoprotein that enters arterial walls at sites of endothelial damage can be remobilized in the form of high-density lipoprotein (HDL). However, it may become oxidized and be taken up by macrophages as part of atherogenesis (see below).

There have been no satisfactory subprimate animal models of atheroma until recently, but the advent of transgenic mice deficient in specific key enzymes and receptors in lipoprotein metabolism is rapidly transforming this fast-moving field. None the less, most of our understanding of atheroma comes from human pathology (dating

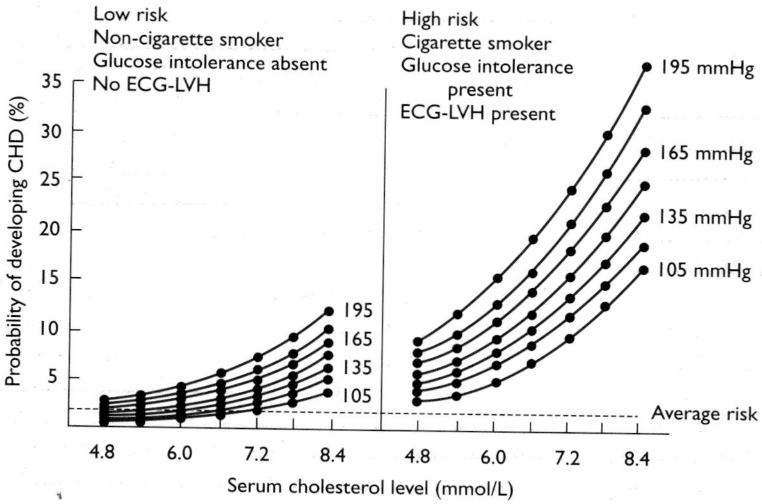

Figure 26.1: Probability of developing coronary heart disease in 6 years: 40-year-old men in the Framingham Study during 16 years follow up. The numbers to the right of the curves show the systolic blood pressure (mmHg).

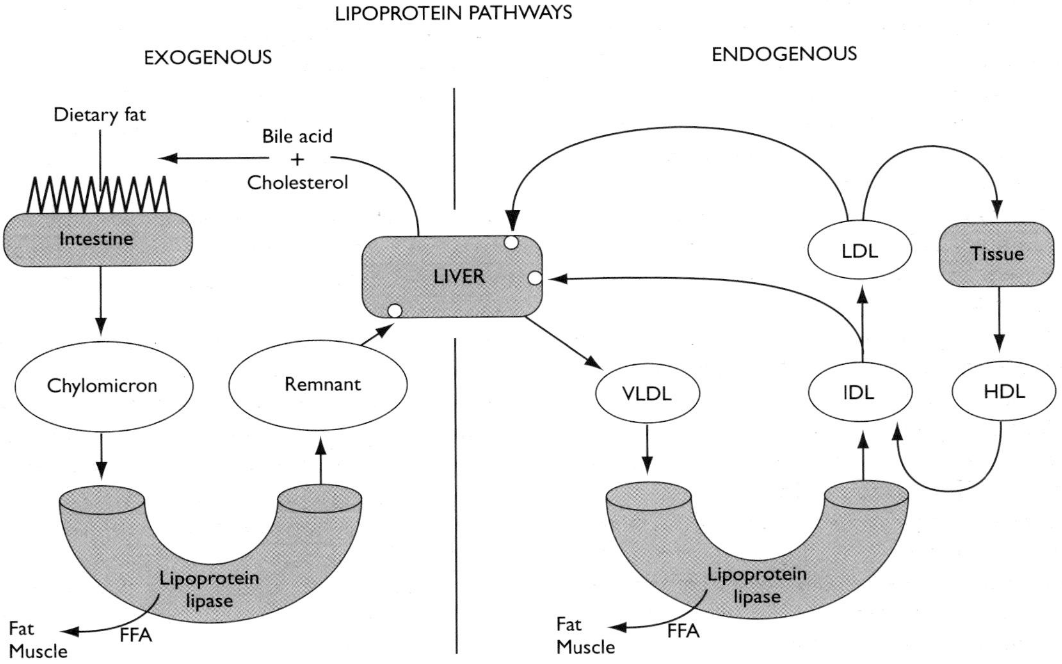

Figure 26.2: Lipoprotein transport. FFA = free fatty acids, VLDL = very-low-density lipoprotein, IDL = intermediate-density lipoprotein, HDL = high-density lipoprotein.

from the classical studies of Rokitanski, Duguid and Florey) and from experimental studies in primates (especially those of Ross). Intimal injury is believed to initiate the atheromatous process. This process shares many of the cellular and biochemical features (e.g. adhesion molecules, cytokines) of chronic inflammation and tissue repair. The nature of the initial injury is not known. Several infectious agents (including viruses and *Helicobacter pylori*) have been mooted as of possible aetiological significance, and recently *Chlamydia pneumonii* has been identified in atheromatous lesions. If these organisms prove to be important in pathogenesis, this will open up a whole new range of potential preventive and therapeutic opportunities. Rheological factors (e.g. turbulence) are believed to be responsible for the striking predilection for certain sites (e.g. at the low-shear side of the origin of arteries branching from the aorta). The injury may initially be undetectable morphologically, but results in focal endothelial cell dysfunction. Blood monocytes adhere to receptors expressed by injured endothelium, and migrate into the vessel wall where they become macrophages. These possess receptors for oxidized (but not native) LDL, which they ingest to become 'foam cells'.

Lesions become infiltrated with extracellular as well as intracellular cholesterol. Platelets also adhere to the injured intima. Macrophages and platelets both secrete growth factors, including platelet and macrophage-derived growth factors and transforming growth factor β, which cause migration, proliferation and differentiation of vascular smooth muscle cells and fibroblasts from the underlying media and adventitia. These processes result in the formation of fibro-fatty plaques.

Atheromatous lesions are not necessarily irreversible. There is currently considerable interest in the possibility that the combination of diet and drugs causes regression of atheroma, and evidence to support this. Cholesterol is mobilized from tissues in the form of HDL particles. These are not atherogenic – indeed, epidemiological studies have identified HDL as being strongly negatively correlated with risk of coronary heart disease. There is great interest in the connection between hyperlipidaemia and thrombosis, and it has been found that there is a close relationship between one of the apolipoproteins and plasminogen. Apo(a) is present in a lipoprotein known as Lp(a) which was first identified as a blood-group variant responsible for occasional transfusion reactions. The plasma concentration of Lp(a) varies over a 100-fold range and is strongly genetically determined. Apo(a) is very large and contains multiple repeats of one of the kringles of plasminogen (a kringle is a doughnut-shaped loop of amino acids held together by three internal disulphide bonds). It is likely that this homology leads to interference by Lp(a) with the function of plasminogen, which is the precursor of the endogenous fibrinolytic plasmin, and hence to a predisposition to thrombosis on atheromatous plaques.

Key points

Atherogenesis

- Endothelial injury initiates the process. The distribution of lesions is influenced by turbulence (e.g. at branch points) in the arterial circulation.
- Monocytes in blood stick to injured endothelium and migrate into the vessel wall, where they become macrophages.
- LDL is oxidized by free radicals generated by activated cells (including macrophages and endothelial cells). Oxidized LDL is taken into macrophages via scavenger receptors.
- This sets up a chronic inflammatory process in which chemical messengers are released by lipid-laden macrophages ('foam cells'), T-lymphocytes and platelets. These interleukins and growth factors cause the migration and proliferation of vascular smooth muscle cells and fibroblasts, which form a fibro-fatty plaque.
- Cigarette smoking promotes several of these processes (e.g. platelet activation). An infectious agent (*Chlamydia pneumonii*) is often present in the fatty lesions, but its role in pathogenesis is uncertain.
- If the plaque ruptures, thrombosis occurs on the subendothelium, and may occlude the vessel, causing stroke, myocardial infarction, etc., depending on the anatomical location.

Prevention of atheroma

Modifiable risk factors for the genesis of atheromatous plaque are potentially susceptible to therapeutic intervention. These include smoking, obesity, sedentary habits, dyslipidaemia, glucose intolerance (see Chapter 36) and systemic arterial hypertension (see Chapter 27). Male sex is a strong risk factor for coronary artery disease, and there is good epidemiological evidence that oestrogen replacement reduces cardiac disease in post-menopausal women. There was concern that progestogen treatment may attenuate this benefit, but this possibility has recently been ruled out. Prevention of coronary disease can thus be added to the other benefits of hormone replacement treatment in post-menopausal women (see Chapter 40).

Smoking

Cigarette smoking (see chapter 52) is a strong risk factor for vascular disease. It causes vasoconstriction via activation of the sympathetic nervous system and platelet activation with a consequent increase in thromboxane A_2 biosynthesis, although the precise mechanism whereby smoking promotes atheroma is unknown. Stopping smoking is of substantial and rapid benefit. Smoking causes considerable physical and psychological dependence, and attempts to give up are often unsuccessful. Much of the dependence is due to the pharmacological effects of nicotine, and nicotine chewing gum or 'patches' for transdermal administration (which are available in the UK as over-the-counter products, see Chapter 4) are sometimes helpful. They reduce the dysphoria during the first few weeks of stopping smoking, and approximately double the number of people who succeed in remaining free from the habit, although the proportion who relapse is depressingly high. Individuals must not smoke while using nicotine patches, and these patches should not be used in pregnancy or within 6 weeks of a myocardial infarction or stroke. In any case, they should not be used for longer than 3 months, as it is unclear how many of the long-term adverse effects of smoking on vascular disease are in fact mediated by nicotine.

Diet and habits

Obesity is increasingly common, probably because humans have evolved mechanisms for storing energy during periods of plenty against the future likelihood of famine. It is a strong risk factor for atheromatous disease, especially in individuals with a predominantly abdominal distribution of excess fat (i.e. a high waist:hip ratio). The influence of obesity on cardiovascular risk is partly accounted for by its association with other risk factors, such as hypertension and hypercholesterolaemia. Weight reduction in obese individuals restores life expectancy toward normal.

Treatment of obesity (see Chapter 33, p. 386–7) is notoriously difficult, and the list of grotesquely inappropriate therapies that have been employed is a testament to human folly.* Surgical treatments, including wiring the jaws, stapling the stomach and 'apronectomies', have little role. Bulk agents such as methylcellulose have been used in an attempt to produce feelings of satiety, but there is little evidence that they are effective, and they cause bloating, flatulence and, rarely, oesophageal or intestinal obstruction. They are less palatable than high-fibre foods such as baked ('jacket') potatoes. Centrally acting appetite suppressants have been used, but there is no evidence that they improve the long-term outlook, and their history is not reassuring. **Amphetamines** cause dependence as well as a range of neuropsychiatric symptoms (e.g. euphoria, nervousness, irritiability, drowsiness, insomnia, tiredness, dizziness, hallucinations, paranoia and depression), and gastrointestinal (e.g. dry mouth, nausea, vomiting, constipation or diarrhoea) and cardiovascular (e.g. palpitations, arrhythmias) side-effects, and use of amphetamine-like drugs (e.g. **diethylpropion**) is not justified. **Fenfluramine** is structurally related to amphetamine, but has a sedative rather than a stimulant effect. Abuse has occurred, and depression sometimes develops when the drug is abruptly discontinued. It should not be used in patients with epilepsy or a history of psychiatric illness or drug abuse. Some physicians use fenfluramine or **dexfenfluramine** (the active dextro-isomer) as adjunctive treatment in severe obesity. They have been associated with pulmonary hypertension. These drugs should not be used in patients who are only mildly or moderately overweight, and should not be used long term. Increasing basal metabolic rate by treatment with **thyroxine** is justified only in patients with hypothyroidism. Selective β_3-agonists that exert an effect on thermogenesis have been developed that increase energy expenditure and cause weight loss during short-term treatment. There is no evidence of long-term efficacy, and they cause muscle tremor in a large proportion of patients, although more selective drugs of this class appear promising. Currently, there is considerable interest among basic scientists and in the pharmaceutical industry in the role of a newly discovered peptide hormone (*leptin*) which signals from peripheral fat to central appetite control centres where another peptide (*neuropeptide Y*, NPY) is involved as a neurotransmitter. It is to be hoped that this interest will translate into a clinically safe and effective means of combating obesity.

Meanwhile, dietary restraint (coupled if possible with increased exercise) remains the only sensible therapeutic strategy. The desirable range of weight for height in adults is defined by body mass index (BMI):

$$\text{BMI} = \text{weight (kg)}/(\text{height})^2\ (\text{m})^2.$$

The BMI should be between 20 and 25 kg/m^2. Each kilogram of excess weight represents approximately 7000 kcal of stored energy. Dietary restriction of energy intake to create a negative energy balance is the only practicable way to use up the excess stores. Life-long alteration of dietary habits is needed to maintain ideal body weight, so advice on a suitable and acceptable diet is essential. Patients need to be given a target weight and advised of a realistic rate of weight loss that they should attempt to achieve. Very-low-calorie and formula diets cause an excessive loss of non-fat body mass, do nothing to improve eating habits in the long term, and are not recommended. Instead, advice should centre on the importance of small regular meals, reduced fat and increased fibre, with a total energy intake of 800 kcal/day or more. An energy deficit of 1000 kcal/day will result in a loss of about 1 kg of body weight per week, which is the maximum useful rate of weight loss. Behavioural modification is essential, and psychological support (e.g. from groups such as Weight Watchers) can be valuable.

* 'There is a sucker born every minute, and one born to take him' (Barnum).

Diet is important for factors other than weight alone. In most studies, people who eat relatively large amounts of fruit, vegetables and grains have been found to have substantially lower risks of death from cardiovascular disease (and also from cancer). Anti-oxidant vitamins may account for some of this benefit. Saturated fats are important determinants of plasma cholesterol levels (see below). Conversely, mono- or polyunsaturated fatty acid intake can *lower* plasma cholesterol. Among polyunsaturated fatty acids there may be important differences (e.g. between natural *cis*-isomers and potentially atherogenic *trans*-isomers present in some margarines). There is epidemiological evidence that eating modest amounts of fish regularly reduces cardiovascular risk independent of providing natural polyunsaturated fatty acids. There is also epidemiological evidence that eating food rich in natural anti-oxidants, such as salads (rich in vitamin C) and nuts (rich in vitamin E), reduces cardiovascular risk. This is certainly less likely to cause adverse effects than are drugs such as **probucol,** which is anti-oxidant but which lowers HDL and has marked toxic effects in animals. Controlled trials (as opposed to epidemiological observation) of the vascular effects of anti-oxidant vitamins are scarce. One study based at Cambridge (the 'CHAOS' Study) suggested a marked effect of vitamin E in cardiac events, but was not designed to detect an effect on mortality. Larger trials are currently in progress.

Sedentary habits are a risk factor for atheromatous disease, and regular exercise improves cardiovascular risk. This appears to be independent of any effect on obesity, but perhaps relates to favourable effects on systolic blood pressure, HDL (which is increased by exercise) and fibrinolysis. Exercise also improves one's sense of well-being and reduces stress.

Dyslipidaemia

Individuals at increased risk of atherosclerosis because of high circulating LDL levels relative to HDL have dyslipidaemia. Marked elevation of LDL or triglyceride (TG) can cause other problems, such as pancreatitis, eruptive xanthomas or other stigmata of hypercholesterolaemia, but these are uncommon, in contrast to premature atherosclerotic coronary (and other) arterial disease. Reducing the total plasma cholesterol concentration reduces the risk of coronary heart disease, and can cause regression of atheroma. The potential benefits of lowering plasma cholesterol levels can be viewed from either an individual or a public health perspective. Individuals with the highest plasma cholesterol concentrations have most to gain from cholesterol-lowering measures, especially if they also have other risk factors. However, to achieve maximum impact on the prevalence of coronary artery disease in a country such as the UK, it is essential to reduce the average plasma cholesterol concentration of the whole community, not just those at highest individual risk. This is because most vascular events occur in individuals without marked elevation of plasma cholesterol levels, because the total number of such people is so much greater than the few with very high values. Consequently, a shift of the population distribution curve towards lower values with a quite modest reduction in the average value would have a very substantial effect on the prevalence of coronary artery disease. These two perspectives are not mutually exclusive, and general dietary advice directed at the population as a whole should be combined with opportunistic screening of individuals, especially those with additional risk factors for vascular disease. More aggressive measures (including the use of drugs) can be targeted at individuals at greatest risk. The top priority in this regard are individuals who have clinical evidence of atheromatous disease (e.g. angina, history of myocardial infarction, symptomatic carotid stenosis, claudication). Such individuals should generally receive treatment, usually with a statin for *secondary prevention*, as their risk of coronary events is high (approximately 3–6% per annum).

Screening/primary prevention

The most cost-effective method of screening for general practitioners and hospital physicians is to determine serum cholesterol opportunistically when the occasion presents itself, provided that the patient is not suffering from an acute illness such as influenza or myocardial infarction (since this transiently but profoundly lowers the circulating cholesterol concentration), or from a chronic disease (e.g. dementia, malignant disease or cor pulmonale) that would render treatment inappropriate. The presence of additional risk factors for coronary disease or, even more strongly, of a personal history of vascular disease (e.g. angina, previous myocardial infarction) renders such screening even more appropriate. Physical signs of vascular disease or of hyperlipidaemia (e.g. tendon, eruptive or palmar xanthomas, early arcus, xanthelasma) occasionally alert the physician to the possibility of hypercholesterolaemia. In patients without clinical evidence of atheromatous disease, the decision as to whether to initiate drug treatment at any given level of serum lipids should be informed by the *risk of coronary events*. This is calculated from tables of risk factors such as the New Zealand guidelines.

APPROACH TO THERAPY

An approach to therapy is summarized in Figure 26.3.

1 Measure height and weight, and determine the ideal body weight. Advice regarding healthy eating habits, particularly with a view to attaining ideal body weight and avoidance of excessive intake of saturated fats, as well as general advice about smoking and regular exercise, should be given to everyone.
2 Since the risk of coronary disease rises smoothly with cholesterol concentration, recommendations regarding actions that are justified at specified concentrations are arbitrary. As with arterial blood pressure, 'lower is better' but, again as for hypertension, in practice physicians need an arbitrary framework (such as that recommended by the European Atherosclerosis Society) within which to make individual clinical judgements. If the screening cholesterol is < 5.2 mM, dietary advice should be reinforced, but blood sampling need not be repeated unless there are multiple coexisting risk factors, and then probably not for a year or more.
3 A further blood sample should be obtained in the fasted state from individuals with total cholesterol of > 5.2 mM on the initial screen. This is used to determine total cholesterol (TC), triglycerides (TG) and HDL. (TC is little influenced by whether or not blood is sampled during fasting, but TG concentration is elevated by the presence of chylomicra during fat absorption.) From these values, LDL can be calculated using the Friedwald equation:

$$\text{LDL} = \text{TC} - (\text{HDL} + \text{TG}/2.2)\ \text{mM}.$$

This second sample reduces the probability of acting on a value that was elevated due to laboratory variation. It also identifies individuals (often women) with total cholesterol > 5.2 mM but with relatively high levels of HDL (e.g. > 1.8 mmol/L) and LDL < 3.8 mM, who are *not* at increased risk of coronary disease and can be reassured.
4 Consider the possibility of secondary hypercholesterolaemia (see Table 26.1). It is important

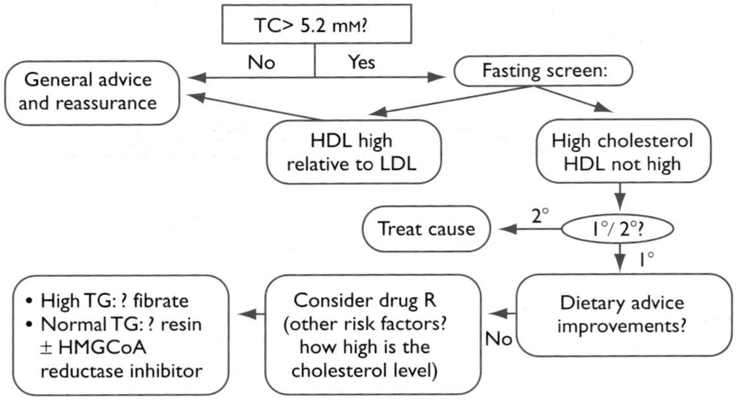

Figure 26.3: Approach to dyslipidaemia. TC = total cholesterol, HDL = high-density lipoprotein, TG = triglyceride, 1° = primary dyslipidaemia, 2° = secondary dyslipidaemia, HMGCoA 5 β-hydroxy-β-methylglutaryl coenzyme A.

Table 26.1: Secondary dyslipidaemia

Disorder	Main lipid disturbance
Diabetes	Mixed
Hypothyroidism	Cholesterol
Alcohol excess	Triglyceride
Nephrotic syndrome	Cholesterol
Renal failure	Mixed
Primary biliary cirrhosis	Cholesterol

to exclude *hypothyroidism*, which can be asymptomatic and commonly causes hypercholesterolemia. Hypertriglyceridemia raises the possibility of excessive alcohol consumption, and further history and laboratory evidence such as elevated γ-glutamyl transpeptidase activity or raised mean corpuscular volume may be informative. Underlying disorders should be treated if present.

5 A detailed dietary history is obtained, and more detailed dietary advice is given to individuals with total cholesterol > 5.2 mM. This should include advice to reduce intake of egg yolks (which are rich in cholesterol), and items high in saturated fat, including red meat, sausages, bacon, offal, butter, full-cream milk and fried foods together with advice to trim fat from food before cooking, use of grilling, poaching or microwave cooking methods, and a relative increase (through substitution) of vegetables, fish, chicken and corn or olive oil. Reasonable recommendations are as follows: total fat < 30% of calories; ratio of unsaturated to saturated fat > 1.0; cholesterol < 300 mg daily; and calories to achieve/maintain ideal body weight. It is important to try to give advice that will be acceptable to each individual in the long term. Effects of diet vary depending on the enthusiasm and time spent by both physician and dietitian. Response to diet is assessed by measuring total serum cholesterol after 4–8 weeks, with further encouragement and follow-up as needed.

6 Drug treatment is considered for individuals in whom total cholesterol fails to fall below the individual target (e.g. 5.2 mM) despite dietary advice. The higher the cholesterol concentration, the greater the potential absolute individual benefit from such treatment. However, the decision to start drug treatment also needs to take into account the presence or otherwise of additional risk factors. The gradient of the function relating coronary risk to plasma cholesterol concentration is smooth, the slope of the line being determined by the presence or absence of other risk factors (see Figure 26.1), and lipid-lowering drugs are not without adverse effects. Decisions about the concentration of cholesterol at which the benefit of treatment outweighs the risks, inconvenience and expense are still contentious, and what follows is based on our current practice. A personal history of coronary artery disease (i.e. secondary as opposed to primary prevention) or of familial hypercholesterolaemia are the strongest indications for drug intervention. In the absence of other risk factors we initiate drug treatment only if the total cholesterol concentration is persistently > 7.5 mM despite adherence to dietary advice, and then only in selected patients.

7 With regard to choice of drug, resins decrease the plasma cholesterol concentration and reduce the risk of coronary artery disease, but the magnitude of their effect is modest and there is a high incidence of gastrointestinal side-effects. They are useful in combination with HMGCoA reductase inhibitors, in patients with very severe disease. Since they are not absorbed and have been used extensively, they are also a rational choice in children with severe familial hyperlipidaemias in whom they may prevent disease progression and buy time while the safety and efficacy of some of the newer agents and strategies (e.g. HMGCoA reductase inhibitors and gene therapy) are explored. Resins increase plasma triglyceride levels, so they should not be used in patients with hypercholesterolaemia and coincident marked hypertriglyceridaemia. If triglycerides are elevated as well as cholesterol, the possibility of excessive alcohol intake is reviewed, and appropriate advice is given if necessary. If the patient is obese, calorie restriction is intensified. Fibrates are effective in lowering cholesterol levels in patients with high cholesterol together with markedly elevated triglycerides.

DRUGS USED TO TREAT DYSLIPIDAEMIA

The three main classes of drugs used to treat dyslipidaemia are the *statins*, *exchange resins* and *fibrates*. Additional drugs (see Table 26.2) are useful in special situations.

HMGCoA reductase inhibitors

USE

Simvastatin, **pravastatin** and **antorvastatin** are available in the UK, and many similar drugs are being developed. They are generally similar, although simvastatin is more widely distributed in the body as it is less polar than pravastatin, which is distributed selectively to the liver (its site of action) by virtue of a specific uptake mechanism. These drugs are highly effective in lowering LDL cholesterol, especially in patients with heterozygous familial hypercholesterolaemia, in whom they are particularly useful. Large-scale studies have not only shown that statins reduce the incidence of coronary events and prolong life, but have also demonstrated excellent safety. The dose (10–40 mg of simvastatin or pravastatin at bedtime) is adjusted on the basis of repeated plasma lipid determinations.

MECHANISM OF ACTION

HMGCoA reductase is the rate-limiting step in cholesterol biosynthesis from acetate. Inhibition of this enzyme results in reduced cytoplasmic cholesterol levels in hepatocytes, which respond by increasing the synthesis of LDL receptors that are expressed on their surface membranes. This in turn increases hepatic LDL uptake from the plasma, reducing the plasma LDL concentration. HMGCoA reductase inhibitors have little effect on plasma concentrations of triglycerides or of HDL.

ADVERSE EFFECTS AND CONTRAINDICATIONS

HMGCoA reductase inhibitors are generally very well tolerated. Mild and infrequent side-effects include nausea, constipation, diarrhoea, flatulence, fatigue, insomnia and rash. More serious adverse events are rare, but include rhabdomyolysis, hepatitis and angioedema. Liver function tests should be performed before starting treatment and at intervals thereafter, and patients should be warned to stop the drug and report at once for determination of creatine kinase levels if they develop muscle aches. HMGCoA reductase inhibitors should not be used in alcoholics or in patients with active liver disease, or during pregnancy. In contrast to their great usefulness in patients with heterozygous familial hypercholesterolaemia, HMGCoA reductase inhibitors are not very effective in patients with the extremely rare *homozygous* form of familial hypercholesterolaemia, who are unable to synthesize LDL receptors. (These patients may present with symptomatic coronary artery disease in childhood or adolescence, and liver transplantation is a therapeutic option.) Antorvastatin is an exception, and is licensed for this indication.

PHARMACOKINETICS

Statins are well absorbed from the intestine, extracted by the liver (their site of action) and are subject to extensive presystemic metabolism. Simvastatin is an inactive lactone prodrug which is metabolized in the liver to its active form, the corresponding β-hydroxy fatty acid.

DRUG INTERACTIONS

- The potential for rhabdomyolysis and consequent acute renal failure may be increased by concurrent use of an HMGCoA reductase inhibitor with a fibrate, and close monitoring is mandatory if such a combination is employed.
- The efficacy of HMGCoA reductase inhibitors is substantially increased by concurrent use of a bile acid-binding resin, and this may prove useful in treating severely affected individuals, especially those with established disease.

Anion-exchange resins

USE

Cholestyramine or **colestipol** are used to treat patients with hypercholesterolaemia. The American Lipid Research Clinics trial of middle-aged men with primary hypercholesterolaemia showed that addition of such a resin to dietary treatment resulted in a fall of approximately 13% in plasma cholesterol concentration, and that this was associated with a 20–25% reduction in coronary heart disease over a 7.5-year follow-up period. Cholestyramine and colestipol are similar in their safety and efficacy, but cholestyramine consists of

Table 26.2: Drugs used in dyslipidaemia

Class/drug	Biochemical effect	Effect on coronary artery disease	Effect on longetivity	Adverse effects	Special situations
Statin/simvastatin, pravastatin	LDL↓↓	↓↓	↑ (4S, WOSCOPS)	Rare: myositis ↑ liver transaminase	Contraindicated in pregnancy, caution in children
Resin/cholestyramine	LDL↓TG↑	↓	NP	Constipation, flatulence, nausea	Contraindicated in biliary obstruction
Fibrate/gemfibrizil, bezafibrate	TG↓↓LDL↓ HDL↑	↓	NP	Myositis; gastro-intestinal symptoms	Contraindicated in alcoholics, renal/liver impairment
Nicotinic acid derivatives/high-dose nicotinic acid, acipimox	TG↓↓LDL↓ HDL↑	↓	NP	Flushing (PGD_2-mediated; diarrhoea; uriticaria; epigastric pain; hyperuricaemia; hyperglycaemia	Useful in familial hypercholesterolaemia; PG-related adverse effects ameliorated by aspirin before the dose
Probucol	LDL↓HDL↓ Anti-oxidant	NP	NP	QT prolongation on ECG	Contraindicated during and up to 6 months before pregnancy
Fish oil/eicosapentanoic acid-rich supplements	TG↓	NP	NP	Belching with a fishy after-taste	Used in patients with pancreatitis caused by raised TG. Contraindicated in patients with familial hypercholesterolaemia, in whom it increases cholesterol levels

NP = not proven

much coarser particles, and individual patients may prefer one or the other drug for this reason. Resins are taken as a suspension, and are more palatable if dispersed in fruit juice than in water. Some patients prefer to make up the following day's supply the night before and leave it in the refrigerator. This results in a soft suspension rather than a gritty one. The dose of cholestyramine is 8–24 g daily given as a single dose or divided 8-hourly immediately before meals. Other uses of these resins include the following:

- diarrhoea due to ileal resection or Crohn's disease;
- diarrhoea after vagotomy or in diabetic autonomic neuropathy;
- pruritus in incomplete biliary obstruction.

MECHANISM OF ACTION

Bile acid-binding resins (see Figure 26.4) are not absorbed from the intestine, and they bind bile acids in the gut lumen, disrupting micelles and thereby inhibiting reabsorption of bile salts and cholesterol. This lowers plasma cholesterol levels in two ways.

1 A larger proportion of cholesterol synthesized by the liver is converted into bile salts, and less enters the circulation as cholesterol and its esters.
2 Bile acids inhibit the rate-limiting 7-hydroxylation step in cholesterol oxidation, so the resins increase cholesterol breakdown.

However, cytoplasmic cholesterol exerts negative feedback inhibition on HMGCoA reductase, which is rate limiting in cholesterol *synthesis*. Lowering plasma cholesterol by means of a resin removes this inhibition and accelerates cholesterol production. Accelerated cholesterol synthesis therefore limits the magnitude of the effect of resins on plasma cholesterol. This accounts for the marked synergy between resins and HMGCoA reductase inhibitors which block cholesterol synthesis.

ADVERSE EFFECTS AND CONTRAINDICATIONS

Since resins are not absorbed, the major side-effects relate to the gut, and consist of bloating, wind, abdominal discomfort and distension, constipation or diarrhoea, and anorexia. These affect around one-third of patients. Absorption of vitamins D, K and folic acid is reduced, and supplements may be needed, especially in children,

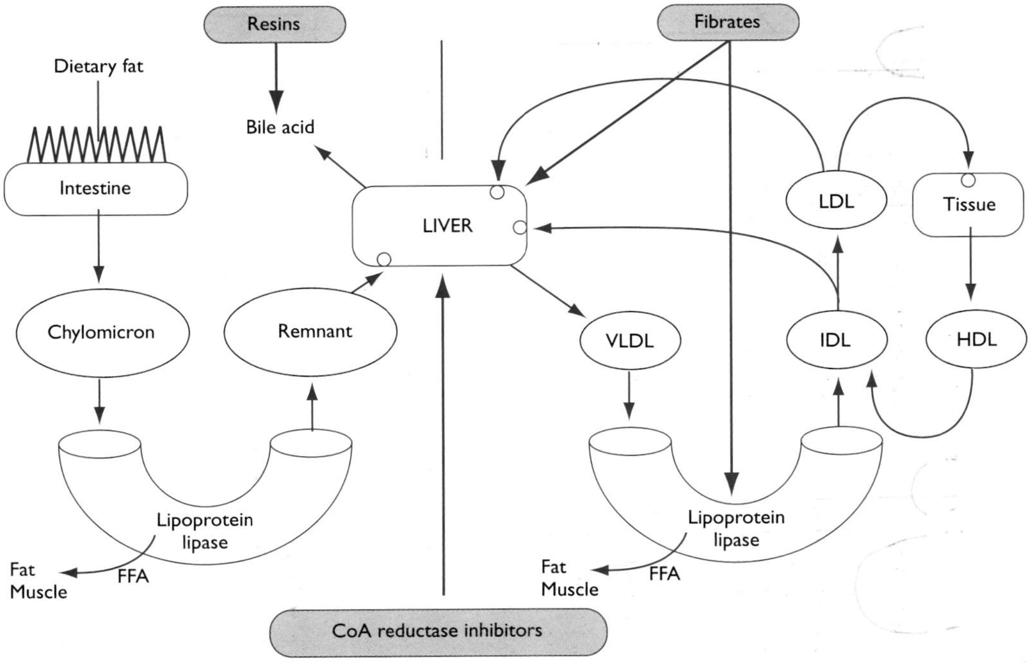

Figure 26.4: Sites of action of lipid-lowering drugs (see Figure 24.2 for abbreviations).

pregnant women and nursing mothers. If uncorrected, prolonged use can predispose to haemorrhage due to reduced synthesis of vitamin K-dependent coagulation factors. Resins are contraindicated in patients with complete biliary obstruction, in whom they will be ineffective.

DRUG INTERACTIONS

Bile acid-binding resins give rise to several clinically important interactions due to interference with absorption of other drugs (e.g. thiazides, antibiotics, warfarin, thyroxine and digoxin). Drugs should be taken at least 1 h before or 4–6 h after a dose of resin. The potentially useful interaction between resins and HMGCoA reductase inhibitors has been described above.

Fibrates

USE

Several fibrates, including **bezafibrate** and **gemfibrozil**, are in common clinical use. **Fenofibrate** has similar actions, but in addition it has a uricosuric effect; hyperuricaemia and gout commonly coexist with hypertriglyceridaemia, so this is of some clinical utility in such patients. **Clofibrate** – which was used in a World Health Organization (WHO) trial – is less often used because it increases biliary cholesterol secretion and predisposes to gallstones. Its use is therefore limited to patients who have had a cholecystectomy. Furthermore, while it reduced the number of myocardial infarctions in the WHO trial, this was offset by an increased number of cancers of various kinds. The meaning of this has been extensively debated, but remains obscure. This issue is clouded by the effect of malignancy in lowering serum cholesterol levels. The original observations with clofibrate may have been a statistical accident, and there is no excess of cancers in patients treated with gemfibrozil in other trials (e.g. the Helsinki Heart Study). These studies have shown that fibrates have a marked effect in lowering plasma TG, with a modest (*c.* 10%) reduction in LDL and a similar increase in HDL. Coronary heart disease was reduced by about one-third. The dose of gemfibrozil is 600 mg twice daily. Bezafibrate is available in a slow-release preparation that is administered as a single night-time dose of 400 mg.

MECHANISM OF ACTION

The mechanism of the fibrates (see Figure 26.4) is incompletely understood. They stimulate lipoprotein lipase (hence their marked effect on TG) and also increase LDL uptake by the liver. In addition to their effects on plasma lipids, the fibrates lower fibrinogen levels and improve glucose tolerance, although it is not known whether these potentially advantageous changes are clinically important.

ADVERSE EFFECTS

All fibrates can cause myositis, especially in alcoholics (in whom they should not be used) and in patients with impaired renal function (in whom elimination is prolonged and protein binding is reduced). They can also further reduce renal function in such patients. In addition, they cause a variety of gastrointestinal side-effects, including nausea and abdominal discomfort. Headache, impotence and urticaria have also been reported.

CONTRAINDICATIONS

Fibrates should be used with caution, if at all, in patients with renal or hepatic impairment. They should not be used in patients with gall-bladder disease or with hypoalbuminaemia (e.g. from nephrotic syndrome). They are contraindicated in pregnancy and in alcoholics (this is particularly important because alcohol excess causes hypertriglyceridaemia; see Table 26.1).

PHARMACOKINETICS

Both bezafibrate and gemfibrozil are completely absorbed when given by mouth, highly protein bound, and excreted mainly by the kidneys.

DRUG INTERACTIONS

Fibrates potentiate oral anticoagulants, and bezafibrate (although not gemfibrozil) potentiates the hypoglycaemic effect of the sulphonylureas. Concurrent use with an HMGCoA reductase inhibitor may increase the risk of myositis.

Treatment of dyslipidaemia at extremes of age and during pregnancy

The elderly

The value of drug treatment of hyperlipidaemia in the elderly has not been formally tested, but advancing age is a strong risk factor for vascular disease and (as with hypertension; see Chapter 27) the absolute benefit of treatment in terms of events prevented per year of treatment is expected to be greatest in the elderly. This is reflected in current

Key points

Treatment of dyslipidaemia

- Treatment goals must be individualized according to absolute risk. Patients with established disease need a lower target LDL cholesterol level than do healthy individuals.
- Dietary measures involve maintaining ideal body weight (by caloric restriction if necessary) and reducing consumption of saturated fat – both animal (e.g. red meat, dairy products) and vegetable (e.g. coconut oil) – as well as cholesterol (e.g. egg yolk).
- Drug treatment is usually with a statin (taken once daily at night) which is effective, well tolerated and reduces mortality. Consider the possibility of hypothyroidism before starting treatment.
- Resins are inconvenient, unpalatable and cause gastrointestinal upset. They are a useful adjunct to a statin in severely dyslipidaemic patients who show an inadequate response to a statin alone.
- Fibrates are useful as a first-line treatment in patients with primary mixed dyslipidaemias with high triglyceride levels as well as high LDL (and often low HDL). Consider the possibility of alcohol excess in this setting, and treat accordingly.
- Other reversible risk factors for atheroma (e.g. smoking, hypertension) should be sought and treated. Oestrogen replacement should be considered in post-menopausal women.
- Consideration should be given to the possible use of aspirin as an antiplatelet/antithrombotic drug.

Case history

A 36-year-old primary-school teacher was seen because of hypertension at the request of the surgeons following bilateral femoral bypass surgery. His father had died at the age of 32 years of a myocardial infarct, but his other relatives, including his two children, were healthy. He did not smoke or drink alcohol. He had been diagnosed as hypertensive 6 years previously, since which time he had been treated with slow-release nifedipine, but his serum cholesterol level had never been measured. He had been disabled by claudication for the past few years, relieved temporarily by angioplasty 1 year previously. There were no stigmata of dyslipidaemia, his blood pressure was 150/100 mmHg, and the only abnormal findings were those relating to the peripheral vascular disease and vascular surgery in his legs. Serum total cholesterol was 12.6 mmol/L, triglyceride was 1.5 mmol/L and HDL was 0.9 mmol/L. Creatinine and electrolytes were normal. The patient was given dietary advice and seen in clinic 4 weeks after discharge from hospital. He had been able to run on the games field for the first time in a year, but this had been limited by the new onset of chest pain on exertion. His cholesterol level on the diet had improved to 8.0 mmol/L. He was readmitted.

Questions

Decide whether each of the following statements is true or false.

(a) This patient should receive a statin.
(b) Coronary angiography is indicated.
(c) Renal artery stenosis should be considered.
(d) The target for total cholesterol should be 6.0 mmol/L.
(e) A resin would be contraindicated.
(f) An α_1-blocker for his hypertension could coincidentally improve his dyslipidaemia.
(g) His children should be screened.

Answer

(a) True.
(b) True.
(c) True.
(d) False.
(e) False.
(f) True.
(g) True.

Comment

It was unfortunate that this young man's dyslipidaemia was not recognized earlier. Coronary angiography revealed severe inoperable triple-vessel disease. The target total cholesterol level should be < 5.0 mmol/L, and was achieved with a combination of diet, a statin at night and a resin in the morning. Renal artery stenosis is common in the setting of peripheral vascular disease, but renal angiography was negative. This patient's relatively mild hypertension was treated with doxazosin (a long-acting α_1-blocker, see Chapter 27, p. 271) which increases HDL as well as lowering blood pressure. He probably has heterozygous monogenic familial hypercholesterolaemia, and his children should be screened. One of his sons is hypercholesterolaemic, and is currently being treated with a combination of diet and a resin.

guidelines (e.g. those shown in Table 26.1). We treat otherwise healthy individuals with established atheromatous disease aggressively.

The young

Children with evidence of familial hyperlipidaemia represent a difficult management problem, and specialist advice should be sought. Experience of long-term safety of the most effective class of drug for treating heterozygous familial hypercholesterolaemia, namely the HMGCoA reductase inhibitors, has not been established, and there is a case for dietary modification combined with treatment with an anion-exchange resin as a temporizing measure in such children while experience of these drugs accumulates and other promising therapeutic modalities (notably replacement of the gene encoding the LDL receptor) are evaluated.

In pregnancy

The safety of hypolipidaemic drugs during pregnancy has not been established, and drugs that are eliminated from the body very slowly (e.g. probucol) should not generally be given to young women for this reason. Treatment by diet alone is preferable.

Further reading

Durrington PN. 1989: *Hyperlipidaemia. Diagnosis and management*. London: Butterworth and Co.

Feher MD, Richmond W. 1991: *Lipids and lipid disorders*. London: Gower Medical Publishing.

Ross R. 1993: The pathogenesis of atherosclerosis: a perspective for the 1990s. *Nature* **362,** 801–9.

Scandinavian Simvastatin Survival Study Group. 1994: Randomised trial of cholesterol lowering in 4444 patients with coronary heart disease: the Scandinavian Simvastatin Survival Study (4S). *Lancet* **344**, 1383–9.

Shepherd J, Cobbe SM, Ford I *et al.* 1995: Prevention of coronary heart disease with pravastatin in men with hypercholesterolaemia. *New England Journal of Medicine* **333**, 1301–7.

CHAPTER TWENTY-SEVEN

HYPERTENSION

- Introduction
- Pathophysiology
- General principles of management
- Drugs used to treat hypertension
- Special situations

INTRODUCTION

Systemic arterial hypertension is one of the strongest known modifiable risk factors for ischaemic heart disease. It is also responsible for considerable potentially preventable disability from stroke, renal failure and heart failure. Despite this, it continues to be underdiagnosed and undertreated in the UK. This is probably partly because hypertension is difficult to define. Usual arterial pressure has a continuous distribution in the population, and it is arbitrary to divide this into discrete 'hypertensive' and 'normotensive' groups. In addition, doctors frequently underestimate the magnitude of the excess risk attributable to hypertension over a time-scale that is long in relation to clinical trials but relevant to the individual patient, and are sometimes unduly pessimistic about the benefit that treatment confers. To put this in perspective, Beevers and MacGregor (1987) estimate that a 35-year-old man with a blood pressure of 150/100 mmHg has an odds-on chance of dying before the age of 60 years unless active steps are taken to reduce his blood pressure. Insurance companies pay close attention to blood pressure for good reason!

Figure 27.1 shows the relationship between usual mean diastolic blood pressure and the risks of coronary heart disease and of stroke redrawn from an overview by an Oxford group of epidemiologists. Over this range of blood pressure, the lower the diastolic pressure the lower the risk of each complication, the relationships being approximately log-linear (i.e. the risk rises steeply with increasing blood pressure). The same group performed a meta-analysis of published trials of antihypertensive drug treatment, and showed that the reduction in diastolic blood pressure achieved by drug treatment reduced the risk of stroke by the full extent predicted, and reduced the risk of coronary disease by about 50% of the maximum predicted, within approximately 2.5 years. These effects are impressive, and form a secure scientific basis for the clinical value of diagnosing and treating hypertension.

PATHOPHYSIOLOGY

Hypertension is occasionally secondary to some distinct disease (see Table 27.1). However, most patients with persistent arterial hypertension have essential hypertension.

Arterial blood pressure is determined by both cardiac output and peripheral vascular resistance. Peripheral resistance is determined by the calibre and total cross-sectional area of the resistance vessels (small arteries and arterioles) in the various tissues (see Figure 27.2). One or more of a 'mosaic' of interconnected predisposing factors (including

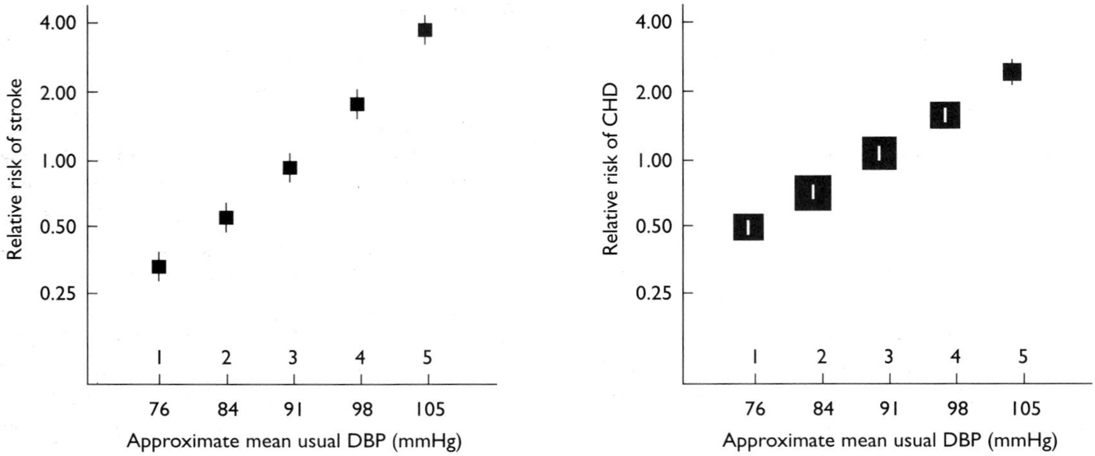

Figure 27.1: Risks of stroke and coronary heart disease (CHD) in relation to diastolic blood pressure (DBP). (Redrawn with permission from MacMahon *et al.* 1990: *Lancet* **335**, 765–74.) © The Lancet Ltd.

Table 27.1: Secondary hypertension

Coarctation of aorta
Renal artery stenosis
Renal disease (parenchymal or obstructive)
Conn's syndrome
Cushing's syndrome
Phaeochromocytoma

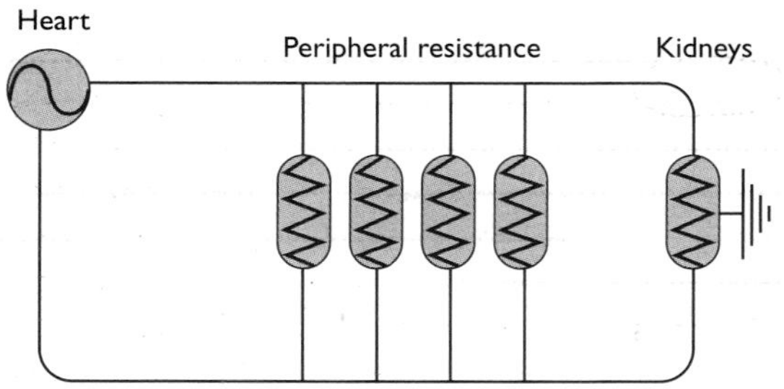

Figure 27.2: Arterial blood pressure is controlled by the force of contraction of the heart and the peripheral resistance (resistances in parallel though various vascular beds). The fullness of the circulation is controlled by the kidneys, which play a critical role in essential hypertension.

positive family history, obesity, insulin resistance and stress, among others) are commonly present in patients with essential hypertension. The importance of intrauterine factors (the 'Barker hypothesis') has recently been emphasized by the finding that hypertension in adult life is strongly associated with low birth weight, although this hypothesis remains controversial.

Cardiac output may be increased in children or young adults during the earliest stages of essential hypertension. However, by the time hypertension is established, the predominant haemodynamic abnormality is usually elevated peripheral resistance. Peripheral resistance is determined by the number and luminal diameters of the resistance vessels. Structural alterations, such as a reduction in vessel numbers ('pruning') or vessel-wall hypertrophy with consequent encroachment on the lumen, as well as functional abnormalities (e.g. increased vasoconstriction or reduced vasodilatation), are believed to be important in determining the increased peripheral resistance in patients with essential hypertension. The genesis of such changes is poorly understood.

The kidney plays a key role in the control of blood pressure and in the pathogenesis of hypertension. Excretion of salt and water controls intravascular volume, which in turn influences the force of contraction of the heart by the Starling mechanism. Secretion of renin influences vascular tone and electrolyte balance. Renal disease (vascular, parenchymal or obstructive) is a cause of arterial hypertension (see Table 27.1). Conversely, severe hypertension causes glomerular sclerosis, manifested clinically by proteinuria and reduced glomerular filtration, leading to a vicious circle of worsening blood pressure and progressive renal impairment. Renal cross-transplantation experiments in several animal models of hypertension, as well as observations following therapeutic renal transplantation in humans, both point to the importance of the kidney in the pathogenesis of hypertension.

Non-renal mechanisms are also important in the control of the circulation and in the pathogenesis of hypertension. These include neuronal mechanisms, especially the sympathetic nervous system, and endocrine and autocrine/paracrine mechanisms. The blood pressure of an individual varies widely at different times, and this can cause a diagnostic problem. The activity of the sympathetic nervous system causes a continual background of vasoconstrictor tone that varies rapidly to adjust for changes in cardiovascular demand with alterations in posture and physical activity. It is also activated by emotional states such as anxiety, and this can result in 'white-coat' hypertension.

There has been considerable debate as to the possible importance of tonically active vasodilator mechanisms in opposing sympathetically mediated vasoconstriction. There is little evidence for tonically active vasodilator *nerves*, except in a few highly specialized vascular beds, or for tonically active blood-borne vasodilator hormones. However, recent evidence points to a tonically active *paracrine* vasodilator mechanism. Inhibition of biosynthesis of nitric oxide (now believed to be the endothelium-derived relaxing factor described by Furchgott) causes vasoconstriction. This implies that basal release of nitric oxide by endothelial cells provides a background vasodilator tone. Conversely, inhibiting the action of endothelin, a vasoconstrictor peptide synthesized by endothelial cells, causes vasodilation. This implies that basal release of endothelin contributes to background vasoconstrictor tone. Abnormalities of these paracrine mechanisms may contribute to the pathogenesis of hypertensive vascular disease.

Clinically important consequences of hypertension ('end-organ damage') include damage to both large and small blood vessels, as well as left ventricular hypertrophy. It is easy to understand how increased arterial pressure causes an increased risk of arterial rupture and bleeding from a weak spot in the arterial wall (e.g. from a Charcot–Bouchard aneurysm, causing a cerebral haemorrhage). The close link between hypertension and atherogenesis is less well understood, but may be related to vascular injury (believed to initiate atherogenesis; see Chapter 26). Damage to small vessels occurs most floridly in the vasculitis (fibrinoid necrosis) that is the hallmark of accelerated or malignant hypertension, and also underlies the glomerular sclerosis and consequent proteinuria and progressive renal impairment that complicate severe essential hypertension.

Key points

Pathophysiology of hypertension

- Few patients with persistent systemic arterial hypertension have a specific aetiology (e.g. renal disease, endocrine disease, coarctation of aorta). Most have essential hypertension (EH), which confers increased risk of vascular disease (e.g. thrombotic or haemorrhagic stroke, myocardial infarction). Reducing blood pressure reduces the risk of such events.
- The cause(s) of EH is/are ill-defined. Polygenic influences are important, as are environmental factors including salt intake and obesity. The intrauterine environment (determined by genetic/environmental factors) may be important in determining blood pressure in adult life.
- Increased cardiac output may occur before EH becomes established
- Established EH is characterized haemodynamically by normal cardiac output but increased total systemic vascular resistance. This involves both structural (remodelling) and functional changes in resistance vessels.
- EH is a strong independent risk factor for atheromatous disease, and interacts supra-additively with other such risk factors.

GENERAL PRINCIPLES OF MANAGEMENT

1 Make sure that you measure the blood pressure accurately, using an appropriately sized cuff (bladder at least two-thirds of arm circum-

ference) and recording Korotkov sounds 1 (systolic) and 5 (diastolic). Repeat the reading.

2 Consider the possibility of an underlying cause. Many forms of secondary hypertension, including coarctation of the aorta and endocrine tumours, are managed surgically. Renal artery stenosis merits consideration of angioplasty.

3 Seek evidence of end-organ damage. Cotton-wool spots, retinal haemorrhages, papilloedema and/or microscopic haematuria in the setting of severe hypertension suggest accelerated or malignant hypertension which is a medical emergency requiring immediate admission to hospital (see below). Such evidence of microvascular damage is rare in modern practice, and in its absence the appropriate tempo of evaluation and treatment is much less precipitate. Other evidence of end-organ damage, including symptoms or signs of atheromatous disease, cardiac hypertrophy (with or without a fourth heart sound), cardiac failure, or evidence of renal impairment, indicate that long-term treatment will be essential. The most sensitive measure of ventricular hypertrophy is provided by two-dimensional echocardiography. If this is unavailable, an electrocardiogram should be obtained, but this is less sensitive. It is important to appreciate that the *absence* of evidence of end-organ damage does *not* indicate that treatment is unnecessary.

4 Confirm (or refute) the persistence of clinically significant hypertension by establishing a number of accurate readings on separate occasions. Blood pressure varies in everyone, and it is probably the average of several readings of pressure that is important. Automated ambulatory and/or home readings are sometimes helpful in deciding on the need for treatment in borderline cases, especially in patients with marked sympathetic activation when confronted with doctors ('white-coat' hypertension).

5 Consider the possibility that hypertension is caused by alcohol withdrawal, or by some other drug. Heavy drinkers develop marked hypertension after drinking, even when they are not otherwise obviously in an acute state of alcohol withdrawal. Withdrawal from narcotics also causes hypertension, but the cause is usually obvious. Oral contraceptives can cause hypertension that usually settles when the drug is stopped. Vasoconstrictors including ergotamine and ephedrine as well as amphetamine, cocaine and related drugs of abuse (e.g. 'ecstasy') can cause acute hypertension, as can ingestion of fermented foods or drink containing tyramine in patients receiving monoamine oxidase inhibitors (see Chapters 13 and 19). Mineralocorticoids (including liquorice intoxication) can cause hypertension.

6 Evaluate the patient for other cardiovascular risk factors, and attend to these if present. Risk factors interact positively and are usually supra-additive with hypertension in determining the risk of cardiovascular disease (Figure 26.1). Knowledge of these factors should therefore inform the decision as to whether or not to initiate drug treatment in any individual patient. The higher the absolute risk of vascular disease, the greater the benefit (per unit time) of treatment.

7 Dietary factors – apart from avoiding excessive alcohol intake, it is important to treat obesity and avoid excessive salt consumption. Some individuals are very sensitive to salt restriction, whereas unfortunately others are not. Statistically, Afro-Caribbeans are more likely to be salt sensitive than whites. Individuals with the highest initial pressures tend to show the greatest falls in blood pressure in response to a salt-restricted diet whereas, disappointingly, mild hypertensives on average show much more modest responses. However, there is considerable individual variation in response, and English physicians often pay less attention than they should to this harmless intervention, perhaps because it is time-consuming to educate patients effectively to achieve a worthwhile reduction in salt intake. It is reasonable to measure 24-h sodium ion excretion in suitably motivated patients, and to individualize therapeutic endeavours by attempting to achieve an excretion rate of less than 50 mmol/24 h (low by UK standards, but substantially greater than the salt intake of our hunter-gatherer forebears, or of some rural societies with low blood pressure today) while monitoring the blood pressure and urinary sodium excretion. Input from a skilled dietitian is invaluable.

8 Consider other forms of non-drug treatment, (e.g. relaxation techniques) in patients with mild elevation of blood pressure and stressed lifestyle. These approaches may usefully be combined with other dietary and 'lifestyle' advice during a run-in phase of repeated observation over several months or longer, depending on the pressure.

9 Current guidelines of the British Hypertension Society suggest that a patient will derive more benefit than harm from drug treatment when diastolic pressure is consistently > 100 mmHg or is 90–100 mmHg and there are additional risk factors or target organ damage, or in elderly patients with systolic pressure > 160 mmHg. If one or more of these conditions is met, explain this and seek the patient's agreement to long-term treatment, explaining the importance of compliance and the need for regular monitoring. It is important to emphasize that hypertension is not an illness but a risk factor for illness, and that the object of treatment is not to feel better here and now, but rather to remain healthy.

10 Before starting drug treatment, review the possibility of coexisting disease that would limit the choice of drug. A history of gout is a relative contraindication to the use of a diuretic and obstructive airways disease or peripheral vascular disease contraindicate the use of beta-blockers.

11 Whenever possible, choose a class of drug that has been shown to be effective in terms of clinical end-points such as stroke reduction. Thiazide diuretics or beta-blockers are relatively inexpensive and their adverse effects are well known and reversible on stopping treatment. Of the two, we recommend a thiazide if all other things are equal, especially if the patient is Afro-Caribbean. Some authorities prefer to initiate treatment with a converting-enzyme inhibitor or calcium channel antagonist.

12 Start with a low dose and, except in emergency situations, titrate this upward gradually. Almost every category of antihypertensive drug that has been introduced into clinical practice has been used initially in too high a dose, with resultant toxicity (hydralazine, thiazide diuretics, propranolol and captopril all exemplify this). One reason is that physicians are impatient to see a rapid reduction in pressure, which has become elevated as a result of slow processes that initially probably took many months to assert themselves and may require at least as long to regress. The converse is that if antihypertensive medication is discontinued, perhaps because it was initiated before adequate demonstration of persistent hypertension, the hypertension may reassert itself after only a few months of normal blood pressure. Close and continued monitoring in such circumstances is therefore mandatory.

13 If control is not established by a single agent, consider the possibility of non-compliance. If this is excluded, consider either substitution of a drug of a different category, or addition of a second drug. There is no hard and fast rule about this, but if a drug has had minimal or no effect on its own, it may be more reasonable to substitute a different agent, whereas if it has had a real but insufficient effect it is more reasonable to add a second drug with a complementary mechanism of action. In this context thiazides and beta-blockers combine well, as do diuretics and converting enzyme inhibitors, beta-blockers and calcium-channel blockers, alpha-blockers with converting-enzyme inhibitors and a number of other rational combinations. In patients with severe hypertension, three and occasionally four drugs may be needed. Try to keep such regimes as simple as possible, using once daily or twice daily dosing when possible.

14 Loss of control – if blood pressure control, having been well established, is lost, there are several possibilities to be considered.

- *Non-compliance* – this is the most common cause of loss of control. It is conceptually the simplest, but in practice often the most difficult to pin down. Hospital admission may be warranted, and if the problem is faced frankly but non-confrontationally, the outcome is often surprisingly good.
- *Drug interaction* – the commonest cause with modern antihypertensive treatment is concurrent use of non-steroidal anti-inflammatory drugs (NSAIDs). NSAIDs increase blood pressure in hypertensive patients receiving antihypertensive drugs, irrespective of the particular category of drug used, by inhibiting the renal biosynthesis

of vasodilator/natriuretic prostaglandins (including prostaglandin E_2 and prostacyclin). All NSAIDs possess this property to some extent, but sulindac (which has relatively little effect on renal prostaglandin synthesis) is less potent than others in this regard, as is aspirin. Paracetamol and opiates such as codeine do *not* exhibit this pharmacodynamic interaction, and may be useful in patients with severe hypertension coexisting with painful osteoarthrosis.

- *Intercurrent disease* – patients with hypertension frequently have atheromatous disease. If a plaque in a renal artery progresses to cause haemodynamically significant stenosis, hyperreninaemia may cause a rapid increase in arterial pressure, and even precipitate malignant hypertension. Other possible intercurrent disease includes progressive renal impairment, renal infarction and progressive obstructive uropathy in an ageing man with prostatic hypertrophy.

DRUGS USED TO TREAT HYPERTENSION

There are five main classes of drugs for the treatment of essential hypertension, namely diuretics, β-adrenoceptor antagonists, angiotensin-converting enzyme inhibitors (ACEI) and angiotensin-receptor antagonists, calcium-channel antagonists and α_1-adrenoceptor antagonists. A sixth class, consisting of centrally acting drugs, had **clonidine** as its prototype. This is a mixed agonist that stimulates both α_2- and imidazoline (I_1)-receptors. Recently there has been some resurgence of interest in this class of drug with the introduction of moderately selective I_1-agonists (e.g. **moxonidine**). These are imperfect, but show the way to more selective centrally acting drugs for the future.

Diuretics (see also Chapters 30 and 35)

USE IN HYPERTENSION

Diuretics remain the logical first choice for treating patients with mild hypertension, unless contraindicated by some coexistent disease. They are also valuable for more severe cases, combined with other drugs. Diuretics have been shown to reduce the risk of stroke in several large clinical trials, and indeed in the Medical Research Council (MRC) trial they did so significantly more effectively than did beta-blockade, although this may have been a statistical quirk. The dose–response curve of diuretics on blood pressure is remarkably flat. However, the adverse metabolic effects described below are dose related. Thiazides (e.g. **bendrofluazide**, **hydrochlorothiazide**) are preferable to loop diuretics for the treatment of uncomplicated hypertension, and are given by mouth as a single morning dose. They begin to act within 1–2 h and work for 12–24 h. Treatment should be started using a low dose (e.g. bendrofluazide, 2.5 mg each morning). Loop diuretics are useful in hypertensive patients with moderate or severe renal impairment, and in patients with hypertensive heart failure.

MECHANISM OF ACTION

Thiazide diuretics inhibit reabsorption of sodium and chloride ions in the early part of the distal convoluted tubule. Excessive salt intake or a low glomerular filtration rate interferes with their antihypertensive effect, and thiazides are ineffective in anephric patients. Natriuresis is therefore probably important in determining their hypotensive action. However, it is not the whole story, since although plasma volume falls when treatment is started, it returns to normal with continued treatment, despite a persistent effect on blood pressure, suggesting an additional mode of action. During chronic treatment, total peripheral resistance, which is raised initially, slowly falls, suggesting an action on resistance vessels. This could be an autoregulatory change in response to the altered blood volume, or it could be due to an effect of the drug in reducing arteriolar tone. Such an effect might be indirect, perhaps involving release of a vasodilator mediator from the kidneys in view of the obligatory requirement of functioning kidneys for thiazide diuretics to be able to exert their hypotensive effect. Vascular responses to pressor agents (including angiotensin II and noradrenaline) are reduced during chronic treatment with thiazides.

ADVERSE EFFECTS

1. *Impotence* – analysis of the reasons for withdrawal from randomized blind treatment with thiazide from the MRC trial showed a higher rate of impotence than in placebo-treated or beta-blocker-treated patients. This may have been exaggerated by the unnecessarily high dose of bendrofluazide (10 mg) used in that study.
2. *Increased plasma renin* – the contraction of plasma volume caused acutely by diuretics results in increased plasma renin levels, which limits the magnitude of the effect of diuretics on blood pressure.
3. *Metabolic and electrolyte changes* – Thiazide diuretics have several metabolic effects. These are seldom clinically important, provided that the dose is low:
   - *hyponatremia* – this is sometimes severe;
   - *hypokalaemia* – thiazides are kaliuretic as well as natriuretic, an inevitable consequence of increased sodium ion delivery to the distal nephron where sodium and potassium ions are exchanged. This results in mild hypokalaemia in many subjects. Despite this, total body potassium may be little affected during chronic treatment, and as long as plasma potassium remains at 3.0 mmol/L or greater, there is little reason to add potassium supplements (which are unlikely to be effective at tolerable doses) or potassium-sparing diuretics (which have toxicities of their own);
   - hypomagnesaemia;
   - hyperuricaemia – most diuretics reduce urate clearance. They therefore increase the plasma urate concentration and can precipitate gout in predisposed individuals;
   - hyperglycaemia – thiazides reduce glucose tolerance, and can cause hyperglycaemia in non-insulin-dependent diabetics;
   - hypercalcaemia – thiazides reduce urinary calcium ion clearance (unlike loop diuretics, which increase it), and can therefore precipitate clinically significant hypercalcaemia in hypertensive patients with hyperparathyroidism;
   - hypercholesterolaemia – thiazide diuretics cause a small increase in plasma cholesterol concentration, which may not persist during prolonged treatment. This is of uncertain significance, and does not account quantitatively for the failure of clinical trials to show as large an effect of treatment of hypertension on coronary disease as on stroke. To put it in perspective, MRC trial patients randomized to bendrofluazide actually experienced a fall in total cholesterol concentration during treatment, albeit of significantly smaller magnitude than in those randomized to placebo. The possible importance of this modest metabolic effect has been overemphasized by sales forces eager to promote newer, relatively expensive, drugs.
4. Idiosyncratic reactions – including rashes (which may be photosensitive) and purpura, which may be thrombocytopenic or non-thrombocytopenic.

CONTRAINDICATIONS

The effects of thiazide diuretics described above contraindicate their use in patients with severe renal impairment (in whom they are unlikely to be effective), and in patients with a history of gout, and suggest that caution is needed when using these drugs in patients with mild hypertension but severe hypercholesterolaemia. They should not be used in pre-eclampsia, which is associated with a contracted intravascular volume. Diuretics should be avoided in men with prostatic symptoms. It is prudent to discontinue diuretics temporarily in patients who develop intercurrent diarrhoea and/or vomiting, to avoid exacerbating fluid depletion.

DRUG INTERACTIONS

In addition to the non-specific adverse interaction with NSAIDs mentioned above, all diuretics interact with lithium. Li^+ is similar to Na^+ in many respects, and is reabsorbed mainly in the proximal convoluted tubule (see Chapter 19). Diuretics indirectly increase Li^+ reabsorption in the proximal tubule, by causing volume contraction. This results in an increased plasma concentration of Li^+, and hence increased likelihood of toxicity. Diuretic-induced hypokalaemia and hypomagnesaemia can increase the toxicity of digoxin (see

Chapters 30 and 31). Combinations of a thiazide with a potassium-sparing diuretic such as amiloride (co-amilozide) or triamterene are widely prescribed, and are especially useful in patients who require simultaneous treatment with digoxin, sotolol or other drugs that prolong the electrocardigraphic QT-interval.

Potentially useful interactions with other antihypertensive drugs abound. Useful interactions include thiazide/beta-blocker, thiazide/angiotensin-converting enzyme inhibitor and thiazide/alpha-blocker. An unexpected exception to this is provided by most calcium-channel blockers, whose hypotensive actions are *not* enhanced, and may even be attenuated, by concurrent use of diuretics. This is particularly disappointing as one of the most troublesome adverse effects of dihydropyridine calcium-channel blockers is ankle swelling, which is *not* however reduced by diuretics.

β-Adrenoceptor antagonists

USE (SEE ALSO CHAPTER 31 FOR USE IN ARRHYTHMIAS)

Examples of β-adrenoceptor antagonists currently in clinical use are shown in Table 27.2. **Atenolol** and **metoprolol** are currently the beta-blocking drugs most widely used to treat hypertension in the UK. Beta-blockers lower blood pressure and reduce the risk of stroke in patients with mild essential hypertension. Statistically they are less effective in Afro-Caribbean patients than in white people. In contrast, ethnic Chinese are usually more sensitive to the effects of beta-blocking drugs than are whites. Treatment is started with a small dose (e.g. atenolol, 25 mg, metoprolol, 50 mg) and the daily dose increased gradually measuring blood pressure, pulse and, especially in the case of partial agonists (see below), pulse following exercise. Doses of atenolol greater than 100 mg or of metoprolol greater than 200 mg daily are seldom needed, so dose titration is simpler than with propranolol.

Beta-Blockers are usually well tolerated and, although more expensive than thiazide diuretics, are much less expensive than calcium-channel blockers, converting-enzyme inhibitors or alpha-blockers. Unless contraindicated (see below), they are appropriate first-line drugs for patients with essential hypertension who do not tolerate thiazides, or as an additional drug in patients whose response to thiazides is inadequate. They are particularly useful in hypertensive patients who have angina pectoris or who have survived myocardial infarction. The negative inotropic effect of beta-blocking drugs may be particularly useful for stabilizing patients with dissecting aneurysms of the thoracic aorta, in whom it is desirable not only to lower the mean pressure but also to reduce the rate of rise of the arterial pressure wave.

CLASSIFICATION OF β-ADRENOCEPTOR ANTAGONISTS

Adrenoceptors are classified α or β, based on the effects of different agonists and antagonists. A further subdivision has been made into β_1-receptors, mainly in the heart, β_2-receptors in blood vessels, bronchioles and other cells and tissues and, more recently, β_3-receptors, which mediate metabolic effects (e.g. in brown fat). Non-selective β-adrenoceptor antagonists (e.g. propranolol) do not distinguish between these subtypes.

Cardioselective beta-blockers These drugs (e.g. atenolol, metoprolol) inhibit β_1-receptors but exert little influence on bronchial and vascular β_2-receptors when employed in low doses in experiments on isolated tissues *in vitro*. However, such selectivity is relative rather than absolute, and in clinical practice cardioselectivity is of little relevance. Even cardioselective β_1-antagonists (at least those currently available) are hazardous for patients with asthma or obstructive airways disease. Metabolic differences between selective and non-selective beta-blockers also appear to be of only marginal importance in clinical practice. Beta-blockers are generally best avoided in insulin-requiring diabetics, and there are usually acceptable alternatives available. The popularity of atenolol among clinicians is due largely to its convenience for the patient, rather than to its selectivity for the β_1-receptor subtype. This convenience relates to its duration of action, which enables it to be administered once daily.

Some beta-blockers (e.g. **oxprenolol**, **pindolol**) are *partial agonists* and possess intrinsic sympathomimetic activity. Partial agonists antagonize full agonists because they occupy a substantial

Table 27.2: Examples of β-adrenoceptors in clinical use

Drug	Selectivity	Pharmacokinetic features	Comment
Propranolol	Non-selective	Non-polar; substantial presystematic metabolism; variable dose requirements; multiple daily dosing	First beta-blocker in clinical use
Atenolol	β_1-selective	Polar; renal elimination; once daily dosing	Widely used; avoid in renal failure
Metoprolol	β_1-selective	Non-polar; cytochrome P_{450} (2D6 isoenzyme)	Widely used
Esmolol	β_1-selective	Short acting given by IV infusion; renal elimination of acid metabolite	Used in intensive-care unit/theatre (e.g. dissecting aneurysm)
Sotalol	Non-selective (L-isomer)	Polar; renal elimination	A racemate: the D-isomer has class III anti-arrhythmic actions (see Chapter 31)
Labetolol	Non-selective	Hepatic glucuronidation	Additional alpha-blocking and partial β_2-agonist activity. Used in the latter part of pregnancy
Oxprenolol	Non-selective	Hepatic hydroxylation/glucuronidation	Partial agonist

fraction of the receptors to produce their modest effect, and therefore compete successfully with the more efficacious full agonists, which occupy only a small fraction of the receptors to produce a maximal effect (see Chapter 2). Pure antagonists such as atenolol often cause mild bradycardia (heart rate typically around 60 beats/min) because of unopposed vagal activity. By contrast, partial agonists such as oxprenolol cause some β-adrenoceptor stimulation and the resting heart rate is often 70–80 beats/min. However, during increased sympathetic activity (e.g. on exercising), tachycardia is blunted. Theoretically, drugs with intrinsic sympathomimetic activity might be less likely to induce cardiac failure, peripheral vasoconstriction, depressed atrioventricular conduction or marked bradycardia. This does not generally seem to be important in practice.

Vasodilating beta-blockers, β_2-Receptor activation causes vasodilatation, and acute administration of non-selective beta-blocking drugs typically causes mild vasoconstriction. However, some beta-blockers have additional actions that cause vasodilatation, which is theoretically an advantage in treating patients with hypertension. The mechanisms of these so-called vasodilating beta-blockers vary. Some (e.g. **labetolol**, **carvedilol**) have additional alpha-blocking activity. **Celiprolol** is a relatively selective β_1-antagonist which has additional *agonist* activity at β_2-receptors. **Nebivolol** releases endothelium-derived nitric oxide, and is the most cardioselective β_1-antagonist available.

MECHANISM OF ACTION

Despite their efficacy in lowering blood pressure, the mechanism by which beta-blocking drugs achieve this is by no means obvious. As explained above, they actually increase peripheral vascular resistance in acute-dose studies, although this effect is transient, and is offset by the fall in cardiac output. They *reduce renin secretion* by the kidney. However, β-adrenoceptor antagonists are effective in some patients with low plasma renin as well in those with high renin hypertension, and their effects are additive with those of converting-enzyme inhibitors, so inhibition of renin secretion is unlikely to be the full explanation for their hypotensive action.

Propranolol has *central effects* and *reduces* sympathetic output from the central nervous system, but again this appears to be inadequate as an explanation, since more polar beta-blockers, such as atenolol, which penetrate the blood–brain barrier much less readily than does propranolol, are as effective as propranolol in lowering blood pressure. The hypotensive action of these drugs is therefore attributed, somewhat unsatisfactorily, to their actions on the heart. Patients on long-term β_1-antagonists do not usually have a low cardiac output, and it seems likely that additional mechanisms, perhaps involving baroreceptors or other homeostatic adaptations, must also be involved.

ADVERSE EFFECTS AND CONTRAINDICATIONS

1 *Intolerance* – β-adrenoceptor antagonists cause a variety of symptoms in apparently healthy individuals, some of whom may not tolerate them in consequence. Of these, fatigue, cold extremities, sexual dysfunction and loss of motivation and *joie de vivre* are common. Less often, β-adrenoceptor antagonists (especially, but not invariably, non-polar ones such as propranolol that readily cross the blood–brain barrier) cause hallucinations or vivid and sometimes nightmare-like dreams.

2 *Airways obstruction* – β-adrenoceptor antagonists, whether non-selective or cardioselective, can cause catastrophic airways obstruction in patients with pre-existing obstructive airways disease, especially asthma, but also emphysema and chronic bronchitis, and are contraindicated in these conditions. Patients with asthma sometimes tolerate a small dose of a selective drug when first prescribed, only to suffer an exceptionally severe attack subsequently, and such drugs should ideally be avoided altogether in asthmatics.

3 *Heart failure* – the negative inotropic action of β-adrenoceptor antagonists renders them potentially dangerous in patients with heart failure. However, recent evidence suggests that when used in very low doses under close supervision, these drugs prolong survival in such patients (see Chapter 30)

4 *Peripheral vascular disease and vasospasm* – β-adrenoceptor antagonists predictably worsen symptoms of claudication in patients with symptomatic atheromatous peripheral vascular disease. Patients with peripheral vasospasm

should also not be prescribed beta-blockers which worsen Raynaud's phenomenon. The rather small number of patients with angina in whom coronary artery vasospasm contributes significantly to their 'variant' or 'Printzmetal' angina may also experience a 'paradoxical' worsening of their symptoms if they are prescribed beta-blockers.

5 *Hypoglycaemia* – the propensity of β-adrenoceptor antagonists to mask symptoms of hypoglycaemia (which, apart from sweating, which is largely cholinergically mediated, are caused mainly by adrenergic pathways) renders them hazardous in patients with insulin-dependant diabetes mellitus. Not only are symptoms of hypoglycaemia masked, but also the rate of recovery from hypoglycaemia is slowed, especially by non-selective beta-blockers, because adrenaline stimulates gluconeogenesis via β_2-adrenoceptors.

6 *Heart block* – β-adrenoceptor antagonists are contraindicated in patients with minor degrees of heart block, because of the risk of precipitating complete block.

7 *Metabolic disturbance* – β-adrenoceptor antagonists cause several subtle biochemical or metabolic changes of uncertain clinical significance. They cause a small increase in serum triglyceride concentration and a small fall in serum high-density lipoprotein. They cause a small rise in serum potassium levels because of inhibition of renin release (and hence reduction of aldosterone release) in some individuals, but this is not usually clinically important. Some studies have documented deterioration of glycaemic control in patients with non-insulin-dependent diabetes, which may be additive with the effect on blood glucose of thiazide diuretics in such patients.

PHARMACOKINETICS

β-Adrenoceptor antagonists are well absorbed when administered orally, and are only given intravenously to control blood pressure in rare emergency situations (e.g. dissecting aortic aneurysm) or, occasionally, peri-operatively. (They are sometimes also used to treat supraventricular arrhythmias; see Chapter 31.) **Esmolol** is a relatively cardioselective β-adrenoceptor antagonist with a very short duration of action which is given by intravenous infusion for these indications, usually in the dose range 50–200 μg/kg/min.

Polarity is an important determinant of the pharmacokinetics of different beta-blocking drugs. Propranolol, oxprenolol and metoprolol are among the least polar, and atenolol and sotolol are among the most polar. The less polar (and more lipophilic) the drug, the more extensive and rapid is absorption from the gut, but also the higher is presystemic metabolism in the gut wall and liver. The dose of propranolol required to cause beta-blockade when given intravenously is therefore only a small fraction of that needed when it is given orally (approximately 1 mg, compared to 40 mg or more).

Propranolol has an active metabolite (4-hydroxypropranolol), and metoprolol is metabolized by the enzyme that hydroxylates debrisoquine, the activity of which varies between individuals as a balanced polymorphism in the UK population (see Chapter 5). However, these potentially complicating factors have little bearing on the dose requirements for these drugs in ordinary clinical practice. Lipophilic beta-blockers enter the brain more readily than do polar drugs. Central nervous system side-effects such as nightmares and hallucinations occur more commonly with non-polar beta-blockers. Polar (water-soluble) beta-blockers tend to be excreted by the kidneys without metabolism, to have longer half-lives, and to accumulate in renal failure.

Non-polar (lipophilic) beta-blockers are usually highly protein bound. For example, propranolol is 85–95% bound largely to α_1-acidic glycoprotein (which carries 75% at therapeutic plasma concentrations) and also albumin and lipoproteins. Polar (hydrophilic) beta-blockers have low protein binding. For example, atenolol is less than 5% bound. Increased plasma concentrations of acute-phase proteins, evidenced by a raised erythrocyte sedimentation rate, cause increased plasma concentrations of highly protein-bound beta-blockers (e.g. metoprolol, propranolol), but not of drugs such as atenolol.

The antihypertensive effects of beta-blockers outlast plasma levels, and for this reason atenolol is given once daily despite having an elimination half-life of less than 24 h. Slow-release preparations are sometimes employed to optimize control over 24 h with a single daily dose.

DRUG INTERACTIONS

Pharmacokinetic interactions β-Adrenoceptor antagonists inhibit drug metabolism indirectly *by decreasing hepatic blood flow* secondary to decreased cardiac output. This causes accumulation of drugs such as lignocaine that have such a high hepatic extraction ratio that their clearance reflects hepatic blood flow, if given concurrently with beta-blocking drugs. Cimetidine causes accumulation of propranolol, and may precipitate toxicity, by inhibiting its metabolism by hepatic cytochrome P_{450}–related oxidation.

Pharmacodynamic interactions Increased negative inotropic and atrioventricular (AV) nodal effects occur with verapamil (giving both intravenously can be fatal), lignocaine and other negative inotropes. Exaggerated *hypoglycaemia* with insulin and oral hypoglycaemic drugs may be caused by β-antagonists. The antihypertensive effect of beta-blockers is antagonized by NSAIDs.

Diuretic/beta-blocker combinations

Many beta-blockers marketed in the UK are available as combined preparations with a diuretic. These may be useful for improving compliance if the appropriate dosage ratio of diuretic and beta-blocker is available. They are also cheaper for the patient, although not for the National Health Service. Dose inflexibility limits their use. They should not be used as first-line therapy, nor should their dose be titrated upwards to obtain a large dose of beta-blocker.

DRUGS THAT INTERRUPT THE RENIN–ANGIOTENSIN SYSTEM

Angiotensin-converting enzyme inhibitors

USE

Several angiotensin-converting enzyme inhibitors (ACEI) are in clinical use (see Table 27.3 for examples). These drugs are a useful addition to a diuretic in patients with moderate or severe hypertension that is not controlled by diuretic alone. Several of them are also licensed for use as single agents in patients with mild essential hypertension. Large-scale comparative studies with thiazide diuretics and beta-blockers are urgently needed, as there are theoretical reasons to believe that converting-enzyme inhibitors might perform either worse or better than these proven therapies. Such a study is planned – the Anglo-Scandinavian Cardiac Outcome Trial (ASCOT).

ACEI are more expensive than thiazide diuretics or beta-blockers, but are well tolerated by most patients and provide a useful alternative for patients in whom thiazide diuretics and beta-blockers are contraindicated, or who do not tolerate them. Their beneficial effect in patients with heart failure (see Chapter 30) makes them particularly useful in hypertensive patients with this complication. A case has been made that ACEI have a distinctive and favourable effect on the progression of diabetic nephropathy over and above their effect in lowering blood pressure. Larger controlled studies are needed to confirm

Table 27.3: Examples of angiotensin-converting enzyme inhibitors (ACEI) in clinical use

Drug	Special features	Comments
Captopril	-SH group	First ACEI in clinical use; more than once daily dosing; high doses can cause side effects related to -SH group
Enalapril	Prodrug (active metabolite: enalaprilat)	Intermediate duration of action
Lisinopril	Lysine derivative of enalaprilat	Intermediate duration of action
Trandolapril	Slow elimination	Long (> 24 h) duration of action: once daily use

this and to determine whether the effect is is clinically important.

Treatment is initiated using a small dose given last thing at night, because of the possibility of first-dose hypotension. If possible, diuretics should be withheld for 1 or 2 days before the first dose for the same reason. However, first-dose hypotension is much less problematic than starting treatment with a converting-enzyme inhibitor in patients with heart failure (see Chapter 30) in whom blood pressure is usually lower, circulating plasma renin activity is often higher, and diuretic therapy is less safe to withhold. The dose is subsequently usually given in the morning and increased gradually if necessary, while monitoring the blood-pressure response.

MECHANISM OF ACTION

ACE (also known as kininase 2) catalyses the cleavage of a pair of amino acids from the carboxy terminus of short peptides, thereby 'converting' the inactive decapeptide angiotensin I to the potent vasoconstrictor angiotensin II. As well as *activating* the vasoconstrictor angiotensin in this way, it also *inactivates* bradykinin and some other vasodilator peptides. Converting enzyme is widely distributed in the body, and is present on the luminal surface of vascular endothelial cells. The enzyme has a short tail anchoring it inside the cytoplasm, a transmembrane domain, and a large portion which extends extracellularly, where it encounters angiotensin I and other potential substrates in the circulating plasma. This portion contains two active sites, each with a zinc atom. The lung is rich in ACE because of its huge surface area of endothelial cells, and was the first organ identified as containing the enzyme, but other tissues (including heart, kidney, striated muscle and brain) also contain high activities of ACE both on the endothelial cells and elsewhere.

Converting-enzyme inhibitors lower blood pressure by reducing angiotensin II, and perhaps also by increasing vasodilator peptides such as bradykinin. The relative contributions to the lowering of blood pressure made by inhibition of the circulating renin–angiotensin system and of local renin–angiotensin systems in individual vascular beds have not yet been established. Both are almost certainly important in different physiological circumstances. Angiotensin II increases noradrenaline release from sympathetic nerve terminals, so ACE inhibitors reduce sympathetic activity. This probably explains why their use is not associated with reflex tachycardia, despite causing arteriolar and venous dilatation. Angiotensin II causes aldosterone secretion from the zona glomerulosa of the adrenal cortex, and inhibition of this contributes to the antihypertensive effect of converting-enzyme inhibitors. Angiotensin II is a growth factor for vascular smooth muscle and some other cells, and in some but not all animal models of hypertension, converting-enzyme inhibitors influence the arteriolar and left ventricular remodelling that is believed to be important in the pathogenesis of human essential hypertension.

METABOLIC EFFECTS

The ACE inhibitors do not have effects on concentrations of plasma cholesterol or triglycerides. They cause a mild increase in plasma potassium concentration which is usually unimportant, but may sometimes be either desirable or problematic depending on renal function and the other drugs being used (see section on adverse effects and drug interactions below).

ADVERSE EFFECTS AND CONTRAINDICATIONS

Converting-enzyme inhibitors are generally well tolerated. **Captopril** has fared especially well when evaluated formally by 'quality of life' questionnaires. Adverse effects include:

1. *First-dose hypotension* – steps to minimize this are described above in the section on use.
2. *Dry cough* – this is the most frequent symptom (5–30% of cases) during chronic dosing, and is often (but not always) mild. The cause is unknown, but it may be due to kinins accumulating and stimulating cough afferents, perhaps via stimulation of prostaglandin production. The latter possibility was raised by a small study which showed that ACE-inhibitor cough could be reduced by treatment with **sulindac**, which inhibits prostaglandin biosynthesis. Inhaled **cromoglycate** (see Chapter 32 p. 348–9) also suppresses ACEI cough in some patients. **Losartan** (an angiotensin II receptor antagonist, see below) does not potentiate bradykinin and does not cause cough.
3. *Functional renal failure* – this occurs *predictably* in patients with haemodynamically significant *bilateral renal artery stenosis*, and in patients with

renal artery stenosis in the vessel supplying a single functional kidney. Converting-enzyme inhibitors are therefore contraindicated in such patients. Plasma creatinine and potassium levels should be monitored before and during the early weeks of therapy with ACEI, and the possibility of renal artery stenosis considered in patients in whom there is a marked rise in creatinine levels. Provided that the drug is stopped promptly, such renal impairment is reversible. The explanation of acute reduction in renal function in this setting is that glomerular filtration in these patients is critically dependent on angiotensin-II-mediated efferent arteriolar vasoconstriction, and when angiotensin II synthesis is inhibited, glomerular capillary pressure falls and glomerular filtration ceases. This should be borne in mind particularly in ageing patients with atheromatous disease, which often involves one or both renal arteries.

4 *Hyperkalaemia* – a modest increase in plasma potassium concentration occurs as a result of reduced aldosterone secretion. This may usefully counter the small reduction in potassium ion concentration caused by thiazide diuretics. However, increased plasma potassium is potentially hazardous in patients with renal impairment, and great caution must be exercised in this setting. This is even more important when such patients are also prescribed potassium supplements and/or potassium-sparing diuretics, including those marketed for hypertension as fixed-dose combinations with a thiazide (e.g. co-amilozide) in patients receiving converting-enzyme inhibitors.

5 *Fetal injury* – renal failure occurs in the fetus if converting enzyme is inhibited, resulting in oligohydramnios. ACEI are therefore contraindicated in late pregnancy, and other drugs are preferred in women of childbearing potential with essential hypertension.

6 *Urticaria and angioneurotic oedema* – increased kinin concentrations have been invoked to explain the urticarial reactions and angioneurotic oedema sometimes caused by ACEI, although the evidence for this is incomplete.

7 *–SH-group-related effects* – when it was first introduced into clinical use, captopril was found to cause a cluster of adverse effects, including heavy proteinuria, neutropenia, rash and taste disturbance, which were identified as being related to its sulphydryl group. Similar effects occur with penicillamine, another drug that contains a sulphydryl group (see Chapter 25). These dose-related effects seldom occur with the maximum doses of captopril that are now regarded as useful for treating hypertension (i.e. usually no more than 50 mg twice daily).

PHARMACOKINETICS

Currently available converting-enzyme inhibitors are all active when administered orally, but are highly polar and are eliminated in the urine. Some of them (e.g. **fosinopril**) are also metabolized by the liver. A number of these drugs (e.g. captopril, **lisinopril**) are active *per se*, while others (e.g. **enalapril**, **quinapril**) are prodrugs, and require metabolic conversion to active metabolites (e.g. enalaprilat, quinaprilat). In practice this is of little or no importance. None of the currently available ACE inhibitors penetrate the central nervous system particularly well, and none of them penetrate to inhibit the testicular enzyme. There is only a weak correlation between inhibition of plasma-converting enzyme and chronic hypotensive effect, possibly because of the importance of converting enzyme in various key tissues rather than in the plasma.

DRUG INTERACTIONS

The useful interaction with diuretics has already been alluded to above. Diuretic treatment increases plasma renin activity, and the consequent activation of angiotensin II and aldosterone limits their efficacy. ACEI interrupt this loop and so enhance the hypotensive efficacy of diuretics, as well as reducing thiazide-induced hypokalaemia. Conversely, ACEI have a potentially adverse interaction with potassium-sparing diuretics and potassium supplements, leading to hyperkalaemia, especially in patients with renal impairment, as mentioned above. As with other antihypertensive drugs, NSAIDs increase blood pressure in patients treated with converting-enzyme inhibitors.

Angiotensin-receptor antagonists

Most of the effects of angiotensin II, including vasoconstriction and aldosterone release, are mediated by the angiotensin II subtype 1 (AT_1) receptor. Many years ago, peptide analogues of angiotensin (e.g. **saralasin**) were synthesized and studied experimentally, but were not used extensively clinically. More recently, non-peptide antagonists have become available, and several of them are now marketed for treatment of hypertension in the UK. Their pharmacology differs predictably from that of converting-enzyme inhibitors, since unlike these drugs they do not potentiate bradykinin. **Losartan** (25–100 mg once daily) has a similar clinical profile of efficacy in hypertension and of adverse effects and cautions to converting enzyme inhibitors, with the exception of cough, which occurs no more frequently than with placebo in patients who have experienced this symptom with a converting-enzyme inhibitor. AT_1-blockers do not block the AT_2-receptor, which is exposed to high concentrations of angiotensin II during treatment with an AT_1-blocker. The effects (if any) of this are unknown, but should be borne in mind before prescribing the newer drugs rather than an alternative and more established drug such as an ACE inhibitor.

Calcium-channel blockers

Drugs that block voltage-dependent Ca^{2+} channels are used to treat angina (see Chapter 28) and supraventricular tachyarrhythmias (see Chapter 31) as well as hypertension. There are three chemically distinct classes of calcium-channel blockers in clinical use, namely *dihydropyridines, benzothiazepines* and *phenylalkylamines*. Examples are listed in Table 27.4.

USE

Dihydropyridine calcium-channel blockers lower blood pressure and are a useful addition to a β-adrenoceptor antagonist in patients with moderate or severe hypertension who are not adequately controlled by a beta-blocker alone. Some of these drugs (e.g. **nifedipine**, **amlodipine**) are also licensed for use alone in patients with mild essential hypertension. As with the converting-enzyme inhibitors, large-scale comparative studies with thiazide diuretics and beta-blockers are urgently needed, as there are theoretical reasons to believe that calcium-channel blockers might perform either worse or better than these proven therapies. These uncertainties have been highlighted (but not illuminated) by recent high-profile debates on possible adverse effects (see below) of these drugs identified by meta-analyses and case–control and cohort studies. The Systeur trial has been reassuring. A randomized controlled trial (the ASCOT Study) to determine their effect on clinical end-points is planned.

Calcium-channel blockers provide a useful alternative for patients in whom thiazide diuretics and beta-blockers are contraindicated, or who do

Table 27.4: Examples of calcium-channel-blocking drugs in clinical use

Class	Drug	Effect on heart rate	Adverse effects	Comment
Dihydropyridine	Nifedipine	↑	Headache, flushing, ankle swelling	Slow-release preparations for once/twice daily use
	Amlodipine	↑	Ankle swelling	Once daily use in hypertension, angina
	Nimodipine	±	Flushing, headache	Prevention of cerebral vasospasm after subarachnoid haemorrhage
Benzothiazepine	Diltiazem	±	Generally mild	Prophylaxis of angina, hypertension
Phenylalkylamine	Verapamil	↓	Constipation; marked negative inotropic action	See Chapter 31 for use in arrhythmias. Slow-release preparation for hypertension, angina

not tolerate them, although they have several distinct side-effects of their own. Amlodipine has a long half-life, and is taken once daily. Because of its long half-life, the daily dose of amlodipine should not be increased too rapidly. In any event it has a relatively small useful dose range of 5–10 mg.

There has been a vogue in the UK for the use of nifedipine sublingually for the treatment of hypertensive emergencies. A capsule is bitten into and the liquid allowed to remain in the mouth. When administered in this way it has been shown that most of the absorbed nifedipine is in fact swallowed, and that this method causes unpredictable and sometimes catastrophic hypotension with consequent watershed infarction of the brain. The drug is not licensed to be used in this way, and advice to use it thus (especially when anonymous, as in one regrettable editorial published in an influential medical journal) is to be deplored. Slow-release preparations of nifedipine (10–40 mg twice daily) do not have these problems, and a longer-acting preparation for once daily use is also available (30–60 mg).

MECHANISM OF ACTION

Calcium-channel blockers inhibit the influx of Ca^{2+} through voltage-dependent L-type calcium channels. Calcium entry through such channels in vascular smooth muscle controls the contractile state of actomyosin. Calcium-channel blockers therefore relax arteriolar smooth muscle, reduce peripheral vascular resistance and lower arterial blood pressure. Their ability to relax vascular smooth muscle also underlies their use in coronary artery spasm, cerebral vasospasm following subarachnoid haemorrhage (where **nimodipine** is used) and Raynaud's phenomenon. Calcium-channel blockers are negatively inotropic because they inhibit Ca^{2+} entry into cardiac tissue.

METABOLIC EFFECTS

Calcium-channel blockers do not affect the concentrations of plasma cholesterol or triglycerides or extracellular calcium homeostasis.

ADVERSE EFFECTS

Calcium-channel blocking drugs are usually reasonably well tolerated.

1 The commonest adverse effects of the dihydropyridines are flushing and headache which are directly related to arteriolar vasodilatation. This activates baroreflexes, activating the sympathetic nervous system and causing tachycardia. This can worsen angina and possibly accounts for adverse effects on mortality identified by meta-analysis of controlled trials of their use in the setting of acute myocardial infarction. These effects are most severe when treatment is started, and are related to peak plasma concentration. Consequently they are most marked with short-acting drugs such as nifedipine, less marked with slow-release formulations, and least marked with a long-half-life drug such as amlodipine, with which the frequency of these complaints in double-blind trials is similar to that for placebo.
2 Ankle swelling is common with all of the dihydropyridines, and often takes some time to become manifest. The reason for the particular propensity of dihydropyridines (as distinct from other calcium-channel blockers and most other vasodilators) to cause this side-effect is not completely understood. It has been suggested that dihydropyridines preferentially relax arteriolar smooth muscle, thereby exposing the capillaries in the feet to unphysiologically high pressures, causing exudation of fluid by the Starling mechanism.
3 The negative inotropic effect of the calcium-channel blockers can exacerbate cardiac failure. This propensity is most marked with **verapamil** and least marked in the case of the dihydropyridines, because of their relative selectivity for vascular smooth muscle, and the tendency for the reduction in cardiac afterload caused by arteriolar dilatation to offset the direct negative inotropic effect of the heart. However, caution is needed when treating patients with even mild degrees of heart failure with any calcium-channel blocking drug.
4 Constipation is an undesired effect of phenylalkylamines such as verapamil on gastrointestinal smooth muscle.
5 Case–control and cohort studies have raised the possibility that, in elderly people, calcium-channel antagonists may increase the risk of gastrointestinal bleeding and of neoplasia. These possibilities will be addressed in randomized controlled trials. Meanwhile, these theoretical hazards do not preclude the use of

these drugs in cases where alternatives are less effective or less well tolerated.

PHARMACOKINETICS

Calcium-channel antagonists are absorbed when given by mouth. Nifedipine has a short half-life, and many of its adverse effects (e.g. flushing, headache) relate to the peak plasma concentration. Slow-release preparations improve its performance in this regard, but are limited by the transit time of the bowel. Amlodipine has a half-life of 2–3 days and produces a smooth effect, as well as only requiring once daily administration. Slow-release nifedipine is preferred to amlodipine in urgent situations, as it permits more rapid dose titration.

DRUG INTERACTIONS

The favourable interaction of dihydropyridine calcium-channel-blocking drugs with β-adrenoceptor antagonists when used orally to treat patients with moderately severe hypertension uncomplicated by cardiac failure has already been mentioned. It contrasts with the potentially catastrophic interaction with β-antagonists of intravenous verapamil when used intravenously to treat patients with tachyarrhythmias.

α-Adrenoceptor antagonists

There are two main subtypes of α-receptor, termed α_1- and α_2. α_1-Agonists (including endogenous noradrenaline) cause vasoconstriction and hypertension, and α-adrenoceptor antagonists lower blood pressure.

USE

Non-specific alpha-blockade causes profound postural hypotension and reflex tachycardia. The use of such drugs is very limited and specialized. **Phenoxybenzamine** is distinctive in irreversibly alkylating the receptors. It is still uniquely valuable in preparing patients with phaeochromocytoma for surgery, but has no place in the management of essential hypertension. **Prazosin** was the first selective reversible α_1-blocker to become available clinically. Unlike phenoxybenzamine, it does not block presynaptic α_2-receptors that are normally stimulated by released noradrenaline and which inhibit further transmitter release. Thus there is no interference with this negative feedback pathway, and consequently relatively little tachycardia. Alpha-blockers reduce plasma low-density lipoprotein (LDL) cholesterol and increase high-density lipoprotein (HDL) cholesterol, effects that could be of particular value in treating patients with coexisting dyslipidaemia. However use of prazosin is limited by the occurrence of severe hypotension and collapse, especially following the first dose. It has a short elimination half-life and is given at least twice daily. Because of these problems, alpha-blockers were not widely used. This has changed with the introduction of **doxazosin** and **terazosin**. These drugs are structurally closely related to prazosin. They possess similar α_1–selectivity, but have substantially longer elimination half-lives, permitting once daily use and causing fewer problems with first-dose hypotension.

Long-acting α_1-adrenoceptor antagonists are useful additions to diuretics, β-adrenoceptor antagonists, Ca^{2+}-antagonists or converting-enzyme inhibitors in patients with moderate hypertension. Doxazosin is also licensed for use as a single agent in patients with mild essential hypertension, although so far there have been no controlled clinical trials to demonstrate that α_1-adrenoceptor antagonists reduce the risk of stroke or other clinically important events in such patients. Large-scale comparative studies with thiazide diuretics and/or beta-blockers are needed, since there are theoretical reasons to believe that α_1-blockers might perform either worse or better (e.g. because of their effects on plasma lipids) than these proven therapies.

It is prudent to start treatment with a long-acting α_1-blocker with a small dose (1 mg of either doxazosin or terazosin) given before going to bed, and to warn patients about the possibility of postural hypotension if they get up during the night. Nevertheless, postural hypotension is less of a problem than with prazosin. The dose may be titrated to up to 16 mg (doxazosin) or 20 mg (terazosin) if necessary. Despite the elimination half-life of 10–12 h the daily dose should not be escalated too rapidly, and the effect on erect as well as supine blood pressure should be monitored. Since α_1-antagonists reduce cardiac afterload and, unlike β-antagonists and calcium-channel antagonists, have no direct negative inotropic effect, they are particularly useful as an addition to a converting-enzyme inhibitor or diuretic in hypertensive patients with cardiac failure. They also reduce symptoms of bladder outflow tract obstruction (see Chapter 35), and are useful in men with mild symptoms from benign prostatic hypertrophy who do not desire surgery but who do not tolerate thiazide diuretics because of urinary urgency or nocturia.

MECHANISM OF ACTION

The sympathetic nervous system is tonically active, and noradrenaline released from postganglionic nerve terminals activates α_1-receptors on vascular smooth muscle, causing tonic vasoconstriction via release of Ca^{2+} from intracellular stores by inositol trisphosphate and by influx of Ca^{2+} through receptor-operated as well as voltage-dependent channels. (Voltage-dependent channels are opened indirectly via depolarization of the smooth muscle membrane.) α_1–Blockers cause vasodilatation by antagonizing this tonic action of noradrenaline.

ADVERSE EFFECTS

1. First-dose hypotension and postural hypotension have been mentioned above.
2. Other effects, including nasal stuffiness, headache, dizziness, dry mouth, impotence and pruritus, have also been reported, but are relatively infrequent.
3. Alpha-blockers can cause urinary incontinence, especially in women with pre-existing pelvic pathology. This is uncommon, but it is important to be aware of the possibility, since this effect is reversible on stopping the drug.

METABOLIC EFFECTS

α_1–Adrenoceptor antagonists have a mild favourable effect on plasma lipids, with an increase in HDL and a reduction in LDL cholesterol. Whether these desirable biochemical effects translate into a clinically useful reduction in ischaemic heart disease is not yet known.

PHARMACOKINETICS

The mean elimination half-life of prazosin is approximately 3 h. Doxazosin and terazosin have elimination half-lives of approximately 10–12 hours and provide acceptably smooth 24-h control if used once daily.

Key points

Drugs used in essential hypertension

- Diuretics – thiazides (in low dose) are preferred to loop diuretics unless there is renal impairment. They may precipitate gout and worsen glucose tolerance or dyslipidaemia, but they reduce the risk of stroke and other vascular events. Adverse effects include hypokalaemia, which is seldom problematic, and impotence. They are suitable first-line drugs, especially in black patients, who often have low circulating renin levels and respond well to salt restriction and diuretics.
- Beta-blockers reduce the risk of vascular events, but are contraindicated in patients with obstructive pulmonary disease. Adverse events (dose related) include fatigue and cold extremities. Heart failure, heart block or claudication can be exacerbated in predisposed patients. They are first-line drugs and are particularly useful in patients with another indication for them (e.g. angina, post-myocardial infarction). Black patients tend to respond poorly to them as single agents.
- ACE inhibitors are particularly useful as an addition to a thiazide in moderately severe disease. Research data on their effects on vascular events are awaited. The main adverse effect on chronic use is cough; losartan, an angiotensin-II receptor antagonist, lacks this effect but is otherwise similar to ACE inhibitors.
- Calcium-channel antagonists are useful additions to beta-blockers in moderately severe disease. Long-acting drugs/preparations are preferred. Research data on effects on vascular event rates are awaited. The main adverse effect in chronic use is ankle swelling.
- α_1-Blockers are useful additional agents in patients who are poorly controlled on one or two drugs. Long-acting drugs (e.g. doxazosin, terazosin) are preferred. Effects on vascular event rates are unknown. Unlike other antihypertensives, they improve the lipid profile.
- α-Methyldopa is useful in patients with hypertension during pregnancy
- Other drugs that are useful in occasional patients with severe disease include minoxidil, hydralazine and nitroprusside.

Other drugs used in hypertension

In addition to the five main classes of antihypertensive drugs described above, there are several older drugs that have distinct uses in special situations. These include **minoxidil**, **nitroprusside**, **hydralazine** and **α-methyldopa**. Some of the more important properties of these drugs are summarized in Table 27.5.

SPECIAL SITUATIONS

Elderly

Most vascular events occur in elderly people who therefore have most to gain from antihypertensive treatment provided that they are otherwise in good health. Evidence for this view comes from several controlled trials including the European Working Party on Hypertension in the Elderly (EWPHE) Study and the Systolic Hypertension in Elderly Persons (SHEP) Study, which demonstrated significant reductions in myocardial infarction with treatment in this age group. However, elderly people are also at greatest risk of adverse effects, and treatment should be mild and dose titration gradual. There are no hard and fast rules about the choice of drug. Diuretics (e.g. Dyazide™, which was used in the EWPHE Study) are often successful, but should be avoided in men with symptoms of prostatism or women with incontinence. They may need to be withheld temporarily in the event of intercurrent desalinating illness (e.g. with fever, vomiting and diarrhoea). β-Adrenoceptor antagonists are also sometimes effective and well tolerated. It is important to obtain an electrocardiogram and to ensure that there is no evidence of heart block or suggestion of sick sinus syndrome. Converting-enzyme inhibitors are usually well tolerated by elderly people, as are calcium-channel antagonists. α-Adrenoceptor antagonists are best avoided unless there is an extra indication in the form of prostatism from benign prostatic hypertrophy, because even healthy elderly people often experience some degree of postural hypotension, and lack the homeostatic mechanisms to compensate for additional causes of postural hypotension. Centrally acting drugs (e.g. α-methyldopa) were used as add-on treatment in the EWPHE trial.

Pregnancy

MANAGEMENT OF ECLAMPSIA/PRE-ECLAMPSIA

Eclampsia is a leading cause of fetal and maternal mortality. Pre-eclampsia (its forerunner) occurs from the twentieth week of pregnancy and consists of hypertension, proteinuria and oedema, often with elevation of plasma urate and liver enzymes, and thrombocytopenia and other evidence of consumptive coagulopathy. It can progress rapidly to eclampsia, which is characterized by convulsions. The pathophysiology is poorly understood, but the primary abnormality is believed to be in the placenta (hydatidiform mole commonly causes pre-eclampsia). In normal pregnancy there is vasodilation and resistance to vasoconstrictor stimuli which is lost in pre-eclampsia. Earlier hopes that the condition could be prevented by low-dose aspirin have not been confirmed, and prevention is not possible at present.

Women with pre-eclampsia should be admitted to hospital. Pre-eclampsia resolves rapidly (usually within a few days) after delivery of the placenta, although occasionally late postpartum eclampsia develops up to 10 days after delivery. Near term the baby should therefore be delivered promptly. Earlier in gestation, attempts to prolong the pregnancy by treating blood pressure may be worthwhile, although they seldom do more than buy a little extra time, and the risks of eclampsia are considerable. If headache or epigastric pain, hyper-reflexia, deterioration of renal function or development of consumptive coagulopathy develop, or if the fetus is in jeopardy, delivery should be undertaken promptly whatever the gestational age. Glucocorticoids may be used to accelerate maturation of the fetal lung and reduce the risk of respiratory disease in the newborn baby.

From this it is evident that drugs have only a secondary role to play in the management of established pre-eclampsia/eclampsia. When drug treatment is indicated, α-methyldopa is given by mouth. The starting dose is 250 or 500 mg two or three times daily, and the dose can be increased rapidly if necessary to a maximum of 3–4 g daily in divided doses. If this fails to control the blood pressure, hydralazine can be added in doses up to

Table 27.5: Additional antihypertensive drugs used in special situations

Drug	Mechanism of action	Uses	Side-effects/limitations
Minoxidil	Minoxidil sulphate (active metabolite) is a K^+-channel activator	Very severe hypertension that is resistant to other drugs	Fluid retention; reflex tachycardia; hirsutism; coarsening of facial appearance. Must be used in combination with other drugs (usually a loop diuretic and β-antagonist)
Nitroprusside	Breaks down chemically to NO, which activates guanylyl cyclase in vascular smooth muscle	Given by intravenous infusion in intensive-care unit for control of malignant hypertension	Short term IV use only: prolonged use causes cyanide toxicity (monitor plasma thiocyanate levels); sensitive to light; close monitoring to avoid hypotension is essential
Hydralazine	Direct action on vascular smooth muscle; biochemical mechanism not understood	Previously used in 'stepped-care' approach to severe hypertension; β-antagonist in combination with diuretic. Retains a place in severe hypertension during pregnancy	Headache; flushing; tachycardia; fluid retention. Long-term high-dose use causes systemic lupus-like syndrome in susceptible individuals
α-Methyldopa	Taken up by noradrenergic nerve terminals and converted to α-methyl-noradrenaline, which is released as a false transmitter. This acts centrally as an α_2-agonist and reduces sympathetic outflow	Hypertension during pregnancy. Occasionally useful in patients who cannot tolerate other drugs	Drowsiness (common); depression; hepatitis; immune haemolytic anaemia; drug fever.

200 mg daily by mouth. In more urgent situations (i.e. when the clinical picture suggests that eclampsia is imminent) blood pressure should be controlled by intravenous hydralazine, ideally given as a constant-rate infusion or, if an infusion pump is not available, as a series of small intravenous boluses, starting with a 5-mg dose followed by 5–10 mg every 20–30 min as needed, with continuous monitoring of blood pressure.

Until recently, the best strategy for preventing seizures was unknown, with US practice favouring parenteral magnesium sulphate and UK practice favouring phenytoin or diazepam. A large multinational controlled trial has demonstrated unequivocally that magnesium sulphate is superior in preventing recurrent seizures in this setting (approximately half as many recurrent seizures as on diazepam, and a two-thirds reduction compared to phenytoin). The dose used was large (4 g, i.e. approximately 16 mmol of Mg^{2+}, IV over 5–20 min, as a loading dose, followed by 1 g/h for 24 h as an IV infusion; some centres used an intramuscular regime after the loading dose, but this is painful). Additional boluses (2–4 g) can be given if fits recur. Blood pressure should be measured frequently, and ECG monitoring is advisable. The fetal heart rate should be monitored until delivery. Mg^{2+} is eliminated in the urine, and adverse effects of Mg^{2+} occur more commonly if there is renal impairment. Plasma creatinine levels should be checked, and the magnesium concentration should be monitored closely if possible. Symptoms of Mg^{2+} toxicity include nausea, flushing, diplopia, dysarthria and weakness of limb muscles. Signs include loss of tendon reflexes. In severely hypertensive women (especially with hyper-reflexia) it is reasonable to measure plasma magnesium levels and give replacement treatment with intravenous magnesium sulphate if the concentration is low, even if a fit has not occurred, although this is of unproven efficacy.

PRE-EXISTING HYPERTENSION

Most women with pre-existing hypertension have essential hypertension, although of course secondary hypertension is also encountered in pregnant women. Among secondary causes, it is especially important to keep the possibility of phaeochromocytoma in mind, as this can present during pregnancy in a manner that is clinically indistinguishable from pre-eclampsia, yet its successful management is very different to that of either pre-eclampsia or essential hypertension, and failure to make this diagnosis accounts for a disproportionate number of maternal deaths.

Women with essential hypertension are at increased risk of pre-eclampsia, but more than 85% of such women have uncomplicated pregnancies, so it is appropriate to provide general reassurance. If treatment is *initiated* during pregnancy it is appropriate to use methyldopa, which has the longest record of use and follow-up in children born to mothers following treatment. Information on the use of first-line antihypertensive drugs during pregnancy is decidedly sparse. One has to balance the risk of stopping such a drug against uncertainties about the possible adverse effects on the fetus.

Angiotensin-converting enzyme inhibitors are absolutely contraindicated in later stages of pregnancy, as they cause oligohydramnios and neonatal renal failure. The use of diuretics during pregnancy is controversial. It is generally agreed that they should not be used to treat established pre-eclampsia or eclampsia (unless left ventricular failure has supervened), but some authorities recommend continuing them if they were being taken before conception. Beta-blockers are not recommended because they have been associated with reduced fetal blood flow and growth retardation. In contrast, the combined alpha- and beta-blocker labetalol has been used successfully in pregnancy, although concerns have been expressed about maternal hepatotoxicity. Trials of Ca^{2+}-antagonists have been promising, but experience of their long-term use during pregnancy is limited.

Accelerated and malignant hypertension

Malignant hypertension is diagnosed on the basis of high blood pressure accompanied by papilloedema and, usually, microscopic haematuria with red-cell casts. Hypertension with grade III retinopathy (cotton-wool spots and/or haemorrhages) is sometimes called accelerated hypertension. Both conditions are associated with a vasculitis characterized by fibrinoid necrosis in arterioles in brain and kidneys, and with progression to death within 1 year in 90% of cases if untreated. These are emergency situations that require immediate hospitalization. There are two principles for successful treatment:

1 to lower the blood pressure promptly; but
2 to avoid lowering it too much.

The reason why excessive lowering of the blood pressure is so dangerous in this situation is that cerebral autoregulation is severely impaired in these circumstances, so that reducing the pressure to values which would be well tolerated in normotensive individuals causes an excessive reduction in blood flow in patients with malignant hypertension (see Figure 27.3). Inadequate cerebral blood flow causes infarction in watershed areas of the brain, and blindness or disconnection syndromes and other forms of stroke can follow a precipitate fall in blood pressure.

In most patients blood pressure should therefore be reduced over a period of days rather than hours. The main indications for parenteral drugs are left ventricular failure with pulmonary oedema or hypertensive encephalopathy. If these are absent, the patient should be confined to bed and oral treatment commenced with a beta-blocker or slow-release preparation of a calcium-channel antagonist such as a slow-release preparation of nifedipine. It is important to note that unpredictable and sometimes catastrophic (i.e. causing blindness or stroke) falls in blood pressure have been reported following intravenous boluses of antihypertensive drugs and after nifedipine (e.g. following biting into a capsule of the liquid formulation of this drug).

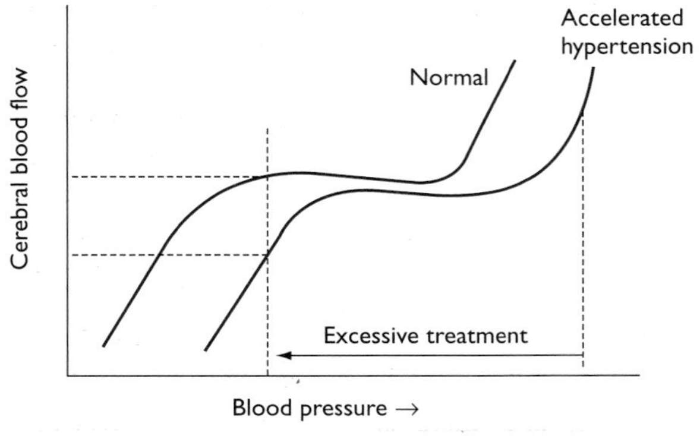

Figure 27.3: Cerebral blood flow in accelerated hypertension. The autoregulation curve is shifted to the right. Cerebral blood flow is increased before treatment, but if blood pressure is reduced by treatment to a value that would be well tolerated in a normal subject, this will cause a potentially catastrophic fall in cerebral blood flow in a patient with accelerated hypertension.

Frusemide is used for left ventricular failure complicating malignant hypertension. More severe failure is an indication for sodium **nitroprusside** by constant-rate infusion in an intensive-care unit. If intensive-care facilities are unavailable, an oral drug regime may be safer for the patient. Encephalopathy is present if convulsions or a fluctuating level of consciousness or changing focal neurological signs occur. It is rare, and optimal management depends on intensive-care-unit facilities. Neurological features in hypertensive patients often result from cerebral infarction or haemorrhage due to thrombosis of a large vessel or rupture of a Charcot–Bouchard aneurysm, rather than to encephalopathy. These are contraindications to rapid blood pressure reduction, which may exacerbate the neurological deficit. Sodium nitroprusside administered by constant-rate infusion (0.5 μg/kg/min increasing to 8 μg/kg/min) is the best drug for treating hypertensive encephalopathy, but it is mandatory to monitor the response frequently, and oral treatment with conventional agents should be started as soon as possible.

Once the immediate emergency is past, the possibility of secondary hypertension should be considered, particularly renal artery stenosis, which is present in about one-third of such patients.

Acute aortic dissection

Aortic dissection is extended by a wide pulse pressure and by a rapid rate of rise in arterial pressure (dP/dt). Vasodilators such as hydralazine which increase pulse pressure and dP/dt should therefore be avoided in the first instance. A fast-acting parenteral β-receptor antagonist (e.g. esmolol) can be infused intravenously, supplemented by sodium nitroprusside once beta-blockade has been achieved. Following stabilization, the anatomy of the tear is defined and a surgical plan is established. If operation is not indicated, medical therapy should include an oral beta-blocker if possible.

Case history

A 72-year-old woman sees her general practitioner because of an *E.coli* urinary infection. Her blood pressure is 196/86 mmHg. She had had a small stroke 2 years previously, which was managed at home, and from which she made a complete recovery. At that time, her blood pressure had been recorded as 160/80 mmHg. She looks after her husband (who has mild dementia) and enjoys life, particularly visits from her grandchildren. She smokes 10 cigarettes/day, does not drink alcohol and takes no drugs. The remainder of the examination is unremarkable. Serum creatinine is normal, total cholesterol is 5.6 mmol/L and HDL is 1.2 mmol/L. The urinary tract infection resolves with a short course of amoxycillin. This patient's blood pressure on two further occasions is 176/84 and 186/82 mmHg, respectively. An ECG is normal. She is resistant to advice to stop smoking (on the grounds that she has been doing it for 55 years and any harm has been done already) and the suggestion of drug treatment (on the grounds that she feels fine and is 'too old for that sort of thing').

Questions

Decide whether each of the following statements is true or false.

(a) This patient's systolic hypertension is a reflection of a 'stiff' circulation, and drug treatment will not improve her prognosis.
(b Drug treatment of the hypertension should not be contemplated unless she stops smoking first.
(c) If she agrees to take drugs for her hypertension, she will be at greater risk of adverse effects than a younger woman.
(d) Attempts to discourage her from smoking are futile
(e) An α_1–blocker would be a sensible first choice of drug, as it will improve her serum lipid levels.
(f) Aspirin treatment should be considered.

Answer

(a) False.
(b) False.
(c) True.
(d) False.
(e) False.
(f) True.

Comment

Treating elderly patients with systolic hypertension reduces their excess risk of stroke and myocardial infarction. The absolute benefit of treatment is greatest in elderly people (in whom events are common). Treatment is particularly desirable as this patient made a good recovery from a stroke. She was strongly discouraged from smoking (by explaining that this would almost immediately reduce the risk of a further vascular event), but she was unable to stop. Continued smoking puts her at increased risk of stroke, and she agreed to take bendrofluazide 2.5 mg daily with the goal of staying healthy so that she could continue to look after her husband and enjoy life. She tolerated this well and her blood pressure fell to around 165/80 mmHg. The addition of a long-acting ACE inhibitor (trandolapril, 0.5 mg in the morning) led to a further reduction in blood pressure to around 150/80 mmHg. α_1-Antagonists can cause postural hypotension, which is particularly undesirable in the elderly.

Diabetes

Diabetes and hypertension often coexist. Hypertension is a risk factor for many of the complications of diabetes, and diabetics who are also hypertensive have a particularly high incidence of myocardial infarction, stroke and renal failure. The progression of renal impairment in diabetics can be slowed by treatment with antihypertensive drugs. It is therefore especially worth treating hypertension in diabetic patients. The target blood pressure should be 140/80 (i.e. more aggressive than in non-diabetics).

Diuretics and β-adrenoceptor antagonists each have disadvantages in diabetic patients. High doses of Thiazides worsen glucose tolerance in diabetics on oral agents or diet, and β-adrenoceptor antagonists may mask symptoms of hypoglycaemia in patients who are treated with insulin. Low doses of thiazides are recommended. Each of these classes of agent have mild but potentially adverse effects on plasma lipid profiles that are theoretically particularly undesirable in diabetic patients. Ca^{2+}-antagonists and converting-enzyme inhibitors are useful in diabetic patients, and there is evidence that converting-enzyme inhibitors have a unique ability to reduce albumin excretion (a marker of diabetic glomerular injury) in such patients, and thus perhaps to reduce the rate of progression of renal damage.

Renal impairment

Although most patients with hypertension have normal or near-normal renal function, hypertension is a common cause and effect of renal failure. Although good control of blood pressure is not easy in many patients with renal failure, it should be sought vigorously, as uncontrolled hypertension accelerates the deterioration of renal function and good control may delay the need for dialysis although, disappointingly, in some patients renal functional deterioration is inexorable despite apparently good control of blood pressure.

Thiazides are not effective in patients with renal failure and, in contrast to patients with normal renal function, a loop diuretic (e.g. frusemide) is preferable in individuals with substantial degrees of renal dysfunction. Potassium-retaining diuretics such as amiloride or triamterene should be *avoided* in renal failure because of the risk of hyperkalaemia (especially in patients receiving converting-enzyme inhibitors).

Mild hypertension in patients with reduced renal function may respond to a β-adrenoceptor antagonist, calcium-channel blocker, α_1–adrenoceptor antagonist or converting-enzyme inhibitor. Renal function should be monitored closely when starting treatment with any of these drugs, because a reduction in mean arterial pressure may cause a further reduction in glomerular filtration. Converting-enzyme inhibitors are a special case, as these drugs predictably cause functional renal failure in patients with bilateral renal artery stenosis (or renal artery stenosis in an artery supplying a single functioning kidney). This is due to the loss of efferent arteriolar tone, on which glomerular filtration in these individuals depends. It is reversible if it is recognized promptly and the drug discontinued. More severe hypertension often requires the use of combinations of drugs, as in patients with normal renal function.

The blood pressure of patients on chronic dialysis can often be controlled by slow removal of water and salt during dialysis, and by restriction of dietary salt and water between dialyses, supplemented with drug treatment if necessary.

FURTHER READING

Eclampsia Trial Collaborative Group. 1995: Which anticonvulsant for women with eclampsia? Evidence from the collaborative eclampsia trial. *Lancet* **345**, 1455–63.

Fletcher AE, Bulpitt CJ. 1992: How far should blood pressure be lowered? *New England Journal of Medicine* **326**, 251–4.

Goodfriend TL, Elliott ME, Catt KJ. 1996: Angiotensin receptors and their antagonists. *New England Journal of Medicine* **334**, 1649–54.

Setaro JF, Black HR. 1992: Refractory hypertension. *New England Journal of Medicine* **327**, 543–7.

Sibai BM. 1996: Treatment of hypertension in pregnant women. *New England Journal of Medicine* **335**, 257–65.

Swales JD (ed.) 1994: *Textbook of hypertension*. Oxford: Blackwell Science.

van Zwieten PA. 1997: Central imidazoline (I_1) receptors as targets of centrally acting antihypertensives: moxonidine and rilmenidine. *Journal of Hypertension* **15**, 117–25

CHAPTER TWENTY-EIGHT

ISCHAEMIC HEART DISEASE

- Pathophysiology
- Management of stable angina
- Management of unstable coronary disease
- Drugs used in ischaemic heart disease

PATHOPHYSIOLOGY

Ischaemic heart disease is nearly always caused by *atheroma* (see Chapter 26) in one or more of the coronary arteries. Such disease is very common in western societies, and is often asymptomatic. When the obstruction caused by an uncomplicated atheromatous plaque exceeds a critical value, myocardial oxygen demand during exercise exceeds the ability of the stenosed vessel to supply oxygenated blood, resulting in chest pain brought on predictably by exertion and relieved within a few minutes on resting ('angina pectoris'). Drugs that alter *haemodynamics* can reduce angina.

Most patients with angina pectoris experience attacks of pain in a constant stable pattern, but in some patients attacks occur at rest, or they may occur with increasing frequency and severity on less and less exertion ('unstable angina'). Unstable angina may be a prelude to myocardial infarction, which can also occur unheralded. Both unstable angina and myocardial infarction occur as a result of fissuring of an atheromatous plaque in a coronary artery. Platelets adhere to the underlying subendothelium and white thrombus, consisting of platelet/fibrinogen/fibrin aggregates, extends into the lumen of the artery. *Myocardial infarction results when thrombus occludes the coronary vessel.*

In addition to mechanical obstruction caused by atheroma, with or without adherent thrombus, *spasm* of smooth muscle in the vascular media can contribute to ischaemia. The importance of such vascular spasm varies both among different patients and at different times in the same patient, and its contribution is often difficult to define clinically. The mechanism of spasm also probably varies, and has been difficult to establish. Possible mediators include vasoconstrictors released from formed elements of blood (e.g. platelets or white cells) or from nerve terminals. 5-Hydroxytryptamine (5HT, serotonin), thromboxane A_2 and various neuropeptides and endothelium-derived peptides (e.g. angiotensin II and endothelin) may each contribute either alone or in combination in different circumstances. A relative deficiency of endothelium-derived vasodilators, including nitric oxide and prostacyclin, may be as important as release of vasoconstrictors. Several of these mediators influence platelet function as well as vascular smooth muscle contraction. 5HT and thromboxane A_2 are pro-aggregatory, while several vasodilators, including prostacyclin and nitric oxide, are anti-aggregatory. Consequently, thrombosis as well as spasm is likely to be favoured in situations characterized by an imbalance of these vasoactive mediators. There is currently considerable interest in these issues, but the importance or otherwise of spasm in the majority of patients with acute coronary syndromes is unknown.

Treatment of patients with ischaemic heart disease is directed at the three pathophysiological elements identified above, namely *atheroma*, *haemodynamics* and *thrombosis*. Such treatment not only improves symptoms but also prolongs life.

Management of stable angina

Modifiable risk factors

Modifiable risk factors include *smoking*, *hypertension*, *hypercholesterolaemia*, *diabetes mellitus*, *obesity* and *lack of exercise*. The object of defining these factors is to improve them in individual patients, thereby preventing progression (and hopefully causing regression) of coronary atheroma. This is discussed in Chapters 26, 27 and 36.

Pain relief

Angina is relieved by **glyceryl trinitrate (GTN)**. However, in patients with chronic stable angina, pain usually resolves within a few minutes of stopping exercise even without treatment, so prophylaxis is usually more important than relief of an attack.

Prophylaxis

Antithrombotic therapy with **aspirin** reduces the incidence of myocardial infarction. Prophylaxis is also directed at reducing the frequency of attacks of angina. In this context, GTN is best used for 'acute' prophylaxis. A dose is taken immediately before undertaking activity that usually brings on pain (e.g. climbing a hill), in order to prevent pain. Alternatively, long-acting nitrates (e.g. **isosorbide mononitrate**) may be taken regularly to reduce the frequency of attacks. **Nicorandil** has been introduced in the UK (having been used for several years in Japan). It combines nitrovasodilator with K^+-channel-activating properties, and relaxes veins and arteries. It is used in acute and long-term prophylaxis of angina, but its place in treatment is still being defined. Headache is common, and this drug is probably best reserved for patients who do not respond adequately to isosorbide mononitrate. Beta-blockers or calcium-channel blockers are also useful for chronic prophylaxis (see below).

Consideration of surgery/ angioplasty

Cardiac catheterization identifies patients who would benefit from coronary artery bypass graft (CABG) surgery or angioplasty. Coronary artery disease is progressive, and there are two roles for such interventions:

1 symptom relief;
2 to improve outcome.

CABG and angioplasty are both excellent treatments for relieving symptoms of angina, although they are not a permanent cure, and symptoms may recur if there is restenosis, if the graft becomes occluded, or if the underlying atheromatous disease progresses. Angioplasty as currently performed does not improve the final outcome in terms of survival or myocardial infarction, whereas CABG can benefit some patients. Those with significant disease in the left main coronary artery survive longer if they are operated on, and so probably do patients with severe triple-vessel disease. Patients with strongly positive stress cardiograms have a relatively high incidence of such lesions, but unfortunately there is no foolproof method of making such anatomical diagnoses non-invasively, so the issue of which patients to subject to the low risks of invasive study remains one of clinical judgement and of cost.

Surgical treatment consists of coronary artery grafting with saphenous vein or, preferably, internal mammary artery to bypass diseased segment(s) of coronary artery. Angioplasty has yet to be shown to prolong life, but can be valuable as a less demanding alternative to surgery in patients with accessible lesions whose symptoms are not adequately controlled by medical therapy alone, despite a risk of acute thrombosis or subacute restenosis and concerns about possible long-term adverse functional effects of de-endothelializing the arterial segment subjected to dilatation. Restenosis is reduced by the use of prosthetic devices ('stents'), and prevention of thrombosis and restenosis by means of such devices is currently evolving rapidly. Several antiplatelet drugs, including (e.g. **ticlopidine Cloridognel and Tirofiban**; (see Chapter 29), are used increasingly for short periods in this setting. This field is developing rapidly.

Management of unstable coronary disease

Unstable angina

Patients with unstable angina must stop smoking. This is more urgent than in other patients with coronary artery disease, because of the acute prothrombotic effect of smoking. Such patients require *urgent antiplatelet/antithrombotic therapy*, in the form of aspirin and heparin (often low-molecular-weight heparin administered subcutaneously; see Chapter 29). This approximately halves the likelihood of myocardial infarction, and is the most effective known treatment for improving outcome in pre-infarction syndromes. By contrast, GTN, while more effective than aspirin in relieving *pain* associated with unstable angina, does not improve *outcome*. It is usually given as a constant-rate intravenous infusion for this indication. A β-adrenoceptor antagonist is prescribed if not contraindicated. If β-adrenoceptor antagonists are contraindicated, a long-acting Ca^{2+} antagonist is a useful alternative. **Diltiazem** is often used as it does not cause reflex tachycardia, and is less negatively inotropic than **verapamil**. β-adrenoceptor antagonists and Ca^{2+}-antagonists are often prescribed together, but there is disappointingly little evidence that their effects are synergistic or even additive. Nicorandil is now often added as well, but again there is not much evidence of added benefit. Emergency angiography may be indicated in patients who do not stabilize, with a view to urgent surgery or angioplasty. Once the patient has stabilized, attention to modifiable risk factors and consideration of angiography and possible surgery are considered.

Myocardial infarction

Acute management

Oxygen

This is given in the highest concentration available (unless there is coincident pulmonary disease with carbon dioxide retention) delivered by face mask (FIO_2 approximately 60%) or by nasal prongs if a face mask is not tolerated.

Pain relief

This usually requires an intravenous opiate (morphine or diamorphine; see Chapter 24) and concurrent treatment with an anti-emetic (e.g. promethazine or metaclopramide; see Chapter 33).

Infarct limitation

Antithrombotic/fibrinolytic treatment is extremely important. Aspirin and thrombolytic therapy both reduce infarct size and improve survival – each to a similar extent. Their beneficial effects are additive (Fig 28.1), and early fears about potentially unacceptable toxicity of the combination proved unfounded, so they are used together. Heparin is needed to maintain patency of a vessel opened by aspirin plus thrombolysis when recombinant tissue plasminogen activator is used for thrombolysis; it should not be used routinely after streptokinase.

Haemodynamic treatment has less impact than antithrombotic drugs, but is also potentially important. The use of beta-blockers within the first few hours of infarction has a modest short-term benefit. The International study of Infarct Survival (ISIS-I) (in patients who did *not* receive thrombolytic treatment, which is now standard) showed that the 7-day mortality in treated patients was 3.7%, compared to 4.3% in controls. This small benefit was not maintained (there were more deaths in the atenolol group than in the control group at 1 year) and does not warrant routine use of beta-blockers for this indication (as opposed to their use in secondary prevention 5 days or more after acute infarction, which is discussed below). A rationale has been developed for the use of angiotensin-converting enzyme inhibitors (ACEI) in acute myocardial infarction, in terms of possible improvements in cardiac work load and prevention of deleterious cardiac remodelling. Trials with ACEI have mainly been positive: **ramipril** (1.25–5 mg twice daily) reduced mortality from 23% (in controls) to 17% in patients with clinical evidence of heart failure 3–10 days after myocardial infarction in the Acute Infarction Rampril Efficacy (AIRE) study (average follow-up period of 15 months). **Captopril** (6.25–50 mg three times daily) reduced all-cause mortality with asymptomatic left ventricular dysfunction from 24.6% (in controls) to 20.4% after a mean follow-up of 3.5 years (Survival and Venticular

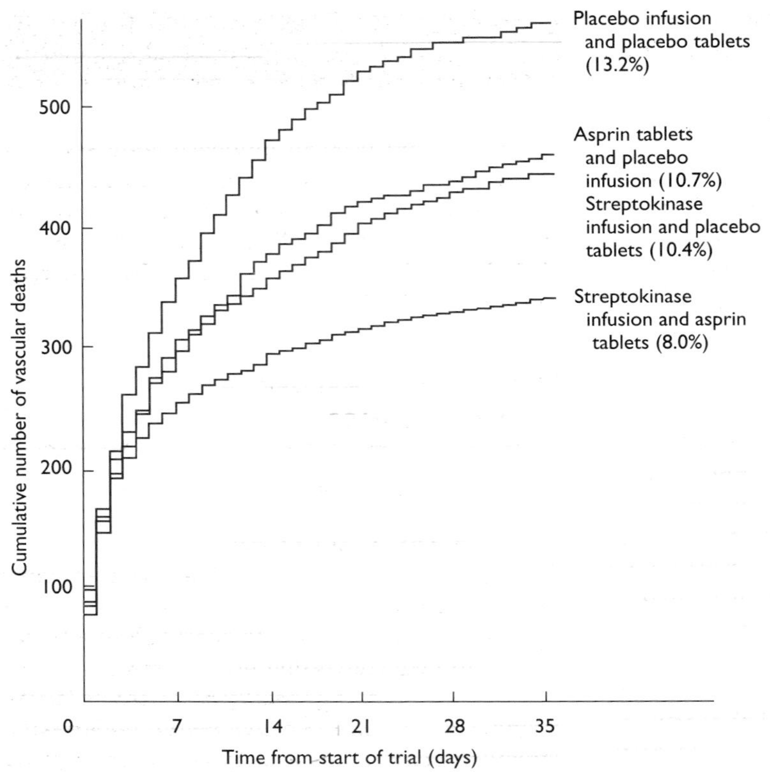

Figure 28.1: Summary graphs of ISIS-II. (Adapted from ISIS-2 trial 1988: *Lancet* ii, 350–60.) © The Lancet Ltd.

Enlargement (SAVE) study), and reduced mortality at 6 months by about 0.65% in another large study (International Study of Infarct Survival-IV, ISIS-IV). **Lisinopril** (2.5–10 mg once daily) reduced the 6-week mortality from 7.1% (in controls) to 6.3% in patients treated within 24 h of admission to hospital with myocardial infarction (GISSI-3). **Trandolapril** (1–4 mg once daily) given 3–7 days after infarction to patients with left ventricular dysfunction (ejection fraction by echo < 35%) for 2–4 years reduced mortality from 42.3% (in controls) to 34.7% (Trandolapril Cardiac Evaluation, TRACE). In contrast, early administration of **enalapril** in patients without clinical evidence of heart failure, and presenting within 24 h of onset of symptoms, showed a small trend toward an unfavourable effect on survival (Co-operative New Scandinavian Enalapril Survival Study-II, CONSENSUS II). Overall, the message appears to be that there is a small benefit from early treatment with ACEI in patients with even minor degrees of left ventricular dysfunction (this represented approximately 25% of infarct patients screened in the TRACE study), that the magnitude of this benefit increases with increasing ventricular dysfunction, but that it is not useful to treat patients with normal left ventricular ejection. Clinical decision-making is made more difficult by technical differences between the various methods of non-invasive quantitation of the ejection fraction (echo/nuclear medicine).

TREATABLE COMPLICATIONS

These may occur early in the course of myocardial infarction, and are best recognized and managed with the patient in a coronary-care unit. Transfer from the admission room should therefore not be delayed by obtaining X-rays, as a portable film can be obtained on the unit if necessary. Complications include *cardiogenic shock* (see Chapter 30) as well as acute tachy- or brady-*arrhythmias* (see Chapter 31). Prophylactic treatment with anti-arrhythmic drugs (i.e. before significant arrhythmia is documented) has *not* been found to improve survival.

Long-term measures

Drugs are used prophylactically following recovery from myocardial infarction to prevent sudden death or recurrence of myocardial infarction. Aspirin and β-adrenoceptor antagonists each reduce the risk of recurrence or sudden death. Meta-analysis of the many clinical trials of aspirin has demonstrated an overwhelmingly significant effect of modest magnitude (an approximately 30% reduction in risk of reinfarction), and several individual trials of β-adrenoceptor antagonists have also demonstrated conclusive benefit. In addition, long-term use of ACEI, although controversial, may also reduce the risk of recurrent myocardial infarction.

RISK FACTORS

Modifiable factors should be sought and attended to as for patients with angina (see above). It is important to use lower 'target' levels of serum cholesterol than in primary prevention, and most such patients are candidates for treatment with a statin after recovery from myocardial infarction, with a target total cholesterol concentration of < 5 mmol/L.

CONSIDERATION OF SURGERY/ANGIOPLASTY

Ideally all patients who are potentially operative candidates would have angiography at some stage. In practice, the same considerations apply as for patients with angina (see above), and in the UK angiography is currently usually undertaken on the basis of a clinical judgement based on age, coexisting disease, presence or absence of post-infarction angina and often on a stress test performed after recovery from the acute event.

PSYCHOLOGICAL AND SOCIAL FACTORS

After recovery from myocardial infarction, patients require an explanation of what has happened, advice about activity in the short and long term, and about work, driving and sexual activity, and help in regaining self-esteem. Cardiac rehabilitation includes attention to secondary prevention as well as to psychological factors. A supervised graded exercise programme is often valuable. Neglect of these unglamorous aspects of management may cause prolonged and unnecessary unhappiness.

DRUGS USED IN ISCHAEMIC HEART DISEASE

Drugs that are used to influence atherosclerosis are described in Chapter 26. In the present chapter we briefly describe those drugs that are used to treat ischaemic heart disease either because of their haemodynamic properties or because they inhibit thrombosis.

DRUGS THAT INFLUENCE HAEMODYNAMICS

Organic nitrates

USE AND ADMINISTRATION

GTN is used to relieve anginal pain (organic nitrates are also used in combination with **hydralazine** in patients with heart failure who are unable to take converting enzyme inhibitors; see Chapter 30). GTN is generally best used as 'acute' prophylaxis, i.e. immediately before undertaking strenuous activity. It is usually given sublingually (0.3- or 0.5-mg tablets, or a 0.4-mg spray), thereby ensuring rapid absorption and avoiding presystemic metabolism (see Chapter 5), but in patients with unstable angina it may be given as an intravenous infusion (5–200 μg/min). The spray has a somewhat more rapid onset of action and a much longer shelf-life than tablets, but is more expensive. GTN is absorbed transdermally, and is available in a patch preparation for longer prophylaxis than the short-term benefit provided by a sublingual dose. Alternatively, a longer-acting nitrate such as **isosorbide mononitrate** may be used to reduce the frequency of attacks; it is less expensive than GTN patches and is taken by mouth (usually 20–40 mg twice daily). In patients whose pattern of pain is predominantly during the daytime, it is prescribed to be taken in the morning and at lunch-time, thereby 'covering' the day but avoiding development of tolerance by omitting an evening dose. Longer-acting controlled-release preparations (e.g. 'Imdur') are available for once daily use.

GTN is volatile, so the tablets have a limited shelf-life (around 6 weeks after the bottle is opened), and they need to be stored in a cool place in a tightly capped dark container, without cotton wool or other tablets. Adverse effects can be minimized by swallowing the tablet after strenuous activity is completed (a more genteel alternative to spitting it out!), because of the lower systemic bioavailability from gut than from buccal mucosa.

MECHANISM OF ACTION

GTN works by relaxing vascular smooth muscle (Figure 28.2). It is metabolized by smooth-muscle cells with generation of nitric oxide (NO). This combines with a haem group in guanylyl cyclase, activating this enzyme and thereby increasing the cytoplasmic concentration of the second messenger cGMP. cGMP causes sequestration of Ca^{2+} within the sarcoplasmic reticulum, thereby relaxing smooth muscle. NO is also synthesized from endogenous substrate (L-arginine) under physiological conditions by a constitutive enzyme in vascular endothelial cells, and is the 'endothelium-derived relaxing factor' originally described by Furchgott. This endogenous NO is responsible for resting vasodilator tone present in human resistance arterioles under basal conditions. Nitrovasodilator drugs provide NO in an endothelium-*independent* manner, and are therefore effective even if endothelial function is severely impaired, as in many patients with coronary artery disease.

HAEMODYNAMIC EFFECTS

For reasons that are still uncertain, GTN is relatively selective for venous rather than arteriolar smooth muscle. Venodilatation reduces cardiac preload. Reduced venous return results in reduced ventricular filling and hence a reduction in ventricular chamber diameter. Ventricular wall tension is directly proportional to chamber diameter (the Laplace relationship), so wall tension is reduced by GTN, which thereby reduces cardiac work and oxygen demand. In addition, coronary blood flow improves due to the decreased left ventricular end-diastolic pressure. This improves forward flow in the coronary arteries (which occurs during diastole), and any spasm of the diseased vessel is opposed by NO-mediated coronary artery relaxation. The mild reduction in arterial tone reduces afterload and thus also reduces myocardial oxygen demand. Nitrates also relax some non-vascular smooth muscles,

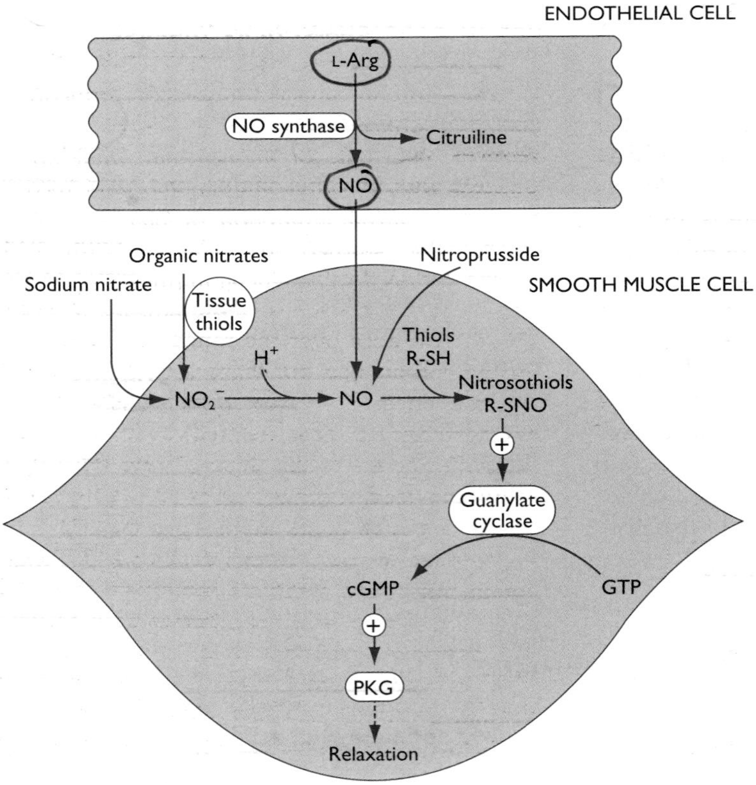

Figure 28.2: Mode of action of nitrates. (Adapted with permission from Rang HP, Dale MM, Ritter JM. 1995: Pharmacology, 3rd edn. Edinburgh: Churchill Livingstone.)

and therefore sometimes relieve the pain of oesophageal spasm and biliary or renal colic, causing potential diagnostic confusion.

ADVERSE EFFECTS

Organic nitrates are generally very safe, although they can cause hypotension in patients with diminished cardiac reserve. *Headache* is common, and GTN patches have not fared well when evaluated by 'quality of life' questionnaires for this reason. Tolerance is another problem. This can be minimized by omitting the evening dose of isosorbide mononitrate (or by removing a patch at night).

β-Adrenoceptor antagonists (see also Chapters 27 and 31)

USE IN ISCHAEMIC HEART DISEASE

The main uses of beta-blockers in patients with ischaemic heart disease are in *prophylaxis of angina*, and in *reducing the risk of sudden death or reinfarction following myocardial infarction* ('secondary prevention').

Angiotensin-converting enzyme inhibitors (ACEI) (see also Chapters 27 and 30)

USE IN ISCHAEMIC HEART DISEASE

As well as their well established uses in hypertension (see Chapter 27) and in heart failure, including chronic heart failure caused by ischaemic heart disease (see Chapter 30), there is also substantial evidence to support the use of ACEI in the early stages of myocardial infarction (see above). The evidence suggests that any benefit is very small (or non-existent) in patients with completely normal ventricular function, but that with increasing ventricular dysfunction there is increasing benefit. Treatment should be started with small doses with dose titration up to doses that have been demonstrated to improve survival.

Calcium antagonists (see also Chapters 27 and 31)

USE IN ISCHAEMIC HEART DISEASE

The main use of calcium-channel antagonists in patients with ischaemic heart disease is for prophylaxis of angina. They are particularly useful in patients in whom beta-blockers are contraindicated. Disappointingly, despite having quite different pharmacological actions to beta-blockers, these classes of drugs do not appear to act synergistically in angina, and should not be routinely co-administered as prophylaxis to such patients. They may be particularly useful in uncommon patients in whom spasm is particularly prominent (spasm can be worsened by beta-blockers). Short-acting dihydropyridines should be avoided because they cause reflex tachycardia. Diltiazem or a long-acting dihydropyridine (e.g. amlodipine or a controlled-release preparation of nifedipine) are often used in this setting. Unlike β-adrenoceptor antagonists and ACEI, Ca^{2+} antagonists have *not* been found to prolong survival when administered early in the course of myocardial infarction.

DRUGS THAT INFLUENCE THROMBOSIS

Aspirin

The use of aspirin as a mild analgesic is described in Chapter 24, and its antiplatelet effect is also referred to in Chapter 29.

USE IN CARDIOVASCULAR DISEASE

The use of aspirin in cardiovascular disease depends on its effects on platelet function. It *improves survival in acute myocardial infarction* and reduces the risk of myocardial infarction in patients with unstable angina and after recovery from myocardial infarction. It has not been so extensively studied in patients with stable angina, but is also beneficial in this group as well. There is no evidence that the efficacy of aspirin varies with dose over the range 75–320 mg/day during chronic use, but there is evidence that the adverse effect of major upper gastrointestinal haemorrhage is dose related over this range. Accordingly, the lower dose (75 mg once daily) should be used routinely for chronic prophylaxis. At the onset of acute myocardial infarction it is appropriate to use a higher dose (e.g. 300 mg) to obtain rapid and complete inhibition of platelet cyclo-oxygenase. It has sometimes been assumed (on spurious grounds) that enteric-coated or buffered preparations will be safer than the regular formulation, but this has not been confirmed, and in general regular aspirin is to be preferred. Aspirin *reduces the risk of stroke* in patients with transient cerebral ischaemic attacks. It also reduces the risk of venous thrombosis, and of thrombo-embolism in patients with atrial fibrillation and following valve replacement, but conventional anticoagulation with warfarin is more effective, and is preferred for these indications. Aspirin also reduces the risk of myocardial infarction in apparently healthy middle-aged men, but is *not* recommended as prophylaxis in asymptomatic men, because in this setting its benefits are probably outweighed by its adverse effects on the stomach and possibly also an increased risk of haemorrhagic stroke.

MECHANISM OF ACTION

Aspirin (acetylsalicylic acid) irreversibly inhibits fatty acid cyclo-oxygenase (COX), a key enzyme in the biosynthesis of prostaglandins and thromboxanes. It achieves this by acetylation of a serine residue in the constitutive enzyme, COX_1, thereby preventing access of substrate (arachidonic acid) to the active site by steric hindrance. Thromboxane (TX) A$_2$ is the main cyclo-oxygenase product of activated platelets, and is pro-aggregatory and a vasoconstrictor. TXA_2 therefore acts as a positive feedback, recruiting more platelets to sites of platelet activation. When platelets adhere to thrombogenic material in a ruptured atheromatous plaque, they become activated and synthesize TXA_2, which causes further platelets to stick to one another ('aggregation'), resulting in propagation of the thrombus and ultimately occlusion of the artery. Aspirin inhibits platelet TXA_2 biosynthesis and thus opposes thrombus extension. The pharmacological effects of aspirin are explained by inhibition of COX. These include anti-inflammatory, antipyretic and mild analgesic effects in addition to its effect on platelet function, which is manifested by a mild prolongation of bleeding time. Many of the adverse effects of aspirin are also caused by inhibition of COX (see below). Although NSAIDs such as ibuprofen and indomethacin also inhibit COX, they are much less effective than aspirin in inhibiting platelet TXA_2 biosynthesis, possibly because, unlike aspirin, they are *reversible* inhibitors of the enzyme. It should not therefore be assumed that patients who are receiving such drugs for another indication are thereby necessarily receiving adequate antiplatelet therapy.

PHARMACOKINETICS

Aspirin is rapidly absorbed from the gastrointestinal tract, and is rapidly deacetylated to yield salicylate, which has anti-inflammatory but little if any antiplatelet activity at ordinary doses. Salicylate is metabolized further (see Figure 24.2, p. 216), and its metabolites, together with some unchanged salicylate, are excreted in the urine. There has been considerable interest in the possibility that very low doses of aspirin (40 mg/day or less) may selectively inhibit platelet TXA_2 biosynthesis without reducing prostacyclin (PGI_2) biosynthesis in blood vessels. Aspirin acetylates platelet COX as platelets circulate through portal venous blood (where the acetylsalicylic acid concentration is high during absorption of aspirin from the gastrointestinal tract), whereas systemic endothelial cells are exposed to much lower concentrations because at low doses hepatic esterases result in little or no aspirin entering systemic blood. This has been demonstrated experimentally, but the strategy has yet to be shown to result in increased antithrombotic efficacy of very low doses. In practice, even much higher doses given once daily or every other day achieve considerable selectivity for platelet vs. endothelial COX, because platelets (being anucleate) do not synthesize new COX after their existing supply has been irreversibly inhibited by covalent acetylation by aspirin, whereas endothelial cells regenerate new enzyme rapidly (within 6 h in healthy human subjects). Consequently, there is selective inhibition of platelet COX for most of the dose interval if a regular dose of aspirin (e.g. 75–320 mg) is administered every 24 or 48 h.

ADVERSE EFFECTS AND CONTRAINDICATIONS IN RELATION TO USE FOR ISCHAEMIC HEART DISEASE

Dose-related adverse effects ('type A') consequent on the pharmacological effect of aspirin on COX are common (approximately 25% of UK physicians were intolerant of the drug in a trial that required regular prolonged use). Furthermore, although it has been available over the counter for nearly a century, some of its adverse effects are serious. The commonest severe adverse effect is upper gastrointestinal haemorrhage, and the commonest symptom is dyspepsia. These relate to inhibition of PGE_2 biosynthesis in the stomach. PGE_2 is the main COX product of the stomach, and has a number of effects that help to protect this organ from ulceration, including mucus secretion, inhibition of acid secretion, vasodilatation of microvessels in the submucosa which carry away hydrogen ions that have diffused back through the mucosal barrier, and possibly a cytoprotective effect on the mucosal cells themselves. Inhibition of PGE_2 biosynthesis consequently predisposes to ulceration. Should such an ulcer occur, bleeding is exacerbated because of inhibition of platelet TXA_2 biosynthesis. Active ulcer disease contraindicates the use of aspirin. A history of previous ulcer disease also argues against its use, although if the indication is strong enough the risk may be judged to be clinically acceptable. In such cases coincident treatment with an H_2 antagonist (e.g. cimetidine) and/or with a stable PGE analogue (misoprostol) may be useful, although in patients with rheumatoid arthritis the prescription of misoprostol with NSAIDs has not been shown to reduce haematemesis, despite the fact that it reduces other serious upper gastrointestinal complications of NSAID use, so such a strategy is by no means proven. Constipation is less well recognized as an unwanted effect of aspirin than are upper gastrointestinal symptoms, but it is not uncommon. It may also relate to inhibition of PGE_2 biosynthesis, since PGE_2 increases gastrointestinal motility and causes a secretory diarrhoea when administered therapeutically.

Other adverse effects of aspirin are described in Chapter 24.

Fibrinolytic drugs

Several fibrinolytic drugs are used in acute myocardial infarction, including **streptokinase** (an enyme from streptococci that breaks down fibrin), **anistreplase** (APSAC – a prodrug that liberates streptokinase) and **alteplase** (human tissue plasminogen activator made in bacteria by recombinant DNA technology). In addition, **urokinase** (from human urine), although unlicensed for use in myocardial infarction, is sometimes used to dissolve blood clots in extracorporeal shunts or in the anterior chamber of the eye complicating hyphema. Streptokinase works indirectly, combining with plasminogen to form an activator complex that converts the remaining free plasminogen to plasmin which dissolves fibrin clots. Alteplase is a direct-acting plasminogen activator.

USE IN MYOCARDIAL INFARCTION

Streptokinase has been available for many years, but its efficacy in reducing myocardial damage and mortality in myocardial infarction has only been appreciated during the last 15 years. This realization has revolutionized the management of acute myocardial infarction. The credit for this is due to two large clinical trials (GISSI and ISIS-II). Subsequent trials have confirmed and extended their findings. Fibrinolytic therapy is indicated for patients with severe pain lasting for more than 20 min and ST-segment elevation or bundle-branch block on the ECG. The maximum benefit is obtained if treatment is given within 90 min of the onset of pain.

Treatment using streptokinase with aspirin is effective, safe and relatively inexpensive. Alteplase, which does not produce a generalized fibrinolytic state, but selectively dissolves recently formed clot is also safe and effective. The Global Use of Strategies to Open Occluded Coronary Arteries (GUSTO) study demonstrated superiority of alteplase over streptokinase when it is given more rapidly than previous standard practice (over 30 min instead of over 3 h) and immediately followed by heparin – a saving of approximately one extra life per 100 cases treated early. The additional cost of alteplase has not been universally judged to justify the fairly small additional benefit, at least in the UK. It is worth noting that greater benefit could result from steps to ensure earlier treatment than from routine use of tissue plasminogen activator instead of streptokinase. Alteplase also has a place in treatment of the increasing number of patients in whom streptokinase is contraindicated because of previous use.

ADMINISTRATION

Fibrinolytic drugs are given intravenously. Streptokinase is given as an infusion of 1.5 mega-units over 60 min with regular monitoring of blood pressure, and reduction of the infusion rate if necessary. Anistreplase, 30 units, being a prodrug, is given over a shorter period (4–5 min). Alteplase can be given over 3 h – adults over 67 kg in weight are given a bolus dose of 10 mg followed by 50 mg over the next hour and 40 mg over the following 2 h (total dose 100 mg). Individuals with lower body weight are given a total of 1.5 mg/kg divided in the same proportions, i.e. 10% as a bolus, 50% infused over the next hour and 40%

over the subsequent 2 h. There is a case (from GUSTO) for giving the drug over 90 min rather than 3 h, especially in early anterior infarction.

ADVERSE EFFECTS AND CONTRAINDICATIONS

Bleeding may occur with any of the fibrinolytic drugs, especially in patients who have received invasive monitoring, such as Swann–Ganz catheterization, which should therefore be avoided if possible. The intramuscular route of injection (for any drug) must be avoided because of the risk of haematoma. Many of the contraindications to fibrinolytics relate to conditions that increase the risk of bleeding. These exclusions were originally applied more stringently than is now current practice, as increasing use has shown that early fears were exaggerated. Patients are not generally treated with fibrinolytic drugs if they have recently (within the last 3 months) undergone surgery, are pregnant, have evidence of recent active gastrointestinal bleeding, symptoms of active peptic ulcer disease or evidence of severe liver disease (especially if complicated by the presence of varices), have recently suffered a stroke or head injury, have severe uncontrolled hypertension, have a significant bleeding diathesis, have suffered recent substantial trauma (including vigorous chest compression during resuscitation) or require invasive monitoring (e.g. for cardiogenic shock). The position regarding diabetic or other proliferative retinopathy is controversial. If ophthalmological advice is locally and immediately available, this is no longer universally regarded as an absolute contraindication to fibrinolysis.

With regard to streptokinase and its prodrug, anistreplase, immune reactions are important. Streptokinase is a streptococcal protein, so individuals who have been exposed to it synthesize antibodies that can cause allergic reactions or loss of efficacy due to binding to and neutralization of the drug. Individuals who have received either of these drugs within the previous year should not be retreated with them if they reinfarct. The situation regarding previous streptococcal infection is less certain. Such infections (usually in the form of sore throats) are quite common and often go undiagnosed. Despite this, ISIS-III demonstrated similar efficacy of streptokinase and alteplase, so it seems unlikely that such mild infections substantially reduce the efficacy of streptokinase. It is therefore reasonable to exclude patients from treatment with streptokinase only if they have a history of bacteriologically proven severe streptococcal infection such as cellulitis or septicaemia.

Hypotension may occur during infusion of streptokinase, partly as a result of activation of kinins and other vasodilator peptides. The important thing is tissue perfusion rather than the blood pressure *per se*, and as long as the patient is warm and well perfused, hypotension is not an absolute contraindication to the use of fibrinolytic therapy,

Key points

Ischaemic heart disease: pathophysiology and management

- Ischaemic heart disease is caused by atheroma in coronary arteries. Primary and secondary prevention involves attention to dyslipidaemia, hypertension and other modifiable risk factors.
- Stable angina is caused by narrowing of a coronary artery leading to inadequate myocardial perfusion during exercise. Symptoms may be relieved or prevented (prophylaxis) by drugs that alter the balance between myocardial oxygen supply and demand by influencing haemodynamics. Organic nitrates and Ca^{2+}-antagonists do this by relaxing vascular smooth muscle, whereas β-adrenoceptor antagonists slow the heart.
- In most cases the part played by coronary spasm is uncertain. Organic nitrates and Ca^{2+}-antagonists oppose such spasm.
- Unstable angina is caused by fissuring of an atheromatous plaque leading to thrombosis. It is treated with aspirin and heparin, which improve outcome, and with intravenous glyceryl trinitrate if necessary for relief of anginal pain.
- Myocardial infarction is caused by occlusion of a coronary artery by thrombus arising from an atheromatous plaque. It is treated with aspirin, fibrinolytic drugs (with or without heparin), inhaled oxygen, or opoids. Angiotensin-converting-enzyme inhibitors improve outcome in patients with ventricular dysfunction.
- After recovery from myocardial infarction, secondary prophylaxis is directed against atheroma, thrombosis (aspirin) and arrhythmia (β-adrenoceptor antagonists), and in some patients is used to improve haemodynamics (angiotensin-converting-enzyme inhibitors).

Case history

A 46-year-old advertising executive complains of exercise-related pain when playing his regular daily game of squash for the past 3 months. Ten years ago he had a gastric ulcer which healed with ranitidine, and he had experienced intermittent indigestion subsequently, but was otherwise well. His father died of a myocardial infarct at the age of 62 years. He smokes 20 cigarettes per day and admits that he drinks half a bottle of wine a day plus 'a few gins'. Physical examination is notable only for obesity (body mass index 30 kg/m^2) and a blood pressure of 152/106 mmHg. Resting ECG is normal, and exercise ECG shows significant ST depression at peak exercise, with excellent exercise tolerance. Serum total cholesterol is 6.4 mmmol/L, triglycerides are 3.8 mmol/L and HDL is 0.6 mmol/L. γ-Glutamyl transpeptidase is elevated, as is the mean corpuscular volume (MCV). Cardiac catheterization shows a significant narrowing of the left circumflex artery but the other vessels are free from disease.

Question

Decide whether each of the following statements is true or false.

Immediate management could reasonably include:

(a) a converting-enzyme inhibitor;
(b) GTN spray to be taken before playing squash;
(c) no reduction in alcohol intake, as this would be dangerous;
(d) referral for angioplasty;
(e) isosorbide mononitrate;
(f) a low dose of aspirin;
(g) nicotine patches;
(h) dexfenfluramine.

Answer

(a) False.
(b) False.
(c) False.
(d) False.
(e) True.
(f) True.
(g) False.
(h) False.

Comment

This patient has single-vessel disease and should be started on medical management with advice regarding diet, smoking and reduction of alcohol consumption. He should continue to exercise, but would be wise to switch to a less extreme form of exertion. Taking a GTN spray before playing squash could have unpredictable effects on his blood pressure. A long-acting nitrate may improve his exercise tolerance, and low-dose aspirin will reduce his risk of myocardial infarction. In view of the history of ulcer and indigestion, consideration should be given to checking for *Helicobacter pylori* (with treatment if present) and/or reinstitution of prophylactic acid suppressant treatment. His dyslipidaemia is a major concern, especially the low HDL despite his high alcohol intake and regular exercise. It will almost certainly necessitate some form of drug treatment in addition to diet. His blood pressure should improve with weight reduction and reduced alcohol intake. However, if it does not, and if the angina persists despite the above measures, a β-adrenoceptor antagonist may be useful despite its undesirable effect on serum lipids. If angina is no longer a problem, but hypertension persists, a long-acting alpha-blocker (which increases HDL) would be worth considering.

although it does indicate the need for paticularly careful monitoring, and sometimes for slowing down or temporarily halting the infusion.

DRUG INTERACTIONS

Two useful interactions are important. As explained above, aspirin has an additive effect with streptokinase. Secondly, heparin is needed after treatment with alteplase (but not streptokinase) to prevent early reocclusion of the thrombosed artery.

FURTHER READING

Anderson HV, Willerson JT. 1993: Thrombolysis in acute myocardial infarction. *New England Journal of Medicine* **329**, 703–9.

Fibrinolytic Therapy Trialists (FTT) Collaborative Group. 1994: Indications for fibrinolytic therapy in suspected acute myocardial infarction: collaborative overview of early mortality and major morbidity results from all randomised controlled trials of more than 1000 patients. *Lancet* **343**, 311–22.

Hennekens CH, Albert CM, Godfried SL, Gaziano JM, Buring JE. 1996: Adjunctive drug therapy of acute myocardial infarction – evidence from clinical trials. *New England Journal of Medicine* **335**, 1660–7.

Kelly RA, Smith TW. 1996: Nitric oxide and nitrovasodilators: similarities, differences and interactions. *American Journal of Cardiology* **77**, 2C–7C (see also other articles on nitrovasodilators in this supplement).

Ridker PM, Hebert PR, Fuster V, Hennekens CH. 1993: Are both aspirin and heparin justified as adjuncts to thrombolytic therapy for acute myocardial infarction? *Lancet* **341**, 1574–7.

CHAPTER TWENTY-NINE

ANTICOAGULANTS *and* ANTIPLATELET DRUGS

- Introduction
- Pathophysiology of thrombosis
- Anticoagulants
- Antiplatelet drugs
- Anticoagulants in pregnancy and puerperium

INTRODUCTION

The treatment and prevention of thrombosis involves three classes of drugs, namely *anticoagulants, antiplatelet drugs* and *fibrinolytics*. Aspirin (the main antiplatelet drug in clinical practice) and fibrinolytics are discussed in Chapter 28. The clinical pharmacology of the anticoagulants and other antiplatelet drugs is described in the present chapter. Anticoagulants inhibit the coagulation cascade. Their main use is to treat and prevent venous thrombosis ('red thrombus') and its major complication, pulmonary embolism, whereas antiplatelet and fibrinolytic drugs are mainly used in the treatment of platelet-rich coronary and other arterial thrombi ('white thrombus'). Nevertheless, there are many links between platelet activation and the coagulation cascade, so it is not surprising that anticoagulants can also have beneficial effects in the prevention of coronary artery disease, or that antiplatelet drugs have some effect on venous thrombosis.

PATHOPHYSIOLOGY OF THROMBOSIS

Thrombosis can be defined as haemostasis occurring in the wrong place. Haemostasis is achieved by an exquisitely balanced series of interlocking control systems involving both positive feedbacks – permitting very rapid responses to the threat of haemorrhage following sharp injury – and negative feedbacks – to prevent the clotting mechanism from running out of control and causing thrombus to propagate throughout the circulation following haemostasis at a site of injury. In addition there is an endogenous fibrinolytic system that dissolves thrombus that has done its job. Not surprisingly, these systems sometimes go wrong, resulting in bleeding disorders such as haemophilia or thrombocytopenic purpura, or in thrombosis.

Thrombosis is caused by injury to the vessel wall, stasis and activation of coagulation processes (platelets and the coagulation cascade), these three processes being referred to as Virchow's triad. Coagulation involves the sequential activation of a cascade of clotting factors which amplifies a small initial event to produce a macroscopic plug of fibrin. Each factor is present in blood as an inactive zymogen. Several of these factors (II, VII, IX and X) are glycoproteins which contain γ-carboxyglutamic acid residues that are the result of post-translational modification. This process requires vitamin K. After activation (indicated by the letter 'a' after the Roman numeral that designates the zymogen), several of the factors acquire proteolytic activity. Thrombin and factors IXa, Xa, XIa and XIIa are all serine proteases. Oestrogens increase the activity of the coagulation pathway, and there is an increased risk of venous thrombosis associated with pregnancy, oral contraception (especially preparations containing higher doses of oestrogen), and even with postmenopausal hormone replacement therapy (albeit to only a small extent).

There are two coagulation pathways (intrinsic and extrinsic) that converge on factor X (Figure 29.1), and there are several possible entry points to the cascade. Blood vessels are lined with a continuous layer of endothelial cells that possess an array of mechanisms (e.g. the capacity to synthesize prostacyclin and nitric oxide, and the presence of heparan and thrombomodulin – a receptor that binds thrombin and prevents its procoagulant effect while enabling it to activate anticoagulant protein C) whereby blood is preserved in a fluid state. Damage to the endothelium exposes platelets to collagen and other subendothelial material, to which they adhere and become activated. Activated platelets express glycoprotein receptors (IIb/IIIa) on their surface membranes that are dormant in quiescent platelets. Glycoprotein IIb/IIIa binds fibrinogen which links adjacent activated platelets in an aggregate. Activated platelets also synthesize thromboxane A_2 from arachidonic acid liberated from their membranes by phospholipase, and secrete adenosine diphosphate and other preformed mediators that recruit further platelets and cause the aggregate to propagate. They also secrete clotting factors, including factor Va, and negatively charged phospholipids (e.g. phosphatidyl serine) become exposed on their outer membranes and act as surface catalysts for factor Xa. Another way in which endothelial damage initiates coagulation is by exposure of the blood to tissue factor in underlying fibroblasts. Tissue factor interacts with factor VII to initiate the extrinsic pathway.

Activated factor X catalyses the conversion of prothrombin (factor II) to thrombin, which is the most important enzyme of the cascade. It cleaves small peptides from the N-terminal region of fibrinogen dimers, allowing them to polymerize to form strands of insoluble fibrin. It also acts on receptors on platelet surface membranes, thereby causing platelet activation. Thrombus consists of platelets and other formed elements of the blood enmeshed within a fibrin network. Thrombus structure is not homogeneous, even in the red thrombus that forms in veins. Typically there is a platelet-rich head attached to the vessel wall, and a tail of gelatinous material containing large num-

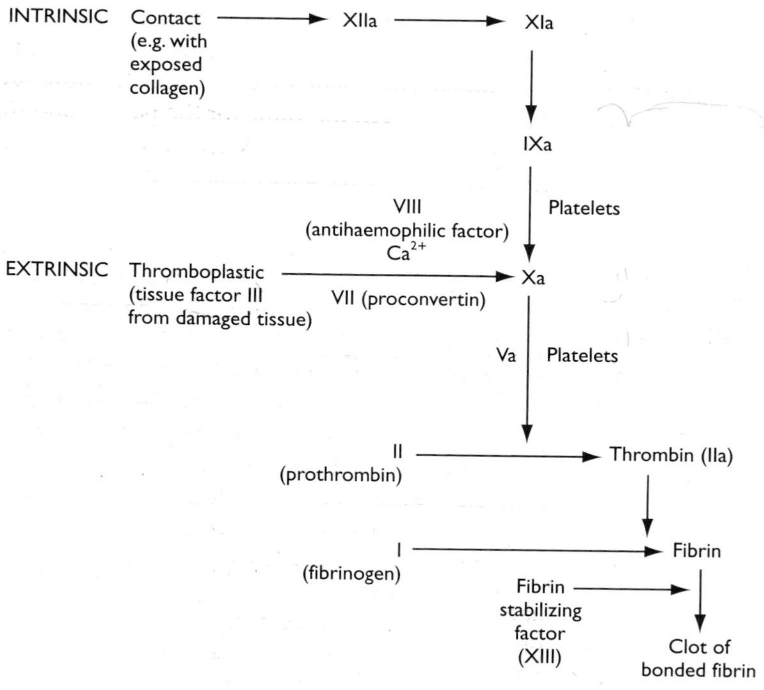

Figure 29.1: Simplified clotting factor cascade. 'a' indicates activation of appropriate clotting factor.

Key points

Thrombosis

- Thrombosis can be defined as haemostasis occurring in the wrong place. Virchow defined the following predisposing factors:
  - reduced flow (e.g. in leg veins during cramped travel);
  - damaged blood vessels (e.g. when an atheromatous plaque ruptures);
  - increased coagulation factor or platelet activity (e.g. during pregnancy and in some malignancies)
- Thrombi are structured (unlike clot *in vitro*), and consist of platelets and fibrin.
- Platelet-rich ('white') thrombi form in the arterial circulation. Aspirin inhibits platelet function and is important in prophylaxis against arterial thrombosis (e.g. myocardial infarction, stroke).
- Fibrin-rich thrombi containing red cells and with fewer platelets ('red' thrombi) form in veins and can break off and cause pulmonary emboli. Heparin and oral anticoagulants (e.g. warfarin) are important in their prevention (prophylaxis) and treatment.

bers of red cells similar to the clot that forms when blood is allowed to coagulate in a glass tube *in vitro*.

ANTICOAGULANTS

Heparin

Heparin is a sulphated acidic mucopolysaccharide present in the granules of mast cells. It was discovered in liver (hence the name 'heparin') by McLean, who was undertaking a vacation project as a medical student at the Johns Hopkins Hospital. Currently it is prepared from lung or intestine of ox or pig, and is a mixture of polymers of varying molecular weights. Since the structure is variable, the dosage is expressed in terms of units of biological activity.

USE

Heparin is available as either the sodium or calcium salt. It is administered either as an intravenous infusion (to treat established disease) or by subcutaneous injection (as prophylaxis). Intramuscular injection must not be used because it causes haematomas. Intermittent bolus intravenous injections cause a higher frequency of bleeding complications than does constant intravenous infusion, and are no longer recommended for this reason. For prophylaxis, 5000 units in 0.2 mL are injected via a fine (25-gauge) needle into the fatty layer of the lower abdomen 8- or 12-hourly. An inch or so of skin is pinched up and pressure applied after the injection to minimize bruising. Coagulation times are not routinely monitored when heparin is used prophylactically in this way, but such monitoring may be appropriate if long-term prophylaxis is contemplated using this method. Continuous intravenous infusion is initiated with a bolus of 5000 units for a 70-kg adult (and proportionately less for a child on a weight basis) followed by 25 000 or 30 000 units in saline or 5% glucose infused over 24 h. Therapy is monitored by measuring the activated partial thromboplastin time (APTT) 4–6 h after starting treatment and then every 6 h until two consecutive readings are within the target range, and thereafter at least daily. The pharmacokinetics of heparin are complex (see below), and this in turn complicates monitoring. It is essential that the APTT is measured without delay after the blood has been sampled, as otherwise there is a predictable prolongation of the APTT *in vitro* which will lead to inappropriate dose reduction. Dose adjustments are made to keep the APTT ratio (i.e. the ratio between the value for the patient and the value of a control) in the range 1.5–2.5. Table 29.1 gives guidelines for dose adjustment.

Table 29.1: Dose adjustment guidelines for maintaining APPT ratio in the range 1.5–2.5 (modified from *Drug and Therapeutics Bulletin*, Vol. 30, Number 20, 1994)

APPT ratio	Change in heparin dose
> 7.0	Stop for 1 h and reduce by 10 000 U/24 h
5.1–7.0	Reduce by 10 000 U/24 h
4.1–5.0	Reduce by 5000 U/24 h
3.1–4.0	Reduce by 2000 U/24 h
2.6–3.0	Reduce by 1000 U/24 h
1.5–2.5	No change
1.2–1.4	Increase by 5000 U/24 h
< 1.2	Increase by 10 000 U/24 h

APTT = activated partial thromboplastin time

The main indications for heparin are as follows:

1 to prevent formation of thrombus (e.g. thromboprophylaxis during surgery);
2 to prevent extension of thrombus (e.g. treatment of deep-vein thrombosis);
3 prevention of thrombosis in extracorporeal circulations (e.g. haemodialysis, haemoperfusion, membrane oxygenators, artificial organs) and intravenous cannulae;
4 to maintain patency of the vessel following thrombolysis with anistreplase (recombinant human tissue plasminogen activator);
5 arterial embolism;
6 disseminated intravascular coagulation (DIC). This is produced by a heterogeneous group of disorders, and treatment is aimed at the underlying cause (e.g. prostate cancer, sepsis, eclampsia). Heparin is sometimes used as an adjunct, although it occasionally worsens the situation and is mainly used when DIC is associated with clinical thrombosis. Its use for this indication demands specialist input and meticulous laboratory control.

MECHANISM OF ACTION

The main action of heparin is on the coagulation cascade. It works by binding to antithrombin III, a naturally occurring inhibitor of thrombin and other serine proteases (factors IXa, Xa, XIa and XIIa), and enormously potentiating its inhibitory action. Consequently it is effective *in vitro* as well as *in vivo*, but is ineffective in (rare) patients with inherited or acquired deficiency of antithrombin III. A lower concentration is required to inhibit factor Xa and the other factors early in the cascade than is needed to antagonize the action of thrombin, providing the rationale for low-dose heparin in prophylaxis. Heparin also has complex actions on platelets. As an antithrombin drug it inhibits platelet activation by thrombin, but it can also cause platelet activation and paradoxical thrombosis by an immune mechanism (see below).

ADVERSE EFFECTS AND CONTRAINDICATIONS

These include the following:

1 *bleeding* – this is the chief side-effect, and was one of the commonest drug-induced adverse effects in hospital patients in the Boston Collaborative Drug Surveillance Program. It may occur at any site and may be life-threatening. Risk factors include old age, haemostatic defect (commonly drug induced by aspirin or recent fibrinolytic therapy) and recent trauma. Contraindications generally relate to situations in which the risk of bleeding is judged to be unacceptable, (e.g. following a cerebral bleed, in the presence of bleeding or potential bleeding into an inaccessible space (thorax or abdomen) including recent liver or renal biopsy, lumbar puncture or epidural anaesthesia, recent eye surgery and severe haemostatic disorders);
2 *thrombocytopenia and thrombosis* – a modest decrease in platelet count within the first 2 days of treatment is common (approximately one-third of patients) but clinically unimportant. By contrast, severe thrombocytopenia is rare. It occurs between 2 days and 2 weeks of treatment and is associated with thrombotic as well as haemorrhagic complications. It is now known to be caused by IgG or IgM antibodies directed against a complex of heparin with platelet factor 4, a heparin-binding protein secreted from platelet α-granules. Heparin-like molecules (glycosaminoglycans) on the surface of endothelial cells also bind platelet factor 4, and the antibody can initiate vascular injury by binding to these. Platelet counts should be obtained in patients treated for more than 5 days, and treatment should be stopped if they develop thrombocytopenia;
3 *osteoporosis and vertebral collapse* – this is a rare complication described in young adult patients receiving heparin in doses of 10 000 units or more daily for longer than 10 weeks (usually longer than 3 months);
4 *skin necrosis* at the site of subcutaneous injection after several days treatment;
5 *alopecia*;
6 *hypersensitivity reactions*, including chills, fever, urticaria, bronchospasm and anaphylactoid reactions, occur rarely;
7 *hypoaldosteronism* – heparin inhibits aldosterone biosynthesis. This is seldom clinically significant, but there have been case reports of fatal hyperkalaemia and selective hypoaldosteronism with pathological changes in the zona glomerulosa of the adrenal cortex associated with heparin treatment.

There is no evidence that rebound hypercoagulability on discontinuing heparin (demonstrable *in vitro*) is clinically significant.

MANAGEMENT OF SEVERE HEPARIN-ASSOCIATED BLEEDING

1 Compression of the bleeding site – when this is accessible – should be carried out.
2 Protamine sulphate is given as a slow intravenous injection, as rapid injection can cause anaphylactoid reactions. It is of no value if it is more than 3 h since heparin was administered. The exact dose can be determined from a titration *in vitro*. More commonly, a dose of 1 mg for every 100 units of heparin given over the preceding hour (maximum dose 50 mg, above which protamine itself has anticoagulant properties) can be used empirically.
3 If bleeding is severe and continues despite the above measures, fresh frozen plasma should be given to provide uninhibited coagulation factors.

PHARMACOKINETICS

Heparin is not absorbed from the gastrointestinal tract, and is administered parenterally. Its elimination half-life ($t_{\frac{1}{2}}$) is in the range 0.5–2.5 h and is dose dependent, with a longer $t_{\frac{1}{2}}$ at higher doses and wide inter-individual variation. The short $t_{\frac{1}{2}}$ probably reflects rapid uptake by the reticulo-endothelial system, and there is no reliable evidence of hepatic metabolism. Heparin also binds non-specifically to endothelial cells, and to platelet and plasma proteins, and with high affinity to platelet factor 4, which is released during platelet activation. The mechanism underlying the dose-dependent clearance is unknown. The short $t_{\frac{1}{2}}$ means that a stable plasma concentration is best achieved by a constant infusion rather than by intermittent bolus administration. Both unfractionated and low-molecular-weight varieties (see below) of heparin do not cross the placental barrier or enter milk, and heparin is used in pregnancy because of the teratogenic effects of warfarin and other oral anticoagulants.

SPECIAL GROUPS

Antithrombin III levels are physiologically low in neonates (and even more so in prematurity), rising to adult levels within about 3 months. Acquired antithrombin III deficiency has been described as an unusual problem in some patients with nephrotic syndrome, liver failure and disseminated intravascular coagulation. Such patients are resistant to the anticoagulant effect of heparins, which depend on activation of antithrombin III.

Low-molecular-weight heparins

Low-molecular-weight heparins are making a major impact on the practice of anticoagulation. They preferentially inhibit factor Xa and, when administered as a depot, they release an inhibitor of tissue factor pathway (TFPI). They were developed in the hope of reducing the risk of major haemorrhage that accompanies the use of conventional unfractionated preparations. They do not prolong the APTT, and monitoring (which requires sophisticated factor Xa assays) is not needed in routine clinical practice, because their pharmacokinetics are less unpredictable than those of unfractionated preparations. There is evidence that low-molecular-weight heparins such as **enoxaparin** and **dalteparin** are at least as safe and effective as unfractionated products. They are effective in prophylaxis against deep venous thrombosis. Low-molecular-weight heparins have proved to be more effective than conventional heparin in preventing deep-vein thrombosis (about one-third the incidence of venographically confirmed disease in a meta-analysis of six trials) and pulmonary embolism (about one-half the incidence) in patients undergoing orthopaedic surgery, but with the same incidence of major bleeds. The recommended dose of **tinzaparin** varies according to indication – for thromboprophylaxis in fairly low-risk situations, 50 anti-Xa units per kg body weight, and for prophylaxis in high-risk situations (e.g. patients with prosthetic heart valves in whom warfarin must be discontinued temporarily for some reason) or for treatment of established thrombosis 175 anti-Xa units per kg, each given once daily as a subcutaneous injection. Thrombocytopenia and related thrombotic events and antiheparin antibodies are less common in patients treated with low-molecular-weight rather than unfractionated preparations. Once daily dosage makes them convenient, and although they are more expensive than regular heparin, it is sometimes possible to teach patients to self-administer them at home, with a potential cost saving resulting from shortened hospital stay.

Key points

Heparins

- Heparins are sulphated mucopolysaccharides, administered parenterally, usually by bolus IV injection followed by IV infusion, or by low dose subcutaneous injection twice daily.
- Uses include treatment of established proximal deep-vein thrombosis (DVT) or pulmonary embolus (PE), perisurgical prophylaxis against DVT/PE, extracorporeal circulations, as an adjunct in acute myocardial infarction and unstable angina, and in arterial embolism.
- Adverse effects include bleeding (which can be managed with protamine in severe cases); thrombocytopenia and paradoxical thrombosis are rare but important.
- Monitoring is by measurement of the APTT.
- Low-molecular-weight heparins (e.g. tinzaparin) are effective and convenient. They do not require routine haematological monitoring, but can cause bleeding. Patients can be taught to administer them at home.

Hirudin

Hirudin is the anticoagulant of the leech, and can now be synthesized in bulk by recombinant DNA technology. It is a direct inhibitor of thrombin, and is more specific than heparin. Unlike heparin, it inhibits clot-associated thrombin and is not dependent on antithrombin III. Early human studies showed that the pharmacodynamic response is closely related to plasma concentration, and its pharmacokinetics are more predictable than those of heparin. In one double-blind randomized controlled study, hirudin substantially reduced thrombo-embolism in over 1000 patients undergoing elective hip surgery. Its place in therapeutics is currently being established by further trials.

Warfarin and other anticoagulants

Warfarin, a derivative of 4–hydroxycoumarin, is the most commonly used oral anticoagulant. Unless otherwise specified, the following discussion refers specifically to warfarin, rather than to other oral anticoagulants. **Phenindione**, an indane 1:3 dione derivative, is an alternative, but has a number of severe and distinctive adverse effects (see below), so it is seldom used except in rare cases of idiosyncratic sensitivity to warfarin.

USE

Warfarin is a racemic mixture of R and S stereoisomers. The main indications for oral anticoagulation are as follows:

1. *deep vein thrombosis and pulmonary embolism* – there is evidence that recurrence may be prevented if oral anticoagulants are continued for at least 3 months after a single episode of deep vein thrombosis and for at least 6 months after a single episode of pulmonary embolism. Recurrent deep vein thrombosis probably requires lifelong anticoagulation, and similarly recurrent pulmonary embolism with the attendant risk of secondary pulmonary hypertension may also be an indication for lifelong treatment;
2. *atrial fibrillation* – the morbidity from embolism (especially stroke) is reduced by anticoagulation in patients with atrial fibrillation associated with many conditions, including mitral stenosis, thyrotoxicosis, chronic sino-atrial disease, congestive cardiomyopathy and ischaemic heart disease. Aspirin also reduces the risk of embolic stroke in patients with atrial fibrillation, but is less effective than warfarin. It provides a useful alternative for patients with contraindications to anticoagulation;
3. moderate to severe *mitral stenosis* (with associated left atrial dilatation) in patients in sinus rhythm carries a substantial risk of embolism that is reduced by anticoagulants;
4. patients with *prosthetic valve replacements* require lifelong anticoagulation, but this does not invariably apply to tissue valves (xenografts). Recent evidence suggests that such patients at high risk of thrombosis (i.e. following artificial valve replacement, or tissue valves with atrial fibrillation or a history of embolism) have markedly reduced mortality from vascular causes and reduced risk of embolization if aspirin (100 mg daily) is added to warfarin. The increased risk of bleeding was modest in the setting of careful monitoring, and was more than offset by the benefit. The first generation of *coronary stents* required prolonged anticoagulation, but this is not needed for current devices.

Treatment of deep-vein thrombosis and pulmonary embolus is started with heparin, because of its immediate effect. Heparin is usually continued for 7 days to allow stabilization of warfarin dose. Therapy is monitored by measuring the international normalized ratio (INR). This is the prothrombin time related to an international standard for thromboplastin reagents. Before starting treatment, a baseline value of INR is determined. This is not influenced by concurrent heparin treatment provided that the APTT is < 2.5. If the APTT is > 2.5 the laboratory can correct this by addition of **protamine** *in vitro* to neutralize the heparin before determination of the INR. Provided that the baseline INR is normal, anticoagulation is started by administering two 10-mg doses 24 h apart at the same time of day (most conveniently in the evening). If the baseline INR is prolonged or the patient has risk factors for bleeding (e.g. old age or debility, liver disease, heart failure, or recent major surgery), treatment is started with a lower dose (e.g. 5 mg daily). The INR is measured daily, and on the morning of day 3 about 50% of patients will be within the therapeutic range and heparin can be discontinued. A useful guide for adjusting the warfarin dose (from the *Drug and Therapeutics Bulletin*) is given in Table 29.2.

Once the situation is stable, the INR is checked weekly for the first 6 weeks and then monthly or 2-monthly if control is good. The patient is warned to report immediately if there is evidence of bleeding, to avoid contact sports or other situations that put them at increased risk of trauma, to avoid alcohol (or at least to restrict their intake to a moderate and unvarying amount), to avoid over-the-counter drugs (other than paracetamol), and to check that any prescription drug is not expected to alter their anticoagulant requirement. Women of childbearing age should be warned of the risk of teratogenesis and given advice on contraception. Appropriate target ranges for different indications reflect the relative risks of thrombosis/haemorrhage in various clinical situations. Table 29.3 lists the suggested ranges of INR that are acceptable for various indications.

MECHANISM OF ACTION

Oral anticoagulants prevent hepatic synthesis of the vitamin K-dependent coagulation factors II, VII, IX and X. Preformed factors are present in blood so, unlike heparin, oral anticoagulants are

Table 29.2: Dose adjustment when starting warfarin

Day	INR (9.00–11.00 a.m.)	Dose (mg) (5.00–7.00 p.m.)
1	< 1.4	10
2	< 1.8	10
	1.8	1
	> 1.8	0.5
3	< 2	10
	2.0–2.1	5
	2.2–2.3	4.5
	2.4–2.5	4
	2.6–2.7	3.5
	2.8–2.9	3
	3.0–3.1	2.5
	3.2–3.3	2
	3.4	1.5
	3.5	1
	3.6–4.0	0.5
	> 4.0	0
		Predicted maintenance dose:
4	< 1.4	> 8
	1.4	8
	1.5	7.5
	1.6–1.7	7
	1.8	6.5
	1.9	6
	2.0–2.1	5.5
	2.2–2.3	5
	2.4–2.6	4.5
	2.7–3.0	4
	3.1–3.5	3.5
	3.6–4.0	3
	4.1–4.5	Miss next dose then 2 mg
	> 4.5	Miss two doses then 1 mg

INR = international normalized ratio.

Table 29.3: Suggested acceptable INR ranges for various indications

Clinical state	Target INR range
Prophylaxis of DVT, including surgery on high-risk patients	2.0–2.5
Treatmant of DVT/PE/systemic embolism/mitral stenosis with embolism	2.0–3.0
Recurrent DVT/PE while on warfarin; mechanical prosthetic heart valve	3.0–4.5

not effective *in vitro* and are only active when given *in vivo*. Functional forms of factors II, VII, IX and X contain residues of γ-carboxyglutamic acid. This is formed by carboxylation of a glutamate residue in the peptide chain of the precursor. This is accomplished by cycling of vitamin K between epoxide, quinone and hydroquinone forms. This cycle is interrupted by warfarin, which is structurally closely related to vitamin K, and inhibits vitamin K epoxide reductase.

ADVERSE EFFECTS

1 *Haemorrhage* is the most important adverse reaction. Intracranial bleeding is especially serious, although gastrointestinal bleeding can also be life-threatening. The incidence depends both on predisposing pathology in the patient (note the contraindications listed below) and on the INR. If the INR is > 4.5 but there is no bleeding, warfarin is withheld and the INR is monitored daily, but if there is bleeding, vitamin K is given. It is administerded intravenously over 3–5 min to avoid dysphoric reactions and hypotension, or orally (by which route it is rapidly absorbed in the absence of diarrhoea or malabsorption from liver or other disease). Minor bleeding can be treated with as little as 1 mg of vitamin K, which does not make the patient resistant to subsequent rewarfarinization. For life-threatening bleeding, 5 mg of vitamin K are is given intravenously together with a factor IX concentrate which also contains factors II and X, and a factor VII concentrate is now also available. (It should be noted that recombinant factor IX and very highly purified factor IX concentrates are now becoming available which, although they have the advantage of causing fewer thrombotic complications in patients with haemophilia B, for whom they are intended, are not effective in reversing warfarin toxicity.) Fresh frozen plasma is a less potent alternative.

2 Other adverse actions of warfarin include the following:

- *teratogenesis,* particularly osteodysplasia punctata, optic atrophy and microcephaly and intrauterine death;
- *rashes;*
- *thrombosis* is a rare but severe and well-documented paradoxical effect of warfarin, and can result in extensive tissue necrosis, usually in a fatty structure such as a breast or buttock. Peripheries (feet or penis) may become gangrenous in this way. Pathologically these lesions are associated with extensive thrombosis in venules. Vitamin K is involved in the biosynthesis of anticoagulant proteins C and S as well as of the clotting factors, and deficiencies of these proteins are associated with thrombotic disease. Protein C has a short elimination half-life, and when warfarin treatment is started its plasma concentration declines more rapidly than that of the vitamin K-dependent coagulation factors, so the resulting imbalance can temporarily favour thrombosis.

3 Adverse effects of phenindiones include the following:

- interference with iodine uptake by the thyroid;
- renal tubular damage;
- hepatitis;
- agranulocytosis;
- dermatitis;
- secretion into breast milk.

CONTRAINDICATIONS

Contraindications to oral anticoagulants include the following:

- active bleeding (e.g. peptic ulceration, active ulcerative colitis);
- blood dyscrasias with haemorrhagic diathesis;
- dissecting aneurysm of the aorta;
- recent surgery of the central nervous system (CNS) or eye;
- space-occupying CNS lesion;
- *pregnancy* – first trimester (especially during organogenesis in weeks 6–9), and the final 4 weeks (because of intracranial bleeding in the infant at delivery, and postpartum haemorrhage in the mother).

Relative contraindications to oral anticoagulation include the following:

- history of potential bleeding lesion;
- high risk of head injury (poorly controlled epilepsy, history of recurrent falls);
- severe uncontrolled hypertension;
- diabetes with proliferative retinopathy;
- alcoholism;
- any stage of pregnancy;

- hepatic or renal insufficiency;
- lack of sufficient intelligence or co-operation on the part of the patient;
- elderly or debilitated patients.

PHARMACOKINETICS

Warfarin can be measured in plasma by high-performance liquid chromatography, but separation of the R and S enantiomers requires specialized methods. Following oral administration, absorption is almost complete and maximum plasma concentrations are reached within 2–8 h. Approximately 97% is bound to plasma albumin. Warfarin does gain access to the fetus, but does not appear in breast milk in clinically relevant amounts. The basal rate of warfarin metabolism is under polygenic control. There is substantial variation between individuals in warfarin $t_{\frac{1}{2}}$, the active S enantiomer having a $t_{\frac{1}{2}}$ of 18–35 h and the R enantiomer having a $t_{\frac{1}{2}}$ of 20–60 h. The R and S enantiomers are metabolized differently in the liver. The S enantiomer is metabolized to 7-hydroxywarfarin by a cytochrome P_{450}-dependent mixed function oxidase, while the less active R enantiomer is metabolized by soluble enzymes to RS warfarin alcohol. Hepatic metabolism is followed by conjugation and excretion into the gut in the bile. Deconjugation and reabsorption then occur, completing the enterohepatic cycle.

Knowledge of the plasma concentration of warfarin is not useful in routine clinical practice because the pharmacodynamic response (INR) can be measured accurately, but it is valuable in the investigation of patients with unusual resistance to warfarin, in whom it helps to distinguish poor compliance, abnormal pharmacokinetics and abnormal sensitivity. Since warfarin acts by inhibiting synthesis of active vitamin K-dependent clotting factors, the onset of anticoagulation following dosing depends on the catabolism of preformed factors. Consequently, the delay between dosing and effect cannot be shortened by giving a loading dose. The $t_{\frac{1}{2}}$ of the factors involved are as follows: II, 60 h; VII, 6 h; IX, 20 h; X, 40 h.

DRUG INTERACTIONS

Numerous clinically important drug interactions occur with warfarin, which has a narrow therapeutic range and a steep dose–response curve. It has the potential to cause life-threatening toxicity, but inadequate treatment can also result in death through progression of thrombo-embolic disease. Many reports of drug interactions with warfarin are poorly documented and are based on single case reports. However, it is prudent to minimize the use of other drugs during oral anticoagulation. When additional drugs are deemed essential, it is important to monitor the INR closely over the next 2 weeks. Drugs that are often needed or useful in patients receiving warfarin and that do *not* interact adversely include digoxin, frusemide and paracetamol.

Potentially important *pharmacodynamic* interactions with warfarin include those with antiplatelet drugs. Aspirin, the main such drug in clinical use, not only influences haemostasis by its effect on platelet function but also increases the likelihood of peptic ulceration, displaces warfarin from plasma albumin, and in high doses decreases prothrombin synthesis. Despite these potential problems, recent clinical experience suggests that with close monitoring the increased risk of bleeding when low doses of aspirin (100 mg daily) are taken regularly with warfarin may be more than offset by clinical benefits to patients at high risk of thrombo-embolism following cardiac valve replacement (see above). Broad-spectrum antibiotics potentiate warfarin by suppressing the synthesis of vitamin K_1 by gut flora. Conversely, some enteral feeding solutions antagonize oral anticoagulants because they contain vitamin K.

There are several *pharmacokinetic* interactions with warfarin that are of clinical importance. It was originally thought that the main effect of phenylbutazone was exerted via competition for plasma albumin binding. Certainly competition between warfarin and phenylbutazone for binding to plasma albumin can be demonstrated *in vitro*. However, the mechanism underlying this interaction has turned out to be more interesting, and is a well-documented instance of stereoselective metabolic inhibition (others include co-trimoxazole, metronidazole and erythromycin). Phenylbutazone *increases* the plasma clearance of R-warfarin by approximately twofold but *decreases* S-warfarin clearance. Confusingly, the clearance of racemic warfarin measured by methods that do not distinguish the enantiomers appears to be unchanged, since the decrease in S-warfarin clearance masks the increased R-warfarin clearance. However, the relative amount of the more potent S-warfarin is increased, so anticoagulant potency

Beware (!) Broad spectrum antibiotics.

Key points

Oral anticoagulants

- These work by interfering with the action of vitamin K on factors II, VII, IX and X. Warfarin is the most important oral anticoagulant.
- Uses include treatment of patients with DVT/PE after initial treatment with heparin, atrial fibrillation, mitral stenosis and artificial heart valves.
- Adverse effects include haemorrhage (managed with vitamin K or fresh frozen plasma/clotting factor concentrates in severe cases), teratogenesis (contraindicating its use in early pregnancy) and, rarely, paradoxical thrombosis.
- Monitoring is by measurement of the international normalized ratio (INR). There is very wide variation in individual dosage requirements
- Drug interactions are common and important, and include interactions with anticonvulsants, antibiotics, sulphonylureas and non-steroidal anti-inflammatory drugs.

is enhanced. Restriction of the use of phenylbutazone (to patients with severe ankylosing spondylitis) has reduced the occurrence of this potentially fatal interaction, but some other non-steroidal anti-inflammatory drugs (NSAIDs) and dextropropoxyphene also inhibit warfarin metabolism. The gastrotoxic and platelet-inhibitory actions of the NSAIDs further increase the risk of serious haemorrhage. Cimetidine (but not ranitidine) and amiodarone also potently inhibit warfarin metabolism and potentiate its effect.

Cholestyramine impairs warfarin absorption and interrupts its enterohepatic recirculation. Drugs that induce hepatic microsomal enzymes, including rifampicin, carbamazepine and phenobarbitone, increase warfarin metabolism and increase the dose required to produce a therapeutic effect. Furthermore, if the dose is not reduced when such concurrent therapy is discontinued, catastrophic over-anticoagulation and haemorrhage may ensue.

ANTIPLATELET DRUGS

Aspirin and other drugs acting on the thromboxane pathway

Aspirin is the most important antiplatelet drug in clinical use. It works by inhibiting the synthesis of TXA_2, and its use in the treatment and prevention of ischaemic heart disease is described more fully in Chapter 28. Numerous clinical trials, several of them large-scale studies, have demonstrated its efficacy, with reductions in myocardial infarction and vascular death ranging from approximately 25% following myocardial infarction to approximately 50% in patients with unstable angina. Efficacy has not been clearly related to dose, with doses of 320 mg on alternate days or 150 mg daily being effective. Aspirin also reduces the incidence of stroke in patients with transient ischaemic attacks by approximately 10%. TXA_2 is synthesized by activated platelets and acts on receptors on platelets (causing further platelet activation and propagation of the aggregate) and on vascular smooth muscle (causing vasoconstriction). Figure 29.2 shows the pathway of its biosynthesis from arachidonic acid. Aspirin inhibits thromboxane synthesis – it acetylates a serine residue in the active site of constitutive (type I) cyclo-oxygenase (COX-1) in platelets, irreversibly blocking this enzyme. The most common side-effect is gastric intolerance, and the

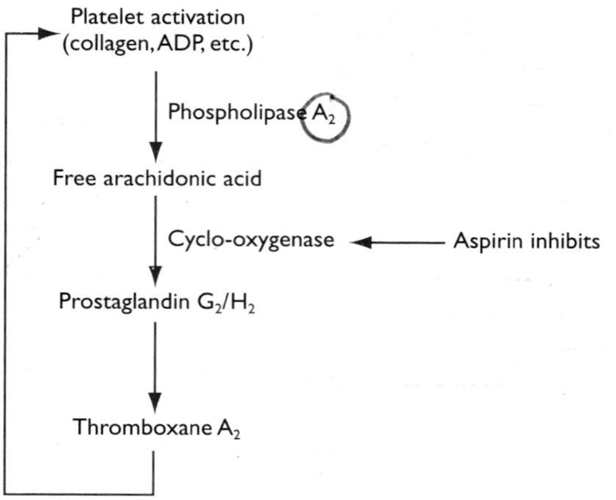

Figure 29.2: Thromboxane A_2 and platelet activation. ADP = adenosine diphosphate.

most common severe adverse reaction is upper gastrointestinal bleeding. Both effects stem from inhibition of COX-1 in the stomach.

Other drugs that act on the thromboxane pathway have considerable therapeutic potential, but have not yet entered clinical use. These include thromboxane-receptor antagonists, which have the potential advantage over aspirin of greater selectivity. Thus they do not inhibit prostaglandin E_2 in the stomach (and so do not cause gastric toxicity of the type caused by aspirin) and do not inhibit prostacyclin (and hence may have greater antithrombotic efficacy than aspirin). Thromboxane synthase inhibitors have the added potential benefit of increasing prostacyclin biosynthesis at the same time as inhibiting thromboxane biosynthesis. Drugs are available that simultaneously inhibit TXA_2 synthesis and action (combined synthase inhibitors/receptor antagonists). They thus avoid one potential problem of pure thromboxane synthase inhibitors, namely that prostaglandin H_2, (the precursor of TXA_2 that accumulates when platelets are activated in the presence of thromboxane synthase inhibition) can also activate thromboxane receptors. Development of these potentially important drugs has been slow, at least partly due to the need to compete commercially with aspirin.

Epoprostenol (prostacyclin)

USE

Epoprostenol is the approved drug name for synthetic prostacyclin, the principal endogenous prostaglandin of large and medium-sized blood vessels such as the aorta and coronary arteries. It is used in the preparation of washed platelet concentrates. Epoprostenol relaxes pulmonary as well as systemic vasculature, and this underpins its use in patients with primary pulmonary hypertension. It has been administered chronically to such patients for periods of months or even years while awaiting heart–lung transplantation. Epoprostenol inhibits platelet activation during haemodialysis. It can be used with heparin, but is also effective as sole anticoagulant in this setting, and is therefore particularly useful for haemodialysis in patients in whom heparin is contraindicated. It has also been used in other types of extracorporeal circuit (e.g. during cardiopulmonary bypass). Epoprostenol has been used with apparent benefit in acute retinal vessel thrombosis and in patients with critical limb ischaemia and with platelet consumption due to multiple organ failure, especially those with meningococcal sepsis. Rigorous proof of efficacy is difficult to provide in such settings. Epoprostenol is dissolved immediately before use in a special alkaline glycine buffer, and is infused intravenously (or, in the case of haemodialysis, into the arterial limb supplying the dialyser). The starting dose is 2 ng/kg body weight/min. This can be increased in stepwise increments of 2 ng/kg/min if necessary to 16 ng/kg/min, with frequent monitoring of blood pressure (usually with an automated indirect method) and heart rate during the period of dose titration. A modest reduction in diastolic pressure with an increase in systolic pressure (i.e. increased pulse pressure) and reflex tachycardia is the expected and desired haemodynamic effect. If bradycardia and hypotension occur, the infusion should be temporarily discontinued and the patient's legs elevated if necessary.

MECHANISM OF ACTION

Prostacyclin acts on specific receptors on the plasma membranes of platelets and vascular smooth muscle. These are coupled by G-proteins to adenylyl cyclase. Activation of this enzyme increases the biosynthesis of the second messenger cyclic adenosine monophosphate (cAMP), which causes inhibition of platelet aggregation to all agonists, and relaxes vascular smooth muscle.

ADVERSE EFFECTS

The vasodilator effect of prostacyclin causes flushing, headache, reduced diastolic blood pressure, increased pulse pressure and reflex tachycardia. Unusually, but of more concern, as mentioned above, vagally mediated bradycardia and hypotension occur. In addition, prostacyclin can cause nausea, abdominal discomfort, diarrhoea and uterine cramps, but these effects are usually mild and much less pronounced than with the E-series prostaglandins. Crushing chest pain is (rarely) experienced by individuals with no evidence of ischaemic heart disease; jaw pain is common during chronic administration. These effects usually resolve within minutes of stopping or reducing the infusion. The bleeding complications which were anticipated have in fact been rare, perhaps because whereas prostacyclin is very potent in inhibiting platelet aggregation, it is much less effective in inhibiting platelet adhesion. Consequently, the haemostastic function of platelets is little influenced by prostacyclin, despite its antithrombotic action.

PHARMACOKINETICS

Prostacyclin is unstable under physiological conditions. It is therefore dissolved in base and infused intravenously. (Stable analogues such as **carbacyclin** and **iloprost** have been developed but have not yet been marketed in the UK.) The half-life of prostacyclin in the circulation is approximately 3 min, so a steady state is achieved rapidly and dose increments can be made safely every 8–12 min. Prostacyclin hydrolyses spontaneously to an inactive product (6-oxo-prostaglandin $F_{1\alpha}$) which is excreted in the urine both unchanged and as inactive enzyme-derived oxidation products, of which the major metabolite is 2,3-dinor-6-oxo-prostaglandin $F_{1\alpha}$.

Dipyridamole

USE

Dipyridamole was introduced as a vasodilator, but is now promoted, often in combination with aspirin, for its effects on platelet function. The combination with aspirin has been effective in reducing the incidence of graft occlusion following coronary artery bypass grafting, but has not been directly compared with aspirin alone. Addition of dipyridamole to warfarin in patients with prosthetic heart valves appeared to reduce the risk of thrombo-embolism in one trial published in 1971, but the incidence of such events in the group treated with anticoagulation alone was unusually high, casting doubt on the reliability of this conclusion. A recent European randomized controlled trial in patients with transient ischaemic attacks ('EPSIM-2') showed that it reduces stroke when used alone. It has a place in the treatment of patients with transient ischaemic attacks who do not tolerate aspirin, or in whom attacks persist despite treatment with aspirin. A completely separate use is as a diagnostic agent in dipyridamole/thallium scanning of the heart. This is used in patients for whom a stress test is clinically indicated, but who are unable to co-operate with an exercise test (e.g. because of severe claudication or osteoarthrosis). In these individuals intravenous dipyridamole can act as a pharmacological stress and enable areas of reversible cardiac hypoperfusion to be identified.

MECHANISM OF ACTION

Dypyridamole influences platelet function. The mechanism of this function, as well as of its vasodilator action, is partly via inhibition of phosphodiesterase which leads to reduced breakdown of cAMP, and partly via inhibition of adenosine uptake with consequent enhancement of the actions of this mediator on platelets and vascular smooth muscle.

DRUG INTERACTIONS

Dipyridamole increases the potency and duration of action of adenosine. This may be clinically important in patients receiving dipyridamole in whom adenosine is considered for treatment of arrhythmia (e.g. following bypass surgery).

Ticlopidine

USE

Ticlopidine is used in North America as prophylaxis against stroke or myocardial infarction in patients at high risk, in peripheral arterial disease, in diabetic microangiopathy and to reduce platelet activation in extracorporeal circulations. It is used by cardiologists following placement of coronary artery stents because of evidence that treatment with aspirin plus ticlopidine for 1 month following stenting reduces cardiac events and haemorrhagic and vascular complications compared to combined anti-coagulant/aspirin treatment. It reduces the risk of recurrence in patients who have recovered from ischaemic stroke, and even appears to be rather more effective than aspirin, 650 mg twice daily, for this indication, but at the expense of a substantial incidence of adverse events, some of them severe. Ticlopidine is also effective in reducing the risk of stroke and myocardial infarction in patients with intermittent claudication. In patients with unstable angina, the addition of ticlopidine to beta-blockers, nitrates and calcium-channel antagonists resulted in an approximately 50% reduction in myocardial infarction. This is similar to the effect of aspirin in unstable angina. Ticlopidine reduces the rate of progression of microaneurysms in patients with diabetes mellitus by about threefold. The clinical importance of this is not known. The drug is given by mouth, 250 mg twice daily. White blood cell counts are checked every 2 weeks for the first 12 weeks (see below).

MECHANISM OF ACTION

Ticlopidine does not inhibit cyclo-oxygenase, and its mechanism is entirely different to that of aspirin. It is an inactive prodrug that is converted in the liver to unstable biologically active metabolite(s) that have not been characterized. Consequently it is inactive when added to platelet-rich plasma *in vitro*, but when platelet-rich plasma is prepared from a subject who has ingested the drug, aggregation to a wide variety of agonists, including ADP, is inhibited. This wide spectrum of activity is explained by inhibition of fibrinogen binding to activated glycoprotein IIb/IIIa receptors. (It is this fibrinogen binding that causes platelets to stick together in response to aggregating agents of all kinds.) Ticlopidine also reduces fibrinogen concentrations by about 10% during chronic treatment, although the importance of this is unknown.

ADVERSE EFFECTS AND CONTRAINDICATIONS

- *Neutropenia* occurs in about 2.4% of patients, usually in the first 12 weeks, and is severe in 0.8% of cases.
- *Thrombocytopenia* and *pancytopenia* have also been described, but are less common than neutropenia.
- *Cholestatic jaundice* has been reported to occur in the first few months, and is reversible on stopping the drug.
- *Gastrointestinal symptoms* are common (around 40% of patients) and include nausea, anorexia, vomiting, epigastric pain and diarrhoea. These symptoms usually occur early and may resolve despite continued treatment, or may not recur on reinstituting treatment.
- *Rashes* occur.
- Plasma lipid concentrations increase by about 10% during chronic treatment, the increases occurring in all fractions, so that the ratio of low-density to high-density lipoprotein (LDL/HDL) remains unchanged.
- Ticlopidine is contraindicated in patients with coagulation or platelet disorders, or with diseases where local bleeding may occur (e.g. haemorrhagic stroke or active peptic ulcer disease).

Key points

Antiplatelet drugs

- Aspirin is clinically the most important antiplatelet drug.
- It is indicated in patients at high risk of arterial thrombosis (e.g. following myocardial infarction, transient ischaemic attack or in other patients with established atheromatous disease).
- Several dosage regimens have proved effective (e.g. 300 mg on alternate days, or 75 mg daily), but it has not been practicable to identify the optimum regime by clinical trial.
- The main adverse effects of aspirin are on the gastrointestinal tract, the most severe of these being gastrointestinal bleeding. These effects are dose related and can be countered by suppression of acid secretion by the stomach if necessary.
- Other antiplatelet drugs have highly specialized uses and include epoprostenol (prostacyclin), dipyridamole, ticlopidine and abciximab.

Clopidrogel

Clopidrogel has recently been licensed for use in the UK. Its mechanism of action is similar to Ticlopidine but it does not cause neutropenia. It is more effective than aspirin (albeit considerably more expensive).

Monocolonal antibodies to glycoprotein IIb/IIIa

USE

Abciximab, a monoclonal antibody to glycoprotein IIb/IIIa, when used as an adjunct to heparin and aspirin reduces occlusion following angioplasty, but can cause bleeding. Its use is currently restricted to patients undergoing angioplasty in whom there is a high risk of acute coronary thrombosis. Hypersensitivity reactions can occur.

ANTICOAGULANTS IN PREGNANCY AND PUERPERIUM

There is an increased risk of thrombo-embolism in pregnancy, and women at risk (e.g. those with

Case history

A 54-year-old barrister had a mitral valve replacement with an artificial prosthesis. He had had rheumatic fever as an adolescent but had subsequently been very fit until he developed symptoms of fatigue and reduced exercise tolerance. He was discharged from hospital on warfarin 4 mg daily and with an INR of 4.2, with instructions to attend his general practitioner within 1 week and to attend the coagulation clinic 2 weeks after that. His GP found him to be well, with an INR of 4.0. The warfarin dose was not changed. Two days later he was brought to hospital at 6.00 p.m. by his wife with severe headache and clouding of consciousness. He had taken two doses of paracetamol the previous night because of low back pain, but had been well that afternoon, playing with a football with his 8-year-old grandson. He had become unwell soon after returning home for tea. On examination, he was drowsy, irritable and the left pupil was larger than the right one. The results of the INR are awaited.

Questions

Decide whether each of the following statements is true or false.

(a) This probably represents a drug interaction between warfarin and paracetamol.
(b) The patient should be given vitamin K before waiting for the INR.
(c) Advice should be sought from the haematologist on call regarding the use of factor concentrates.
(d) This probably resulted from resuming alcohol consumption after leaving hospital.
(e) The patient should be encouraged to take fluids by mouth.
(f) Further history should be sought from the grandson.

Answer

(a) False.
(b) True.
(c) True.
(d) False.
(e) False.
(f) True.

Comment

A target INR of 3.0–4.5 is appropriate in this setting, but it does confer a significant excess risk of haemorrhage. The value obtained by the GP was actually slightly lower than that recorded at discharge, so a pharmacokinetic interaction was unlikely at that time. Paracetamol (which the patient took subsequently) does not interact with warfarin, in contrast to aspirin. The clinical picture strongly suggests an intracranial bleed, a suspicion that was strengthened by the grandson's subsequent account of the patient's demonstration of 'heading' the football. Neurosurgical intervention was life-saving, and both vitamin K and factor concentrates were given despite the inevitable risk of thrombosis on the prosthetic valve.

prosthetic heart valves) must continue to be anticoagulated. However, warfarin crosses the placenta, and when taken throughout pregnancy will result in complications in about one-third of cases (16% of fetuses will be spontaneously aborted or stillborn, 10% will have postpartum complications (usually due to bleeding) and 7% will suffer teratogenic effects).

Heparin (both unfractionated and low-molecular-weight forms) does not cross the placenta, and may be self-administered subcutaneously. Its long-term use may cause *osteoporosis*, and there is an increased risk of *retroplacental bleeding* resulting in fetal death. One approach to the management of pregnancy in women on anticoagulants is to change to *subcutaneous heparin* from the time of the first missed period and remain on this until term, maintaining a high intake of elemental calcium as well as adequate but not excessive intake of vitamin D. Unfractionated heparin is self-administered subcutaneously every 12 h in doses adjusted to maintain the mid-interval APTT at 1.5 × control. Experience with low-molecular-weight heparins is more limited than that with the unfractionated product, but so far the results are encouraging. This may well become the approach of choice for anticoagulation in pregnancy, as it only needs to be administered once daily, and there is less risk of heparin-induced thrombocytopenia with associated thrombosis, and of osteoporosis.

There is a small but definite increased risk of spinal haematoma with regional analgesia in patients on heparin. The latter may be withheld at the start of regular uterine contractions. Some authorities believe that regional analgesia is not contraindicated if the APTT is normal and heparin has not been given within the preceding 4–6 h before delivery, but heparin together with warfarin is restarted immediately postpartum and continued until the full effect of warfarin is re-established. If labour starts suddenly in a woman in whom the APTT is excessively prolonged, protamine can be given. Warfarin does not enter breast milk to a significant extent, and mothers may nurse their babies while anticoagulated in this way (in contrast to those on phenindione).

Further reading

Koopman MM, Prandoni P, Piovella F *et al.* 1996: Treatment of venous thrombosis with intravenous unfractionated heparin administered in the hospital as compared with subcutaneous low-molecular-weight heparin administered at home. The Tasman study group. *New England Journal of Medicine* **334**, 682–7.

Levine M, Gent M, Hirsh J. 1996: A comparison of low-molecular-weight heparin administered primarily at home and administered in the hospital for proximal deep-vein thrombosis. *New England Journal of Medicine* **334**, 677–81.

Salzman EW. 1992: Low-molecular-weight heparin and other new antithrombotic drugs. *New England Journal of Medicine* **326**, 1017–9.

Toglia MR, Weg JG. 1996: Venous thromboembolism during pregnancy. *New England Journal of Medicine* **335**, 108–14.

CHAPTER THIRTY

HEART FAILURE

- Introduction
- Pathophysiology
- Therapeutic objectives
- General measures
- Shock: general principles
- Drugs for cardiac failure

INTRODUCTION

Heart failure occurs when the heart fails to deliver adequate amounts of oxygenated blood to the tissues during exercise or, in severe cases, at rest. Such failure of pump function may be chronic, in which case symptoms of fatigue, ankle swelling, effort dyspnoea and orthopnoea predominate, or it may be acute, with sudden onset of pulmonary oedema and shortness of breath. Both acute and chronic heart failure severely reduce life expectancy.

PATHOPHYSIOLOGY

Heart failure can be caused by diseases of the heart (myocardium – ischaemic heart disease or idiopathic cardiomyopathy; conducting tissue – various arrhythmias; pericardium – constrictive pericarditis, pericardial effusion; or endocardium – valvular disease), hypertension (systemic or pulmonary), congenital defects (atrial or ventricular septal defects or patent ductus arteriosus) or extracardiac disorders, including fluid overload, anaemia and thyrotoxicosis.

Heart failure causes several pathophysiological changes that are 'counter-regulatory', i.e. they make the situation worse, not better. This puzzling situation is probably due to natural selection, as our ancestors probably encountered low cardiac output during haemorrhage rather than as a result of heart failure. Mechanisms to conserve blood volume and maintain blood pressure would therefore have been of selective advantage. However, reflex and endocrine changes that are protective in the setting of haemorrhage are totally inappropriate in patients with low cardiac output due to pump failure rather than volume loss.

An important part of modern treatment of cardiac failure is therefore directed towards reversing these counter-regulatory changes, which include the following.

1 Activation of the renin–angiotensin–aldosterone system and renin release, with consequent increased production of angiotensin II (which increases peripheral resistance both by direct vasoconstriction and indirectly by synergy with the sympathetic nervous system) and aldosterone (which causes salt and water retention). The use of angiotensin-converting-enzyme inhibitors in patients with heart failure has been one of the most important therapeutic advances of the last decade. Its efficacy in prolonging life (see below) has been demonstrated in several large randomized trials.
2 Activation of sympathetic nervous system reflexes leading to increased sympathetic tone, tachycardia and vasoconstriction. The positive

inotropic action of noradrenaline may support the failing heart, so the use of β-adrenoceptor antagonists in heart failure is potentially hazardous. Nevertheless, sustained β-receptor activation may be harmful in this setting. Many years ago a Swedish group reported that β-antagonists were of clinical benefit. Recently, a clinical trial involving titration of low doses of **carvedilol** (a β-antagonist with additional pharmacological effects) in patients receiving digoxin, diuretics and angiotensin-converting-enzyme inhibitor showed reduced mortality and morbidity in the treated group. This has been confirmed in trials of other β-antagonists (e.g. Metoprolol).

Important physiological factors determining cardiac performance include *preload, afterload, myocardial contractility* and *heart rate*. Each of these may be adversely affected by the primary cause of heart failure, and may be exacerbated by the counter-regulatory changes mentioned above.

Preload

The filling pressure of the left ventricle determines the extent of stretch of myocardial fibres at the end of diastole. Up to a point, increased stretch results in increased force of contraction but, in the failing heart, beyond this point further stretch results in reduced contraction (the Frank–Starling relationship). Preload is increased directly if blood (or physiological saline) is infused intravenously too rapidly. The major influences on preload are blood volume, which increases in heart failure due to salt and water retention, and increased capacitance vessel tone due to sympathetic nervous system activation. In heart failure, preload is usually excessive, and cardiac function is improved by drugs that reduce blood volume (diuretics) or reduce capacitance vessel tone (venodilators).

Afterload

This determines the tension that needs to be developed in the ventricular wall to eject the stroke volume. It is principally determined by the systemic vascular resistance, such that: the lower this resistance, the less the impedance to ventricular emptying. Systemic vascular resistance is excessively high in the majority of patients with heart failure, because of inappropriate activation of the renin–angiotensin and sympathetic nervous systems, as explained above. Drugs that reduce afterload (arteriodilators) therefore improve cardiac output in patients with heart failure.

Myocardial contractility

This describes the intrinsic contractility of the heart, and is reduced following myocardial infarction or in idiopathic congestive cardiomyopathy. Cellular/tissue remodelling of the heart is important in the progression of disease. Recent preliminary evidence suggests that treatment with **growth hormone** strikingly improves cardiac performance and the overall functional capacity of patients with idiopathic dilated cardiomyopathy. The results of randomized studies of chronic treatment are eagerly awaited. Selected patients with severe disease may benefit dramatically from cardiac transplantation. Positive inotropes (e.g. digoxin, phosphodiesterase inhibitors, (β_1-adrenoceptor agonists) can improve cardiac performance temporarily by increasing contractility, but at the expense of increased work and oxygen consumption of viable cardiac muscle.

Heart rate

Cardiac output is the product of heart rate and stroke volume, so increased heart rate increases cardiac output in the healthy heart. It does this at the expense of increased cardiac work and oxygen consumption. When there is coronary artery disease, coronary blood flow may be reduced and ischaemia worsened as the rate increases. Furthermore, cardiac function deteriorates as the rate increases beyond an optimum, due to insufficient time for filling during diastole, and positive chronotropes are not useful clinically in the absence of specific bradyarrhythmia. Indeed, the main clinical use of drugs that affect heart rate for heart failure is the use of **digoxin** to *slow* ventricular rate in rapid atrial fibrillation (see below).

THERAPEUTIC OBJECTIVES

Therapy specific for the underlying disease may be available. Surgery (e.g. for valvular or congen-

Key points

Heart failure: pathophysiology and principles of therapeutics

- Heart failure has diverse origins (e.g. congenital or valvular heart disease, systemic or pulmonary hypertension); ischaemic and idiopathic cardiomyopathy are especially important.
- Neurohumoral activation (e.g. of sympathetic and renin–angiotensin systems) may have *adverse* consequences.
- Treatment is sometimes specific (e.g. valve replacement), but more often is directed generally at:

  preload (reduced by diuretics, nitrates and ACE inhibitors);
  afterload (reduced by ACE inhibitors and hydralazine);
  contractility (increased by digoxin and dobutamine);
  heart rate (rapid rates do not permit optimal filling; rapid atrial fibrillation is slowed by digoxin).

ital heart disease), pacing (for symptomatic bradyarrhythmias) or oxygen (for cor pulmonale) may be indicated in addition to drugs to improve haemodynamics by reducing cardiac load or increasing contractility. In addition to correction of specific defects where this is possible, the objectives of management are:

1 to improve symptoms, and
2 to prolong survival.

General measures

These include the following:

1 sitting the patient upright in acute heart failure;
2 oxygen to correct hypoxia if present;
3 withdrawal of drugs that aggravate cardiac failure, i.e. negative inotropes (e.g. calcium-channel blockers), direct cardiac toxins (e.g. daunorubicin) or drugs that cause salt retention (e.g. non-steroidal anti-inflammatory drugs). The role of β-antagonists is controversial (see above). They have been cast both as villains (because of their negative inotropic effects) and also more recently as heroes. They must be introduced at low dose with close monitoring;
4 dietary salt and, less importantly, fluid restriction;
5 anticoagulants – bed rest, vigorous diuresis and low cardiac output predispose to deep venous thrombosis and pulmonary embolism. Anticoagulation reduces this risk. Once patients are up and about anticoagulation may not be needed, provided that they are in sinus rhythm. Aspirin should be considered in patients with ischaemic heart disease, to reduce the risk of reinfarction;
6 bed rest – this improves renal blood flow and is appropriate in acute heart failure, but seldom, if ever, in chronic heart failure.

Shock: general principles

Shock is life-threatening hypoperfusion of vital organs, especially the brain and kidneys. The main types of shock are as follows:

1 *hypovolaemic* – replacement of volume with blood, plasma, colloid (e.g. dextran or gelatin solutions) or crystalloid solutions (e.g. physiological saline) is the main therapeutic approach;
2 *endotoxin* – appropriate antibiotics, in addition to fluids and pressors, are given as needed;
3 *cardiogenic* – this requires augmentation of myocardial contractility, although in many patients the pump is irreversibly damaged and no therapy is effective. A few patients with apparent cardiogenic shock have problems for which there is specific therapy which may be life-saving. These are often readily diagnosed on Swan–Ganz catheterization, and include unrecognized hypovolaemia, right ventricular infarction, cardiac tamponade, ventriculoseptal or papillary muscle rupture.

However, in the majority of patients with cardiogenic shock the problem is due to pump failure. Measurement of pulmonary capillary wedge pressure (a measure of left heart filling pressure) together with arterial blood pressure, cardiac output and urine output should permit optimal use of pressor and vasodilator drugs as well as management of volume status in these patients. Recently, this has been challenged by evidence that Swan–Ganz catheter use is associated with increased mortality, and the precise role of this form of monitoring is currently being revised. Management often involves a combination of **dobutamine** (a positive inotrope that is relatively free of chronotropic effects), low-dose **dopamine** (to improve renal blood flow) and an arterial vasodilator (e.g. sodium nitroprusside or glyceryl trinitrate) to reduce cardiac load and improve tissue perfusion. These short-term measures permit recovery of function in some patients with reversible cardiac dysfunction (e.g. from so-called 'stunned' myocardium).

DRUGS FOR CARDIAC FAILURE

Diuretics (see also Chapters 27 and 35)

USE FOR CARDIAC FAILURE

A diuretic is usually the drug of first choice for controlling symptomatic oedema and dyspnoea in patients with heart failure. In very mild cardiac failure, a thiazide (see Chapters 25 and 33) is sometimes adequate, but more severe cases require a loop diuretic such as frusemide, started at a low dose (e.g. 20–40 mg by mouth and increased if necessary). Acute pulmonary oedema requires treatment with *intravenous* frusemide (e.g. 40 mg, or if needed larger doses given slowly – not faster than 4 mg/min). Slow intravenous infusion of frusemide by syringe pump is useful in resistant severe cases. Combinations of a fixed dose of frusemide with a potassium-sparing diuretic such as amiloride ('co-amilofruse') are marketed aggressively and enjoy considerable popularity, but they are relatively expensive and are not without problems. They should not be prescribed uncritically and automatically in place of frusemide, but are useful in certain circumstances (see below). **Spironolactone** has recently been shown to improve survival in patients with cardiac failure. Concern about containing spironolactone with ACE inhibitors may have been overstated.

MECHANISM OF ACTION

Loop diuretics inhibit $Na^+/K^+/2Cl^-$ cotransport in the thick ascending limb of Henlé's loop, and cause kaliuresis in addition to the desired natriuresis. Increased elimination of salt and water decreases cardiac preload and reduces oedema. Frusemide also has an indirect vasodilator effect (probably via prostaglandin and vasodepressor neutral lipid mediators released from the kidneys), since diuresis begins about 10–20 min after an intravenous dose, whereas dramatic symptomatic improvement in patients with pulmonary oedema can occur more rapidly.

ADVERSE EFFECTS

Diuretics have several electrolyte/metabolic effects of uncertain clinical significance. They cause some degree of hypokalaemia in many subjects, and sometimes also hypomagnesaemia and hyponatraemia. Increased elimination of sodium chloride causes hypochloraemic alkalosis, which can be important in patients with cor pulmonale from obstructive airways disease. Total body potassium levels may be little affected during chronic treatment, but many of the adverse interactions of diuretics with other drugs (see below) are probably mediated by hypokalaemia and/or hypomagnesaemia, although this issue remains controversial. Diuretics reduce urate clearance, thereby increasing the plasma urate concentration and precipitating gout in predisposed individuals. Thiazides impair glucose tolerance, and can cause hyperglycaemia in non-insulin-dependent diabetics.

Frusemide causes idiosyncratic reactions, including rashes and (rarely) bone-marrow depression, evidenced by either neutropenia or thrombocytopenia. These latter reactions require the drug to be stopped, and an alternative loop diuretic (e.g. bumetanide) may be useful in this situation. High doses of frusemide (particularly if given by rapid intravenous injection) are predictably ototoxic, causing deafness and tinnitus, because formation of endolymph in the inner ear involves an $Na^+/K^+/2Cl^-$ transporter.

PHARMACOKINETICS

Absorption of frusemide from the gastrointestinal tract is delayed in severe cardiac failure, due to oedema of the intestinal mucosa (see Chapter 7), and frusemide is more effective when administered intravenously (ideally by syringe pump) than when given by the oral route in these circumstances. When the clinical situation improves, the oral route can then be used.

Frusemide is eliminated in the urine. It is secreted in the proximal tubule and becomes progressively more concentrated as water is reabsorbed in the proximal tubule, so when it reaches its site of action in the ascending limb of the loop of Henlé its concentration in the tubular fluid is much greater than that in the plasma. Since the ion transporter that it inhibits is located on the luminal surface, this explains the selectivity of frusemide for the $Na^+/K^+/2Cl^-$ exchanger in the kidney as opposed to other sites in the body, such as the inner ear.

DRUG INTERACTIONS

Diuretic-induced hypokalaemia increases the toxicity of several important cardiovascular drugs, notably digoxin. It increases the risk of *torsades de pointes* from Class Ia and III anti-arrhythmic drugs that prolong the cardiac action potential (e.g. quinidine, disopyramide, amiodarone, sotolol; see Chapter 31). Potassium supplements can counter this problem, but are unpleasant to take, and are present in totally inadequate amounts in 'combination' tablets. Concurrent use of a potassium-sparing diuretic (e.g. amiloride or triamterene) with frusemide is sometimes justified in the treatment of heart failure, particularly if digoxin or one of the above anti-arrhythmic drugs is also needed. However, K^+-retaining diuretics have important toxicities and can cause severe hyperkalaemia, especially if given with converting-enzyme inhibitors and/or administered to patients with renal impairment, which is a common accompaniment to heart failure. It is therefore important to monitor plasma concentrations of potassium during treatment with diuretics. In modern practice, converting-enzyme inhibitors, which help to conserve potassium, are used earlier than hitherto (see below), and digoxin is usually relegated to third-line treatment, so potassium-sparing diuretics are often unnecessary, and it is unfortunate that expensive fixed-dose combinations are prescribed so uncritically.

Non-steroidal anti-inflammatory drugs (NSAIDs) cause salt and water retention by inhibiting prostaglandin biosynthesis by the kidney (prostaglandin E_2 and prostacyclin are vasodilator and natriuretic in action). The NSAIDs therefore reduce the effectiveness of frusemide and other diuretics. Diuretics also interact with lithium by causing salt depletion, thereby increasing the drug's proximal tubular reabsorption and plasma concentration, and hence the likelihood of toxicity.

Converting-enzyme inhibitors (see also Chapters 27 and 28)

Angiotensin-converting enzyme (ACE) is inhibited by several synthetic peptides and peptide analogues derived originally from the toxin of a South American snake (*Bothrops jacaraca*). Many different ACE inhibitors are now marketed.

USE IN HEART FAILURE

Angiotensin-converting-enzyme inhibitors are a major advance in the treatment of cardiac failure. They reduce mortality as well as improving symptoms, and are superior to other vasodilators that have been used to treat heart failure. When symptoms are mild, diuretics can be temporarily discontinued a day or two before starting an ACE inhibitor, reducing the likelihood of first-dose hypotension. In these circumstances treatment with an ACE inhibitor can be started as an outpatient, as for hypertension (see Chapter 27). A small starting dose is used and the first dose is taken last thing before retiring at night, with advice to sit on the side of the bed before standing if the patient needs to get up in the night. Starting doses of 2.5 mg for enalapril, or of 6.25 mg for captopril, are appropriate. The dose is increased with careful monitoring of blood pressure and signs of heart failure to a maintenance dose that is individualized for each patient (usual doses are enalapril, 5–10 mg twice daily, or captopril, 25–50 mg 2–3 times daily). Baseline evaluation with an objective measure of ventricular function (e.g. ejection fraction by echocardiography) is increasingly needed to detect evidence of subclinical heart failure following myocardial infarction, in view of the evidence of improved survival from treatment of such patients with ACE inhibitors.

MECHANISM OF ACTION

Angiotensin-converting enzyme (also called kininase II) is located on the surface membrane of vascular endothelial cells as well as in other cells and in plasma. The lung (which possesses a huge surface area of endothelium) is particularly rich in ACE, but this enzyme is also present in many other organs, including the heart and systemic resistance vessels. Angiotensin-converting enzyme catalyses the removal of two terminal amino acid residues from angiotensin I and from several other short peptides. This results in the formation of angiotensin II (a potent vasoconstrictor) from its inactive precursor angiotensin I. Angiotensin II releases aldosterone from the zona glomerulosa of the adrenal cortex, as well as constricting vascular smooth muscle, and therefore causes salt and water retention and urinary loss of potassium. In addition to activating the vasoconstrictor/salt-retaining angiotensin mechanism, ACE also inactivates bradykinin, which is an endogenous vasodilator. Angiotensin-converting-enzyme inhibitors therefore reduce angiotensin-mediated vasoconstriction and salt retention, mildly increase plasma potassium, and enhance bradykinin-mediated vasodilatation. They reduce cardiac preload and afterload, thereby improving the function of the failing heart.

ADVERSE EFFECTS

Hypotension can be a problem when starting treatment. Patients with heart failure usually have high concentrations of circulating renin, and this is further increased by treatment with diuretics. The introduction of an ACE inhibitor can therefore cause dramatic 'first-dose' hypotension. This can be minimized as explained above. Patients in whom first-dose hypotension is marked may be those with greatest activation of the renin–angiotensin system, and consequently those most likely to benefit from treatment with ACE inhibitors in the long term. Angiotensin-converting-enzyme inhibitors are usually well tolerated during chronic treatment, although dry cough is common and occasionally unacceptable. This symptom may be caused by kinin accumulation stimulating cough afferents. The same explanation has been offered for the urticarial reactions and angioneurotic oedema that are sometimes caused by ACE inhibitors. Functional renal failure is a predictable effect of ACE inhibitors in patients with haemodynamically significant bilateral renal artery stenoses, or with renal artery stenosis in the vessel supplying a single functional kidney. Angiotensin converting-enzyme inhibitors are contraindicated in pregnancy from the second trimester until term because they cause renal failure in the fetus, oligohydramnios and also birth defects.

Angiotensin-converting-enzyme inhibitors cause a modest increase in plasma potassium levels as a result of reduced aldosterone secretion. This may usefully counter the small reduction in potassium ion concentration caused by diuretics. However, increased plasma potassium is potentially hazardous in patients with renal impairment, and close monitoring of plasma potassium and creatinine levels is essential in this setting. This is particularly important when such patients are also prescribed potassium supplements and/or potassium-sparing diuretics, including those marketed as fixed-dose combinations (e.g. co-amilozide, coamilofruse), or NSAIDs which can reduce renin secretion.

When it was first introduced, captopril caused a cluster of adverse effects including heavy proteinuria, rashes and neutropenia. These were identified as being related to its sulphydryl group. Similar effects occur with penicillamine, another drug that contains a sulphydryl group (see Chapter 25). These dose-related effects seldom occur with the maximum doses of captopril that are now commonly regarded as useful (i.e. usually no more than 50 mg twice daily) and paradoxically, converting-enzyme inhibitors (including captopril) actually *reduce* albuminuria in patients with diabetic nephropathy (see Chapter 36) and other renal glomerular disorders.

PHARMACOKINETICS

See Chapter 27

DRUG INTERACTIONS

The useful interaction with diuretics has already been mentioned. Diuretic treatment increases plasma renin activity, and the consequent activation of angiotensin II and aldosterone limits the efficacy of diuretic treatment. Converting-enzyme inhibitors interrupt this loop and so enhance the efficacy of diuretics.

Adverse interactions with potassium-sparing diuretics and potassium supplements, leading to hyperkalaemia, especially in patients with renal impairment, can be life-threatening. Non-steroidal anti-inflammatory drugs are contraindicated in patients with heart failure, and may cause renal failure and severe hyperkalaemia as well as fluid retention in such patients who are receiving treatment with converting-enzyme inhibitors.

Other vasodilators

Before the introduction of converting-enzyme inhibitors, several other vasodilators were found to be effective in heart failure. These include **hydralazine** and α-adrenoceptor antagonists (see Chapter 27) and organic nitrates (see Chapter 28). The combination of hydralazine (to reduce afterload) with a long-acting nitrate (to reduce preload) improves survival, but less than with a converting-enzyme inhibitor. It should be used in patients in whom converting-enzyme inhibitors are contraindicated or not tolerated. Alternatively, there is increasing evidence that an angiotensin II (AT_1) receptor antagonist, such as losartan, is effective for heart failure.

Cardiac glycosides (see also Chapter 31, p. 323)

William Withering published his description of the use of digitalis (an extract of the foxglove) as a cure for 'dropsy' (congestive cardiac failure) in 1785. 'Digitalis' is the name used for a group of cardiac glycosides that all possess an aglycone ring essential for activity. These share similar pharmacodynamic properties, and differ in their pharmacokinetics. Among digitalis glycosides, **digoxin** is now used almost exclusively, although the faster acting **ouabain** is useful in urgent situations, whereas **digitoxin**, which has a longer elimination half-life, can be useful when drugs have to be given under supervision (e.g. to a mildly demented patient by a visiting nurse who can call only three times a week).

USE

The only undisputed indication for chronic digoxin in heart failure is control of ventricular rate in rapid atrial fibrillation. However, mild persistent haemodynamic benefit has been demonstrated in severely compromised patients in sinus rhythm who are inadequately controlled on diuretics, presumably as a consequence of its positive inotropic effect. And addition of digoxin to diuretics and ACE I reduces hospitalization and improves symptoms, without prolonging life. It is therefore useful for controlling symptoms in such patients. It is usually given orally, but if this is impossible or if a rapid effect is required, it can be given intravenously. Since the half-life ($t_{\frac{1}{2}}$) is approximately 1–2 days, repeated administration of a once daily maintenance dose (usually 0.125–0.5 mg, depending on estimated renal function) results in a plateau concentration in about 5–10 days. The dose may be adjusted based on plasma concentration determinations once steady state has been reached. If clinical circumstances are more urgent, a therapeutic plasma concentration can be obtained more rapidly by administering a loading dose, e.g. a single dose of 0.5 mg followed by 0.25 mg 8-hourly for three doses followed by the estimated once daily maintenance dose. In even more urgent situations digitalization can be initiated by an intravenous loading dose of 0.5 mg.

MECHANISM OF ACTION

Digoxin inhibits membrane Na^+/K^+ adenosine triphosphatase (ATPase), which actively extrudes Na^+ from myocardial as well as other cells. This causes accumulation of intracellular Na^+ which indirectly increases intracellular Ca^{2+} content via reduced Na^+/Ca^{2+} exchange and increased intracellular Ca^{2+} storage. The rise in availability of intracellular Ca^{2+} accounts for the positive inotropic effect of digoxin. Excessive poisoning of Na^+/K^+-ATPase causes numerous non-cardiac as well as cardiac (arrhythmogenic) toxic effects. Ventricular slowing results from several mechanisms, particularly the effect of increased vagal activity on the AV node. Slowing of ventricular rate improves cardiac output in patients with atrial fibrillation by improving ventricular filling during diastole. Clinical progress is assessed by measuring heart rate (at the apex): successful control is usually achieved at apical rates of 70-80 beats/min.

ADVERSE EFFECTS AND CONTRAINDICATIONS

Digoxin has a low therapeutic index. Studies of the prevalence of intoxication have yielded figures of 15–20% for hospital in-patients receiving the drug. As pharmaceutical preparations have become purer the incidence of gastrointestinal symptoms (nausea, vomiting and diarrhoea) as the harbinger of toxicity has decreased, but the initial indication of intoxication can be a fatal cardiac arrhythmia. Before using digoxin it is important to consider the possibility of Wolff–Parkinson–White (WPW) syndrome, in which the drug is usually contraindicated because it can cause ventricular fibrillation in this setting.

PHARMACOKINETICS

Currently available preparations disperse rapidly and uniformly, although this has not always been the case in the past. Approximately 80% of the drug is excreted unchanged in the urine in patients with normal renal function. It is eliminated mainly by glomerular filtration, although a small amount is subject to both tubular secretion and reabsorption. A small amount undergoes metabolism to inactive products or excretion via the bile and elimination in faeces. The proportion eliminated by these non-renal clearance mechanisms increases in patients with renal impairment, being 100% in anephric patients, in whom the $t_{\frac{1}{2}}$ is approximately 4.5 days.

It is sometimes useful to measure the digoxin plasma concentration. Blood should be sampled more than 6 h after an oral dose or immediately before the next dose is due (trough level). The usual therapeutic range is 1–2 ng/mL, although toxicity can occur at concentrations of less than 1.5 ng/mL in some individuals. Plasma concentration determination is useful when toxicity is suspected, and in patients in sinus rhythm in whom there is no simple pharmacodynamic measure of response analogous to apical heart rate in patients with atrial fibrillation.

DRUG INTERACTIONS

Digoxin has a steep dose–response curve and a narrow therapeutic range, and clinically important interactions are common (see Chapters 13 and 31). Pharmacokinetic interactions with digoxin include reduced absorption, which can result in loss of efficacy (e.g. antacid, bile acid-binding resins, tetracyclines), and combined pharmacokinetic effects involving displacement from tissue-binding sites and reduced renal elimination (e.g. digoxin toxicity due to concurrent treatment with verapamil or amiodarone).

Pharmacodynamic interactions with digoxin are also important. In particular, drugs that cause hypokalaemia (e.g. diuretics, β-agonists, glucocorticoids) predispose to digoxin toxicity by increasing its binding to (and effect on) Na^+/K^+-ATPase. Drugs causing hypomagnesaemia (e.g. diuretics, alcohol excess) also predispose to digoxin toxicity. β-adrenoreceptor antagonists, despite their negative inotropic effects such drugs (e.g. carvedilol, metoprolol), have been shown to improve survival in patients with chronic heart failure. They must be introduced slowly, starting with a very low dose, increased over a period of weeks and months.

Sympathomimetic amines

USE IN SHOCK

Sympathomimetic amines are sometimes used in acute severe heart failure with hypoperfusion (shock). Before sympathomimetic amines are employed to treat severe hypotension from any cause, hypovolaemia must be corrected. Sympathomimetic amines are given by a central line. Reliable constant-rate infusion pumps are essential to avoid inadvertent bolus administration with the risk of direct cardiac toxicity (arrhythmia and sudden death). **Adrenaline** is important in the treatment of *cardiac arrest* (see Chapter 31) and *anaphylactic shock* (see Chapter 49). **Noradrenaline** is a potent β_1 – and, especially, α-agonist. When injected parenterally it can precipitate tachyarrhythmias because of its β_1-agonist action, but paradoxically it can also cause secondary reflex bradycardia, initiated by the carotid sinus baroreceptors and mediated by the vagus. Despite causing increased cardiac contractility and increased oxygen demand, it may actually decrease cardiac output, and it is now seldom used in severe cardiac failure, having been supplanted by newer drugs, notably **dobutamine**.

Dobutamine is chemically related to isoprenaline but is predominantly a β_1-receptor agonist. It exerts a more prominent inotropic than chronotropic action. It does not release endogenous catecholamines and is less likely to cause arrhythmias than pressor doses of dopamine. It is the pressor agent of choice in patients with shock caused by myocardial infarction or following cardiac surgery, and is usually given with invasive monitoring on the intensive-care unit in doses of 5–40 μg/kg/min. Although it causes some peripheral vasodilatation, it does not dilate the renal vasculature. Thus in cardiogenic shock, a combination of dobutamine (to increase cardiac output) with low-dose dopamine (for its renal effect, see below), or with low-dose sodium nitroprusside or glyceryl trinitrate (to reduce cardiac load) is often appropriate.

Dopamine is the biochemical precursor of noradrenaline, but also has transmitter functions in its own right in the central nervous system and in the renal vasculature. It releases endogenous catecholamines, including noradrenaline, when given in high pharmacological doses, and it is markedly pro-arrhythmogenic, probably for this reason. However, at low doses it has a selective vasodilator effect on the renal vascular bed mediated via specific dopamine receptors. Low doses, 2–5 μg/kg/min, increase renal perfusion and urine output. This dose is often given with intravenous frusemide to produce diuresis. Cardiac output is slightly increased and peripheral resistance is slightly decreased by dopamine, so the mean blood pressure is little altered.

MECHANISM OF ACTION

Cardiovascular responses to sympathomimetic amines are mediated by α- and β-adrenoceptors which are coupled to intracellular processes via G-proteins. β-Receptors are coupled to adenylyl cyclase, and many effects of β-receptor stimulation are mediated by cyclic AMP (see Chapter 3). The second-messenger systems involved in mediating the effects of α-receptor stimulation are more diverse. Pharmacological effects of α- and β-receptor stimulation include the following:

1 α_1-receptor stimulation leads to vasoconstriction (via activation of phospholipase C increasing intracellular inositol trisphosphate (ITP) and hence intracellular Ca^{2+} concentration).
2 β_1-receptors are located in the heart, and stimulation leads to increased heart rate and contractility.
3 β_2-receptor stimulation dilates peripheral and coronary arteries and arterioles. Recent evidence has shown that some of these effects are mediated by release of nitric oxide from the endothelium.
4 Dopamine receptors selectively vasodilate renal vasculature.

ADVERSE EFFECTS

These include arrhythmias and infarct extension from increased oxygen demand. Extravasation can cause tissue necrosis, and it is essential to establish good venous access.

PHARMACOKINETICS

Dobutamine has a short $t_{\frac{1}{2}}$ (2 min) and is mainly eliminated by hepatic metabolism to glucuronides and 3-O-methyldobutamine. Dopamine also has a short plasma $t_{\frac{1}{2}}$, and is taken up into sympathetic nerves by uptake 1. It may consequently displace endogenous catecholamines from the nerve terminals. It is taken up from the cytoplasm by synaptic vesicles and converted by dopamine β-hydroxylase in the vesicles into noradrenaline, which is subsequently available for release in response to nerve impulses. Alternatively, it may not gain access to vesicles but be metabolized in the nerve terminals to yield vanillyl mandelic acid, which is excreted in the urine.

DRUG INTERACTIONS

The valuable pharmacodynamic interactions between dobutamine and dopamine, and between dobutamine and vasodilators such as sodium nitroprusside have already been mentioned. Adrenoceptor- and dopamine-receptor antagonists (such as chlorpromazine or haloperidol) predictably reduce the potency of these drugs, and patients in cardiogenic shock who have received them may require increased doses of sympathomimetic amines to compete with such antagonists.

Phosphodiesterase inhibitors

Phosphodiesterase (PDE) inactivates cyclic AMP, so it might be anticipated that inhibitors of this enzyme would to some extent mimic the actions of β-agonists, increasing the force of contraction of the heart and relaxing vascular smooth muscle. Such actions might be therapeutically useful, especially since phosphodiesterase inhibitors are active when given orally, unlike the sympathomimetic amines discussed above. Xanthine alkaloids (e.g. **theophylline**) are phosphodiesterase inhibitors, and were used in the past to treat patients with heart failure, but they are toxic and not very effective. Furthermore, some of their pharmacological effects are due to competitive antagonism at adenosine (A_2) receptors and other biochemical actions distinct from their action on cyclic nucleotide phosphodiesterase.

Inhibitors with specificity for different isoenzymes of PDE have been developed, some of which have clinical potential. The most extensively studied isoenzyme is PDE III, and PDE III inhibitors (e.g. **enoximone, amrinone, milrinone**) are positively inotropic vasodilators, and also inhibit platelet aggregation. Short-term administration of amrinone to patients with heart failure increases cardiac output and lowers ventricular filling pressure. However, long-term administration has not been shown to be beneficial, and may indeed shorten survival. Adverse effects include hypotension (secondary to vasodilatation), cardiac arrhythmias (probably secondary to increased cAMP in cardiac cells), thrombocytopenia and, in the case of enoximone, hepatotoxicity. At present these drugs do not play a major role in the treatment of heart failure, although it is possible that more selective PDE III inhibitors currently being developed will do so in future.

Key points

Treatment of chronic cardiac failure

- General measures include dietary salt restriction and reviewing other prescribed drugs which may be negative inotropes (e.g. Ca^{2+} antagonists) or cause salt and water retention (e.g. NSAIDs).
- Initial treatment is with a diuretic (usually a loop diuretic). Frusemide alone (rather than combined with amiloride) is preferred when ACE inhibitor treatment is contemplated.
- An ACE inhibitor (started at low dose and increased to adequate regular dosage), e.g. enalapril twice daily, improves survival. Hypotension should be anticipated when starting treatment ('first-dose hypotension') and diuretics withheld before giving the first dose, usually last thing at night. Serum creatinine and K^+ should be checked soon after starting treatment.
- The combination of nitrate with hydralazine also improves survival, although less so than an ACE inhibitor. It is used when ACE inhibitors are contraindicated or not tolerated.
- Digoxin may be added if the patient remains symptomatic. It is a mainstay of treatment if there is rapid atrial fibrillation. Serum K^+ levels should be checked.
- Promising but controversial newer treatments include growth hormone β-blockers and spironolactone.
- Surgical procedures (e.g. transplantation) are occasionally an option.

Case history

A 62-year-old physician has developed symptoms of chronic congestive cardiac failure in the setting of treated essential hypertension. He had had an angioplasty to an isolated atheromatous lesion in the left anterior descending coronary artery 2 years previously, since when he had not had angina. He also has a past history of gout. He is taking bendrofluazide for his hypertension, takes meclofenamate regularly to prevent recurrences of his gout. He disregarded his cardiologist's advice to take aspirin because he was already taking another cyclo-oxygenase inhibitor (in the form of the meclofenamate). On examination he has a regular pulse of 88 beats/min, blood pressure of 160/98 mmHg, a 4–5 cm raised jugular venous pressure, mild pretibial oedema and cardiomegaly. Routine biochemistry tests are unremarkable except for a serum urate level of 0.76 mmol/L, a total cholesterol concentration of 6.5 mmol/L, a triglyceride concentration of 5.2 mmol/L and γ-glutamyltranspeptidase twice the upper limit of normal. An echocardiogram shows a diffusely poorly contracting myocardium.

Question

Decide whether each of the following would be appropriate as immediate measures.

(a) Digitalization.
(b) Intravenous frusemide.
(c) A detailed personal/social history.
(d) Substitute allopurinol for the meclofenamate.
(e) Hold the bendrofluazide temporarily and start an ACE inhibitor.
(f) Start bezofibrate.

Answer

(a) False.
(b) False.
(c) True.
(d) False.
(e) True.
(f) False.

Comment

The aetiology of the heart failure in this case is uncertain. Although ischaemia and hypertension may be playing a part, the diffusely poorly contracting myocardium suggests the possibility of diffuse cardiomyopathy, and the raised γ-glutamyltranspeptidase and triglyceride levels point to the possibility of alcohol excess. If this is the case, and if it is corrected, this could improve the blood pressure, dyslipidaemia and gout as well as cardiac function. In the long term, allopurinol should be substituted for the NSAID, but if done immediately this is likely to precipitate an acute attack. Aspirin *should* be taken (for its antiplatelet effect, which may not be shared by all other NSAIDs). Treatment with a fibrate would be useful for this pattern of dyslipidaemia, but only after establishing that it was not alcohol-induced.

FURTHER READING

Cleland JGF (ed.) 1993: *The clinician's guide to ACE inhibition*. Edinburgh: Churchill Livingstone.

JN Cohn. 1996: The management of chronic heart failure. *New England Journal of Medicine* **335**, 490–8.

Loh E, Swain E. 1996: Growth hormone for heart failure – cause for cautious optimism. *New England Journal of Medicine* **334**, 856–7.

Pfeffer MA, Stevenson LW. 1996: β-Adrenergic blockers and survival in heart failure. *New England Journal of Medicine* **334**, 1396–7.

Soni N. 1996: Swan-song for the Swan–Ganz catheter? *British Medical Journal* 313, 763–4.

CHAPTER THIRTY-ONE

CARDIAC ARRHYTHMIAS

- Pathophysiology
- Common arrhythmias
- General principles of management
- Classificiation of anti-arrhythmic drugs
- Cardiopulmonary resuscitation: basic life support
- Cardiac arrest: advanced life support
- Treatment of other specific arrhythmias
- Selected anti-arrhythmic drugs

PATHOPHYSIOLOGY

The chambers of the heart contract in a co-ordinated manner, pumping blood efficiently around the body. Co-ordination is achieved by a specialized conducting system. Excitation involves triggering a propagated action potential, which is coupled to contraction by changes in cytoplasmic Ca^{2+} concentration. Cardiac cells share some of the properties of other excitable tissues such as nerve and striated muscle, including:

1 an inside negative 'resting' potential caused by the concentration gradient of K^+ across a relatively K^+-permeable plasma membrane; and
2 a propagated action potential during which the potential inside the cells becomes positive with respect to the outside due to a rapid but transient increase in Na^+ permeability in the presence of high external Na^+ concentration and low cytoplasmic Na^+ concentration.

Cardiac tissues also have distinctive features of their own, including:

1 a prolonged depolarization phase of the action potential during which Ca^{2+} enters through voltage-dependent Ca^{2+} channels; and
2 the capacity of some cardiac tissues to develop spontaneous pacemaker activity.

The most rapid pacemaker, usually the sinoatrial (SA) node, captures the system and determines the heart rate. Action potentials propagate from the SA node to atrial myocytes and also through specialized pathways in the atria to the atrioventricular (AV) node, and then via the bundle of His and Purkinje fibres to the ventricular myocytes. Repolarization follows depolarization, leaving the cells refractory for a brief interval, after which the cycle is repeated. This cycle of orderly propagated depolarization originating in the SA node, followed by repolarization, is known as sinus rhythm. Sinus rhythm is influenced by nervous activity (e.g. it is slowed by the vagus nerve which releases acetylcholine that acts on muscarinic receptors to increase the K^+ permeability of the cardiac membrane, and it is accelerated by sympathetic nerves which release noradrenaline that acts on cardiac β_1–receptors) and by endocrine mechanisms (e.g. circulating catecholamines and thyroxine). These control mechanisms permit the heart rate to adapt appropriately to varying physiological demands, such as exercise.

The cycle of propagated orderly depolarization followed by repolarization is generally extremely reliable, occurring some 2.5–3 $\times$ 10^9 times in a human lifetime. This reliability depends on a 'fall-back' mechanism, whereby if impulse generation in the SA node fails, another pacemaker lower down the conducting system takes over. The cost of this safety net is the innate tendency of cells throughout the heart to initiate independent 'ectopic' (i.e. outside the SA node) pacemakers. Occasional ectopic beats are not sinister. Rarely, however, because of the innate automaticity of cardiac tissue, ectopic beats initiate repetitive activity resulting in an *arrhythmia*. Under pathological circumstances (e.g. in the presence of an abnormal anatomical pathway, or following myocardial infarction, or if there is an abnormal balance of inorganic ions or of chemical mediators) this arrhythmia can temporarily or permanently interrupt sinus rhythm.

COMMON ARRHYTHMIAS

SUPRAVENTRICULAR

Arising from the sinus node

SINUS TACHYCARDIA

In sinus tachycardia the rate is 100–150 beats/min with normal P-waves and PR interval. Treatment is directed at the underlying cause, such as pain, anxiety, left ventricular failure, asthma, thyrotoxicosis, iatrogenic causes (e.g. β-agonists).

SINUS BRADYCARDIA

The rate is less than 60 beats/min with normal complexes. This is common in athletes, in young healthy individuals and patients taking beta-blockers. It also occurs in patients with raised intracranial pressure or SA node disease ('sick-sinus syndrome'), and is common during myocardial infarction. It only requires treatment if it causes or threatens haemodynamic compromise.

Atrial arrhythmias

ATRIAL FIBRILLATION

The atrial rate in atrial fibrillation is > 350 beats/min, with variable AV conduction resulting in an irregular pulse. If the AV node conducts rapidly, the ventricular response is also rapid. Ventricular filling is consequently inadequate and cardiac output falls. The most important methods of treating atrial fibrillation are either to convert it to sinus rhythm, or to slow conduction through the AV node, slowing ventricular rate and improving cardiac output even though the rhythm remains abnormal.

ATRIAL FLUTTER

Atrial flutter has a rate of 250–350/min with fixed ventricular conduction. For example, an atrial rate of 300/min with 3:1 block gives a ventricular rate of 100/min.

Nodal and other supraventricular arrhythmias

ATRIOVENTRICULAR BLOCK

- *First degree* – this consists of prolongation of the PR interval.
- *Second degree* – there are two types, namely Mobitz I, in which the PR interval lengthens progressively until a P-wave fails to be conducted to the ventricles (Wenckebach phenomenon), and Mobitz II, in which there is a constant PR interval with variable failure to conduct to the ventricles.

The importance of first- and second-degree block is that either may presage complete (third-degree) heart block.

- *Third degree* – there is complete AV dissociation with emergence of an idioventricular rhythm (usually < 50/min). Severe cerebral under-perfusion with syncope sometimes followed by convulsions (Stokes–Adams attacks) often results.

Supraventricular tachycardias

Supraventricular tachycardia (SVT) leads to rapid, narrow complex tachycardias at rates of approximately 150/min. Not uncommonly in older patients the rapid rate leads to failure of conduction in one or other bundle and 'aberrant' conduction with broad complexes because of the rate-dependent bundle-branch block. This can be difficult to distinguish from ventricular tachycardia, treatment of which is different in important respects. SVT can be *intranodal* or *extranodal*.

INTRANODAL SUPRAVENTRICULAR TACHYCARDIA

Fibre tracts in the AV node are arranged longitudinally, and if differences in refractoriness develop between adjacent fibres then an atrial impulse may be conducted antegradely through one set of fibres and retrogradely through another, leading to a re-entry ('circus') tachycardia.

EXTRANODAL SUPRAVENTRICULAR TACHYCARDIA

An anatomically separate accessory pathway is present through which conduction is faster and the refractory period shorter than in the AV node. The cardiogram usually shows a shortened PR interval (because the abnormal pathway conducts more rapidly from atria to ventricle than does the AV node), sometimes with a widened QRS complex with a slurred upstroke or delta wave, due to arrival of the impulse in part of the ventricle where it must pass through unspecialized slowly conducting ventricular myocytes instead of through specialized Purkinje fibres (Wolff–Parkinson–White or WPW syndrome). Alternatively, there may be a short PR interval but a normal QRS complex (Lown–Ganong–Levine syndrome) if the abnormal pathway connects with the physiological conducting system distal to the AV node.

Ventricular arrhythmias

1 *Ventricular ectopic beats* – abnormal QRS complexes originating irregularly from ectopic foci in the ventricles.
2 *Ventricular tachycardia* – the cardiogram shows rapid, wide QRS complexes (> 0.14 s), and the patient is usually, but not always, hypotensive and poorly perfused. This rhythm may presage ventricular fibrillation.
3 *Ventricular fibrillation* – the cardiogram is chaotic, and circulatory arrest occurs immediately.

GENERAL PRINCIPLES OF MANAGEMENT

1 Anti-arrhythmic drugs are among the most dangerous at the clinician's disposal. Always think carefully before prescribing one.
2 If the patient is acutely ill on account of a cardiac arrhythmia, the most appropriate treatment is almost never a drug. In bradyarrhythmia, consider pacing, and in tachyarrhythmia consider DC cardioversion. Consider the possibility of hyperkalaemia or other electrolyte disorder, especially in renal disease, and treat accordingly.
3 It is important to treat the patient, not the cardiogram. Remember that several anti-arrhythmic drugs can themselves cause arrhythmias and shorten life. When arrhythmias are prognostically poor, this often reflects severe underlying cardiac disease which is not improved by an anti-arrhythmic drug but which may be improved by, for example, a converting-enzyme inhibitor (for heart failure), aspirin or oxygen (for ischaemic heart disease) or operation (for left main coronary artery disease and valvular heart disease).
4 In an acutely ill patient consider the possible immediate cause of the rhythm disturbance. This may be within the heart (e.g. myocardial infarction, ventricular aneurysm, valvular or congenital heart disease) or elsewhere in the body (e.g. pulmonary embolism, infection or pain, for example from a distended bladder in a stuporose patient).
5 Look for reversible processes that contribute to the maintenance of the rhythm disturbance (e.g. hypoxia, acidosis, pain, electrolyte disturbance including Mg^{2+} as well as K^+ and Ca^{2+}, thyrotoxicosis, excessive alcohol or caffeine intake or pro-arrhythmic drugs), and correct them.
6 Avoid 'cocktails' of drugs.

Key points

Cardiac arrhythmias: general principles

- In emergencies consider:
  - DC shock;
  - pacing.
- Correct pro-arrhythmogenic metabolic disturbances:
  - electrolytes (especially K^+, Mg^{2+})
  - hypoxia/acid-base
  - drugs
- Clinical trials have shown that correcting an arrhythmia does *not* necessarily improve the prognosis – anti-arrhythmic drugs can themselves *cause* arrhythmias.

Classification of anti-arrhythmic drugs

The classification of anti-arrhythmic drugs is not very satisfactory. The Singh–Vaughan–Williams classification (classes I–IV; see Table 31.1), which is based on effects on the cardiac action potential, is widely used, but unfortunately does not reliably predict which rhythm disturbances will respond to which drug. Consequently, selection of the appropriate anti-arrhythmic drug to use in a particular patient remains largely empirical. Furthermore, this classification does not include some of the most clinically useful anti-arrhythmic drugs, some of which are listed in Table 31.2.

Class I

Class I drugs block fast Na^+ channels, thereby slowing the upstroke of the cardiac action potential just as local anaesthetics affect nerve conduction. However, they are selective for open or refractory (rather than resting) channels, so they suppress premature beats or tachyarrhythmias more effectively than they suppress sinus rhythm. They are subdivided into classes Ia, Ib and Ic (see Table 31.3). Class Ia are quinidine-like drugs which also slow repolarization, hence slightly prolonging the action potential; **disopyramide** is an example that is used clinically. Class Ib drugs dissociate very rapidly from the Na^+ channels, and do not prolong repolarization. **Lignocaine** is the most important of these, but has to be given intravenously. Attempts to discover an 'orally active lignocaine' have yielded several drugs with superficially similar electrophysiological effects, such as **tocainide** and **mexilitene**, but despite being 'class Ib' agents they differ from lignocaine in their clinical effect. **Phenytoin** has anti-arrhythmic effects on the heart as well as on the brain, and is also a class Ib drug. However, it is seldom used for its cardiac properties, although it has been used in patients with digoxin-induced arrhythmias. Class Ic drugs (e.g. **flecainide**, **encainide**, **propafenone**) dissociate slowly from Na^+ channels and inhibit conduction in the His–Purkinje system, thereby prolonging the QRS interval. Class Ic drugs predispose to polymorphic ventricular tachycardia which can degenerate into ventricular fibrillation, and clinical trials indicate that they shorten life in some patients. They are now mainly used, under specialist supervision, for prophylaxis of paroxysmal atrial fibrillation.

Table 31.1: Anti-arrhythmic drugs: the Vaughan–Williams/Singh classification

Class	Example	Definition	Comment
I		Rate-dependent block of Na^+ conductance	
a	Quinidine	Intermediate kinetics between b and c	Prolongs cardiac action potential
b	Lignocaine	Rapid dissociation from Na^+ channel	Useful in ventricular tachyarrhythmias
c	Flecainide	Slow dissociation from Na^+ channel	Prolongs His–Purkingje conduction: worsens survival in some instances
II	Atenolol	Slow pacemaker depolarization	Improves survival following myocardial infarction
III	Amiodarone D-Sotalol	Prolong cardiac action potential	Effective in supra- as well as ventricular tachyarrhythmias. Predispose to *torsade de pointes* (a form of ventricular tachycardia); D-sotalol worsens survival in some patients
IV	Verapamil	Block cardiac voltage-dependent Ca^{2+} conductance	Used in prophylaxis of recurrent SVT. Superseded by adenosine for treating attacks. Negatively inotropic

Table 31.2: Drugs/ions not classified primarily as anti-arrhythmic but used to treat important arrhythmias

Digoxin (rapid atrial fibrillation)
Atropine (symptomatic sinus bradycardia)
Adenosine (supraventricular tachycardia)
Adrenaline (cardiac arrest)
Calcium chloride (ventricular tachycardia caused by hyperkalaemia)
Magnesium chloride (ventricular fibrillation)

Class II

Class II drugs are β-adrenoceptor antagonists which reduce the rate of increase of the pacemaker potential. Use of these drugs after myocardial infarction (see Chapter 28) reduces the risk of sudden death and improves survival.

Class III

These drugs prolong the plateau phase of the cardiac action potential, thereby prolonging the QT interval and increasing the absolute refractory period (i.e. the time that must elapse after an action potential before the tissue is again capable of generating an action potential). Such drugs reduce the likelihood of an ectopic pacemaker capturing the system, or of a re-entrant pathway becoming perpetuated, and **amiodarone** and **sotalol** are effective against both ventricular and supraventricular arrhythmias. However, as with other drugs that prolong the QT interval, they predispose to ventricular tachycardia.

Class IV

Class IV drugs are Ca^{2+}-antagonists which block voltage-dependent L-type Ca^{2+} channels. **Verapamil**, a phenylalkylamine, is particularly effective in blocking such channels in AV conducting tissues, and was used acutely to terminate SVT. This use has decreased with the availability of adenosine. Verapamil (given by mouth) remains useful in chronic prophylaxis against recurrent supraventricular tachycardia. In conjunction with digoxin it controls the ventricular rate in patients with rapid atrial fibrillation who are inadequately responsive to digoxin alone.

Cardiopulmonary resuscitation: basic life support

The European Resuscitation Council provides guidelines for basic and advanced life support. When a person is found to have collapsed, make a quick check to ensure that no live power lines are in the immediate vicinity. Ask them, 'Are you all right?', and if there is no response, call for help. Do not move the patient if neck trauma is suspected. Otherwise roll them on their back (on a firm surface if possible) and loosen the clothing around the throat. Assess **A**irway, **B**reathing and **C**irculation (ABC).

Tilt the head and lift the chin, and sweep an index finger through the mouth to clear any obstruction (e.g. dentures). Tight-fitting dentures need not be removed, and may help to maintain the mouth sealed during assisted ventilation.

Table 31.3: Class I anti-arrhythmic drugs

Class	Drug	Comment
Ia	Quinidine	Atropine-like side-effects
	Procainamide	Drug-induced lupus; hypersensitivity
	Disopyramide	Atropine-like side-effects; negative inotrope
Ib	Lignocaine	IV use; see main text
Ic	Flecainide	Predisposes to ventricular tachycardia; used in patients with Wolf–Parkinson–White syndrome with re-entrant tachycardias. Negative inotrope; can cause heart block

If the patient is not breathing spontaneously, start mouth-to-mouth (or, if available, mouth-to-mask) ventilation. Inflate the lungs with two expirations (1–1.5 s), and check that the chest falls between respirations. If available, 100% oxygen should be used.

Check for a pulse by feeling carefully for the carotid or femoral artery before diagnosing cardiac arrest. If the arrest has been witnessed, administer a single thump to the precordium. Start cardiac compression two finger breadths above the xiphisternum at a rate of 60–80/min and an excursion of 1.5–2 in. For a single operator allow two breaths per 15 chest compressions, and if there are two operators give one breath every five compressions. Drugs can cause fixed dilated pupils, so do not give up on this account if drug overdose is a possibility. Hypothermia is protective of tissue function, so do not abandon your efforts too readily if the patient is severely hypothermic (e.g. after being pulled out of a freezing lake). Mobilize facilities for active warming.

Cardiac arrest: advanced life support

Basic cardiopulmonary resuscitation is continued throughout as described above, and it should not be interrupted for more than 10 s (except for administration of DC shock, when personnel apart from the operator must stand well back). 'Advanced' life support refers to the treatment of cardiac arrhythmias in the setting of cardiopulmonary arrest. The electrocardiogram is likely to show *asystole*, severe *bradycardia* or *ventricular fibrillation*. Occasionally narrow complexes are present, but there is no detectable cardiac output (*'electromechanical dissociation'*). The doses given below are for an average-sized adult. During the course of an arrest, other rhythm disturbances are frequently encountered (e.g. sinus bradycardia), and these are considered in the next section on other specific arrhythmias. If intravenous access cannot be established, the administration of double doses of adrenaline (or other drugs as appropriate) via an endotracheal tube can be life-saving.

Asystole

Make sure ECG leads are attached properly, and that the rhythm is not ventricular fibrillation, which is sometimes mistaken for asystole if the fibrillation waves are of low amplitude. If there is doubt, DC counter-shock (200 J). Once the diagnosis is *definite*, administer adrenaline, 1 mg intravenously, followed by atropine, 2 mg intravenously. If P-waves (or other electrical activity) are present, consider pacing.

Ventricular fibrillation

The following sequence is used until a rhythm (hopefully sinus) is achieved that sustains a cardiac output. DC countershock (200 J) is delivered as soon as a defibrillator is available and then repeated (200 J, then 360 J) if necessary, followed by adrenaline, 1 mg intravenously, and further defibrillation (360 J) repeated as necessary. Consider varying the paddle positions, and also consider other anti-arrhythmic drugs (see below), notably amiodarone, 300 mg, intravenously or **bretylium**, 500–1000 mg, if ventricular fibrillation persists. During prolonged resuscitation, adrenaline (1 mg IV) every 5 min is recommended.

Electromechanical dissociation

When the pulse is absent but the ECG shows QRS complexes, this is known as electromechanical dissociation. It may be the result of severe global damage to the left ventricle, in which case the outlook is bleak. If it is caused by some potentially reversible pathology such as hypovolaemia, pneumothorax, pericardial tamponade or pulmonary embolus, volume replacement or other specific measures may be dramatically effective. Adrenaline, 1 mg intravenously, followed by calcium chloride, 10 mL of 10% solution, should be considered. Calcium salts should not be given into the same line as sodium bicarbonate, as this combination results in precipitation of calcium carbonate in the line.

Treatment of other specific arrhythmias

Tachyarrhythmias

Supraventricular

ATRIAL FIBRILLATION

Acute DC cardioversion is the treatment of choice when the patient is hypotensive and poorly perfused (i.e. haemodynamically shocked). Digoxin is useful if the patient is not in shock. It slows ventricular rate by increasing AV block and about 50% of such patients revert to sinus rhythm. Intravenous verapamil (given slowly) is an effective alternative, but is a negative inotrope and can precipitate acute heart failure.

DC shock can cause dangerous arrhythmias in patients who are overdigitalized. To avoid this, the plasma concentration of digoxin should be measured, and if possible more than 24 h should elapse after the last dose of digoxin, unless cardioversion is required as an emergency. Low-energy countershock can be used in this situation, followed by higher-energy shocks only if necessary.

Long-term treatment Patients who have not been in atrial fibrillation for too long and in whom the left atrium is not irreversibly distended may 'spontaneously' revert to sinus rhythm. If this does not occur, such patients benefit from elective DC cardioversion, following which many remain in sinus rhythm. The main hazard is embolization of cerebral or peripheral arteries from thrombus that may have accumulated in the left atrial appendage. Patients should therefore be anticoagulated before elective cardioversion (usually for 4–6 weeks) to prevent new and friable thrombus from accumulating and to permit any existing thrombus to organize, thereby reducing the risk of embolization. An alternative currently undergoing controlled clinical trials is to perform early cardioversion following acute anticoagulation, *provided that transoesophageal echocardiography shows no evidence of thrombus* in the left atrial appendage, anticoagulation being continued for 1 month if the patient remains in sinus rhythm. Anticoagulation should be continued long-term if fibrillation persists or intermittent episodes of arrhythmia recur.

In patients in whom cardioversion is inappropriate (e.g. those with a chronically enlarged left atrium caused by mitral stenosis, in whom sinus rhythm is unlikely to persist even if it can be achieved), digoxin (given by mouth) is the drug of choice. Digoxin is not always adequate to control ventricular rate, and verapamil or a beta-blocker may be added. Amiodarone is very effective, but is only used when other drugs have failed, because of its toxicity (see below).

ATRIAL FLUTTER

Atrial flutter is treated with the same drugs as are effective in atrial fibrillation, but tends to be more resistant to drug treatment. However, it is very responsive to DC cardioversion. Furthermore, in contrast to atrial fibrillation, systemic embolization is unlikely because the regular atrial activity does not predispose to thrombosis in the atrial appendage.

PAROXYSMAL SUPRAVENTRICULAR TACHYCARDIAS

Vagal stimulation (e.g. by carotid sinus massage, facial immersion in cold water, Valsalva manoeuvre or pressure on the eyeballs) may be effective in terminating the arrhythmia. If vagal manoeuvres are ineffective, the next choice is adenosine, given as a rapid intravenous bolus (in increasing doses if necessary). Although it is negatively inotropic, it is cleared rapidly and this effect is brief. Verapamil (10 mg administered intravenously over 5–10 min) is also a negative inotrope, and is cleared much less rapidly than adenosine. It is still sometimes used to terminate SVT in the absence of haemodynamic compromise, although it must be avoided if the patient has been treated with a β-adrenoceptor antagonist, as this combination causes circulatory collapse. β-Adrenoceptor antagonists are themselves effective in terminating SVT, but are *contraindicated* in the presence of haemodynamic compromise or following treatment with verapamil, and are now seldom used.

Patients with underlying heart disease may be haemodynamically compromised by SVT. The best treatment in such cases is usually DC cardioversion, as most drugs used to terminate SVT are negatively inotropic and can be disastrous in this setting. Cardiac glycosides are an important exception, and intravenous ouabain (the most rapidly acting glycoside) or digoxin can be considered in circumstances where DC shock is relatively contraindicated (e.g. post-operatively in cardiac patients who have undergone sternotomy). The decision is often not easy, first because of the extra risk of DC shock if this has to be undertaken in a patient after administration of a glycoside mentioned above, and secondly because of the possibility of previously undiagnosed WPW syndrome. Supraventricular tachycardia in WPW may be worsened by cardiac glycosides or by verapamil because these drugs may dangerously accelerate anterograde conduction in this situation and thus increase ventricular rate. Delta-waves are not present on the ECG in patients with WPW during attacks when conduction through the pathological pathway is retrogradal, so the syndrome can be very difficult to recognize. The rapidity of the ventricular response may warn the clinician of this possibility. Amiodarone is effective in SVT as well as in VT, and can be given slowly intravenously. It is less negatively inotropic than verapamil or β-adrenoceptor antagonists, but is not without risks. If it is used, blood pressure should be monitored carefully.

Recurrence of SVT may not occur. Overindulgence in caffeine or alcohol should be avoided, and smoking should be prohibited. If attacks do recur frequently and do not respond to simple vagal manouevres, prophylactic treatment with an oral β-adrenoceptor antagonist (e.g. atenolol) or verapamil may be effective.

VENTRICULAR ARRHYTHMIAS

Ventricular ectopic beats Electrolyte disturbance, smoking, alcohol abuse and excessive caffeine consumption should be sought and corrected if present. The only justification for treating patients with anti-arrhythmic drugs in an attempt to reduce the frequency of ventricular ectopic beats (VE) in a chronic setting is if the ectopic beats cause intolerable palpitations, or if they precipitate attacks of more serious tachyarrhythmia (e.g. ventricular tachycardia or fibrillation). If palpitations are so unpleasant as to warrant treatment despite the suspicion that this may shorten rather than prolong life, an oral class I agent such as disopyramide may be considered. Sotalol with its combination of class II and III actions is an alternative, although a clinical trial with the D-isomer (which is mainly responsible for its class III action) showed that this worsened survival (the 'SWORD' trial).

In an acute setting (most commonly the immediate aftermath of myocardial infarction), treatment to suppress ventricular ectopic beats may be warranted if these are running together to form brief recurrent episodes of ventricular tachycardia, or if frequent ectopic beats are present following cardioversion from ventricular fibrillation. Lignocaine is used in such situations, and is given as an intravenous bolus followed by an infusion in an attempt to reduce the risk of sustained ventricular tachycardia or ventricular fibrillation.

Ventricular tachycardia If the differential diagnosis from a supraventricular broad complex tachycardia (above) is not in doubt, treatment is usually by DC cardioversion. As an alternative, a bolus of 50–100 mg lignocaine followed by an infusion (1–4 mg/min) with constant monitoring in an intensive-care unit may be considered if the rate is less than 170/min and the blood pressure is well maintained. If the tachycardia is refractory or poorly tolerated, DC cardioversion followed by lignocaine infusion is indicated. Intravenous amiodarone is used for patients who are refractory to lignocaine.

Ventricular fibrillation See above under 'Cardiac arrest: Advanced life support'.

BRADYARRHYTHMIAS

Asystole

See above under 'Cardiac arrest: advanced life support'.

Sinus bradycardia

1 Raising the foot of the bed may be successful in increasing cardiac output and cerebral perfusion.
2 Give atropine (see below).
3 *Discontinue* digoxin, beta-blockers, verapamil or other drugs that exacerbate bradycardia.

4 Pacemaker insertion is indicated if bradycardia is unresponsive to atropine and is causing significant hypotension.

Sick sinus syndrome (tachycardia–bradycardia syndrome)

Treatment is difficult. Drugs that are useful for one rhythm often aggravate the other, and a pacemaker is often needed.

Atrioventricular conduction block

- *First-degree* heart block by itself does not require treatment.
- *Second-degree* Mobitz type I block (Wenckebach block) is relatively benign and often transient. If complete block occurs, the escape pacemaker is situated relatively high up in the bundle so that the rate is 50–60/min with narrow QRS complexes. Atropine (0.6–1.2 mg intravenously) is usually effective. Mobitz type II block is more serious, and may progress unpredictably to complete block with a slow ventricular escape rate. The only reliable treatment is a pacemaker.
- *Third-degree* heart block (complete AV dissociation) can cause cardiac failure and/or attacks of unconsciousness (Stokes–Adams attacks). Treatment is by electrical pacing; if delay in arranging this is absolutely unavoidable, isoprenaline is sometimes used as a temporizing measure. Congenital complete heart block, diagnosed incidentally, does not usually require treatment.

SELECTED ANTI-ARRHYTHMIC DRUGS

Lignocaine and other class I drugs

USE

Lignocaine is important in the treatment of ventricular tachycardia and fibrillation, often as an adjunct to DC cardioversion. An effective plasma concentration is rapidly achieved by giving a bolus of 50–100 mg intravenously over 1 min followed by an infusion of 4 mg/min for 1 h, reducing to 2 mg/min for 2 h and to 1 mg/min thereafter for a period not usually exceeding 36–48 h. Lower doses are required in patients with shock or severe hepatic dysfunction, in whom the initial infusion should not exceed 1 mg/min.

MECHANISM OF ACTION

Lignocaine is a class Ib agent that blocks Na^+ channels, reducing the rate of increase of the cardiac action potential and increasing the effective refractory period. It selectively blocks open or inactivated channels (causing use-dependent block) and dissociates very rapidly.

ADVERSE EFFECTS

These include the following:

1 *central nervous system* – drowsiness, twitching, paraesthesia, nausea and vomiting; focal followed by generalized seizures;
2 *cardiovascular system* – bradycardia, cardiac depression (negative inotropic effect), and asystole.

PHARMACOKINETICS

Oral bioavailability is poor (30%) and lignocaine is given intravenously. It is metabolized in the liver, its clearance being limited by hepatic blood flow. Heart failure reduces lignocaine clearance, predisposing to toxicity unless the dose is reduced. The therapeutic plasma concentration range is 1.5–4.0 mg/L. The difference between therapeutic and toxic plasma concentrations is small. Monoethylglycylxylidide (MEGX) and glycylxylidide (GX) are active metabolites with less anti-arrhythmic action than lignocaine, but with central nervous system toxicity. The mean half-life of lignocaine is approximately 2 h in healthy subjects, with an apparent volume of distribution of approximately 1.5 L/kg.

DRUG INTERACTIONS

Negative inotropes reduce lignocaine clearance by reducing hepatic blood flow, and consequently predispose to accumulation and toxicity.

OTHER CLASS I DRUGS

Other class I drugs have been widely used in the past, but are now used much less frequently. Some of these drugs are shown in Table 31.3.

β-Adrenoreceptor antagonists

see also Chapter 27 p. 262–66)

USE

Anti-arrhythmic properties of β-adrenoceptor antagonists are useful in the following clinical situations:

1. patients who have survived myocardial infarction (irrespective of any ECG evidence of arrhythmia); β-adrenoceptor antagonists prolong life in this situation;
2. inappropriate sinus tachycardia (e.g. in association with panic attacks);
3. paroxysmal supraventricular tachycardias that are precipitated by emotion or exercise;
4. rapid atrial fibrillation that is inadequately controlled by digoxin;
5. tachyarrhythmias of thyrotoxicosis;
6. tachyarrhythmias of phaeochromocytoma, after adequate α-receptor blockade.

Atenolol, 2.5 mg administered over 2.5 min, repeated at 5-min intervals as needed to a maximum total dose of 10 mg is available for intravenous use after myocardial infarction. Esmolol is a cardioselective β-adrenoceptor antagonist for intravenous use with a short duration of action (its elimination half-life, $t_{\frac{1}{2}}$, is approximately 10 min). β-Adrenoceptor antagonists are given more commonly by mouth when used for the above indications. Oral doses of atenolol greater than 100 mg or of metoprolol greater than 200 mg are seldom needed.

CONTRAINDICATIONS

Beta-blocking drugs, whether non-selective or of the currently available partially cardioselective variety, can cause catastrophic airways obstruction in patients with pre-existing obstructive airways disease – whether asthma, emphysema or chronic bronchitis – and are relatively contraindicated in these conditions. Their negative inotropic action renders them potentially hazardous in patients with heart failure (although low doses are currently sometimes used by cardiologists in selected patients with heart failure and sympathetic overactivity). They also predictably worsen symptoms of claudication in patients with symptomatic atheromatous peripheral vascular disease, and symptoms of Raynaud's phenomenon in susceptible patients.

DRUG INTERACTIONS

- Beta-blockers inhibit drug metabolism indirectly by decreasing hepatic blood flow secondary to decreased cardiac output. This causes accumulation of drugs such as lignocaine that have such a high hepatic extraction ratio that their clearance reflects hepatic blood flow.
- Pharmacodynamic interactions – increased negative inotropic effects occur with verapamil (if given intravenously this can be fatal), lignocaine, disopyramide or other negative inotropes. Exaggerated and prolonged hypoglycaemia occurs with insulin and oral hypoglycaemic drugs.

Amiodarone

USE

Amiodarone is highly effective, but its use is limited by the severity of its adverse effects during chronic administration. It is effective in a wide variety of arrhythmias, including:

1. *supraventricular arrhythmias* – resistant atrial fibrillation or flutter, re-entrant tachycardias (e.g. WPW syndrome);
2. *ventricular arrhythmias* – recurrent ventricular tachycardia or fibrillation.

Amiodarone does not preclude the use of DC cardioversion, and may be used to maintain sinus rhythm if cardioversion is successful. It is given intravenously via a central line to avoid thrombophlebitis. Initially 5 mg/kg in 250 mL of 5% glucose is infused over a period 20 min to 2 h (to avoid hypotension), and may be repeated as needed up to 15 mg/kg/24 h. In cardiac arrest with refractory or recurrent ventricular fibrillation it is given as a slow injection of 150–300 mg over 1–2 min. Oral treatment is started when a response is established. For patients who have not received intravenous treatment, 200 mg three times a day for 7 days followed by 200 mg twice daily for a week and 200 mg once daily for a week (or until the desired effect is achieved) helps to establish adequate tissue levels reasonably quickly. The lowest effective dose, usually 100–200 mg daily, is used for maintenance.

MECHANISM OF ACTION

Amiodarone is a class III agent, prolonging the duration of the action potential but with no effect on its rate of rise, and prolonging repolarization by reducing the permeability of the cell membrane to outward potassium current. It also reduces the slope of diastolic depolarization (i.e. the pacemaker potential), and at the sinus node this action reduces the resting heart rate. It delays atrial and AV nodal conduction but has no effect on ventricular conduction.

ADVERSE EFFECTS AND CONTRAINDICATIONS

Adverse effects are many and varied, and are common when the plasma amiodarone concentration exceeds 2.5 mg/L.

1 *Cardiac effects* – the ECG may show prolonged QT, U-waves or deformed T-waves, but these are not in themselves an indication to discontinue treatment. Amiodarone can cause ventricular tachycardia of the variety known as *torsades de pointes*. Care is needed in patients with heart failure, and the drug is contraindicated in the presence of sinus bradycardia or AV block.

2 *Eye* – Amiodarone eventually causes corneal microdeposits in almost all patients. Electron microscopy shows deposits (possibly of drug or metabolite) in tissue macrophages. These deposits form linear opacities that radiate in a fan-like manner throughout the corneal epithelium from a point below the centre of the cornea (described as '*une image de la moustache du chat*'). Patients may report coloured haloes without a change in visual acuity. The deposits are only seen on slit-lamp examination, and gradually regress if the drug is stopped.

3 *Skin* – photosensitivity rashes occur in 10–30% of patients. They are a phototoxic response to wavelengths in both the long ultraviolet (UVA) and visible parts of the spectrum, so ordinary sunscreens (which only protect against UV below 320 nm in wavelength) are ineffective. Topical compounds which reflect both UVA and visible light are needed (e.g. zinc oxide), and patients should be advised to avoid exposure to direct sunlight and to wear a broad-brimmed hat in sunny weather. Patients sometimes develop blue-grey pigmentation of exposed areas. This is a separate phenomenon to phototoxicity.

4 *Thyroid* – amiodarone contains 37% iodine by weight, and may precipitate hyperthyroidism in susceptible individuals, or conversely cause hypothyroidism. It alters thyroid function tests, and specific methods must be used. Usually there is a rise in thyroxine (T_4) and reverse 3,5,3′-tri-iodothyronine (rT_3) with a normal or low T_3 and a flat thyroid-stimulating hormone (TSH) response to thyroid-relaxing hormone (TRH). Thyroid function (T_3, T_4 and TSH) should be assessed before starting treatment and annually thereafter, or more often if the clinical picture suggests thyroid dysfunction.

5 *Pulmonary fibrosis* – (evidenced by dyspnoea with interstitial infiltrates on chest X-ray) may develop with prolonged use. This usually but not always improves on stopping the drug. Improvement may be accelerated by prednisolone.

6 *Hepatitis* – transient elevation of hepatic enzymes may occur, and occasionally severe hepatitis develops.

7 *Peripheral neuropathy* – this occurs in the first month of treatment, and reverses on stopping dosing. Proximal muscle weakness, ataxia, tremor, nightmares, insomnia and headache are also reported.

8 *Gastrointestinal intolerance and cardiac failure* – these are unusual, but can be severe.

PHARMACOKINETICS

Amiodarone is variably absorbed (20–80%) when administered orally. However, both the parent drug and its main metabolite, desethyl amiodarone (the plasma concentration of which exceeds that of the parent drug), are highly lipid soluble. This is reflected in a very large volume of distribution (approximately 5000 L). It is highly plasma protein bound (> 90%) and accumulates in all tissues, particularly the heart. It is only slowly eliminated via the liver, with a $t_{\frac{1}{2}}$ of 28–45 days. Consequently, anti-arrhythmic activity may continue for several months after dosing has been stopped. The therapeutic plasma concentration range is 0.5–1.5 mg/L.

DRUG INTERACTIONS

Amiodarone potentiates warfarin by inhibiting its metabolism. It can precipitate digoxin toxicity (the digoxin dose should be reduced by 50% when amiodarone is added), and can cause severe bradycardia if used with β-adrenoceptor antagonists or verapamil.

Sotalol

USE

Sotalol has a different spectrum of adverse effects to amiodarone. The usual dose is 120–240 mg as a single daily dose by mouth. In urgent situations it can be given by slow intravenous injection, 20–60 mg over 3 min or longer with ECG monitoring, repeated if necessary after 10 min. The plasma K^+ concentration should be monitored during chronic use, and corrected if it is low in order to reduce the risk of *torsades de pointes* (see below).

MECHANISM OF ACTION

Sotalol is unique among β-adrenoceptor antagonists in possessing substantial class III activity. It is a racemate, the D-isomer possessing exclusively class III activity. A clinical trial of D-sotalol (the 'SWORD' study) indicated that it *reduces* survival in patients with ventricular ectopic activity, so the racemate is used.

ADVERSE EFFECTS AND CONTRAINDICATIONS

Sotalol has a different spectrum of adverse effects to amiodarone, but since it does prolong the cardiac action potential (detected on the ECG as a prolonged QT interval) it can cause ventricular tachycardia of the *torsade de pointes* variety, like amiodarone. Hypokalaemia predisposes to this effect, since it is the inward K^+ current that causes repolarization. The beta-blocking activity of sotolol contraindicates its use in patients with obstructive airways disease, heart failure, peripheral vascular disease or heart block.

PHARMACOKINETICS

Sotalol is extremely polar and is excreted unchanged in the urine. The dose should be reduced in patients with renal impairment (glomerular filtration rate < 20 mL/min).

DRUG INTERACTIONS

Diuretics predispose to *torsades de pointes* by causing electrolyte disturbance (hypokalaemia/ hypomagnesaemia). Similarly, other drugs that prolong the QT interval should be avoided. These include class Ia anti-arrhythmic drugs (quinidine, disopyramide), which slow cardiac repolarization as well as depolarization, and several important psychotropic drugs, including tricyclic antidepressants and phenothiazines. Histamine H_1-antagonists (terfenadine, astemizole) should be avoided for the same reason.

Verapamil

USE

Verapamil is used as an anti-arrhythmic:

1. prophylactically to reduce the risk of recurrent SVT by mouth (40–120 mg three times daily);
2. to reduce the ventricular rate in patients with atrial fibrillation who are not adequately controlled by digoxin alone;
3. to terminate SVT in patients who are not haemodynamically compromised. In this setting it is given intravenously over 5 min. Adenosine is generally preferred, but verapamil may be useful in patients in whom adenosine is contraindicated (e.g. asthmatics).

Intravenous verapamil is given during continuous electrocardiographic monitoring; 10 mg may be given over 5 min, followed if necessary by a further 5 mg after 5 min. The oral dose is 40–120 mg three times daily. This is about 10 times the intravenous dose, the difference being due to extensive presystemic metabolism (see below). A sustained-release preparation (240 mg once daily) is convenient, but may be less effective as an anti-arrhythmic because of high presystemic hepatic clearance of the isomer responsible for its effect on cardiac conducting tissue. Intravenous verapamil must not be given to patients who are receiving beta-blockers, as this combination can cause severe AV block and asystole. Oral verapamil is used as an alternative to a β-adrenoceptor antagonist for patients in whom digoxin alone has failed to control ventricular rate in atrial fibrillation. This requires care, because verapamil reduces digoxin excretion, and the dose of digoxin should therefore be halved when these drugs are combined. For the same reason, verapamil is contraindicated in patients with digoxin toxicity, especially as these drugs also have a potentially fatal additive effect on the AV node.

MECHANISM OF ACTION

Verapamil blocks L-type voltage-dependent Ca^{2+} channels. It is a class IV drug and has greater effects on cardiac conducting tissue than other Ca^{2+} antagonists. In common with other calcium antagonists, it relaxes the smooth muscle of peripheral arterioles and veins, and of coronary arteries. It is a negative inotrope, as cytoplasmic Ca^{2+} is crucial for cardiac contraction. As an anti-arrhythmic drug its major effect is to slow intracardiac conduction, particularly through the AV node. This reduces the ventricular response in atrial fibrillation and flutter, and abolishes most re-entry nodal tachycardias. Mild resting bradycardia is common, together with prolongation of the PR interval.

ADVERSE EFFECTS AND CONTRAINDICATIONS

1 *Cardiovascular effects* – Verapamil is contraindicated in cardiac failure because of the negative inotropic effect. It is also contraindicated in sick sinus syndrome or intracardiac conduction block. It can cause hypotension, AV block or other bradyarrhythmias (calcium gluconate, atropine and/or isoprenaline may be useful in emergency situations precipitated by verapamil toxicity). It is contraindicated in WPW syndrome complicated by supraventricular tachycardia, atrial flutter or atrial fibrillation, as it can increase the rate of conduction through the accessory pathway. Verapamil is ineffective in ventricular arrhythmias, and its negative inotropic effect makes its inadvertent use in such arrhythmias extremely hazardous.

2 *Gastrointestinal tract* – about one-third of patients experience constipation, although this can usually be prevented or managed successfully with advice about increased dietary intake of fibre and use of laxatives if necessary.

3 *Other adverse effects* – headache, dizziness and facial flushing are related to vasodilatation (compare with similar or worse symptoms caused by other calcium-channel blockers). Drug rashes, pain in the gums and a metallic taste in the mouth are uncommon.

PHARMACOKINETICS

Verapamil is a racemic mixture of (−) and (+) isomers. The (−) isomer is much more potent than the (+) isomer. Although verapamil is well absorbed after oral administration, its bioavailability is only 10–20%, due to presystemic elimination which is stereoselective, the (−) isomer being preferentially metabolized. This explains the observation that even when equivalent total verapamil concentrations are achieved, the effect on the PR interval is greater for the same total plasma concentration after intravenous than after oral dosing. This is due to higher concentrations of the more active (−) isomer after an intravenous dose. Verapamil is highly protein bound in plasma. It is metabolized by the liver, one of the metabolites (norverapamil) being active. Its mean $t_{\frac{1}{2}}$ is 3–7 h in healthy individuals, but is significantly prolonged in patients with liver disease. Sustained-release preparations permit the use of once daily dosing.

DRUG INTERACTIONS

The important pharmacodynamic interaction of verapamil with β-adrenoceptor antagonists, which occurs especially when one or other member of the pair is administered intravenously, contraindicates their combined use by this route. The pharmacokinetic interaction whereby it increases digoxin concentration and the pharmacodynamic interaction with digoxin was described at the beginning of this section.

Adenosine

USE

Adenosine is used to terminate SVT. In addition to its use in regular narrow complex tachycardia, it is useful diagnostically in patients with regular broad complex tachycardia which is suspected of being SVT with aberrant conduction. If adenosine terminates the tachycardia, this implies that the AV node is indeed involved. However, if this diagnosis is wrong (as is not infrequently the case) and the patient actually has VT, little or no harm results, in contrast to the use of verapamil in VT. Adenosine is administered into a peripheral vein as a bolus followed by a saline flush. The starting dose is 0.05 mg/kg, increasing in increments of 0.05 mg/kg at intervals of 1 min or more until the SVT terminates or a total dose of approximately 20 mg has been given.

MECHANISM OF ACTION

Adenosine acts on specific adenosine receptors. A_1-receptors block AV nodal conduction. Adenosine also constricts bronchial smooth muscle by an

A_1 effect, especially in asthmatics. It relaxes vascular smooth muscle, stimulates nociceptive afferent neurones in the heart and inhibits platelet aggregation via A_2-receptors.

ADVERSE EFFECTS AND CONTRAINDICATIONS

Chest pain, flushing, shortness of breath, dizziness and nausea are common but short-lived. Chest pain can be alarming if the patient is not warned of its benign nature before the drug is administered. Adenosine is contraindicated in patients with asthma or heart block (unless already paced), and should be used with care in patients with WPW syndrome in whom the ventricular rate during atrial fibrillation may be accelerated as a result of blocking the normal AV nodal pathway and hence favouring conduction through the abnormal pathway. This theoretically increases the risk of ventricular fibrillation; however, this risk is probably small, and should not discourage the use of adenosine in patients with broad complex tachycardias of uncertain origin.

PHARMACOKINETICS

Adenosine is rapidly cleared from the circulation by uptake into red blood cells and by enzymes on the luminal surface of endothelial cells. It is deaminated to inosine. The circulatory effects of a bolus therapeutic dose of adenosine last for 20–30 s, although effects on the airways in asthmatics persist for longer.

DRUG INTERACTIONS

Dipyridamole blocks cellular adenosine uptake, and potentiates its action. Theophylline blocks adenosine receptors, and inhibits its action.

Digoxin

See also Chapter 30.

USE

The main use of digoxin as an anti-arrhythmic drug is to control the ventricular rate (and hence improve cardiac output) in patients with atrial fibrillation. Digoxin is usually given orally, but if this is impossible, or if a rapid effect is needed, it can be given intravenously (0.5 mg given over 30 min). Since the $t_{\frac{1}{2}}$ is approximately 1–2 days in patients with normal renal function, repeated administration of a maintenance dose results in a plateau concentration within about 3–6 days. This is acceptable in many settings, but if clinical circumstances are more urgent, a therapeutic plasma concentration can be achieved more rapidly by administering a loading dose (e.g. 0.5 mg followed by 0.25 mg 8-hourly for three doses followed by a maintenance dose of 62.5–500 μg daily). The dose is adjusted according to the response, sometimes supplemented by plasma concentration measurement.

MECHANISM OF ACTION

1 Digoxin inhibits membrane Na^+/K^+-adenosine triphosphatase (ATPase), which is responsible for the active extrusion of Na^+ from myocardial as well as other cells. This results in accumulation of intracellular Na^+, which indirectly increases the intracellular Ca^{2+} content via Na^+/Ca^{2+} exchange and intracellular Ca^{2+} storage. The rise in availability of intracellular Ca^{2+} accounts for the positive inotropic effect of digoxin. Excessive poisoning of Na^+/K^+-ATPase is responsible for numerous non-cardiac as well as cardiac (arrhythmogenic) toxic effects of digoxin.

2 Slowing of the ventricular rate results from several mechanisms, particularly increased vagal activity:
- delayed conduction through the atrioventricular node and bundle of His. This is particularly important in atrial fibrillation, where the atria discharge at very high rates (350/min) and the ventricles follow irregularly with some degree of block. Delaying AV conduction increases the degree of block and slows the ventricular response;
- increased cardiac output due to the positive inotropic effect of digoxin reduces reflex sympathetic tone;
- small doses of digitalis sensitize the sinoatrial node to vagal impulses.

Atropine

USE

Atropine is administered intravenously (0.3–0.6 mg doses, repeated if necessary up to a maximum of 2.4 mg) to patients with haemodynamic compromise due to inappropriate sinus bradycardia. (It is also used for several other non-cardiological indications, including anaesthetic premedication, topical application to the eye to produce mydriasis, and for patients who have been poisoned with organophosphorous anticholinesterase drugs; (see Chapter 53).

MECHANISM OF ACTION

Acetylcholine released by the vagus nerve acts on muscarinic receptors in atrial and cardiac conducting tissues. This increases K^+ permeability, thereby shortening the cardiac action potential and slowing the rate of increase of pacemaker potentials and cardiac rate. Atropine is a selective antagonist of acetylcholine at muscarinic receptors, and it thereby counters these actions of acetylcholine, accelerating the heart rate in patients with sinus bradycardia by inhibiting excessive vagal tone.

ADVERSE EFFECTS AND CONTRAINDICATIONS

Parasympathetic blockade by atropine produces widespread effects, including reduced salivation, lachrymation and sweating, decreased secretions in the gut and respiratory tract, tachycardia, urinary retention in men, constipation, pupillary dilatation and ciliary paralysis. It is contraindicated in patients with narrow-angle glaucoma. Many of the acetylcholine receptors in the brain are antagonized by atropine (atropine-like drugs are used to prevent motion sickness and to treat some of the manifestations of Parkinsonism). Atropine can cause central nervous system effects, including hallucinations. (Atropine is the active alkaloid in deadly nightshade, and is named after Atrope, the Fate responsible for cutting the lifeline in Greek mythology.)

PHARMACOKINETICS

Although atropine is completely absorbed after oral administration, it is administered intravenously to obtain a rapid effect when treating sinus bradycardia when this is causing haemodynamic compromise following myocardial infarction.

Adrenaline

USE

Although not usually classed as an 'anti-arrhythmic' drug (it is, of course, powerfully pro-arrhythmogenic in healthy individuals), adrenaline is used in the emergency treatment of patients with cardiac arrest (whether due to asystole, electromechanical dissociation or ventricular fibrillation). For these indications it is administered intravenously (or sometimes directly into the heart or down an endotracheal tube) (see the above section on cardiac arrest). It has important uses other than in cardiac arrest, being essential for treatment of *anaphylactic shock* (see Chapter 49) and useful in combination with local anaesthetics to reduce their rate of removal from their injection site (see Chapter 23).

MECHANISM OF ACTION

Adrenaline is a potent and non-selective agonist at both α- and β-receptors. It causes an increased rate of depolarization of cardiac pacemaker potential, in addition to increasing the force of contraction of the heart and intense α_1-mediated peripheral vasoconstriction (thereby producing a very marked pressor response), which is partly offset by β_2-mediated arterial vasodilation.

ADVERSE EFFECTS

Adrenaline is powerfully pro-arrhythmogenic, and increases the work of the heart (and hence its oxygen requirement). Its peripheral vasoconstrictor effect can reduce tissue perfusion. For these reasons it is only used systemically in emergency situations.

PHARMACOKINETICS

Adrenaline is rapidly eliminated from the circulation by a high-affinity/low-capacity uptake process into sympathetic nerve terminals ('uptake 1'), and by a lower-affinity/higher-capacity process into a variety of tissues ('uptake 2'). It is subsequently metabolized by monoamine oxidase and catechol-O-methyl transferase, and is excreted in the urine as inactive metabolites, including vanillyl mandelic acid (VMA). The latter is measured as a screening test in patients in whom phaeochromocytoma (a tumour that secretes noradrenaline or adrenaline) is suspected (see Chapter 39).

DRUG INTERACTIONS

Tricyclic antidepressants block uptake 1, and so may potentiate the action of adrenaline. Adrenoceptor antagonists, both α and β, block its actions at these receptors.

Isoprenaline

USE

Isoprenaline is used to speed up the heart in those few patients who are haemodynamically compromised because of complete heart block, and in whom pacing is impractical. It is a temporizing measure while pacing facilities are mobilized. Although it can speed the idioventricular rhythm in such patients, thereby improving cardiac output, the disadvantage is increased oxygen demand and hence possible extension of myocardial infarction and increased risk of serious ventricular tachyarrhythmia. It therefore tends to be used as a last resort. It is given by intravenous infusion (starting dose 1 μg/min, increasing if necessary by 1 μg/min increments up to a maximum of 5 μg/min). It is also sometimes used after myocardial infarction or cardiac arrest when complicated by other severe bradyarrhythmias that are unresponsive to atropine. In addition, it may be useful in managing patients poisoned with β-adrenoceptor antagonists, with verapamil or with disopyramide.

Calcium chloride

USE

Calcium chloride is uniquely valuable for treating the broad complex ('sine-wave') ventricular tachycardia that is a pre-terminal event in patients with severe hyperkalaemia (often secondary to renal failure; see Chapter 35). Its use may 'buy time' during which other measures to lower the plasma potassium concentration (e.g. glucose with insulin, ion-binding resins, dialysis) can take effect or be mobilized. Calcium chloride is given as a slow intravenous injection of 5–10 mL (not more than 2 mL/min of 10% solution of the dihydrate, which is what is provided in prefilled syringes in most cardiac arrest boxes: 10 mL contain 6.8 mmol calcium). It is also used in patients with cardiac arrest due to electromechanical dissociation. In addition calcium chloride is used in patients with hypocalcaemia, but these usually present with tetany rather than with cardiac arrhythmia. It may be useful for treating patients who have received an overdose of Ca^{2+}-antagonists such as verapamil or diltiazem.

MECHANISM OF ACTION

Ca^{2+} is a divalent cation. Divalent cations are involved in maintaining the stability of the membrane potential in excitable tissues, including the heart. The outer aspects of cell membranes contain fixed negative charges that influence the electric field in the membrane, and hence the state of activation of voltage-dependent ion channels (Na^+ and Ca^{2+}) in the membrane. Divalent cations bind to the outer membrane, neutralizing the negative charges and in effect hyperpolarizing the membrane. Conversely, if the extracellular concentration of Ca^{2+} falls, Ca^{2+} dissociates from the membrane, rendering it more unstable. Consequently, a single stimulus to a nerve axon can give rise to a train of action potentials (tetany), and presumably similar instability underlies the cardiac arrhythmias that can accompany hypocalcaemia and hypomagnesaemia.

ADVERSE EFFECTS AND CONTRAINDICATIONS

Calcium phosphate can precipitate in the kidneys of patients with hyperphosphataemia, worsening renal function. However, this consideration is irrelevant when one is faced with a hyperkalaemic patient with broad complex tachycardia.

DRUG INTERACTIONS

Calcium carbonate precipitates if calcium chloride solution is mixed with sodium bicarbonate. Therefore these two drugs should not be given simultaneously through the same line, or consecutively without an intervening saline flush. Calcium increases digoxin toxicity, and calcium chloride must not be administered if this is suspected.

Magnesium

USE

Magnesium sulphate (10 mL of a 50% solution over 1 h) is used in broad complex tachycardia in the peri-arrest situation, in conjuction with other treatment (DC shock, lignocaine and correction of hypokalaemia). Intravenous magnesium sulphate is sometimes effective in treating arrhythmias caused by digoxin, and in drug-induced *torsades de pointes*. One clinical trial suggested that it was of value when administered prophylactically in patients with acute myocardial infarction, but this was not born out by the larger ISIS-IV study (see Chapter 28). It is invaluable in eclampsia in prevention of further convulsions (see Chapter 27). The precise place of magnesium therapy for arrhythmia in the context of acute myocardial infarction is still being worked out, and the optimum dose is uncertain. One recommendation is for 50 mmol magnesium added to 5% dextrose and infused over 12 h in patients following acute myocardial infarction. In urgent situations 8 mmol may be given intravenously by slow injection. Magnesium chloride may be particularly useful in settings where magnesium deficiency is common. These include prior chronic diuretic treatment, hypocalcaemia, hypokalaemia, alcoholism, diarrhoea, vomiting, drainage from a fistula, pancreatitis, hyperaldosteronism or prolonged infusion of intravenous fluid without magnesium supplementation. There is no simple test currently available to detect total body magnesium deficiency, since Mg^{2+} is predominantly an intracellular cation. However, serial plasma magnesium determinations may be useful in preventing excessive dosing with accumulation and toxicity.

MECHANISM OF ACTION

Mg^{2+} is a divalent cation, and at least some of its beneficial effects are probably due to the consequent neutralization of fixed negative charges on the outer aspect of the cardiac cell membranes. In addition, Mg^{2+} is a vasodilator and releases prostacyclin from damaged vascular tissue *in vitro*. Unlike Ca^{2+}, Mg^{2+} does *not* trigger transmitter release or excitation contraction coupling, and indeed it blocks excitatory actions of glutamate on central N-methyl D-aspartate (NMDA) receptors by preventing Ca^{2+} entry.

ADVERSE EFFECTS AND CONTRAINDICATIONS

Excessively high extracellular concentrations of Mg^{2+} can cause neuromuscular blockade. Magnesium chloride should be used with great caution in patients with renal impairment or hypotension, and in patients receiving drugs with neuromuscular blocking activity, including aminoglycoside antibiotics. Mg^{2+} can cause AV block.

PHARMACOKINETICS

Magnesium salts are not well absorbed from the gastrointestinal tract, accounting for their efficacy as osmotic laxatives when given by mouth. Mg^{2+} is eliminated in the urine, and therapy with magnesium salts should be avoided or the dose reduced (and frequency of determination of plasma Mg^{2+} concentration increased) in patients with glomerular filtration rates of < 20 mL/min.

DRUG INTERACTIONS

Magnesium salts form precipitates if they are mixed with sodium bicarbonate and, as with calcium chloride, magnesium salts should not be administered at the same time as sodium bicarbonate, or through the same line without an intervening saline flush. Hypermagnesaemia increases neuromuscular blockade caused by drugs with nicotinic-receptor-antagonist properties (e.g. pancuronium, aminoglycosides).

Bretylium

USE

Bretylium is used to treat recurrent ventricular fibrillation or ventricular tachycardia after DC cardioversion and lignocaine have failed. Amiodarone may be preferable in this situation, although there are no controlled data to support this view. In a controlled comparison with lignocaine in 147 patients with out-of-hospital cardiac arrest, bretylium and lignocaine were found to be similarly effective. Bretylium tosylate is given as a rapid intravenous bolus (5 mg/kg) in cardiac arrest, and this dose can be repeated once if necessary.

MECHANISM OF ACTION

Bretylium is taken up rapidly by the uptake 1 mechanism in adrenergic nerve terminals. It causes release of endogenous noradrenaline, followed by blockade of further release ('adrenergic neurone blockade'), probably because the high concentration in the nerve terminal acts as a local anaesthetic, preventing propagation of action potentials in the sympathetic nerve axons into the terminals. This latter property underlies its hypotensive effect (it used to be given by mouth to treat hypertension, but often caused unacceptable postural hypotension). It is also said to have a class III action on Purkinje fibres and to a lesser extent on ventricular myocytes. The precise mechanism of its action in terminating ventricular fibrillation or tachycardia is unknown. A type II action (i.e. anti-adrenergic) has been invoked, but seems unlikely, as it can have a rapid effect on ventricular fibrillation whereas its adrenergic neurone-blocking action is delayed, and because its behaviour is so different qualitatively from that of other class II agents. *Release of endogenous noradrenaline*, perhaps combined with a class III action, is probably responsible for the therapeutic effect.

ADVERSE EFFECTS

Nausea and vomiting are common after rapid intravenous injection, and subsequent hypotension is inevitable.

Case history

A 66-year-old man made a good recovery from a transmural (Q-wave) anterior myocardial infarction complicated by mild transient left ventricular dysfunction, and was sent home taking aspirin, atenolol, enalapril and simvastatin. Three months later, when he is seen in out-patients, he is feeling reasonably well but is worried by palpitations. His pulse is irregular, but there are no other abnormal findings on examination and his ECG shows frequent multifocal ventricular ectopic beats.

Question

Decide whether management might appropriately include each of the following.

(a) Consideration of cardiac catheterization.
(b) Invasive electrophysiological studies, including provocation of arrhythmia.
(c) Adding flecainide.
(d) Stopping atenolol.
(e) Adding verapamil.
(f) Adding amiodarone.

Answer

(a) True.
(b) False.
(c) False.
(d) False.
(e) False.
(f) False.

Comment

It is important to continue a beta-blocker, which will improve this patient's survival. It is appropriate to consider cardiac catheterization to define his coronary anatomy and to identify whether he would benefit from some revascularization procedure. Other classes of anti-arrhythmic drugs have not been demonstrated to prolong life in this setting. If the symptom of palpitation is sufficiently troublesome, it would be reasonable to consider switching from atenolol to regular (i.e. racemic) sotolol.

Case history

A 16-year-old girl is brought to the Accident and Emergency department by her mother having collapsed at home. As a baby she had cardiac surgery, and was followed up by a paediatric cardiologist until the age of 12 years, when she rebelled. She was always small for her age, and did not play games but went to a normal school and was studying for her GCSE examinations. On examination, she is ill and unable to give a history, and has a heart rate of 160 beats/min (regular) and blood pressure of 80/60 mmHg. There are cardiac murmurs which are difficult to characterize. The ECG shows a broad complex regular tachycardia which the Resident Medical Officer (RMO) is confident is an SVT with aberrant conduction.

Question

Decide whether initial management might reasonably include each of the following.

(a) IV verapamil.
(b) DC shock.
(c) IV adenosine.
(d) IV lignocaine.

Answer

(a) False.
(b) True.
(c) True.
(d) False.

Comment

This patient clearly has underlying heart disease and is acutely haemodynamically compromised by the dysrhythmia. It is difficult to distinguish SVT with aberrant conduction from ventricular tachycardia, but if the RMO is correct, then lignocaine will not be effective. Verapamil, while often effective in SVT, is potentially catastrophic in this setting, but a therapeutic trial of adenosine could be considered because of its short duration of action. Alternatively (or subsequently if adenosine is not effective, which would suggest that the rhythm is really ventricular), direct current (DC) shock is appropriate.

Case history

A 24-year-old medical student arrives at the Accident and Emergency department complaining of rapid regular palpitations coming on abruptly while he was studying in the library for his final examinations which start next week. There is no relevant past history. He looks pale but otherwise well, his pulse is 155 beats/min and regular, his blood pressure is 110/60 mmHg and the examination is otherwise unremarkable. The cardiogram shows a supraventricular tachycardia.

Question

Decide whether initial management might reasonably include each of the following.

(a) IV amiodarone.
(b) Vagal manoeuvres.
(c) IV digoxin.
(d) Reassurance.
(e) DC shock.
(f) Overnight observation.
(g) Specialized tests for phaeochromocytoma.

Answer

(a) False.
(b) True.
(c) False.
(d) True.
(e) False.
(f) True.
(g) False.

Comment

Students who are studying for examinations often consume excessive amounts of coffee, and a history of caffeine intake should be sought. The rhythm is benign and the patient should be reassured. Vagal manoeuvres may terminate the dysrhythmia but, if not, overnight observation may see the rhythm revert spontaneously to sinus. Intravenous amiodarone or initial DC shock would be inappropriate, and IV digoxin (while increasing vagal tone) could render subsequent DC shock (if necessary) more hazardous.

PHARMACOKINETICS

Bretylium is secreted rapidly into the tubular lumen and excreted entirely by the kidneys. The half-life is normally 7–9 hours, and this is much prolonged in renal failure.

DRUG INTERACTIONS

Prior treatment with drugs that block uptake 1 (e.g. tricyclic antidepressants) is likely to render bretylium ineffective. Conversely, an uptake-1 blocker (protriptyline, 5 mg given 6-hourly) has been used to treat the hypotension that follows successful use of the drug. Noradrenaline infusion has also been used in this situation.

FURTHER READING

Ben-David J, Zipes DP. 1993: *Torsades de pointes* and proarrhythmia. *Lancet* **341**, 1578–82.

Pritchett EL. 1992: Management of atrial fibrillation. *New England Journal of Medicine* **326**, 1264–71.

Roden DM. 1994: Risks and benefits of antiarrhythmic therapy. *New England Journal of Medicine* **331**, 785–91.

Shenasa M, Borggrefe M, Haverkamp W *et al.* 1993: Ventricular tachycardia. *Lancet* **341**, 1512–9.

Singh BN, Opie LH, Harrison DC, Marcus FI. 1987: Antiarrhythmic agents. In Opie LH, Chatterjee K, Gersh BJ *et al.* (eds), *Drugs for the heart*, 2nd edn. Orlando, FL: Grune and Stratton, 54–90.

Waldo AL, Wit AL. 1993: Mechanisms of cardiac arrhythmias. *Lancet* **341**, 1189–93.

PART V

THE RESPIRATORY SYSTEM

CHAPTER THIRTY-TWO

THERAPY *of* ASTHMA, COAD *and* OTHER RESPIRATORY DISORDERS

- Pathophysiology of asthma
- Principles of management of asthma and COAD
- Drugs used to treat asthma
- Future directions in drug therapy of asthma
- Respiratory failure
- Cough
- Pulmonary surfactants
- α_1-Antitrypsin deficiency
- Respiratory stimulants
- Drug-induced pulmonary disease

PATHOPYHSIOLOGY OF ASTHMA

Asthma is characterized by fluctuating airways obstruction, with a diurnal variation and a nocturnal nadir. This manifests as a triad of wheeze, cough and breathlessness. These symptoms are due to a combination of constriction of bronchial smooth muscle, oedema of the mucosa lining the small bronchi, and plugging of the bronchial lumen with viscous mucus and inflammatory cells (Figure 32.1). Asthma is broadly categorized into two types, namely non-allergic and allergic, but there is considerable overlap between them. In allergic asthma, which is usually of early onset, extrinsic allergens produce a type I allergic reaction in atopic subjects (see Chapter 49). Type I reactions are associated with the presence of reaginic antibodies (IgE) on the surface of mast cells and probably other immune effector cells (eosinophils and lymphocytes). However, the airways are hyper-responsive to a variety of stimuli, so immunotherapy directed at a specific allergen is disappointing. Patients with non-allergic (late-onset) asthma do not appear to be sensitive to any well-defined antigen, although infection (usually viral) often precipitates an attack. These acute inflammatory processes can ultimately lead to irreversible lung damage. Inflammatory mediators that have been implicated include histamine, 5-hydroxytryptamine (5HT, serotonin), prostaglandin D_2, platelet-activating factor (PAF), neuropeptides, kinins and several leukotrienes (LTs; see below). Increased parasympathetic tone also causes bronchoconstriction. These mediators interact with and can substitute for one another, so the precise role of each is difficult to define.

PRINCIPLES OF MANAGEMENT OF ASTHMA AND COAD

MANAGEMENT OF ACUTE SEVERE ASTHMA

Management includes the following:

1 assessment for possible hospital admission. Severity and response to therapy are monitored clinically (e.g. pulse rate, respiratory rate, pulsus paradox) and by objective measures of

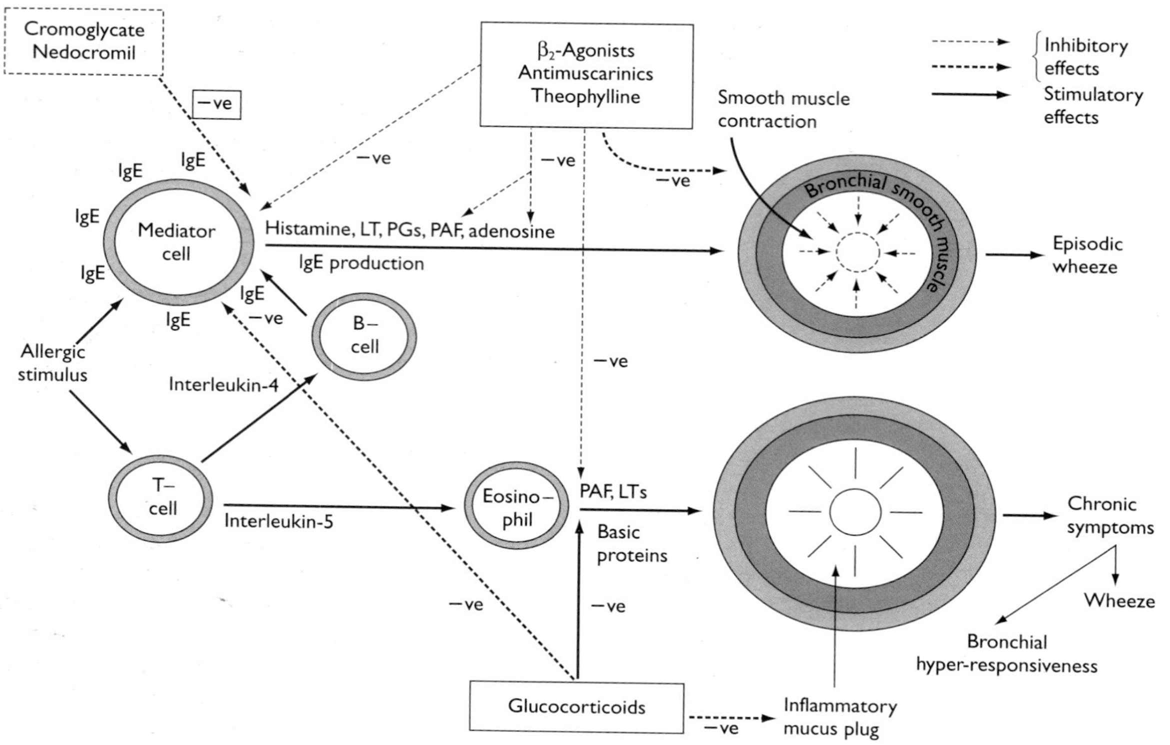

Figure 32.1: Pathophysiology of asthma and sites of drug action. PAF = platelet-activating factor, LTs = leukotrienes, PGs = prostaglandins.

respiratory function (e.g. spirometry, peak expiratory flow rate, blood gases or pulse oximetry);

2 high-percentage oxygen (60% F_iO_2);

3 hydrocortisone intravenously, followed by prednisolone by mouth;

4 a β_2-agonist is inhaled as a mist formed from a solution of the drug in a device called a *nebulizer*. If the patient does not respond, treatment with an antimuscarinic drug (nebulized **ipratropium**) and/or intravenous therapy (with a β_2-agonist or with **aminophylline**) is considered. Paradoxically, bronchodilators can cause a transient *fall* in arterial oxygen tension by worsening ventilation/perfusion mismatching. This, together with their direct actions on the heart, predisposes to cardiac arrhythmias. Arterial hypoxaemia must therefore be prevented by nebulizing β_2-agonists or ipratropium *in oxygen*;

5 5% glucose may be infused intravenously to correct dehydration;

6 serum potassium is monitored, as hypokalaemia may be caused both by corticosteroids and by β_2-agonists;

7 an antibiotic (e.g. **amoxycillin**, **co-amoxiclav** or **clarithromycin**) is given if bacterial infection is suspected;

8 *if the patient fails to respond and develops a rising pulse, with increasing respiratory rate and a fall in PaO_2 to < 8 kPa or a rise in $PaCO_2$ to > 6 kPa, assisted ventilation will probably be needed;*

9 *no sedation should be given* (except with assisted ventilation), as even small doses can cause fatal respiratory depression in this situation.

(This approach is based on management guidelines developed by the British Thoracic Society.)

Chronic Asthma

1 Bronchodilators are used to treat chronic wheeziness and to abort acute episodes. Metered dose inhalers of β_2-agonists are conve-

nient, and with correct usage little drug enters the systemic circulation. Fluorohydrocarbons have been (and currently still are) used as propellants, but are being phased out in accordance with international treaty, because of their adverse effect on the ozone layer and hence on the environment. Aerosols are particularly useful for treating an acute episode of breathlessness, and recent studies suggest that 'on-demand' medication (i.e. taken only when symptomatic) may be more beneficial in the long term rather than regular β_2-agonist therapy. Oral preparations of β_2-agonists or theophylline have a role in paediatric practice, because young children cannot co-ordinate inhalation with depression of the canister in a metered-dose inhaler, but children over 5 years can use these inhalers with a plastic 'spacer' device. These have valved ports that permit a dose to be loaded into the chamber, from which it is breathed by the patient without the need to co-ordinate activation of the device with inspiration. There are several alternative approaches, including breath-activated devices and devices that administer the dose in the form of a dry powder that is sucked into the airways.

2 Patients should be warned to contact the physician promptly if their clinical state deteriorates and the frequency of inhalations is rising.

3 Patients, particularly children, with asthma provoked by allergy, exercise or physical agents (e.g. cold air, sulphur dioxide) sufficient to need bronchodilator drugs may be given a trial of **cromoglycate**. Occasional patients with intrinsic asthma also respond to this drug.

4 Steroids are used in chronic asthma when:
   - *regular* (rather than occasional, as needed) doses of bronchodilator are required;
   - repeated attacks interfere with work or school;
   - the growth of a child is impaired due to chronic asthma.

Systemic side-effects are minimized by using inhaled medication (e.g. **beclomethasone** or **budesonide**). Severely affected patients (e.g. forced expiratory volume in 1 s < 1.5 L for adults) may require oral **prednisolone**, despite its systemic adverse effects. During a chest infection, 30–40 mg prednisolone may be required daily until a response is obtained. The drug is then either discontinued abruptly or reduced rapidly after such short-term treatment. Some very severely affected patients need continuous steroid therapy with increased dosage during exacerbations. If such a patient eventually improves sufficiently for steroids to be withdrawn, this should be done much more gradually. A large dose of glucocorticosteroid administered on alternate days causes less adrenal suppression than daily or more frequent administration of the same total dose (see Chapter 39).

5 Hypnotics and sedatives should *not* be used, as for acute asthma.

6 Patients can perform home peak flow monitoring first thing in the morning and last thing at night, as soon as asthmatic symptoms develop or worsen. With a knowledge of their best peak flow, this allows adjustment of inhaled medication, or appropriate urgent medical assessment if the peak flow rate falls to less than 50% of normal, or diurnal variation (morning 'dipping') exceeds 20%.

Late-onset asthma

This is often difficult to treat, and long-term steroid treatment – with its attendant adverse effects – may be unavoidable. Nevertheless, bronchodilators, inhaled corticosteroids or sodium cromoglycate can be tried. If prolonged treatment with an oral steroid is contemplated, *bisphosphonate treatment* to limit osteoporosis should be considered (see Chapter 38).

Acute bronchitis

Acute bronchitis is a condition that commonly presents to general practitioners. There is little evidence that antibiotics confer benefit in otherwise fit patients presenting with cough and purulent sputum, and usually the most important step is to stop smoking. In the absence of fever or evidence of pneumonia it seems best to avoid antibiotics for this self-limiting condition.

Chronic bronchitis and emphysema

Chronic simple bronchitis is associated with a chronic or recurrent increase in the volume of mucoid bronchial secretions sufficient to cause expectoration. At this stage there need be no disability, and measures such as giving up smoking (which may be aided by the use of nicotine patches or gum; see Chapter 52) and avoidance of air pollution improve the prognosis. Simple hypersecretion may be complicated by infection or the development of airways obstruction. Bacterial infection is usually due to commensal organisms, including *Haemophilus influenzae*, although pneumococci, staphylococci or occasionally branhamella or coliforms may also be responsible. The commonly encountered acute bronchitic exacerbation is due to bacterial infection in only about one-third of cases. In the rest, other factors – such as increased air pollution, environmental temperature changes or viruses – are presumably responsible. *Mycoplasma pneumoniae* infections may be responsible for some cases, and these respond to erythromycin or tetracyclines. Antibiotic therapy is considered when there is increased breathlessness, increased sputum volume and, in particular, increased sputum purulence. Rational antibiotic choice is based on adequate sputum penetration and the suspected organisms. The decision is seldom assisted by sputum culture or Gram stain, in contrast to the treatment of pneumonia. It is appropriate to vary the antibiotic used for different attacks, since effectiveness presumably reflects the sensitivity of organisms resident in the respiratory tract. Commonly used drugs include the following:

1 amoxycillin – which produces sputum concentrations twice those from the same dose of **ampicillin**;
2 **doxycycline**;
3 **trimethoprim**;
4 **cefuroxime** – which penetrates sputum poorly but has some role in the management of bronchitis because of its activity against *H. influenzae*;
5 co-amoxiclav (amoxycillin with clavulanate) is effective against β-lactamase-producing organisms,
6 **erythromycin** or newer macrolides (e.g. clarithromycin/azithromycin);
7 **ciprofloxacin** (a quinolone).

In the absence of respiratory disability, antibiotics alone may be sufficient treatment. Increased respiratory difficulty may be caused by sputum retention. Physiotherapy is traditional and possibly effective in this situation. Prophylactic subcutaneous **heparin** should be considered for patients admitted with an acute exacerbation complicated by respiratory failure or cor pulmonale.

Prevention of acute exacerbations is difficult. *Stopping smoking* is beneficial. Patients should be given a supply of antibiotic to take as soon as their sputum becomes purulent. Despite recovery from an acute attack, patients are at greatly increased risk of death or serious illness from intercurrent respiratory infections, and *administration of influenza and pneumococcal vaccines is important*.

Airways obstruction is invariably present in chronic bronchitis, but is of variable severity. Bronchodilators, either β_2-adrenoreceptor agonists or **aminophylline**, frequently fail because much of the obstruction is irreversible. However, in some patients there is a reversible element, and a

Key points

Therapy of chronic obstructive airways disease

Acute exacerbation

- Controlled oxygen therapy (e.g. FiO_2 24–28%).
- Nebulized β_2 agonists (salbutamol 5 mg 2- to 4-hourly) – intravenously if needed.
- Nebulized anticholinergics – ipratropium bromide (500 μg 6- to 8-hourly).
- Antibiotics (e.g. amoxycillin, ciprofloxacin).
- Short-term prednisolone – 30 mg/day for 1 week.

Chronic disease

- Stop smoking cigarettes.
- Optimize inhaled bronchodilators (salbutamol/ipratropium bromide) and their administration.
- Consider oral theophylline and/or inhaled glucocorticosteroids.
- Treat infection early and aggressively with antibiotics.
- Long-term oxygen therapy (LTOT) 2 L/min (for 12–15 h per day) for severe COPD with cor pulmonale.
- Diuretics for peripheral oedema.
- Consider venesection for severe secondary polycythaemia.
- Exercise, within limits of tolerance.

Table 32.1: Comparative pharmacology of some β_2-agonists other than salbutamol

Drug	Dose Formulations available	Standard dosing regimen	Pharmacokinetics/ Pharmacodynamics	Other comments
Eformoterol	Dry powder inhaler	12–24 μg twice daily	Long acting	Paradoxical bronchospasm may occur
Salmeterol	Metered-dose inhaler (25 μg/puff) Dry powder (50 μg)	25–50 μg at night 25–50 μg twice daily	Onset slow; 12 h duration of action. Hepatic metabolism	Prophylaxis and exercise-induced asthma. *Not for relief of acute bronchospasm*
Terbutaline	Metered-dose inhaler (250 μg/puff) Dry powder (500 μg) Nebulizer solution Tablets/syrup Slow-release tablets	Metered-dose inhaler (250–500 μg 4-hourly) Nebulizer 10 mg 2- to 4-hourly 5 mg 8-hourly 7.5 mg twice daily	Plasma $t_{\frac{1}{2}}$ is 3–4 h. Gastrointestinal and hepatic metabolism	Similar to sulbutamol

trial of these drugs is usually justified to assess whether a benefit will be obtained. Similarly, a short therapeutic trial of corticosteroids, with objective monitoring of the response, may be appropriate.

Intermittent or erratic use of oxygen by patients at home is ineffective, dangerous and expensive. In contrast, long-term oxygen therapy (LTOT), 12–15 h daily, in severely disabled bronchitics with pulmonary hypertension decreases mortality and morbidity. The mortality of such patients is related to pulmonary hypertension, which is increased by chronic hypoxia. Relief of hypoxia on a long-term basis by increasing the concentration of inspired oxygen reverses the vasoconstriction in the pulmonary arteries and decreases pulmonary hypertension. *Long-term oxygen therapy cannot be safely offered to patients who continue to smoke because of the hazards of fire and explosion.*

DRUGS USED TO TREAT ASTHMA

β_2-AGONISTS

USE

β_2-Agonists (e.g. **salbutamol**, **terbutaline** or the long-acting **salmeterol**; see below and Table 32.1) are used to treat the symptoms of asthma both in an acute attack and as maintenance therapy. (Intravenous salbutamol is also used in obstetric practice to inhibit premature labour.) For asthma, β_2-agonists are given via inhalation where possible.

1 Inhalation methods – these include:
   - metered-dose inhaler – aerosol (e.g. salbutamol 100 μg/puff), usual dose one to two puffs up to six times daily. Some patients cannot master this technique;
   - aerosol administered via a nebulizer – 2.5–5 mg salbutamol in sterile saline are given over 5–15 min between 2- and 6-hourly;
   - as a dry powder – almost all patients can use a dry-powder inhaler correctly.

2 Oral methods, including slow-release preparations.

3 Subcutaneous delivery.

4 Intravenous administration.

The increase in FEV_1 after inhaling 200 μg salbutamol begins within 15 min and peaks at 1 h, persisting for 4–6 h. Following intravenous injection of 100–300 μg over 5 min, airways resistance usually falls to a minimum in 5–10 min, although in severely affected patients the response may be delayed by 30 min.

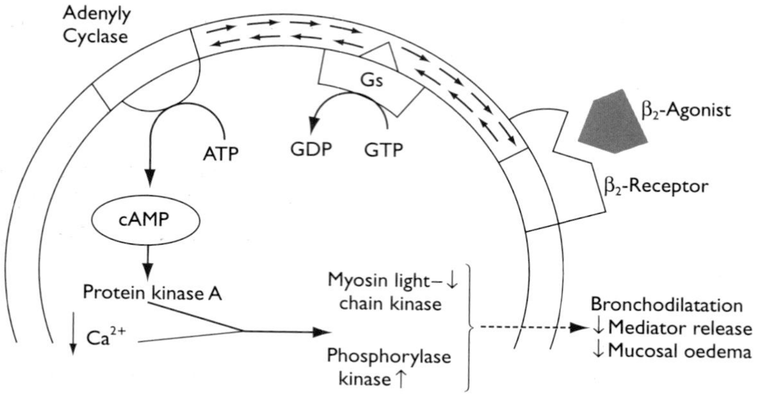

Figure 32.2: Membrane and intracellular events triggered when β_2-agonists stimulate β_2-receptors. Gs = stimulating G-protein, GDP = guanosine diphosphate, GTP = guanosine triphosphate, cAMP = 3′,5′-cyclic adenosine monophosphate.

PHARMACOLOGICAL EFFECTS, MECHANISM OF ACTION AND ADVERSE EFFECTS

Agonists occupying β_2-adrenoceptors increase cyclic adenosine monophosphate (cAMP) by stimulating adenylyl cyclase via membrane-bound coupled G-proteins. Cyclic AMP phosphorylates a cascade of enzymes (see Figure 32.2). This causes a wide variety of actions in different tissues, some of which are desired, but others cause adverse effects, including the following:

1 relaxation of bronchial smooth muscle;
2 inhibition of release of inflammatory mediators;
3 increased mucociliary clearance;
4 relaxation of uterine smooth muscle;
5 increase in heart rate, force of myocardial contraction, speed of impulse conduction and enhanced production of ectopic foci in the myocardium and automaticity in pacemaker tissue. This can cause arrhythmias and symptoms of palpitations;
6 muscle tremor;
7 vasodilatation in muscle. Part of this effect is indirect, via activation of endothelial NO biosynthesis;
8 Metabolic effects:
   - hypokalaemia (via redistribution of K^+ into cells);
   - raised free fatty acid concentrations;
   - increased insulin secretion but also increased glycogenolysis, which has the overall effect of increasing blood sugar.
9 Tolerance of β_2-agonists can occur, but is not a major clinical problem in asthmatic patients.

PHARMACOKINETICS

Salbutamol undergoes pronounced presystemic metabolism in the intestinal mucosa (sulphation) and hepatic conjugation to form an inactive metabolite that is excreted in the urine. Most (80%) of the dose administered by aerosol is swallowed, but the fraction which is inhaled (10–20%) largely remains as free drug in the airways. The plasma elimination half-life ($t_{\frac{1}{2}}$) is 2–4 h.

Salmeterol

Salmeterol is long acting, with a duration of action of at least 12 h, allowing twice daily administration. The lipophilic side-chain of salmeterol binds firmly to an exo-site that is adjacent to but distinct from the β_2-agonist binding site. Consequently, salmeterol functions as an essentially irreversible agonist. The onset of bronchodilatation is slow (3–4 h). Salmeterol should not therefore be used to treat acute attacks of bronchospasm. It is used as prophylactic therapy, especially overnight, with additional 'top-ups' with shorter-acting β_2-agonists. It is expensive.

MUSCARINIC RECEPTOR ANTAGONISTS

USE

Inhaled muscarinic receptor antagonists are most effective in older patients. **Atropine** has a bronchodilator action in bronchitics and asthmatics, with some benefit in patients with exercise-induced asthma (Osler recommended stramonium – which contains atropine – in the form of cigarettes for asthmatics!). Atropine causes systemic side-effects, and modern drugs of this type are quaternary ammonium analogues of atropine that are minimally absorbed because of their positive charge.

Ipratropium bromide

USE

Ipratropium is given as 1–2 puffs (20 or 40 μg) three or four times daily from a metered-dose inhaler. It can be given via a nebulizer (stock solution 0.25 mg/mL; 2 mL (500 μg) diluted with 2 mL saline, nebulized and inhaled). The degree and rate of onset of bronchodilatation are somewhat less than those of salbutamol or terbutaline, but the duration of response is longer. Ipratropium has a place in maintenance therapy and in the treatment of acute severe attacks of asthma. Some benefit for patients with exercise-induced asthma has also been demonstrated, but its slower onset of action makes it most useful in maintenance therapy, especially in chronic bronchitis. It is useful for patients with heart disease or thyrotoxicosis in whom β_2-agonists are unsuitable. It is compatible with β_2-agonists, and such combinations are additive.

MECHANISM OF ACTION

There is increased parasympathetic activity in patients with reversible airways obstruction, resulting in bronchoconstriction through effects of acetylcholine on the M_1, M_2 and M_3 muscarinic cholinoreceptors in the bronchi. The final common pathway is via a membrane-bound G-protein which leads to a fall in cAMP and increased intracellular calcium, with consequent bronchoconstriction. Ipratropium is an antagonist at the M_2 and M_3 cholinoreceptors.

ADVERSE EFFECTS

These include the following:

1 bitter taste (this may compromise compliance);
2 acute urinary retention may be precipitated by high doses in patients with prostatic hypertrophy;
3 rarely, acute glaucoma has been precipitated when nebulized doses are given via a face-mask;
4 paradoxical bronchoconstriction has occasionally been reported due to sensitivity to benzalkonium chloride, which is the preservative in the nebulizer solution.

PHARMACOKINETICS

When administered by aerosol, plasma concentrations of ipratropium are about 1000 times lower than when the same degree of bronchodilatation is produced by systemic administration. Plasma $t_{\frac{1}{2}}$ = 3–4 h

OXITROPIUM

Oxitropium is similar to ipratropium, but with a longer duration of action ($t_{\frac{1}{2}}$ is approximately 12 h), allowing twice daily dosing of 200 μg via a metered-dose inhaler.

METHYLXANTHINES

Theophylline and its derivatives

These are the only phosphodiesterase inhibitors currently in common therapeutic use for asthma. Aminophylline is a mixture of 80% theophylline (the pharmacologically active component) and 20% ethylene diamine, which increases theophylline solubility but is also the likely culprit in occasional allergic reactions.

USE

Aminophylline is used intravenously in patients with severe asthma or severe chronic obstructive airways disease (COAD), and is used orally in less severe cases or to reduce symptoms, especially at night. Oral theophylline is available as sustained-release preparations that allow twice daily dosing.

1 Intravenous aminophylline:
- a loading dose of 5 mg/kg *given over 20–30 min*, followed by;
- a continuous maintenance infusion of 0.5 mg/kg/h. *Infusion rates must be reviewed and adjusted frequently according to plasma theophylline concentrations* (see Chapter 8), and if rapid theophylline determinations are unavailable this substantially reduces the safety of the drug. In patients with impaired liver function or heart failure, the dose should be halved. It should also be reduced in the elderly. It is essential to enquire about

oral theophylline administration prior to intravenous injection. If the patient is receiving oral theophylline, the plasma concentration should be measured, the loading dose omitted until the result is known, and the maintenance dose modified accordingly.

2 Oral theophylline – sustained-release preparations can provide effective therapeutic levels for up to 12 h following a single dose. Because of their slow release rate they have a reduced incidence of gastrointestinal side-effects. Oral theophylline given at night is useful in patients whose airways obstruction increases in the early hours of the morning (morning 'dippers'), although theophylline (like caffeine) can interfere with sleep.

MECHANISM OF ACTION AND PHARMACOLOGICAL EFFECTS

It is still not clear exactly how theophylline produces bronchodilation. Its pharmacological actions include the following:

1 relaxation of airway smooth muscle and inhibition of mediator release (e.g. from mast cells). Theophylline raises intracellular cAMP by inhibiting phosphodiesterase. However, the extent of inhibition is modest at therapeutic concentrations of theophylline;
2 antagonism of adenosine (a potent bronchoconstrictor) at A_2-receptors;
3 anti-inflammatory activity on T-lymphocytes by reducing release of platelet-activating factor (PAF);
4 reduced calcium entry via receptor-operated channels, and inhibition of calcium release from stores by inositol trisphosphate;
5 increased force of contraction of respiratory muscles;
6 central stimulation of respiration.

ADVERSE EFFECTS

The adverse effects of theophylline are generally related to its plasma concentration.

1 *Gastrointestinal tract* – nausea and vomiting are common, are related both to stimulation of the medullary emetic centre and to a local gastric effect, and can occur with plasma concentrations of 10–15 mg/L.
2 *Cardiovascular system* – some adverse effects resemble those of catecholamines, as both drugs raise intracellular cAMP concentrations. These include tachycardia and cardiac arrhythmias (atrial and ventricular), and occur at plasma concentrations of 20–40 mg/L.
3 *Central nervous system* – insomnia, anxiety, agitation, hyperventilation, headache and fits (> 40 mg/L, but *severe CNS toxicity can occur at lower concentrations, especially in the elderly*).
4 *Dilatation of vascular smooth muscle* – headache, flushing and hypotension.

PHARMACOKINETICS

Theophylline is well absorbed from the small intestine (oral administration) or rectum (suppos-

Key points

Bronchodilator agents

- β_2 agonists
- Bronchodilate by increasing intracellular cAMP.
- Short-acting, rapid-onset agents (e.g. salbutamol) are used prn for bronchospasm in asthma.
- Long-acting, slower-onset agents (e.g. salmeterol) are used regularly, once or twice daily.
- Common side-effects include tremor, tachycardias, vasodilatation, hypokalaemia and hyperglycaemia.

Anticholinergics–ipratropium

- Antagonist at the M_2 and M_3 muscarinic receptors in the bronchi, causing bronchodilatation.
- Slow onset of long-lasting bronchodilatation (given 6- to 8-hourly), especially in older patients.
- Bitter taste.
- Little systemic absorption, and side-effects are rare (dry mouth, acute retention, exacerbation of glaucoma).

Theophylline

- Potent bronchodilator (also vasodilator).
- Aminophylline IV for acute severe episodes.
- Slow-release oral preparations for chronic therapy.
- Hepatic metabolism, multiple drug interactions (e.g. clarithromycin, ciprofloxacin).
- Therapeutic drug monitoring of plasma concentrations.
- Side-effects include gastrointestinal disturbances, vasodilatation, arrhythmias, seizures and sleep disturbance.

itories), but intravenous administration is most effective for acute severe asthma. The volume of distribution is about 0.3–0.8 L/kg, and at therapeutic concentrations 60% is bound to plasma proteins. The therapeutic range is 5–20 mg/L, but it is preferable not to exceed 10 mg/L in children. Elimination is mainly (85–90%) by hepatic metabolism, so fixed-dose regimes may lead to high blood levels and toxicity in the presence of liver disease.

DRUG INTERACTIONS

Although synergism between β_2-adrenergic agonists and theophylline has been demonstrated *in vitro*, clinically the effect of this combination is at best additive. Many drugs modify theophylline metabolism (see Table 32.2). Inhibition of theophylline metabolism by erythromycin (and other macrolides) and the fluoroquinolones (e.g. ciprofloxacin) is important because these drugs are commonly used to treat respiratory infections. Concomitant prescription of these agents with theophylline can produce toxicity.

GLUCOCORTICOSTEROIDS

Glucocorticosteroids are used in the treatment of asthma because of their potent anti-inflammatory effect. This is only partly understood, but involves interaction with an intracellular receptor that in turn interacts with nuclear DNA, thereby altering the synthesis of many proteins and factors, including $NF_{\kappa B}$ and lipocortin (which inhibits phospholipase A_2 and hence reduces the availability of arachidonic acid for leukotriene synthesis) (see below and Chapter 39). They are effective both in maintenance therapy (prophylaxis) and in the treatment of the acute severe attack.

Systemic glucocorticosteroids

See also Chapter 39.

Hydrocortisone (200–300 mg) is given intravenously in urgent situations. Improvement (a rise in FEV_1 and forced vital capacity, FVC) does not begin until after 6 h, and is usually maximal 10–12 h following the start of treatment. This

Table 32.2: Factors influencing theophylline clearance (see also p. 105)

Factors decreasing theophylline clearance and suggested initial* dose adjustment (normal dose is 100%)	Factors increasing theophlline clearance and suggested initial* dose adjustment (normal dose is 100%)
Congestive cardiac failure (40%)	Hyperthyroidism (150%)
Hepatic disease, cirrhosis (40%)	Marijuana (150%)
Neonates (60%)	Smoking (150%)
Pneumonia (70%)	Charcoal barbecued meat (130%)
Old age (80%)	
Drugs	Drugs
Azole-antifungals e.g. Ketoconazole, etc. (50%)	Carbamazepine (150%)
Cimetidine (50%)	Phenytoin (150%)
Fluoroquinolones (e.g. ciprofloxacin) (50%)	Rifampicin (150%)
Chloramphenicol (75%)	High-protein, low-carbohydrate diet (150%)
Erythromycin (other macrolides) (75%)	Ethanol (chronic) (120%)
Flu vaccine and interferon (75%)	
Propranolol (70%)	

* Subsequent dose adjustment to be made in the light of plasma concentration monitoring, which should be carried out more frequently in the circumstances listed. The suggested adjustments are obviously very approximate, and depend on the extent of exposure to the various agents.

delay is due to the action of glucocorticosteroids via altered protein synthesis. Oral corticosteroids (e.g. prednisolone 40–60 mg/day) are usually started within 12–24 h.

Inhaled glucocorticosteroids

USE

With modern inhaler devices, delivery to the lung may reach 20–30% of the total dose administered. **Beclomethasone**, 400 μg, is equivalent to 5 mg of prednisolone, and is given at a dose of 250–500 μg twice daily; **budesonide** (200 μg twice daily) is an alternative.

Glucocorticoids can be administered via plastic 'spacer' devices or via metered-dose inhalers or as dry powders. The fluorinated derivatives are extremely powerful anti-inflammatory agents, and mainly exert a local action because they are highly polar and hence only a amall fraction of the dose is absorbed systemically. Approximately 10–20% enters the lungs, the rest being swallowed and then rapidly converted to inactive metabolites by the hepatic cytochrome $P_{450\ 3A4}$ system.

The comparative pharmacology of inhaled glucocorticosteroids is summarized in Table 32.3.

ADVERSE EFFECTS OF INHALED STEROIDS

1 At the lowest recommended daily dose for adults (e.g. beclomethasone 400 μg) there is no prolonged suppression of the hypothalamic–pituitary–adrenal (HPA) axis, although after stopping treatment plasma cortisol is suppressed for 48 h. Higher doses (800–1600 μg) produce more prolonged depression of adrenal function.
2 Candidiasis of the pharynx or larynx occurs in up to 15% of patients. Giving the minimum effective dose, use of a 'spacer', gargling or using mouthwashes after dosing and changing toothbrush regularly all minimize this problem. Occasionally **nystatin** or **amphotericin** lozenges are required.
3 A hoarse voice may develop due to a laryngeal myopathy at high doses. This effect is dose dependent and reversible, and its occurrence is minimized by the use of a 'spacer'.
4 Bruising and skin atrophy may occur at high doses.
5 Reversible inhibition of long bone growth in children can occur at beclomethasone doses of 400–800 μg/day.
6 Posterior subcapsular cataracts may develop following prolonged use.

CROMOGLYCATE AND NEDOCROMIL

USE

Sodium cromoglycate is used to prevent asthma (it is also used as a nasal spray for perennial and allergic rhinitis, and as eyedrops in allergic con-

Table 32.3: Comparative pharmacology of inhaled glucocorticosteroids

Drug	Total daily dose (note that this depends on preparation as well as severity)	Relative binding affinity to receptors*	Relative blanching potency*	Comments
Beclomethasone dipropionate	400–1600 μg/day	0.4	600	Equi-effective compared to budesonide. May be used in children
Budesonide	200–1600 μg/day	9.4	980	Nebulized formulation (250 μg/2 mL) available. May be used in children to avoid systemic steroids
Fluticasone	200–2000 μg/day	18	1200	May cause fewer systemic side-effects than others

* Relative to dexamethasone binding to glucocorticosteroid receptors *in vitro* and blanching of human skin *in vitro*.

junctivitis). For asthma, it is administered by inhalation of a powder liberated from a 20-mg capsule and dispersed by devices containing an inspiration-driven propeller or by spinning of the punctured capsule in a plastic chamber. Cromoglycate produces no benefit during an asthmatic attack, but if taken regularly (e.g. 20–40 mg 6-hourly) it diminishes the frequency of attacks of allergic or exercise-provoked asthma. A good response allows the dose of corticosteroid to be minimized. There is no completely reliable method of predicting which patients will benefit, and a therapeutic trial is often warranted. **Nedocromil** sodium is an alternative to cromoglycate, which can be taken twice daily.

MECHANISM OF ACTION

These drugs do not prevent antigen–antibody combinating, but if given before exposure to an antigen they can prevent type I and III allergic reactions. They inhibit mediator release from sensitized mast cells *in vitro*, and used to be called 'mast-cell stabilizers' for this reason. However, this action does not account for their efficacy in allergic disorders, since congeners that are more potent in this regard are without therapeutic efficacy. Cromoglycate reduces firing of sensory C-fibres in response to kinins, but the mechanism underlying its therapeutic efficacy is uncertain.

ADVERSE EFFECTS

1 Sodium cromoglycate is virtually non-toxic. The powder can (very rarely) produce bronchospasm or hoarseness. Nausea and headache have been reported, but are uncommon.
2 Nedocromil has a bitter taste, and nausea and headache have been reported.

PHARMACOKINETICS

Sodium cromoglycate is not appreciably absorbed from the gut, and is given as an inhaled powder. Most of the powder is swallowed, but about 10% reaches the alveoli, where it acts and a small amount is absorbed. It is not metabolized, unchanged drug appearing mainly in the faeces (because it has been swallowed), together with a small amount in the urine. Nedocromil sodium is also poorly absorbed from the gut.

> **Key points**
>
> Anti-inflammatory agents-cromoglycate and glucocorticosteroids
>
> Sodium cromoglycate
> - Mechanism unclear – anti-inflammatory effect.
> - Chronic prophylactic therapy of 'allergic asthma'.
> - Prevents exercise-induced asthma.
> - Inhaled therapy given, 6-hourly via metered-dose inhaler or dry powder.
> - Side-effects are minimal (headache, cough).
>
> Glucocorticosteroids
> - Mechanism is anti-inflammatory.
> - Systemically (IV/PO) in severe acute and chronic asthma.
> - Inhaled in chronic asthma.
> - Well absorbed from gastrointestinal tract–hepatic metabolism.
> - Once daily dosing of oral drugs (prednisolone) and twice daily dosing for inhaled agents (beclomethasone).
> - Topical therapy – side-effects minimal (oral thrush, hoarse) voice, HPA; suppression only at high dose.
> - Systemic therapy – side effects as Cushing's syndrome.

LEUKOTRIENE MODULATORS

These fall into two classes, namely leukotriene receptor antagonists and 5′-lipoxygenase inhibitors.

Leukotrienes (LT) are fatty-acid-derived mediators containing a conjugated triene structure. They are made when arachidonic acid (see Chapter 25) is liberated from the cell membrane of leukocytes (hence 'leuko-') and other cells, as a result of cell activation by allergic or other noxious stimuli. 5′-Lipoxygenase is the enzyme required for the synthesis of LTA_4, which is an unstable epoxide precursor of the biologically important leukotrienes, of which there are two main groups. LTB_4 is a dihydroxy 20-carbon-atom fatty acid which is a potent pro-inflammatory chemoattractant. The other group consists of the cysteinyl leukotrienes, namely LTC_4, LTD_4 and LTE_4. LTC_4 is a conjugate of LTA_4 with glutathione, a tripeptide which combines with LTA_4 via its cysteine residue. LTC_4 is converted to an active metabolite (LTD_4) by the removal of the terminal amino acid in the peptide side-chain. Removal of a second amino acid results in a less active metabolite (LTE_4). LTC_4, LTD_4 and LTE_4, the 'sulphidopeptide leukotrienes' or 'cysteinyl leukotrienes', collectively account for the activity that used to be referred to as 'slow-reacting substance of anaphylaxis' (SRS-A). They all (but especially LTD_4) act on a receptor called the Cys-LT_1 receptor to cause bronchoconstriction, attraction of eosinophils and production of oedema.

Leukotriene C_4 and D_4 antagonists–montelukast

USE

Leukotriene receptor antagonists can be given orally (10 mg at night in adults, 5 mg in children over 6 years old). **Montelukast** was the first of these drugs to become available clinically (others include **zafirlukast**, **pranilukast** and **pobilukast**). It reduces the requirement for glucocorticosteroid and improves symptoms in chronic asthma, and is also useful in the prophylaxis of exercise- or antigen-induced asthma. Like 5′-lipoxygenase inhibitors (see below), it is effective in aspirin-sensitive asthma, which is associated with diversion of arachidonic acid from the cyclo-oxygenase pathway (blocked by aspirin) to the formation of leukotrienes by 5′-lipoxygenase. Montelukast is expensive.

MECHANISM OF ACTION

Montelukast competes with LTD_4 and LTC_4 for the Cys-LT_1 receptor.

ADVERSE EFFECTS

Montelukast is well tolerated, and has a side-effect profile similar to placebo. There have been no reported cases of hepatitis or pulmonary eosinophilia (reported with zafirlukast).

PHARMACOKINETICS

This drug is rapidly absorbed from the gastrointestinal tract, reaching peak plasma concentrations within 3–4 h. The mean plasma $t_{\frac{1}{2}}$ is 2.7–5.5 h. It undergoes hepatic metabolism by cytochrome P_{450} 3A and 2C9, and is mainly excreted in the bile.

DRUG INTERACTIONS

No drug–drug interactions have been demonstrated between montelukast and digoxin, warfarin, prednisone, theophyllline, oestrogen or progesterone, in contrast to zafirlukast, which inhibits hepatic cytochrome P_{450} enzymes. Enzyme inducers such as phenobarbitone do reduce the plasma concentrations of montelukast.

5′-Lipoxygenase inhibitors

Zileuton (available in the USA) is a competitive inhibitor of 5′-lipoxygenase. It is administered orally (600 mg four times daily) and is cleared by hepatic metabolism with a mean $t_{\frac{1}{2}}$ of 2.5 h. It is used in chronic asthma, to reduce steroid or β_2-agonist dose, and may be particularly helpful in aspirin (or NSAID)-sensitive asthmatics where leukotriene biosynthesis is increased. The commonest side-effect is gastrointestinal upset. Hepatitis, while uncommon, necessitates liver enzyme monitoring.

Key points

Leukotriene modulation in asthma

- Leukotriene B_4 is a powerful chemo-attractant (eosinophils and neutrophils), and increases vascular permeability and produces mucosal oedema.
- Leukotrienes C_4, D_4 and E_4 (cysteinyl leukotrienes) are potent spasmogens and pro-inflammatory substances ('SRS-A').
- Clinically available agents that modulate leukotrienes are leukotriene antagonists (which antagonize cysteinyl leukotrienes – LTD_4, LTC_4 at the Cys LT_1 receptor) and 5′-lipoxygenase inhibitors (which reduce formation of leukotrienes B_4, C_4, D_4 and E_4).
- Leukotriene antagonists (e.g. montelukast) are effective as once daily oral maintenance therapy in chronic persistent asthma. Montelukast has anti-inflammatory properties and is a mild, slow-onset bronchodilator.
- 5′-Lipoxygenase inhibitors, (e.g. zileuton), are not bronchodilators but are useful in chronic asthma maintenance therapy and in aspirin-sensitive asthmatics

ANTIHISTAMINES

H$_1$-BLOCKERS

See Chapter 49.

Astemizole. cetirizine and loratidine

Antihistamines are not widely used in the treatment of asthma, but have an adjunctive role in asthmatics with severe hay fever. **Astemizole** is a relatively non-sedating H_1-antagonist with a very long plasma $t_{\frac{1}{2}}$ of 24–144 h. *There is potential for dangerous interactions leading to ventricular tachycardia with drugs that inhibit its metabolism (e.g. erythromycin, ketoconazole) or prolong the QT interval (e.g. amiodarone).* **Cetirizine** and **loraidine** do not cause this potentially fatal drug–drug interaction.

ALTERNATIVE ANTI-INFLAMMATORY AGENTS

Other anti-inflammatory drugs such as **methotrexate**, 7.5–15 mg weekly, or **cyclosporin A** reduce the glucocorticosteroid requirement in chronic asthmatics, but because of their long-term toxicities (see Chapters 25 and 49) they are not used routinely.

FUTURE DIRECTIONS IN DRUG THERAPY OF ASTHMA

Promising new agents currently undergoing early development for asthma therapy include more specific phosphodiesterase IV inhibitors that may be less toxic than theophylline, endothelin-1 antagonists, tachykinin (NK_1) receptor antagonists and monoclonal antibodies targeted against adhesion molecules, or interleukin-5.

RESPIRATORY FAILURE

Respiratory failure is the result of impaired gas exchange. It is defined as a PaO_2 below 8 kPa (60 mmHg). There are two types of respiratory failure.

1. Type I (ventilation/perfusion inequality) is characterized by a low PaO_2 and a *normal or low* $PaCO_2$. Causes include:
   - acute asthma;
   - pneumonia;
   - left ventricular failure;
   - pulmonary fibrosis;
   - shock lung.
2. Type II (ventilatory failure) is characterized by a low PaO_2 and a *raised* $PaCO_2$ (> 6.3 kPa). This occurs in:
   - severe asthma as the patient tires;
   - some patients with chronic bronchitis or emphysema;
   - reduced activity of the respiratory centre (e.g. from drug overdose or in association with morbid obesity and somnolence – Pickwickian syndrome);
   - peripheral neuromuscular disorders (e.g. Guillain–Barré syndrome or myasthenia gravis).

TREATMENT OF TYPE I RESPIRATORY FAILURE

The treatment of ventilation/perfusion inequality is that of the underlying lesion. Oxygen at high flow rate is given by nasal cannulae or mask. Shock lung is treated by controlled ventilation, oxygenation and positive end expiratory pressure (PEEP).

TREATMENT OF TYPE II RESPIRATORY FAILURE

Sedatives must never be used. Benzodiazepines can produce fatal respiratory depression in patients with ventilatory failure.

Supportive measures

PHYSIOTHERAPY

Physiotherapy is used to encourage coughing to remove tracheobronchial secretions and to encourage deep breathing to preserve airway patency.

OXYGEN

Oxygen improves tissue oxygenation, but high concentrations may further depress respiration by removing the hypoxic respiratory drive. A small increase in the concentration of inspired oxygen to 24% using a Venturi-type mask should be tried. If the $PaCO_2$ does not increase, or increases by < 0.66 kPa and the level of consciousness is unimpaired, the inspired oxygen concentration should be increased to 28%, and after further assessment to 35%. If oxygen produces respiratory depression, assisted ventilation may be urgently needed.

Specific measures

Respiratory failure can be precipitated in chronic bronchitis by infection, fluid overload (e.g. as the pulmonary artery pressure increases and cor pulmonale supervenes) or bronchoconstriction. Antibacterial drugs are used if the sputum has become purulent. Dietary salt restriction and/or diuretics may be needed. Bronchospasm may respond to 2.5–5 mg salbutamol given 2- to 4-hourly in a nebulizer via a tight-fitting mask (often supplemented by nebulized ipratropium, 250–500 μg 6- to 8-hourly). Hydrocortisone (800–1200 mg/day) is given intravenously. If the PaO_2 continues to fall and the $PaCO_2$ continues to rise, endotracheal intubation with suction and controlled respiration should be considered, especially if consciousness becomes impaired.

Key points

Respiratory failure

- Type I (hypocapnic hypoxaemia) and Type II (hypercapnic hypoxaemia).
- Therapy for Type I is supportive with high-percentage oxygen (FiO_2 40–60%).
- Therapy for Type II is low-percentage oxygen (FiO_2 24–28%), and treatment of reversible factors – infection and bronchospasm (with antibiotics, bronchodilators, corticosteroids).
- Type I or Type II respiratory failure may necessitate mechanical ventilation.
- CNS depressant drugs (e.g. opiates) may exacerbate or precipitate respiratory failure, usually of Type II.
- Sedatives are absolutely contraindicated (unless the patient is already undergoing mechanical ventilation).

COUGH

COUGH SUPPRESSANTS

Cough is a normal physiological reflex that frees the respiratory tract of accumulated secretions and removes particulate matter. The reflex is usually initiated by irritation of the mucous membrane of the respiratory tract and is co-ordinated by a centre in the medulla. Ideally, treatment should not impair elimination of bronchopulmonary secretions. A number of antitussive drugs are available, but critical evaluation of their efficacy is difficult. Cough can be produced in volunteers by inhalation of irritants such as sulphur dioxide or citric acid or capsaicin, and the effect of a potential cough suppressant on such induced cough can be measured. Patients with chronic cough are often poor judges of the effect of drugs on their cough because of spontaneous variation in intensity from day to day. Objective recording methods have demonstrated dose-dependent efficacy for some cough suppressants. However, cough should not be routinely suppressed, because of its protective function. Exceptions include intractable cough in carcinoma of the bronchus, and cases in which an unproductive cough interferes with sleep or causes exhaustion. Bland demulcent syrups containing soothing substances (e.g. simple linctus BPC) provide adequate comfort for many patients. Codeine (10–30 mg given orally, see Chapter 24) depresses the medullary cough centre and is highly effective.

EXPECTORANTS

Difficulty in clearing viscous sputum is often associated with chronic cough. Various expectorants and mucolytic agents are available, but they are not very satisfactory.

1 Mixtures containing a demulcent and an antihistamine, a decongestant such as **pseudoephedrine** and sometimes a cough suppres-

sant such as codeine are often prescribed. This cocktail is less harmful than anticipated, probably because the dose of most of its components is too low to exert much of an effect.

2 Drugs which reduce the viscosity of sputum by altering the nature of its organic components are also available. They are sometimes called mucolytics, and the traditional agents are unhelpful because they reduce the efficacy of mucociliary clearance (which depends on beating cilia being mechanically coupled to viscous mucus). The increased viscosity of infected sputum is due to nucleic acids rather than mucopolysaccharides, and is not affected by drugs such as **bromhexine** or **acetyl cysteine**, which are therefore ineffective. **rhDNAase-Pulmozyme**-(phosphorylated glycosylated recombinant human deoxribonuclease 1 enzyme), given by jet nebulizer, cleaves extracellular bacterial DNA and has been shown to be effective in cystic fibrosis patients, decreasing sputum viscosity and reducing the rate of deterioration of lung function. Its major adverse effects are pharyngitis, voice changes, rashes and urticaria.

PULMONARY SURFACTANTS

Several pulmonary surfactants are available. **Colfosceril palmitate** (synthetic dipalmitoylphosphatidylcholine with hexadecanol and tyloxapol) is used in newborn infants undergoing mechanical ventilation for respiratory distress syndrome (RDS). It reduces complications, including pneumothorax and bronchopulmonary dysplasia, and improves survival. Colfosceril (67.5 mg/kg) is given via the endotracheal tube, repeated after 12 h if still intubated. Heart rate and arterial blood oxygenation/saturation must be monitored. The administered surfactant is rapidly dispersed and undergoes the same recycling as natural surfactant. Its principal adverse effects are obstruction of the endotracheal tubes by mucus, increased incidence of pulmonary haemorrhage, and acute hyperoxaemia due to rapid improvement if not appropriately monitored. The alternative pulmonary surfactants that are available are **beractant** (bovine lung extract providing phospholipids), **poractant alfa** (porcine lung extract providing phospholipids) and **pumactant** (synthetic phospholipids).

α_1-ANTITRYPSIN DEFICIENCY

α_1-Antitrypsin is a serine protease produced by the liver. It inhibits neutrophil elastase in lungs. In patients deficient in α_1-antitrypsin, neutrophil elastase destroys the alveolar wall, leading to early-onset emphysema which is rapidly progressive. Such patients usually die of respiratory failure. Diagnosis is by measurement of α_1-antitrypsin levels in the blood. Replacement therapy with α_1-antitrypsin can be considered. Replacement therapy with heat-treated (HIV and hepatitis virus negative) pooled plasma from donors is given intravenously weekly. The $t_{\frac{1}{2}}$ of α_1-antitrypsin is 5.2 days, and its only adverse effect is post-infusion fever. Plasma concentrations rise into the normal range and several small longitudinal clinical studies with weekly dosing suggest a slowing of the loss of FEV_1 compared to historical controls. Aerosolized administration on a weekly basis also appears to be safe and effective in paediatric patients (the intrapulmonary $t_{\frac{1}{2}}$ of α_1-antitrypsin in normals is 70 h). The use of recombinant α_1-antitrypsin is being investigated, as is the potential of α_1-antitrypsin gene therapy.

RESPIRATORY STIMULANTS

Respiratory stimulants (analeptic drugs) stimulate the central nervous system. Small doses produce respiratory and cardiovascular stimulation, but larger amounts produce convulsions. Analeptic drugs are only of limited short-term value in acute exacerbations of chronic lung disease.

Doxapram

This is a non-specific central nervous system stimulant. The ratio of convulsant to respiratory stimulant dose is 70:1, but large doses of **doxapram** produce general CNS stimulation and tachycardia, palpitations, sweating and tremor. Doxapram is contraindicated in epilepsy, hypertension, cerebral oedema and hyperthyroidism, and should not be used with monoamine oxidase inhibitors or sympathomimetic drugs. It is given intravenously, 0.5–1.5 mg/kg over 30 s followed by a maintenance infusion of 2–4 mg/min. The $t_{\frac{1}{2}}$ is 2.5–4.0 h. Doxapram may be considered in the short term for treating patients with acute exacerbations of chronic bronchitis with accompanying type II respiratory failure (i.e. hypercapnia and hypoxia) when mechanical ventilation is unavailable or deemed unsuitable, but it should only be given under expert supervision.

DRUG-INDUCED PULMONARY DISEASE

The lungs may be adversely affected by drugs in several important ways. Physical irritation by dry powder inhalers can precipitate bronchospasm in asthmatics. Allergy to drugs of the immediate variety (type I) is particularly common in atopic individuals. Specific reaginic antibodies (IgE) to drugs can produce disturbances ranging from mild wheezing to laryngeal oedema or anaphylactic shock. Delayed bronchospasm may be due to drug interactions involving IgG antibodies (type III). Any drug may be responsible for allergic reactions, but several antibiotics are powerful allergens. *β-Receptor antagonists* can produce prolonged and sometimes fatal bronchospasm in asthmatics. Aspirin and other non-steroidal anti-inflammatory drugs (see Chapter 24) cause bronchoconstriction in sensitive individuals (1–2% incidence) with asthma, nasal polyps and urticaria. Parasympathomimetic drugs (e.g. bethanechol) and acetylcholinesterase inhibitors such as physostigmine can promote bronchial secretions and increase airways resistance. *Angiotensin-converting enzyme (ACE) inhibitors* (see Chapters 27 and 28) commonly (in 9–30% of patients) cause a chronic dry cough which is dose dependent.

Pulmonary eosinophilia presents as dyspnoea, cough and fever. The chest X-ray shows widespread patchy changing shadows, and there is usually eosinophilia in the peripheral blood. The pathogenesis of the condition is not fully understood, but several drugs have been implicated, including aspirin, nitrofurantoin, imipramine, isoniazid, penicillin, streptomycin and sulphasalazine. *Polyarteritis nodosa* is sometimes associated with hepatitis B acquired by abuse of amphetamine ('skin popping').

The lungs can be involved by pleuritic reactions, pneumonia-like illness and impaired respiratory function due to small, stiff lungs in drug-induced systemic lupus erythematosus. Examples of drugs that cause this include hydralazine, bromocriptine and procainamide.

Many drugs can produce interstitial pulmonary fibrosis, including amiodarone, bleomycin, busulphan, cyclophosphamide, gold salts, methotrexate and nitrofurantoin.

Case history

A 35-year-old woman with a history of mild asthma in childhood (when she was diagnosed as being sensitive to aspirin) was seen in the Medical Out-patients department because of sinus ache, some mild nasal stuffiness and itchy eyes. She had hay fever. For her asthma she was currently taking prn salbutamol (2 puffs) and beclomethasone 500 μg/day. She was given a prescription for an antihistamine, ketotifen 2 mg (two tablets) twice daily. She took the prescription to her local chemist rather than the hospital chemist, and she started taking the tablets the following morning as prescribed. That evening she was rushed to hospital with acute severe asthma- requiring ventilation, but recovered. Fortunately, on the night of her admission her husband brought in all of the prescribed medications she was taking, and this led to her physicians establishing why she had deteriorated so suddenly that day.

Question

What led to this near fatal asthma attack? How could it have been avoided?

Answer

The admitting medical team treated this patient with oxygen, IPPV, corticosteroids and nebulized bronchodilators. Among her medications they found a bottle of ketoprofen (an NSAID) which she had started that morning (two 100 mg tablets twice a day); 1–2% of asthmatics are aspirin and NSAID sensitive. The pharmacist had not checked for NSAID sensitivity and the patient was not expecting an NSAID prescription after what the hospital doctor had told her about ketotifen. Thus it is always important to check in the case of asthmatics that they are not 'aspirin sensitive'.

On reviewing the prescription, the handwriting could have been thought to read 'ketoprofen', but the practitioner was adamant that she had written 'ketotifen'. The second issue in this case was a poorly written prescription for a drug with which the patient was unfamiliar, namely ketotifen, an antihistamine analogue that is claimed to have additional cromoglycate-like properties, but whose anti-allergic effects have been disappointing in clinical practice. *The importance of clearly written appropriate drug prescriptions cannot be over-emphasized.* Possible 'look-alike' drug pairs which have the potential for confusion if not clearly written include alprazolam and alprostadil, chlorpheniramine and chlorpromazine, digoxin and doxepin, esmolol and ethambutol, fexofenadine and fenfluramine, metoprolol and misoprostol, and omeprazole and astemizole. Proprietary names further multiply the opportunities for confusion.

Further reading

Barnes PJ. 1995: Drug therapy: inhaled glucocorticoids for asthma. *New England Journal of Medicine* **332**, 868–75.

British Thoracic Society. 1997: Guidelines for the management of asthma. *Thorax* **52 (Suppl.1)**, S1–S52.

Sampson A, Holgate S. 1998: Leukotriene modifiers in the treatment of asthma. *British Medical Journal* **316**, 1257–8.

Spector S. 1997: Leukotriene activity modulation in asthma. *Drugs* **54**, 369–84.

Ward MJ. 1997: Nebulisers for asthma. *Thorax* **52** (**Suppl.1**), S45– S48.

PART VI

THE ALIMENTARY SYSTEM

CHAPTER THIRTY-THREE

ALIMENTARY SYSTEM *and* LIVER

- Peptic ulceration
- Oesophageal disorders
- Anit-emetics
- Inflammatory bowel disease
- Constipation
- Diarrhoea
- Irritable bowel syndrome
- Pancreatic disease
- Liver disease
- Gallstones
- Drugs that modify appetite

PEPTIC ULCERATION

PATHOPHYSIOLOGY

Peptic ulcer disease is a chronic disorder characterized by frequent recurrences over a period of many years. It affects approximately 10% of the population of western countries. The incidence of duodenal ulcer (DU) is four to five times higher than that of gastric ulcer (GU). Up to 1 million of the UK population suffer from peptic ulceration in a 12-month period.

Peptic ulceration occurs in a number of clinical settings, and it is unlikely that a single drug will be universally effective. The aetiology of ulceration is not well understood, but there are four major factors of known importance:

1 acid–pepsin secretion;
2 the presence of Helicobacter pylori;
3 mucosal resistance to attack by acid and pepsin;
4 non-steroidal anti-inflammatory drugs (NSAIDs).

Key points

Peptic ulceration

- It affects 10% of the population.
- Duodenal ulcers are more common than gastric ulcers (> 4:1).
- Most ulcers are related to *Helicobacter pylori* or NSAIDs.
- Relapse is common.

Acid–pepsin secretion

Gastric parietal (oxyntic) cells secrete isotonic hydrochloric acid (pH < 1). Figure 33.1 illustrates the mechanisms that regulate gastric acid secretion. Acid secretion is stimulated by gastrin, acetylcholine and histamine. Gastrin is secreted by endocrine cells in the gastric antrum and duodenum. Zollinger–Ellison syndrome is an uncommon disorder caused by a gastrin-secreting adenoma associated with very severe peptic ulcer disease.

Mucosal resistance

Some endogenous mediators suppress acid secretion and protect the gastric mucosa. Prostaglandin E_2 (the principal prostaglandin synthesized in the stomach) is an important gastroprotective mediator. It inhibits secretion of acid, promotes secretion of protective mucus and causes vasodilatation of submucosal blood vessels. The gastric and duodenal mucosa is protected against acid–pepsin digestion by a mucus layer into which bicarbonate

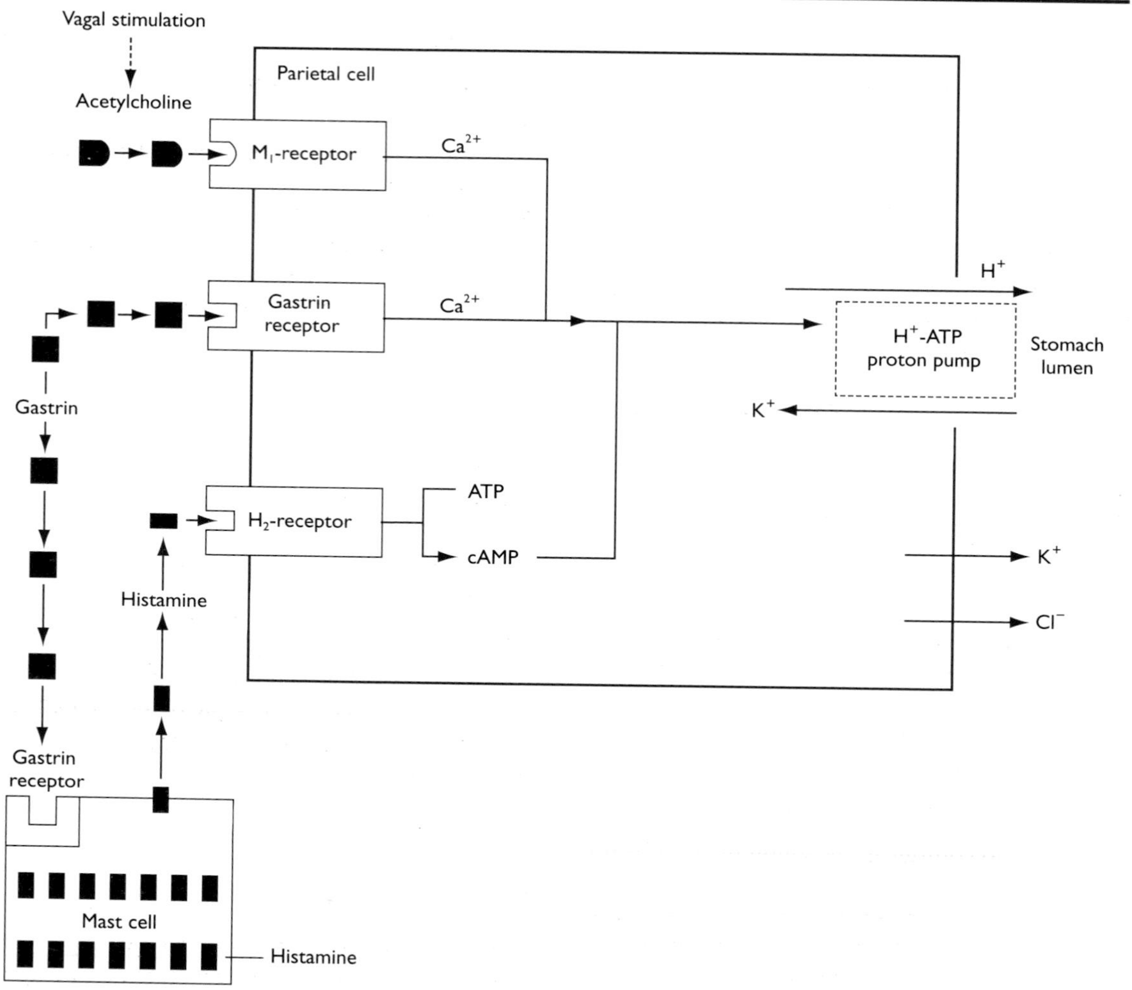

Figure 33.1: Mechanisms regulating hydrochloric acid secretion. Ca^{2+} = calcium, ATP = adenosine triphosphate, cAMP = cyclic adenosine monophosphate, K^+ = potassium, Cl^- = chloride.

is secreted. Agents such as salicylate, ethanol and bile impair the protective function of this layer. Acid diffuses from the lumen into the stomach wall at sites of damage where the protective layer of mucus is defective. The presence of strong acid in the submucosa causes further damage, and persistence of hydrogen ions in the interstitium initiates or perpetuates peptic ulceration. Hydrogen ions are cleared from the submucosa by diffusion into blood vessels, and are then buffered in circulating blood. Local vasodilatation in the stomach wall is thus an important part of the protective mechanism against acid–pepsin damage.

Non-steroidal anti-inflammatory drugs

Aspirin and other NSAIDs inhibit the biosynthesis of prostaglandin E_2 as well as causing direct irritation and damage to the gastric mucosa.

Helicobacter pylori

The presence of the bacterium *Helicobacter pylori* has now been established as a major causative factor in the aetiology of peptic ulcer disease. Although commonly found in the gastric antrum,

Key points

Recommendations for eradication of *Helicobacter pylori*

- Duodenal ulcer
- Gastric ulcer
- Mucosa-associated lymphoid tissue (MALT) lymphoma.
- Severe *H.pylori* gastritis.
- Patients requiring long-term proton-pump-inhibitor treatment (risk of accelerated gastric atrophy).
- Blind treatment with eradication therapy is not recommended.

it may also colonize other areas of the stomach as well as patches of gastric metaplasia in the duodenum. *H.pylori* is present in all patients with active type B antral gastritis, and in 90–95% of those with duodenal ulcers. After exclusion of gastric ulcers caused by non-steroidal anti-inflammatory drug therapy and Zollinger–Ellison syndrome, the incidence of *H.pylori* infection in patients with gastric ulcer approaches 100%. The strongest evidence of a causal relationship between *H.pylori* and peptic ulcer disease is the marked reduction in ulcer recurrence and complications following successful eradication of the organism. It has been shown that the speed of ulcer healing obtained with acid-suppressing agents is accelerated if *H.pylori* eradication is achieved concomitantly. Moreover, eradication of *H.pylori* infection prior to the commencement of NSAID therapy reduces the occurrence of gastro-duodenal ulcers in patients who have not had previous exposure to NSAIDs. *H.pylori* appears to be associated with increased risk of gastric cancer of the corpus and antrum.

PRINCIPLES OF MANAGEMENT

The therapeutic objectives are as follows:

1 symptomatic relief;
2 promotion of ulcer healing;
3 prevention of recurrence once healing has occurred;
4 prevention of complications.

Key points

General management of peptic ulceration

- Stop smoking.
- Avoid ulcerogenic drugs (e.g. NSAIDs, alcohol, corticosteroids).
- Reduce caffeine intake.
- Diet should be healthy (avoid obesity, and foods that give rise to symptoms).
- Test for the presence of *H.pylori*.

Key points

Ulcer-healing drugs

Reduction of acidity:

- antacids;
- H_2-blockers;
- proton-pump inhibitors;
- muscarinic blockers (pirenzapine)

Mucosal protection:

- misoprostol (also reduces gastric acid secretion);
- bismuth chelate (also toxic to *H.pylori*);
- sucralfate;
- carbenoxolone (rarely prescribed).

General management

1 Stopping smoking increases the healing rate of gastric ulcers, and is more effective in preventing the recurrence of duodenal ulcers than H_2-receptor antagonists.
2 Diet is of symptomatic importance only. Patients usually discover for themselves which foods aggravate symptoms.
3 Avoid 'ulcerogenic' drugs, including caffeine (as strong coffee or tea), alcohol, aspirin and other NSAIDs (paracetamol is a safe minor analgesic in these cases) and corticosteroids.
4 With regard to drug therapy, several drugs (see below) are effective. Documented duodenal or gastric ulcerations should be treated with an H_2-blocker or proton-pump inhibitor.
5 Test for the presence of *H.pylori* by using the urease CLO test or antral biopsy at endoscopy.
6 All suspected gastric ulcers should be endoscoped and biopsied to exclude malignancy, with repeat endoscopy following treatment, to confirm healing and for repeat biopsy.

7 The current recommendation in relation to *H.pylori* is summarized above.

The choice of regimen used to eradicate *H.pylori* is based on achieving a balance between efficacy, adverse effects, compliance and cost. Most regimens include a combination of acid suppression and effective doses of one or two antibiotics. A recent survey showed that there are about 145 different regimens for eradication of *H.pylori*! A typical regime is shown in Table 33.1

Eradication should be confirmed, preferably by urea breath test at a minimum of 4 weeks post treatment. As this is a rapidly changing field, the Guidelines issued by the British Society of Gastroenterology should be consulted.

NON-STEROIDAL ANTI-INFLAMMATORY DRUG-ASSOCIATED ULCER

NSAID-related ulcers will usually heal if the NSAID is withdrawn and a proton-pump inhibitor is prescribed for 4 weeks. If the NSAID has to be restarted (preferably after healing), H_2-receptor antagonists or proton-pump inhibitors or misoprostol should be prescribed. The latter is commonly associated with diarrhoea and colic. If *H.pylori* is present it should be eradicated.

Table 33.1: Typical *Helicobacter plyori* eradication regime

Lansoprazole	30 mg bd	all for 1 week
Amoxycillin*	1 g bd	
Metronidazole	400 mg tds	

* Tetracycline 500 mg tds if patient is allergic to penicillin.

DRUGS USED TO TREAT PEPTIC ULCERATION BY REDUCING ACIDITY

Antacids

USE AND ADVERSE EFFECTS

Antacids have a number of actions which include neutralizing gastric acid and thus relieving associated pain and nausea, reducing delivery of acid into the duodenum following a meal, and inactivation of the proteolytic enzyme pepsin by raising the gastric pH above 4–5. In addition, it is thought that antacid may increase lower oesophageal sphincter tone and reduce oesophageal pressure. A number of preparations are available, and the choice will depend on the patient's preference, often determined by the effect on bowel habit. (see Table 33.2).

There are a number of products available on the market which contain a combination of antacids . These are designed:

Table 33.2: Antacids

Antacid	Features	Adverse effects
Sodium bicarbonate	Rapid action	Produces carbon dioxide, causing belching and distension; excess can cause metabolic alkalosis; best avoided in renal and cardiovascular disease
Calcium carbonate	High acid-neutralizing capacity	Acid rebound; excess may cause hypercalcaemia and constipation
Magnesium salts (e.g. dihydroxide, carbonate, triscilicate)	Poor solubility, weak antacids; the trisilicates inactivate pepsin; lower oesophageal sphincter tone, and may be of use in reflux	Diarrhoea
Aluminium hydroxide	Forms an insoluble colloid in the presence of acid, and lines the gastric mucosa to provide a physical and chemical barrier; weak antacid, slow onset of action, inactivates pepsin	Constipation; absorption of dietary phosphate may lead to calcium depletion and negative calcium balance

1 to increase the duration of action (e.g. by coupling a fast-acting antacid such as sodium bicarbonate with a slower-acting agent such as magnesium carbonate);
2 to neutralize the side-effect of one agent with another, (e.g. combining aluminium hydroxide with magnesium hydroxide);
3 to provide a maximal antacid effect by using low doses of several antacids in combination;
4 to reduce flatulence by the addition of dimethicone;
5 to increase relief from reflux by the addition of alginates.

In general terms, antacids should be taken approximately 1 h before or after food, as this maximizes the contact time with stomach acid, and allows the antacid to coat the stomach in the absence of food.

DRUG INTERACTIONS

Magnesium and aluminum salts can bind other drugs in the stomach, reducing the rate and extent of absorption of antibacterial agents such as erythromycin, ciprofloxacin, isoniazid, norfloxacin, ofloxacin, pivampicillin, rifampicin and most tetracyclines, as well as other drugs such as phenytoin, itraconazole, ketoconazole, chloroquine, hydroxychloroquine, phenothiazines, iron and penicillamine. They increase the excretion of aspirin (in alkaline urine).

H_2-receptor antagonists

H_2-receptors stimulate gastric acid secretion and are also present in human heart, blood vessels and uterus (and probably brain). There are a number of competitive H_2-receptor antagonists in clinical use which include **cimetidine** and **ranitidine**. The uses of these are similar and will be considered together in this section. Because each drug is so widely prescribed, separate sections on their individual adverse effects, pharmacokinetics and interactions are given below, followed by a brief consideration of the choice between them.

USE

1 H_2-receptor angonists are effective in healing both gastric and duodenal ulcers. A 4-week course is usually adequate. Nearly all duodenal ulcers and most gastric ulcers that are not associated with NSAIDs are associated with *Heliobacter pylori*, which should be eradicated (see above). Most regimens include an H_2-receptor antagonist or a proton-pump inhibitor. It is essential to exclude carcinoma endoscopically, as H_2-blockers can improve symptoms caused by malignant ulcers. Without gastric acid, the functions of which include providing a barrier to infection, patients on H_2-antagonists and proton-pump inhibitors are predisposed to infection by enteric pathogens, and the rate of bacterial diarrhoea is increased.
2 Oesophagitis may be treated with H_2-antagonists, but proton-pump inhibitors are more effective.
3 In cases of acute upper gastrointestinal haemorrhage and stress ulceration, the use of H_2-blockers is rational, although their efficacy has not been proven.
4 Replacement of pancreatic enzymes in steatorrhoea due to pancreatic insufficiency is often unsatisfactory due to destruction of the enzymes by acid and pepsin in the stomach. H_2-blockers improve the effectiveness of these enzymes in such cases.
5 In anaesthesia, H_2-receptor blockers can be given before emergency surgery to prevent aspiration of acid gastric contents, particularly in obstetric practice (Mendelson's syndrome).
6 The usual oral dose of cimetidine is 400 mg bd or 800 mg nocte, while for ranitidine it is 150 mg bd or 300 mg nocte to treat benign peptic ulceration.

Cimetidine

ADVERSE EFFECTS

Diarrhoea, rashes, dizziness, fatigue, constipation and muscular pain (usually mild and transient) have all been reported. Mental confusion can occur in the elderly. Cimetidine transiently increases serum prolactin levels, but the significance of this effect is unknown. Decreased libido and impotence have occasionally been reported during cimetidine treatment. Chronic cimetidine administration can cause gynaecomastia, which is reversible and appears with a frequency of 0.1–0.2%. Rapid intravenous injection of cimetidine has rarely been associated with bradycardia, tachycardia, asystole or hypotension. There have been rare reports of interstitial nephritis, urticaria and angioedema.

PHARMACOKINETICS

Cimetidine is well absorbed (70–80%) orally, and is subject to a small hepatic first-pass effect. Intramuscular and intravenous injections produce equivalent blood levels. The plasma $t_{\frac{1}{2}}$ is 2 h. Cimetidine is only 15–20% protein bound, and is removed by haemodialysis. It crosses the placenta and the blood–brain barrier, particularly in seriously ill and elderly patients. Elimination is mainly renal as the unchanged compound, but some is excreted as metabolites, mainly the sulphoxide. Renal tubular secretion occurs (by the non-specific base transport carrier; see Chapter 8), so renal clearance exceeds the glomerular filtration rate. Cimetidine blocks the tubular secretion of creatinine, and this explains the transient rise in serum creatinine levels that occurs during the first few weeks of cimetidine treatment. There is a minor excretory pathway into the gut, which may become important in renal failure.

DRUG INTERACTIONS

1 Absorption of ketoconazole (which requires a low pH) and itraconazole is reduced by cimetidine.
2 Metabolism of several drugs is reduced by cimetidine due to inhibition of cytochrome P_{450}, resulting in raised plasma drug concentrations. Interactions of potential clinical importance include those with warfarin, theophylline, phenytoin, carbamazepine, pethidine and other opioid analgesics, tricyclic antidepressants, lignocaine (cimetidine-induced reduction of hepatic blood flow is also a factor in this interaction), terfenadine, amiodarone, flecainide, quinidine and fluorouracil.
3 Cimetidine inhibits the renal excretion of metformin and procainamide, resulting in increased plasma concentrations of these drugs.

Ranitidine

ADVERSE EFFECTS

Ranitidine has a similar profile of minor side-effects to cimetidine. There have been some very rare reports of breast swelling and tenderness in men. However, unlike cimetidine, ranitidine does not bind to androgen receptors, and impotence and gynaecomastia in patients on high doses of cimetidine have been reported to resolve when they were switched to ranitidine. Cardiovascular effects have been even more infrequently reported than with cimetidine. Small amounts of ranitidine penetrate the central nervous system (CNS) and (like but less commonly than cimetidine) it can (rarely) cause mental confusion, mainly in the elderly and in patients with hepatic or renal impairment.

PHARMACOKINETICS

Ranitidine is well absorbed after oral administration, but its bioavailability is only 50%, suggesting that there is appreciable first-pass metabolism. Absorption is not affected by food. Like cimetidine, the $t_{\frac{1}{2}}$ is about 2 h and around 70% is excreted unchanged by the kidneys by tubular secretion and filtration.

In elderly patients the half-life is prolonged by about 50%, probably because of reduced renal excretion. Clearance is only slightly reduced in patients with liver disease, and alteration of the dose is unnecessary. In severe renal failure (creatinine clearance < 20 mL/min), therapeutic levels can be achieved with half the usual dose of ranitidine (75 mg twice daily).

DRUG INTERACTIONS

Ranitidine has a lower affinity for cytochrome P_{450} than cimetidine, and does not inhibit the metabolism of warfarin, phenytoin and theophylline to a clinically significant degree.

CHOICE OF H_2-ANTAGONIST

All of the H_2-receptor antagonists currently available in the UK are effective in peptic ulceration and are well tolerated. Cimetidine and ranitidine are most commonly prescribed, and have been available for the longest time. Cimetidine is the least expensive, but in young men who require prolonged treatment ranitidine may be preferable, due to a lower reported incidence of impotence and gynaecomastia. Ranitidine is also preferable in the elderly, where cimetidine occasionally causes confusion, and also when the patient is on drugs whose metabolism is inhibited by cimetidine (e.g. warfarin, phenytoin or theophylline).

Other H_2-receptor antagonists available for limited use in the UK include **famotidine** and

nizatidine, but they offer no significant advantage over ranitidine.

Proton-pump inhibitors

The proton-pump inhibitors **omeprazole**, **lansoprazole**, **pantoprazole** and **rabeprazole** inhibit gastric acid by blocking the H^+/K^+-adenosine triphosphatase enzyme system (the proton pump) of the gastric parietal cell. The indications for proton-pump inhibitors include the following:

1 benign duodenal and gastric ulcers;
2 NSAID-associated peptic ulcer and gastro-duodenal erosions;
3 in combination with antibacterial drugs to eradicate *H.pylori*;
4 Zollinger-Ellison syndrome;
5 gastric acid reduction during general anaesthesia;
6 gastro-oesophageal reflux disease (GORD);
7 stricturing and erosive oesophagitis where they are the treatment of choice.

Currently there are four licensed proton-pump inhibitors available on prescription in the UK. Of these, the widest clinical experience has been with omeprazole, and so far lanzoprazole and pantoprazole show little significant difference. The main differences, if any, appear to be in relation to possible drug interactions. As yet there do not appear to be any clinically significant drug interactions with pantoprazole, whereas omeprazole inhibits cytochrome P_{450}, and lansoprazole is a weak inducer of cytochrome P_{450}.

Omeprazole

USES

These include the following:

1 duodenal ulcer – at a dose of 20 mg once daily omeprazole heals over 90% of duodenal ulcers after 4 weeks;
2 gastric ulcer – an 8-week course of omeprazole, 20 mg once daily heals 85–90% of gastric ulcers;
3 oesophagitis – omeprazole, 20 mg once daily, heals erosive oesophagitis in approximately 80% of patients after 4 weeks, and is licensed for long-term use in peptic oesophagitis;
4 Zollinger–Ellison syndrome – omeprazole is the drug of choice for suppressing acid secretion in this rare disorder. Such patients may need treatment for long periods at high doses (up to 120 mg daily);
5 other indications – omeprazole may also have a place in the prevention of stress ulceration in acutely ill and burns patients, as well as in the prevention of aspiration syndromes in cases where emergency anaesthesia is necessary. There is as yet no clear evidence that omeprazole reduces morbidity or mortality from upper gastrointestinal bleeding, but the results of further research on this are awaited.

Omeprazole degrades in the presence of moisture, and capsules are supplied in special containers with a desiccant in the lid. Once the container has been opened, the contents should be used within 3 months. To prevent degradation by gastric acid, the granules in each capsule are enteric coated.

MECHANISM OF ACTION

Omeprazole is an irreversible inhibitor of the H^+/K^+ adenosine triphosphatase (ATPase) locus of the gastric parietal cell – the 'proton pump' which secretes acid into the gastric lumen.

ADVERSE EFFECTS

Minor side-effects include diarrhoea and headache (although both may be severe), nausea, constipation and flatulence. Other less common side-effects include muscle and joint pains, skin reactions (some of which are serious), blurred vision, peripheral oedema, gynaecomastia, loss of taste and blood disorders. Severely ill patients may develop reversible mental confusion, depression and hallucinations.

PHARMACOKINETICS

Bioavailability is very variable and depends on the formulation. The time to maximum plasma concentration ranges from 20 min for a solution to over 2 h for enteric-coated granules. The plasma $t_{\frac{1}{2}}$ is between 0.5 and 1.5 h, with a mean value of 1 h. The volume of distribution is 0.3–0.4 L/kg. Omeprazole is 95% plasma protein bound. Although there is a clear dose-related inhibition of gastric acid secretion with omeprazole, peak concentrations of the drug in plasma do not correlate with antisecretory activity.

Omeprazole undergoes rapid and almost complete metabolism, and unchanged drug is not excreted in the urine, although nearly 20% of unchanged drug may be recovered in the faeces. Clearance is not influenced by renal disease or by haemodialysis.

Drug interactions

Omeprazole inhibits cytochrome P_{450} drug metabolism and thereby enhances the effects of warfarin, phenytoin and diazepam.

Antisecretory drugs and gastric cancer

It has been suggested that the chronic use of drugs that suppress gastric acid secretion may cause gastric cancer. The hypothesis is that reduced gastric acidity could allow bacterial colonization of the stomach by nitrate-reducing bacteria. These could produce nitrite from dietary nitrates and could form N-nitroso compounds with food amines. Some N-nitroso compounds are mutagenic and resemble animal carcinogens. All of these steps could theoretically follow any anti-ulcer treatment, and it is certainly the case that carcinoma of the gastric remnant has followed some ulcer operations. Similarly, there is an increased risk of gastric carcinoma with Addisonian pernicious anaemia with associated achlorhydria. However, vagotomy is not associated with this problem, and similarly no causal link has been established between chronic administration of H_2-blocking drugs and gastric cancer in humans or animals. As yet there is also no definite evidence linking omeprazole to gastric cancer in humans or animals. One potentially important problem with regard to the use of antisecretory drugs is their effectiveness in producing transient symptomatic relief in gastric cancer and hence causing delay in diagnosis.

Muscarinic receptor antagonists

Use

Acetylcholine acts on muscarinic receptors in gastrointestinal smooth muscle and stomach to cause contractions and acid secretion. Antimuscarinic drugs are used in the treatment of non-ulcer dyspepsia, irritable bowel syndrome and diverticular disease. Antimuscarinic drugs decrease gastric motility and possibly spasm produced by irritation from ulceration (for this reason they have been termed antispasmodics). Dose is limited by antimuscarinic side-effects and only **pirenzepine**, a selective M_1-receptor antagonist, has significant antisecretory effects at a dose that is tolerated.

Adverse effects and contraindications

The following adverse effects can be predicted from the actions of these drugs on muscarinic receptors:

1. dryness of the mouth (decreased salivation);
2. blurring of vision and photophobia (paralysis of accommodation and dilatation of the pupil), and precipitation of glaucoma;
3. constipation;
4. urinary retention and difficulty with micturition;
5. tachycardia;
6. impotence.

Contraindications include glaucoma, prostatic enlargement, coronary artery disease and pyloric stenosis. Pirenzepine produces fewer such effects than other antimuscarinic drugs because of its higher selectivity for M_1-receptors, but some patients notice mild difficulty with visual accommodation and have a dry mouth. Anticholinergic drugs alter the rate of absorption of other drugs if given concurrently (see Chapter 13).

Drugs that enhance mucosal resistance

Prostagladin analogues

Misoprostol is a synthetic analogue of prostaglandin E_1 which inhibits gastric acid secretion, causes vasodilatation in the submucosa and stimulates the production of protective mucus.

Uses

These include the following:

1. healing of duodenal ulcer and gastric ulcer, including those induced by NSAIDs;

2 the prophylaxis of gastric and duodenal ulceration in patients on NSAID therapy.

ADVERSE EFFECTS

Diarrhoea, abdominal pain, nausea and vomiting, dyspepsia, flatulence, abnormal vaginal bleeding, rashes and dizziness may occur. The most frequent adverse effects are gastrointestinal, and these are usually dose dependent.

CONTRAINDICATIONS

Pregnancy is an absolute contraindication to the use of misoprostol, as the latter causes abortion.

PHARMACOKINETICS

Misoprostol is rapidly absorbed following oral administration, with peak plasma levels of the active metabolite, misoprostol acid, occurring after about 30 min. The plasma elimination $t_{\frac{1}{2}}$ is 20–40 min. It is extensively metabolized to inactive products that are excreted in the urine.

Bismuth chelate

Colloidal tripotassium dicitratobismuthate precipitates at acid pH to form a layer over the mucosal surface and ulcer base, where it combines with the proteins of the ulcer exudate. This coat is protective against acid and pepsin digestion. It also stimulates mucus production and may chelate with pepsin, thus speeding ulcer healing. Several studies have shown it to be as active as cimetidine in the healing of duodenal and gastric ulcers after 4–8 weeks of treatment. It has a direct toxic effect on *H.pylori* and may be used as part of triple therapy.

Bismuth chelate elixir is given diluted with water 30 min before meals and 2 h after the last meal of the day. This liquid has an ammoniacal, metallic taste and odour which is unacceptable to some patients, and chewable tablets can be used instead. Antacids or milk should not be taken concurrently.

Ranitidine bismuth citrate tablets are also available for the treatment of peptic ulcers and for use in *H.pylori* eradication regimes.

ADVERSE EFFECTS

Adverse effects include blackening of the tongue, teeth and stools (causing potential confusion with melena) and nausea. The latter may limit dosing. Bismuth is potentially neurotoxic. Urine bismuth levels rise with increasing oral dosage, indicating some intestinal absorption. Although with normal doses the blood concentration remains well below the toxic threshold, bismuth should not be used in renal failure or for maintenance treatment.

Sucralfate

USE

Sucralfate is used in the management of benign gastric and duodenal ulceration and chronic gastritis. Its action is entirely local, with minimal if any systemic absorption. It is a basic aluminum salt of sucrose octasulphate which, in the presence of acid, becomes a sticky adherent paste that retains antacid efficacy. This material coats the floor of ulcer craters, exerting its acid-neutralizing properties locally, unlike conventional antacid gels which form a diffusely distributed antacid dispersion. In addition it binds to pepsin and bile salts and prevents their contact with the ulcer base. Sucralfate compares favourably with cimetidine for healing both gastric and duodenal ulcers, and is equally effective in symptom relief. The dose is 1 g (1 tablet) four times daily for 4–6 weeks. Antacids may be given concurrently.

ADVERSE EFFECTS

Sucralfate is well tolerated but, because it contains aluminum, constipation can occur, and in severe renal failure accumulation is a potential hazard.

Carbenoxolone

USE

Carbenoxolone is a liquorice derivative used in combination with antacids to treat oesophageal ulceration and inflammation. Its mode of action is complex, and it increases mucosal resistance without affecting acid secretion or motility. There are more effective and better tolerated alternatives.

ADVERSE EFFECTS

Side-effects are frequent and hazardous. Those particularly at risk are the elderly and patients with cardiac, renal and hepatic disease.

Sodium retention is common due to an aldosterone-like action. Headache, oedema, dyspnoea, cardiac failure, hypertension and epilepsy have all been reported.

Case history

A 75-year-old retired greengrocer who presented to the Accident and Emergency department with shortness of breath and a history of melaena is found on endoscopy to have a bleeding gastric erosion. His drug therapy leading up to his admission consisted of digoxin, warfarin and piroxicam for a painful hip, and cimetidine for recent indigestion.

Question

How may this patient's drug therapy have precipitated or aggravated his bleeding gastric erosion?

Answer

NSAIDs inhibit the biosynthesis of prostaglandin E_2 as well as causing direct damage to the gastric mucosa. Warfarin is an anticoagulant and will increase bleeding. Cimetidine inhibits cytochrome P_{450} and therefore inhibits the metabolism of warfarin, resulting in higher blood concentrations and an increased anticoagulant effect.

Hypokalaemia occurs in 30–40% of patients. This can be so severe as to present with muscle weakness, myositis, myasthenia, myoglobinuria and peripheral neuropathy, and a diagnosis of hyperaldosteronism or Guillain–Barré syndrome may be considered. The drug must be stopped and potassium supplements may be needed temporarily.

OESOPHAGEAL DISORDERS

REFLUX OESOPHAGITIS

Reflux oesophagitis is a common problem. It causes heartburn and acid regurgitation and predisposes to stricture formation.

NON-DRUG MEASURES

Non-drug measures which may be useful include the following:

1. sleeping with the head of the bed raised. Most damage to the oesophagus occurs at night when swallowing is much reduced and acid can remain in contact with the mucosa for long periods;
2. avoiding:
   - large meals;
   - alcohol and/or food before bed;
   - smoking, which lowers the lower oesophageal sphincter (LES) pressure, and coffee;
   - aspirin and NSAIDs;
   - constricting clothing around the abdomen;
3. weight reduction;
4. bending from the knees and not the spine;
5. regular exercise.

DRUG THERAPY

Drugs that may be useful include the following:

1. **metoclopramide** or **cisapride** (see below), which raise lower oesophageal sphincter pressure;
2. a mixture of alginate and antacids is symptomatically useful – the alginate forms a viscous layer floating on the gastric contents;
3. a mixture of silicon with an antacid (e.g. dimethicone, aluminum hydroxide and sorbitol). These mixtures are intended to lower surface tension and thus to allow the formation of large gas bubbles that can be easily expelled from the stomach without encouraging reflux. It is not clear why this helps in reflux – possibly the silicon coats the lower oesophagus and 'protects' it from acid/bile. Such mixtures are of uncertain value;
4. symptomatic relief may be obtained with antacids, but there is a risk of chronic aspiration of poorly soluble particles of magnesium or aluminum salts if these are taken at night;
5. H_2-antagonists;
6. Proton-pump inhibitors are the most effective agents currently available for reflux oesophagitis, and are the drugs of choice for erosive reflux oesophagitis.

Cisapride

USE

Cisapride is a motility stimulant that releases acetylcholine in the gut wall. Unlike metoclopramide, it does not have central dopamine antagonist properties. It is costly, and is used in the following:

1 gastroesophageal reflux – cisapride (10 mg three times a day for up to 12 weeks) is more effective than placebo and about as effective as H_2-antagonists in reducing the symptoms and healing reflux oesophagitis;
2 dyspepsia – patients who have dyspeptic symptoms without an identifiable lesion on endoscopy. Cisapride (10 mg three times daily for 2–4 weeks) causes relief of symptoms in more than 80% of such patients, compared to only about 35% of those on placebo;
3 Delayed gastric emptying – this may be due to chronic administration of other drugs such as alcohol, opiates or anticholinergics, or in association with systemic diseases that cause disorders of motility, such as the autonomic neuropathy of diabetes mellitus. A trial of cisapride, 10 mg three times daily for 6 weeks or longer, may prove effective.

ADVERSE EFFECTS

These are predominantly the effects of increased gut motility, such as abdominal cramps, borborygmi, diarrhoea and loose stools. An unpredicted serious adverse effect is prolongation of the QT interval, which predisposes to ventricular arrhythmias. Other minor effects include headache and dizziness, and there have been rare reports of headache and extrapyramidal effects.

PHARMACOKINETICS

There is rapid and extensive absorption (94–96%) following oral administration of cisapride, with a peak concentration at 1–2 h. The plasma $t_{\frac{1}{2}}$ is 7–10 h and it has a volume of distribution of 2.4 L/kg. It is 98% protein bound, predominantly to albumin. The predominant site of metabolism is the liver. The half-life is prolonged in elderly patients and in those with renal failure and cirrhosis, and it is important to reduce the dose in these patients.

DRUG INTERACTIONS

These are mainly a consequence of the increased rate of gastric emptying, which can in turn increase the rate of absorption of other drugs. This is seldom a problem in practice. Other drugs which prolong the QT interval should be avoided.

Case history

A 25-year-old male estate agent complains of intermittent heartburn, belching and sub-xiphisternal pain which has been present on most nights for 2 weeks. It was particularly severe the previous Saturday night after he had consumed a large curry and several pints of beer. The symptoms were not improved by sleeping on two extra pillows or by taking ibuprofen. He smokes 10 cigarettes daily. Examination revealed him to be overweight but was otherwise unremarkable.

Question

Outline your management of this patient.

Answer

Life-style advice – stop smoking, lose weight, adopt a low-fat diet, avoid tight clothing, avoid large meals or eating within 3 h of going to bed. Raise the head of the bed (do not add pillows). Avoid NSAIDs and excessive alcohol.

Prescribe alginate/antacids.

If there is an inadequate response or early relapse, prescribe an H_2-blocker or proton-pump inhibitor for 6 weeks. If symptoms have still not completely resolved, refer the patient for endoscopy.

ANTI-EMETICS

Complex processes underlie nausea and vomiting. Nausea is associated with autonomic effects (sweating, bradycardia, pallor and profuse salivary secretion). Vomiting is preceded by rhythmic muscular contractions of the 'respiratory' muscles of the abdomen (retching), and is a somatic rather than an autonomic function. Central co-ordination of these processes occurs in a group of cells in the dorsolateral reticular formation in the floor of the fourth ventricle of the medulla oblongata in close proximity to the cardiovascular and respiratory centres with which it has synaptic connections. This vomiting centre (Figure 33.2) is not directly responsive to chemical emetic stimuli, but is activated by one or more inputs. The major efferent pathways from the vomiting centre are the phrenic nerve, the visceral efferent of the vagus to the stomach and oesophagus, and the spinal nerves to the abdominal musculature.

An important receptor area for emetic stimuli, namely the chemoreceptor trigger zone (CTZ), is a group of neurones in the area postrema of the

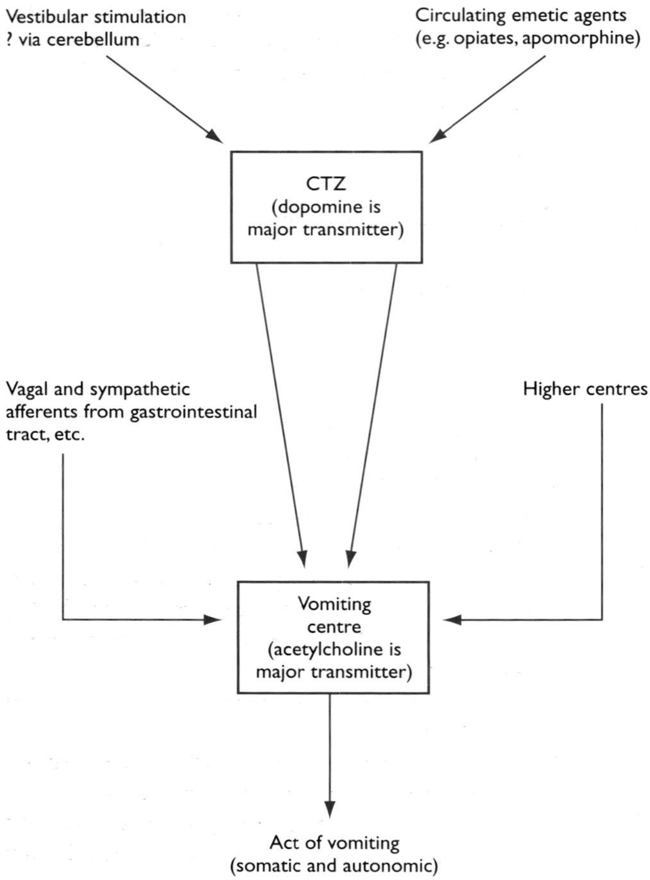

Figure 33.2: The central mechanisms of vomiting.

fourth ventricle which is sensitive to emetic stimuli such as radiation, bacterial toxins and uraemia. Dopamine excites CTZ neurones, which in turn activate the vomiting centre and cause emesis. Emetic stimuli originating in the pharynx, oesophagus and gut are transmitted directly to the vomiting centre via the vagus and glossopharyngeal nerves. Those from the vestibular organs (in travel sickness and Ménière's disease) act indirectly via the CTZ. A histamine pathway is apparently involved in labyrinthine vomiting. **Naloxone**, an opioid antagonist, can block the anti-emetic effect of **nabilone** on the vomiting produced by apomorphine and nitrogen mustard in cats. This and other evidence suggests that opioid receptors may be involved in centrally induced emesis involving higher centres. Drugs may act at more than one site to provoke emesis, for example nitrogen mustard (CTZ, cortex and gut), digitalis (CTZ and gut). Anti-emetic drugs can be classified pharmacologically as shown in Table 33.3.

Anti-emetics should only be used when the cause of nausea or vomiting is known, otherwise the symptomatic relief produced could delay diagnosis of a remediable and serious cause. Nausea and sickness during the first trimester of pregnancy will respond to most anti-emetics, but are rarely treated with drugs because of the possible dangers (currently unquantifiable) of teratogenesis.

Table 33.3: Classification of anti-emetics

Anticholinergics (e.g. hyoscine)
Antihistamines (H_1-blockers) (e.g promethazine)
Dopamine anatagonists (e.g metolopramide)
Phenothiazines (e.g. prochlorperazine)
5-Hydroxytryptamine ($5HT_3$)-receptor antagonists (e.g ondansetron)
Cannabinoids (e.g. nabilone)
Miscellaneous:
Corticosteroids
Benzodiazepines

Key points

Use of anti-emetics

- The cause of vomiting should be diagnosed.
- Symptomatic relief may delay investigation of the underlying cause.
- Treatment of the cause (e.g. diabetic ketoacidosis, intestinal obstruction, intracerebral SOL) usually cures the vomiting.
- The choice of drug depends on the aetiology.

Muscarinic receptor antagonists

These act partly by their antimuscarinic action on the gut, as well as by some central action. **Hyoscine** (0.3 mg) is effective in preventing motion sickness, and is useful in single doses for short journeys, as the anticholinergic side-effects make it unsuitable for chronic use. Hyoscine is an alternative to antihistamines and phenothiazines for the treatment of vertigo and nausea associated with Ménière's disease and middle ear surgery. Drowsiness, blurred vision, dry mouth and urinary retention are more common at therapeutic doses than is the case with antihistamines.

Antihistamines (H_1-blockers)

These are most effective in preventing motion sickness and treating vertigo and vomiting caused by labyrinthine disorders. They have additional anticholinergic actions, and these contribute to their anti-emetic effect. They include cyclizine, promethezine, betahistine and cinnarizine. The main limitations of these drugs are their modest efficacy and common dose-related adverse effects, in addition to antimuscarinic effects.

1 **Cyclizine** given either orally or by injection is effective in opiate-induced vomiting and has been given widely in pregnancy without any untoward effects on the fetus. The main side-effects are drowsiness and a dry mouth.
2 **Promethazine** is also an effective anti-emetic. It is more sedative than cyclizine.
3 **Betahistine** is used in vertigo, tinnitus and hearing loss associated with Ménière's disease.
4 **Cinnarizine** is an antihistamine and calcium antagonist. It has an action on the labyrinth and is effective in the treatment of motion sickness and vertigo.

Dopamine antagonists

Metoclopramide

USE

Metoclopramide is effective for:

1 post-operative vomiting;
2 radiation sickness;
3 drug-induced nausea;
4 migraine (see Chapter 22);
5 diagnostic radiology of the small intestine is facilitated by metoclopramide, which reduces the time required for barium to reach the caecum and decreases the number of films required;
6 facilitation of duodenal intubation and endoscopy;
7 emergency anaesthesia (including that required in pregnancy) to clear gastric contents;
8 symptoms of reflux oesophagitis may be improved, as it prevents nausea, regurgitation and reflux.

The usual effective dose is 10 mg orally three to four times daily. If administered intramuscularly or intravenously, 10 mg are given one to three times daily depending on the severity of the condition. Metoclopramide should be avoided for 3–4 days following gastrointestinal surgery.

ADVERSE EFFECTS

Adverse effects are usually mild but can be severe. Extrapyramidal effects (which occur in about 1% of patients) consist of dystonic effects including akathisia, oculogyric crises, trismus, torticollis and opisthotonos, but Parkinsonian features are absent. These effects are more common in females and in the young. They are treated by stopping metoclopramide and giving benztropine or diazepam acutely if necessary. Overdosage in infants, in whom the maximum dose is 0.5 mg/kg, has produced convulsions, hypertonia and irritability. Milder effects include dizziness, drowsiness, lassitude and bowel disturbances.

MECHANISM OF ACTION

Metoclopramide increases the amount of acetylcholine released at post-ganglionic terminals.

It is a central dopamine antagonist and raises the threshold of the CTZ. It also decreases the sensitivity of the visceral nerves that carry impulses from the gut to the emetic centre. It is relatively ineffective in motion sickness and other forms of centrally mediated vomiting.

High doses of metoclopramide block $5HT_3$ receptors.

PHARMACOKINETICS

Metoclopramide is well absorbed orally, and is also given by intravenous or intramuscular injection. It undergoes metabolism by dealkylation and amide hydrolysis, about 75% being excreted as metabolites in the urine. The mean plasma $t_{\frac{1}{2}}$ is 4 h.

DRUG INTERACTIONS

Metoclopramide potentiates the extrapyramidal effects of phenothiazines and butyrophenones. Its effects on intestinal motility result in numerous alterations in drug absorption, including increased rates of absorption of several drugs such as aspirin, tetracycline and paracetamol.

Domperidone

Domperidone is a dopamine-receptor antagonist similar to metoclopramide. It does not penetrate the blood–brain barrier and it seldom causes sedation or extrapyramidal effects. However, the CTZ lies functionally outside the barrier and thus domperidone is an effective anti-emetic which can logically be given with centrally acting dopamine agonists or levodopa to counter their emetogenic effect (e.g. apomorphine for severe Parkinsonism; see Chapter 20). Domperidone may be administered by mouth, per rectum or by injection.

Phenothiazines

USE

Phenothiazines (see Chapter 18) act on the CTZ, and larger doses depress the vomiting centre as well. The following have established uses as anti-emetics:

1 chlorpromazine, 10–25 mg orally or 25 mg by intramuscular injection; 100 mg by suppository causes sedation (unlicensed);
2 prochlorperazine, 5–25 mg orally, 12.5 mg by intramuscular injection or 25 mg by suppository.
3 perphenazine, 2–5 mg.

These are effective against opioid- and radiation-induced vomiting, and are sometimes helpful in vestibular disturbances. They are least effective in the treatment of motion sickness. All of them carry a risk of extrapyramidal disturbances, dyskinesia and restlessness. Perphenazine is probably the most soporific of this group.

Butyrophenones

See Chapter 18.

Droperidol is used as an anti-emetic. It is given by intramuscular or intravenous injection in a dose of 2.5–10 mg. Its use is largely restricted to opioid-induced vomiting. Extrapyramidal effects and oculogyric crises are a particular risk.

5-HYDROXYTRYPTAMINE ($5HT_3$)-RECEPTOR ANTAGONISTS

The serotonin ($5HT_3$)-receptor antagonists are highly effective in the treatment of acute nausea and vomiting, although they offer little advantage for delayed emesis, occurring secondary to cytotoxic chemotherapy and radiotherapy, as well as the treatment of post-operative nausea and vomiting.

Their exact site of action is uncertain. It may be peripheral at abdominal visceral afferent neurones, or central within the area postrema of the brain, or a combination of both.

Ondansetron

USES

Ondansetron is used for patients who are receiving highly emetogenic chemotherapy at a dose of 8 mg by slow intravenous injection immediately before the chemotherapy, followed by either injections or a constant infusion for maintenance therapy. It is suitable for use in children, the elderly and patients with a renal impairment, although clearance is significantly reduced and the half-life significantly prolonged in patients with moderate or severe impairment of hepatic function. Ondansetron can also be used to treat post-operative nausea and vomiting.

ADVERSE EFFECTS

Serious side-effects are rare. The most common complaint is constipation due to slowing of large bowel transit time. Other effects include headache, a sensation of flushing or warmth, hiccoughs and occasional transient asymptomatic increases in aminotransferases.

PHARMACOKINETICS

Following oral administration absorption is rapid, with peak plasma concentrations reached approximately 1.5 h after an 8-mg dose. The terminal elimination $t_{\frac{1}{2}}$ is approximately 3 h, with a steady-state volume of distribution of about 140 L. Clearance is predominantly by metabolism, with less than 5% excreted unchanged in the urine. The oral bioavailability is about 60%. There is no evidence of induction or inhibition of metabolism of other drugs. The plasma protein binding is approximately 75%.

Other $5HT_3$ antagonists licensed for use in the the UK are **granisetron** and **tropisetron**. The latter carries a caution concerning driving, due to drug-related dizziness and drowsiness affecting the performance of skilled tasks. The rate of metabolism of tropisetron is reduced in slow hydroxylators.

CANNABINOIDS

Cannabis and its major constituent, D-9-tetrahydrocannabinol (THC), have anti-emetic properties and have been used to prevent vomiting caused by cytotoxic therapy. In an attempt to reduce side-effects and increase efficacy, a number of analogues, including nabilone, have been synthesized. The site of action of nabilone is not known, but an action on cortical centres affecting vomiting via descending pathways seems probable. There is some evidence that opioid pathways are involved in these actions. They are only moderately effective.

ADVERSE EFFECTS

Adverse effects include sedation, confusion, incoordination, dry mouth and hypotension. These effects are more prominent in older patients.

MISCELLANEOUS AGENTS

Large doses of corticosteroids exert some anti-emetic action when used with cytotoxic drugs, and the efficacy of the $5HT_3$-antagonists has been shown to be improved when concomitant dexamethasone is given. Their mode of action is not known. Benzodiazepines given before treatment with cytotoxics reduce vomiting, although whether this is a specific anti-emetic action or a reduction in anxiety is unknown.

INFLAMMATORY BOWEL DISEASE

Mediators of the inflammatory response in ulcerative colitis and Crohn's disease include kinins and prostaglandins. The latter stimulate adenylyl cyclase, which induces active ion secretion and thus diarrhoea. Synthesis of prostaglandin E_2, thromboxane A_2 and prostacyclin by the gut increases during disease activity, but not during remission. **Sulphasalazine** and its active metabolite 5-aminosalicylic acid influence the synthesis and metabolism of these eicosanoids, and influence the course of disease activity.

Apart from correction of dehydration, nutritional and electrolyte imbalance (which in an acute exacerbation is potentially life-saving) and other non-specific treatment, corticosteroids, aminosalicylates and immunosuppressive drugs are valuable.

Key points

Inflammatory bowel disease

The cause is unknown.

There is local and sometimes systemic inflammation.

- Correct dehydration, nutritional and electrolyte imbalance.
- Drug therapy: aminosalicylates corticosteroids;
- other immunosuppressive agents.

Corticosteroids

Steroids modify every part of the inflammatory response, and corticosteroids (see Chapter 39) remain the standard by which other drugs are judged. **Prednisolone** and **hydrocortisone** given orally or intravenously are of proven value in the treatment of acute colitis or exacerbation of Crohn's disease. Topical therapy in the form of a rectal drip, foam or enema of hydrocortisone or prednisolone is very effective in milder attacks of ulcerative colitis. Corticosteroid enemas are less effective in Crohn's colitis, and systemic absorption may occur.

Steroids are not useful for maintaining remission in ulcerative colitis. They may have some efficacy in this respect in Crohn's disease, but their associated risks are such that failure to maintain remission below 15 mg prednisolone per day necessitates adoption of alternative steroid-sparing therapy.

Prednisolone is preferred to hydrocortisone as it has less mineralocorticoid effect at equipotent anti-inflammatory doses. The dose, route of administration (oral or rectal) and duration of treatment will vary according to the extent of the disease during relapse and the response to therapy. The usual initial oral dose is 40 mg once daily, and the initial rectal dose is 20 mg once or twice daily.

Recently steroids which are poorly absorbed from the gastrointestinal tract or which have a very high first-pass effect (e.g. **budesonide**) have been licensed for use in this indication as controlled-release capsules and an enema. Their efficacy is equivalent to that of other corticosteroids, but due to extensive hepatic first-pass metabolism they are associated with fewer systemic side-effects.

Aminosalicylates

5-Aminosalicylic acid (5ASA) acts at many points in the inflammatory process and has a local effect on the colonic mucosa. However, as it is very readily absorbed from the small intestine, it has to be attached to another compound or coated in resin to ensure that it is released in the large bowel. Although these drugs are only effective for controlling mild to moderate ulcerative colitis when given orally, they are very effective for reducing the incidence of relapse per year from about 70% to 20%. The aminosalicylates are not effective in small-bowel Crohn's disease. For rectosigmoid disease, suppository or enema preparations are as effective as systemic steroids.

Currently available drugs of this group include sulphasalazine, **mesalazine**, **balsalazide** and **olsalazine**. Sulphasalazine remains the standard agent, but mesalazine, balsalazide and olsalazine avoid the unwanted effects of the sulphonamide carrier molecule of sulphasalazine while delivering 5ASA to the colon. The newer agents are useful in patients who cannot tolerate sulphasalazine, and in men who wish to remain fertile.

Sulphasalazine

See also Chapter 25.

USE

Sulphasalazine is a prodrug which is broken down into the active moiety (5–aminosalicylate) and sulphapyridine. It is used for maintenance treatment of ulcerative colitis, in which it reduces the number of relapses. This effect persists for as long as the drug is taken. Rapid acetylators of sulphapyridine achieve therapeutic levels (20 μg/mL) with 3–4 g of sulphasalazine given orally daily, but slow acetylators are likely to experience side-effects on this dose because their serum level often reaches 50 μg/mL. They usually require only 2.5–3 g per day. Sulphasalazine is best tolerated by all patients if it is started in a small dose of 0.5 g twice daily. It does not help any but the mildest acute attacks for which steroids are the treatment of choice. Sulphasalazine is available as a suppository for use when disease is confined to the rectum, or as an adjunct to oral treatment in total colitis. Enteric-coated tablets are also available. Although it is partially effective in the treatment of acute Crohn's disease, it does not maintain remission. It is not effective in patients with disease confined to the small bowel. The use of aminosalicylates in rheumatological disease is discussed in Chapter 25.

ADVERSE EFFECTS

Nausea, vomiting, epigastric discomfort, headache and rashes (including toxic dermal necrolysis) may occur, but sulphasalazine is generally well tolerated. All of the adverse effects associated with sulphonamides can occur with sulphasalazine, and they are more pronounced in slow acetylators. Toxic effects on the red cells are common (70% of cases) and in some cases lead to haemolysis, anisocytosis and methaemoglobinaemia. Sulphasalazine should be avoided in patients with glucose-6-phosphate dehydrogenase (G6PD) deficiency. Temporary oligospermia with decreased sperm motility and infertility occurs in up to 70% of males who are treated for over 3 years. Uncommon adverse effects include pancreatitis, hepatitis, fever, thrombocytopenia, agranulocytosis, Stevens–Johnson syndrome, neurotoxicity, photosensitization, a systemic lupus erythematosus (SLE)-like syndrome, myocarditis, pulmonary fibrosis, and renal effects including proteinuria, haematuria, orange urine and nephrotic syndrome.

PHARMACOKINETICS

Sulphasalazine is poorly absorbed from the ileum; bacterial flora in the colon reduce the azo link to liberate the active aminosalicylate moiety. This acts locally in the bowel. Patients with an ileostomy lack the appropriate gut flora and cannot cleave sulphasalazine, so it has little place in their management. Sulphapyridine has little therapeutic effect in the context of inflammatory bowel disease, although it is responsible for some of the adverse effects.

Mesalazine

This is 5-aminosalicylic acid coated with a resin which dissolves at the pH found in the terminal ileum and colon. It has only a few side-effects, namely nausea, diarrhoea, abdominal pain and headache, although there have been rare reports of reversible pancreatitis, hepatitis and interstitial nephritis.

Balsalazide

This is mesalazine linked to a carrier molecule (4-aminobenzoyl-β-alanine) via an azo bond. However, bacteria reduce the azo bond releasing mesalazine, the active metabolite, into the colon.

Key points

Aminosalicylates and blood dyscrasias.

- Any patient who is receiving aminosalicylates must be advised to report unexplained bleeding, bruising, purpura, fever or malaise.
- If the above symptoms occur, a blood count should be performed.
- If there is suspicion of blood dyscrasia, stop aminosalicylates.
- Aminosalicylates are associated with agranulocytosis, aplastic anaemia, leucopenia, neutropenia and thrombocytopenia.

Olsalazine

This is a prodrug consisting of a dimer of two 5-aminosalicylic acid (5ASA) molecules linked by an azo bond. Less than 1% is absorbed unchanged from the small bowel. The azo bond is cleaved by colonic bacteria and about 20% of the 5ASA is absorbed, acetylated and then excreted in the urine. Diarrhoea, rash, nausea and abdominal pain cause 20% of patients to stop the drug.

IMMUNOSUPPRESSIVE DRUGS

Although the exact pathogenetic mechanisms involved in inflammatory bowel disease remain unclear, there is abundant evidence that the immune system (both cellular and humoral) is activated in the intestine of patients with inflammatory bowel disease. This forms the rationale for the use of immunosuppressive agents in the group of patients who do not respond to therapy with aminosalicylates or corticosteroids. General indications for their use include patients who have been on steroids for more than 6 months despite efforts to taper them off, those who have frequent relapses, those with chronic continuous disease activity, and those with Crohn's disease with recurrent fistulas. The main agents are **azathioprine** in combination with **6-mercaptopurine**. Other more recently used agents include **methotrexate** (given weekly) and **cyclosporin**.

New therapies under review

Lipoxygenase inhibitors have shown some early promise in ulcerative colitis, and are being investigated further. Other mechanisms currently under review include cytokine modulation (including interleukin I, interleukin II, interferons and tumour necrosis factor), lymphocyte modification (including plasmapheresis) and CD4 antibodies), nutritional therapy (topical short-chain fatty acids and glutamine), transdermal nicotine, heparin, dimethyl sulphoxide (DMSO), and modification of nitric oxide pathways.

Constipation

Bowel function and constipation

Under normal circumstances the rectum is empty and faecal material is stored in the descending and pelvic colon. Under the appropriate stimulation, which may include food or drink, certain surroundings and specific times of day, the colon contracts and faeces enter the rectum. Sensors in the rectal wall are activated by the rise in pressure and also probably by tactile stimuli, and this results in the urge to stool. If this is answered, the rectum and distal portion of the colon are emptied by complex co-ordinated activity consisting of:

1 colonic contraction;
2 relaxation of the anal sphincter;
3 voluntary elevation of the intra-abdominal pressure.

There is considerable variation among healthy people in the frequency of bowel evacuation, and anything between three times weekly and three times daily may be considered the normal range, but a significant *change* in bowel habit is an important symptom that demands investigation. The term 'constipation' when used by patients describes what they consider to be abnormal bowel function, and it is important to determine whether their bowels are indeed behaving abnormally.

Two main mechanisms lead to constipation:

1 decreased colonic activity; and
2 decreased sensitivity of the rectal sensors.

Decreased colonic activity

This causes the bowel contents to pass slowly through the colon and become dehydrated, hard and small in volume. Under these circumstances, emptying of the colon into the rectum is infrequent and rectal stimulation is minimal. This may be due to a variety of factors, including the following:

1 Old age, immobility.
2 Low bulk diet, dehydration.
3 Metabolic disorders – hypercalcemia, myxedema.
4 Depression, confusional states.
5 Various local conditions of the colon large bowel including carcinoma.
6 Drugs (see Table 33.4).

Decreased sensitivity of the rectal sensors

This usually occurs when the 'call to stool' is neglected. After a while the stimulus dies away and the rectum becomes chronically full of faecal material. The condition is called dyschezia. It may occur in an acute form in patients who are too ill to appreciate or to respond to the 'call to stool', or when bowel evacuation is painful, or in a chronic form in which for domestic or other reasons the patient does not have the time, inclination or opportunity to open the bowels at the appropriate time. This is particularly a problem with some children and elderly people.

Table 33.4: Drugs that can cause constipation

Aluminium hydroxide
Amiodarone
Anticholinergics
Disopyramide
Diuretics
Iron preparations
Opioids
Tricyclic antidepressants
Verapamil

Management of constipation

When constipation occurs, it is important first to exclude both local and systemic disease which may be responsible for the symptoms.

In general, patients with constipation present in two ways.

1 Long-standing constipation in otherwise healthy people may be due to decreased colon motility or to dyschezia, or to a combination of both. It is usually sufficient to reassure the patient and to instruct them in the importance of re-establishing a regular bowel habit. This should be combined with an increased fluid intake and increased bulk in the diet. Bran is cheap and often satisfactory. As an alternative, non-absorbed bulk substances such as **methylcellulose** are helpful. The other laxatives described below should only be tried if these more 'natural' treatments fail.
2 Loaded colon or faecal impaction – sometimes it is necessary to evacuate the bowel before it is possible to start re-education, particularly in the elderly or those who are ill. In these cases a laxative such as **senna** combined with **glycerol suppositories** is appropriate.

Laxatives

Laxatives are still widely although often inappropriately used by the public and in hospital. There is now a greater knowledge of intestinal pathophysiology, and of outstanding importance is the finding that the fibre content of the diet has a marked regulatory action on gut transit time and motility and on defecation performance.

As a general rule, laxatives should be avoided. They are employed:

1 if straining at stool will cause damage (e.g. post-operatively, in patients with haemorrhoids or after myocardial infarction);
2 in hepatocellular failure to reduce formation and/or absorption of neurotoxins produced in the bowel;
3 occasionally in drug-induced constipation.

Bulk laxatives

PLANT FIBRE

Plant fibre is the portion of the walls of plant cells that resists digestion in the intestine. The main effect of increasing the amount of fibre in the diet is to increase the bulk of the stools and decrease the bowel transit time; this is probably due to the ability of fibre to take up water and swell. Fibre also binds organic molecules, including bile salts. It does not increase the effective caloric content of the diet, as it is not digested or absorbed.

The main uses of plain fibre (e.g. bran) are as follows:

1 in constipation, particularly if combined with a spastic colon. By increasing the bulk of the intestinal contents, fibre slowly distends the wall of the colon, and this causes an increase in useful propulsive contraction. The main result is a return of the large bowel function towards normal. Similar results are obtained in diverticular disease in which there is colon overactivity associated with a high intraluminal pressure.
2 the proposed effects of fibre in preventing large-bowel carcinoma, piles, appendicitis, coronary artery disease and varicose veins are still speculative.

The starting 'dose' of bran is a dessertspoonful daily, and this can be increased at weekly intervals until a satisfactory result is obtained. It may be mixed with food, as it is difficult to swallow if taken 'neat'.

ADVERSE EFFECTS AND CONTRAINDICATIONS

Bran usually causes some flatulence which is dose related. Phytates in bran could theoretically bind calcium and zinc ions. Bran should be avoided in gluten enteropathy and is contraindicated in bowel obstruction.

OTHER BULK LAXATIVES

Methylcellulose takes up water in the bowel and swells thus stimulating peristalsis. It is a reasonable substitute if bran is not satisfactory.

Osmotic agents

For many years these have been thought to act by retaining fluid in the bowel by virtue of the osmotic activity of their unabsorbed ions. The increased bulk in the lumen would then stimulate peristalsis. However, 5 g of magnesium sulphate would be isotonic in only 130 mL and acts within 1–2 h, well before it could have reached the colon, so mechanisms other than osmotic effects must account for its laxative properties. It has been postulated that, because magnesium ions can also contract the gall-bladder, relax the sphincter of Oddi and increase gastric, intestinal and pancreatic enzyme secretion, they may act indirectly via cholecystokinin. Magnesium ions themselves may also have direct pharmacological effects on intestinal function. **Sodium sulphate** or **magnesium sulphate** (Epsom salts) are commonly used. It should be remembered that a certain amount of magnesium may be absorbed, and accumulation can occur in renal failure. There is little if any rational medical use for these saline purges, apart from in cases of hepatocellular failure, and following activated charcoal in the treatment of overdose (see Chapter 53).

Lactulose

Lactulose is a disaccharide. It passes through the small intestine unchanged, but in the colon is broken down by carbohydrate-fermenting bacteria to unabsorbed organic anions (largely acetic and lactic acids) which retain fluid in the gut lumen and also make the colonic contents more acid. This produces a laxative effect after 2–3 days. It is effective and well tolerated, but relatively expensive. It is of particular value in the treatment of hepatic encephalopathy, as it discourages the proliferation of ammonia-producing organisms and the absorption of ammonia. The usual dose is 30 mL by mouth after breakfast. In patients with liver failure, larger doses are required, usually between 30 and 50 mL three times daily.

Lubricants and stool softeners

These agents were formerly believed to act by softening or lubricating the faeces, but they act at least in part in a similar manner to stimulant purgatives by inhibiting intestinal electrolyte transport.

Dioctyl sodium sulfosuccinate

This is a surface-active agent that acts on hard faecal masses and allows more water to penetrate the mass and thus soften it. Its use should be confined to patients with faecal impaction, and it should not be given over long periods.

Liquid paraffin

Although still available, this treatment is now obsolete and should not be used. The disadvantages of habitual use include malabsorption of fat-soluble vitamins, inhalation pneumonitis, and leakage through the anus. Mineral oil cannot be cleared from the tissues and can cause chronic granulomas.

Chemical stimulants

Many of the agents in this class (e.g. castor oil, phenolphthalein) are now obsolete because of their toxicity, but senna, co-danthramer and bisacodyl are still useful if bulk laxatives are ineffective.

Senna

USE

Senna in the form of pods or leaves has been used as a laxative for many years. The important constituents are glycosides, which are hydrolysed by colonic bacteria to the active principles sennoside A and sennoside B. Their main effect is to enhance the response of the colon to normal stimuli, so it is important to combine them with a high-bulk diet in order to ensure an adequate physiological stimulus. Senna acts directly on the intramucosal plexus of the gut wall and possibly also on electrolyte transport systems. Sennosides are absorbed in the small intestine and secreted into the colon, so senna takes about 8 h to produce an effect. It is taken before retiring to bed.

ADVERSE EFFECTS

Colic (spasm) and diarrhoea occur if the dose is too large. If senna is given to nursing mothers it enters the milk and can cause diarrhoea in the baby. Senna causes a yellow or red discoloration of the urine. Melanosis coli (a benign condition caused by deposition of anthroquinone pigment derived from the drug) may also occur.

Co-danthramer

Co-danthramer has similar properties to senna.

Bisacodyl

Bisacodyl (10 mg by mouth as an enteric-coated preparation) is given at night and an effect is obtained in about 10 h. Suppositories produce bowel evacuation within about 30 min. The drug is deacetylated in the gut and then absorbed, undergoing transformation to the glucuronide in the liver. This is excreted in the bile and converted back to the deacetylated drug, which then acts on the colon. It thus has an enterohepatic cycle.

Glycerol

Glycerol suppositories act as a rectal stimulant due to the local irritant action of glycerol, and are useful if a rapid effect is required.

Phosphate

Phosphate enemas are similarly useful.

Laxative abuse

Persistent use of laxatives, particularly in increasing doses, causes ill health.

After prolonged use of stimulant laxatives, the colon becomes dilated and atonic with diminished activity. The cause is not clear, but this effect is perhaps due to damage to the intrinsic nerve plexus of the colon. The disorder of bowel motility may improve after withdrawing the laxative and using a high-residue diet.

Some people, mainly women, take purgatives secretly. This probably bears some relationship to disorders such as anorexia nervosa that are concerned with weight loss, and is also associated with self-induced vomiting and with diuretic abuse. The clinical and biochemical features can closely mimic Barter's syndrome, and this possibility should always be investigated in patients in whom the diagnosis of this rare disorder is entertained, especially adults in whom true Barter's syndrome almost never arises *de novo*. Features include:

1 sodium depletion – hypotension, cramps, secondary hyperaldosteronism;

> **Case history**
>
> A 70-year-old woman who was previously very active but whose mobility has recently been limited by osteoarthritis of the knees and hips sees her general practitioner because of a recent change in bowel habit from once daily to once every 3 days. Her current medication includes regular co-proxamol for her osteoarthritis, oxybutynin for urinary frequency, aluminium hydroxide PRN for dyspepsia, and bendrofluazide and verapamil for hypertension. Following bowel evacuation with a phosphate enema, proctoscopy and colonoscopy are reported as normal.
>
> *Question*
>
> Which of this patient's medications may have contributed to her constipation?
>
> Answer
>
> - Co-proxamol, which contains dextropropoxyphene (an opioid).
> - Aluminium hydroxide.
> - Bendrofluazide.
> - Verapamil.
> - Oxybutynin (an anticholinergic).

2 Potassium depletion – weakness, polyuria and nocturia and renal damage.

In addition, there may be features suggestive of enteropathy and osteomalacia.

Diagnosis and treatment are difficult; melanosis coli may provide a diagnostic clue. Urinary electrolyte determinations may help, but can be confounded if the patient is also surreptitiously taking diuretics.

Diarrhoea

The most important aspect of the treatment of acute diarrhoea is the maintenance of fluid and electrolyte balance, particularly in children and in the elderly. In non-pathogenic diarrhoea or viral gastroenteritis, antibiotics and antidiarrhoeal drugs are best avoided. Initial therapy should be with oral rehydration preparations (such as 'Dioralyte'® or 'Electrolade'®), which contain electrolytes and glucose. Antibiotic treatment is indicated for patients with systemic illness and evidence of bacterial infection.

Adjunctive symptomatic treatment is sometimes indicated. Two main types of drug may be employed, that either decrease intestinal transit time or increase the bulk and viscosity of the gut contents.

Drugs that decrease intestinal transit time

Opioids

See Chapter 24.

Codeine is widely used for this purpose in doses of 15–60 mg. **Morphine** is also given, usually as a **kaolin** and morphine mixture BPC, which contains 700 μg of anhydrous morphine in every 10-mL dose. **Diphenoxylate** is related to pethidine and also has structural similarities to anticholinergic drugs. It may cause drug dependence and euphoria, and is usually prescribed as 'Lomotil' (diphenoxylate 2.5 mg; atropine sulphate 0.025 mg). Overdose with this drug in children causes features of both opioid and atropine intoxication and may be fatal.

Loperamide

Loperamide is an effective, well-tolerated antidiarrhoeal agent. It antagonizes peristalsis, possibly by antagonizing acetylcholine release in the intramural nerve plexus of the gut, although non-cholinergic effects may also be involved. It is poorly absorbed and probably acts directly on the bowel. The dose is 4 mg initially, followed by 2 mg after each loose stool up to a total dose of 16 mg/day. Adverse effects are unusual, but include dry mouth, dizziness, skin rashes and gastric disturbances. Excessive use (especially in children) is to be deplored.

Drugs that increase bulk and viscosity of gut contents

These are usually satisfactory for milder cases of diarrhoea. Preparations include kaolin compound powder BPC, which contains kaolin (a natural form of aluminum silicate), sodium bicarbonate and magnesium carbonate (2–10 g dose 4-hourly).

Travellers' diarrhoea

This is a syndrome of acute watery diarrhoea lasting for 1–3 days and associated with vomiting, abdominal cramps and other non-specific symptoms, resulting from infection by one of a number of enteropathogens, the commonest being enterotoxigenic *Escherichia coli*. It probably reflects colonization of the bowel by 'unfamiliar' organisms. Because of the variable nature of the pathogen there is no specific treatment.

Doxycycline prevents most episodes of travellers' diarrhoea. There is a risk that widespread use might encourage bacterial antibiotic resistance. Antibacterials can also create problems for the traveller due to their side-effects. Early treatment of diarrhoea with co-trimoxazole or **trimethoprim** alone will control 90% of cases and this, together with oral replacement of salts and water, is the currently preferred approach.

Pseudomembranous Colitis

Broad-spectrum antibacterial drug therapy is sometimes associated with superinfection of the intestine with toxin-producing *Clostridium difficile*. Debilitated and immunosuppressed patients are at particular risk. The infection can be transmitted from person to person. Withdrawal of the antibacterial drug and the introduction of oral **metronidazole** (or **vancomycin**) should be instituted.

Irritable bowel syndrome

This motility disorder of the gut affects approximately 10% of the population. Although the symptoms are mostly colonic, patients with the syndrome have abnormal motility throughout the gut, and this may be precipitated by dietary items such as alcohol or wheat flour. The important management principles are first to exclude a serious cause for the symptoms and then to determine whether exclusion of certain foods or alcohol would be worthwhile. An increase in dietary fibre over the course of several weeks may also reduce the symptoms. Psychological factors may be important precipitants, and counselling may be helpful. Drug treatment is symptomatic and often disappointing.

1 Anticholinergic drugs such as hyoscine have been used for many years, although evidence of their efficacy is lacking. The oral use of better absorbed anticholinergics such as atropine is limited by their side-effects. Pirenzapine is effective in some patients.
2 **Mebeverine** (135 mg before meals three times daily) directly relaxes intestinal smooth muscle without anticholinergic effects. Its efficacy is marginal.
3 **Peppermint oil** relaxes intestinal smooth muscle and is given in an enteric-coated capsule which releases its contents in the distal small bowel. It is given before meals three times daily.
4 Antidiarrhoeal drugs such as loperamide reduce associated diarrhoea.
5 Psychotropic drugs such as antipsychotics and antidepressants with anticholinergic properties have also been effective in some patients. In general, however, they should be avoided for such a chronic and benign condition because of their serious adverse effects (see Chapters 18 and 19).

PANCREATIC DISEASE

Acute pancreatitis has a high mortality, and replacement of fluid and electrolytes can be lifesaving. Pain may be severe and is treated with an opioid (e.g. pethidine). Surgery should usually be reserved for complications (e.g. drainage of a related pseudocyst). Underlying disease (e.g. alcoholism, gallstones, hypertriglyceridaemia or drugs; see Table 33.5) should be sought and treated.

More specific modes of medical management have been disappointing. Drugs recently or currently under investigation include the following:

1 **Aprotinin**, a polypeptide (58 amino acids) extracted from bovine lungs, is a proteolytic enzyme inhibitor. A multicentre trial conducted by the Medical Research Council (MRC) has failed to show that it affects mortality. It is uncertain whether the complication rate is altered. Aprotinin is expensive. It is well tolerated, although being a polypeptide it occasionally produces hypersensitivity and rarely anaphylaxis. (It has an unrelated use in preventing bleeding in repeat cardiac surgery.)

Table 33.5: Drugs that are associated with pancreatis (this is uncommon)

Asparaginase	Oestrogens
Azathioprine	Pentamidine
Corticosteroids	Sodium valporate
Dideoxyinosine (DDI)	Sulphonamides and sulphasalazine
Thiazides	Tetracycline

2 **Glucagon** reduces the volume and enzyme concentration of pancreatic juice. The above-mentioned MRC multicentre trial failed to demonstrate benefit in pancreatitis.
3 Anticholinergic drugs are of no use in pancreatitis as the excess pancreatic enzyme release is not vagally mediated.
4 Corticosteroids have sometimes been advocated as part of treatment for 'shock'. There is no scientific basis for this and they could be harmful.
5 **Octreotide** (a somatostatin analogue) is currently undergoing clinical trials.
6 Bradykinin antagonists have shown activity in animal models.

PANCREATIC INSUFFICIENCY

Exocrine pancreatic insufficiency is an important cause of steatorrhoea. The pancreas has a large functional reserve, and malabsorption does not usually occur until enzyme output is reduced to 10% or less of normal. This type of malabsorption is usually treated by replacement therapy with pancreatic extracts (usually of porcine origin). Unfortunately, although useful, these preparations rarely abolish steatorrhoea. A number of preparations are available, but the enzyme activity varies between preparations – one with a high lipase activity is most likely to reduce steatorrhoea. Unfortunately, less than 10% of the lipase activity and 25% of the tryptic activity is recoverable from the duodenum regardless of the dose schedule. This limited effectiveness of oral enzymes is partly due to acid–peptic inactivation in the stomach and duodenum. H_2-antagonists decrease both acidity and volume of secretion and retard the inactivation of exogenous pancreatic enzymes. They are given as an adjunct to these preparations.

Supplements of pancreatin are given to compensate for reduced or absent exocrine secretion in cystic fibrosis, pancreatectomy, total gastrectomy and chronic pancreatitis. Pancreatin is inactivated by gastric acid, and therefore preparations are best taken with or immediately before or after food. Gastric acid secretion can be reduced by giving an H_2-blocker about 1 h beforehand, or antacids may be given concurrently to reduce acidity.

Pancreatin is inactivated by heat and, if mixed with liquids or food, excessive heat should be avoided. The dose is adjusted according to size, number and consistency of stools such that the patient thrives.

Pancreatin can irritate the perioral skin and buccal mucosa if it is retained in the mouth, and excessive doses can cause perianal irritation. The most frequent side-effects are gastrointestinal ones including nausea, vomiting and abdominal discomfort. Hyperuricaemia and hyperuricuria have been associated with very high doses of the drug.

LIVER DISEASE

PRINCIPLES UNDERLYING DRUG TREATMENT OF HEPATIC ENCEPHALOPATHY AND LIVER FAILURE

In severe liver disease neuropsychiatric changes occur and can progress to coma. The mechanism which produces these changes is not established, but it is known that in hepatic coma and pre-coma the blood ammonia concentration increases. In many patients the progress of encephalopathy parallels the rise in blood ammonia levels. Orally administered nitrogenous compounds (e.g. protein, amino acids, ammonium chloride) yield ammonia in the gut, raise blood ammonia concentrations and provoke encephalopathy. The liver is the only organ that extracts ammonia from the blood and converts it to urea. Bacterial degradation products of nitrogenous material within the gut enter the systemic circulation because of a failure of first-pass hepatic extraction (due to hepatocellular damage), or due to bypass of the hepatocytes by collateral circulation or intrahepatic shunting. Another source is urea, which undergoes enterohepatic circulation and yields about 3.5 g/day of ammonia (see Figure 33.3).

Ammonia diffuses into the blood across the large bowel wall, where it is trapped by becoming ionized due to the lower pH of blood compared to colonic contents. Ammonia is not the only toxin involved, as perhaps 20% of patients with encephalopathy have normal blood ammonia levels and methionine can provoke encephalopathy without causing a significant rise in blood ammonia concentration. Furthermore, ammonia toxicity affects the cortex but not the brainstem, which is also involved in encephalopathy.

Other toxins of potential relevance include the following.

1 Intestinal bacterial decarboxylation produces hydroxyphenyl amines such as octopamine (from tyramine) which could replace normal

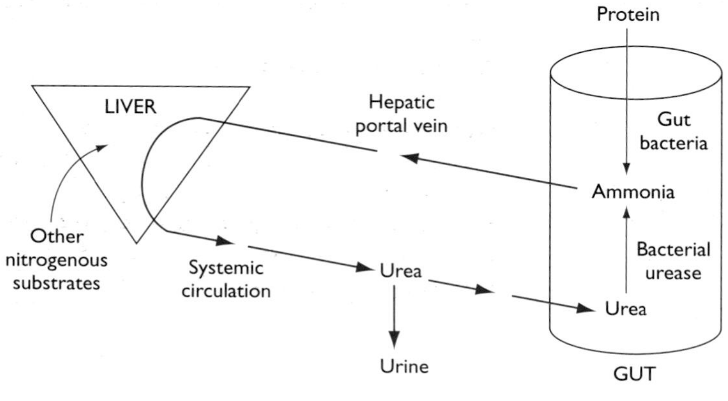

Figure 33.3: Enterohepatic circulation of urea and ammonia.

transmitters at nerve endings in the central and peripheral nervous systems, thus acting as 'false transmitters' and changing the balance of inhibition and excitation at central synapses.

2 Changes in fatty acid metabolism increase plasma free fatty acids, some of which have anaesthetic properties. In addition, these determine the availability of tryptophan to the brain and hence have an effect on 5-hydroxytryptamine.

Glutathione synthesis is impaired in severe liver disease. Cellular damage due to free radical excess can produce multi-organ dysfunction. Intravenous administration of acetylcysteine is used prophylactically in some centres to enhance glutathione synthesis and thereby reduce oxidant (free radical) stresses by scavenging these reactive entities.

Treatment of hepatic encephalopathy includes the following measures:

1 dietary protein restriction to as little as 20 g/day while ensuring an adequate intake of essential amino acids;
2 emptying the lower bowel by means of enemas and purgatives to reduce the bacterial sources of ammonia;
3 oral or rectal administration of non-absorbable antibiotics such as neomycin to reduce the bacterial population of the large bowel. Neomycin, 1–2 g four times daily, is often used. It should be remembered that a 2-g dose produces appreciable absorption and that, if the patient also has renal impairment, neomycin may accumulate and produce toxicity;
4 Oral lactulose, 50–100 g/day, improves encephalopathy. This disaccharide is not a normal dietary constituent and humans do not possess a lactulase enzyme, so lactulose is neither digested nor absorbed but reaches the colon unchanged, where the bacterial flora breaks it down to form lactate, acetate and other acid products. These trap ammonia and other toxins within the lumen by reducing its pH, and in addition they act as a cathartic and reduce ammonia absorption by reducing the colonic transit time;
5 bleeding may occur due to interference with clotting factor synthesis or thrombocytopenia. Vitamin K is given and fresh frozen plasma or platelets are used as required. Ranitidine is often used to prevent gastric erosions and bleeding;
6 sedatives should be avoided as patients with liver disease are extremely sensitive to such drugs. If sedation is essential (e.g. because of agitation due to alcohol withdrawal), small doses of oxazepam are preferred to benzodiazepines with longer-lived metabolites. The hazards of narcotic analgesics to the patient with acute or chronic liver disease cannot be overemphasized;
7 prophylactic broad-spectrum intravenous antibiotics, especially if there is evidence of infection (e.g. spontaneous peritonitis);
8 intravenous acetylcysteine (the value of this has not yet been confirmed).

DRUG THERAPY OF PORTAL HYPERTENSION AND ESOPHAGEAL VARICES

Oesophageal varices form a collateral circulation in response to raised blood pressure in the portal system, and are of clinical importance because of their tendency to bleed. Two-thirds of patients with varices die as a result, and of these, one-third die of the first bleed, one-third rebleed within 6 weeks, and only one-third survive for 1 year.

Key points

Treatment of hepatic encephalopathy

- Supportive.
- Measures to reduce absorption of ammonia from the gut (e.g. low-protein diet, oral antibiotics, lactulose).
- Prompt treatment of infection.
- Prophylactic vitamin K.
- Fresh frozen plasma/platelets as indicated.
- Ranitidine or proton-pump inhibitor (PPI) to prevent gastric erosions and bleeding.
- Avoidance of sedatives, potassium-losing diuretics, opioids, drugs that cause constipation and hepatotoxic drugs whenever possible.

Sclerotherapy and surgical shunt procedures are the mainstay of treatment, and drug therapy must be judged against these gloomy survival figures. In addition to resuscitation, volume replacement and, when necessary, balloon tamponade using a Sengstaken–Blakemore tube, the emergency treatment of bleeding varices may include vasoconstrictor drugs. These reduce portal blood flow through splanchnic arterial constriction.

Drugs currently used for the management of portal hypertension include **octreotide** (the long-acting analogue of somatostatin) and **terlipressin** (a derivative of vasopressin), either of which are used in the acute management of bleeding varices. Terlipressin and octreotide are used to reduce portal pressure urgently, while beta-blockers and vasodilators such as nitrates are used for long-term therapy.

Somatostatin and its long-acting analogue octreotide reduce blood flow and cause a significant reduction in varicocele pressure without effects on the systemic vasculature. To date, a clear cut response in varicocele bleeding has not been demonstrated. Side-effects include vomiting, anorexia, abdominal pain, diarrhoea, headache and dizziness.

New *vaso*-active drugs such as terlipressin appear to have a better therapeutic index and fewer side-effects, although terlipressin has a short half-life and needs to be administered frequently or as an infusion.

A number of trials have demonstrated efficacy of β-adrenergic antagonists in the prevention of gastrointestinal bleeding in patients with portal hypertension, especially in combination with endoscopic sclerotherapy.

Management of chronic viral hepatitis

Chronic viral hepatitis is associated with chronic liver disease, cirrhosis and hepatocellular carcinoma. The carrier rate for hepatitis B in the UK is 0.1–1% (it is particularly prevalent in socially deprived areas of inner cities) and the seroprevalence for hepatitis C is 0.1–0.7%. Chronic viral hepatitis is diagnosed when there is evidence of continuing hepatic damage and infection for at least 6 months after initial viral infection. In hepatitis C the liver function may remain normal for months to years while the patient's blood remains infectious (confirmed by hepatitis C virus RNA detection). The course of the liver damage often fluctuates. While up to 90% of patients with acute hepatitis B clear the virus spontaneously, up to 60% of those with hepatitis C virus do not do so. About 20% of those with chronic active hepatitis progress insidiously to cirrhosis, and about 2–3% go on to develop hepatocellular carcinoma.

Hepatitis B virus is a DNA virus that is not directly cytopathic, and hepatic damage occurs as a result of the host immune response. Hepatocytes infected with hepatitis B virus produce a variety of viral proteins, of which the 'e' antigen (HBeAg) is clinically the most important. HBeAg is a marker for continued viral replication and therefore for infectivity. Hepatitis C virus is a single-stranded RNA virus.

Several controlled trials have shown that **α-interferon** is beneficial in chronic hepatitis B virus infection. The combination of α-interferon and **ribavirin**, a synthetic guanosine analogue, is more effective in chronic hepatitis C than interferon alone.

Drug-induced liver disease

After oral administration the entire absorbed dose of drug is exposed to the liver during the first pass through the body. The drug itself or its metabolites may affect liver function. Metabolic pathways may become saturated at high concentrations and drug or metabolites may accumulate, leading to toxicity. The drugs shown in Table 33.6 predictably cause hepatotoxicity at excessive doses. Although hepatotoxicity is traditionally divided into dose-dependent and dose-independent hepatotoxicity, the relationship is not always clear-cut. For example, even with predictable hepatotoxins there is considerable interindividual variation in susceptibility to hepatic damage. This can sometimes be attributed to genetic polymorphism or to environmental stimuli affecting hepatic microsomal enzymes, or to previous liver disease. Although dose-independent hepatotoxicity is used to classify those reactions that are 'idiosyncratic' and usually unpredictable (Table 33.7), the severity of the resulting liver disease may be related to dose or to duration of therapy. Particu-

Table 33.6: Dose-dependant hepatotoxiticy

Drug	Mechanism	Comment/predisposing factors
Paracetamol	Hepatitis	See Chapter 53
Salicylates	Focal hepatocellular necrosis	Autoimmune disease (especially systemic lupus erythematosus)
	Reye's sydrome	In children with viral infection
Tetracycline	Central and mid-zonal necrosis with fat droplets	–
Azathioprine	Cholestasis and hepatitis	Underlying liver disease
Methotrexate	Hepatic fibrosis	–
Fusidic acid	Cholestasis, conjugated hyperbilirubinaemia	Rare
Rifampicin	Cholestasis, conjugated and unconjugated hyperbilirubinaemia	Transient
Synthetic oestrogens	Cholestasis, may precipitate gallstone disease	Underlying liver disease, rare now that low-dose oestrogens are generally given
HMGCoA reductase inhibitors	Unknown	Usually mild and asymptomatic

Table 33.7: Dose-independant hepatotoxiticy

Drug	Mechanism	Comment/predisposing factors
Chlorpromazine	Cholestatic hepatitis	Estimated incidence 0.5% associated with fever, abdominal pain, pruritus; subclinical hepatic dysfunction is more common
Chlopropamide Tolbutamide	Cholestatic jaundice	–
Isoniazid	Hepatitis	Mild and self-limiting in 20% and severe hepatitis in $< 0.1\%$ of cases. Possibly more common in rapid acetylators
Pyrazinamide	Hepatitis	Similar to isoniazid, but more clearly related to dose
Methyldopa	Hepatitis	About 5% of cases have subclinical, raised transaminases; clinical hepatitis is rare
Phenytoin	Hypersensitivity reaction	Resembles infectious mononucleosis; pharmacogenetic predisposition; cross-reaction with carbamazepine
Isoniazid	Chronic active hepatitis	Associated with prolonged treatment, usually regresses when drug is discontinued
Troglitazone	Hepatic necrosis	No clear risk factors. This (an insulin sensitizer) has been withdrawn in the UK
Nitrofurantoin Dantrolene Halothane Ketoconazole	Hepatitis/hepatic necrosis	See Chapter 23

lar drugs tend to produce distinctive patterns of liver injury, but this is not invariable.

Investigation and management of hepatic drug reactions

Depending on the clinical presentation the most important differential diagnoses are hepatic dysfunction due to viral infection (which may be asymptomatic), malignant disease, alcohol and congestive cardiac failure. The aetiology of a minor elevation of transaminases is often undetermined. If the patient is being treated for a disease associated with hepatic dysfunction, particularly with multiple drugs, identification of the responsible agent is particularly difficult. Minor elevations of transaminase activity are often picked up on routine biochemical profiles. If they are considered to be drug related, but further treatment is indicated, it is reasonable to continue the drug with regular monitoring of liver enzymes if a better alternative therapy is not available. If the transaminases reach twice the upper limit of the normal range it is prudent to stop the drug if the clinical situation permits.

Gallstones

Gallstone dissolution

Chenodeoxycholic acid or ursodeoxycholic acid (which is also used in primary biliary cirrhosis) may be considered in patients who cannot be treated by laparoscopic cholecystectomy or endoscopic biliary techniques, and who have mild symptoms, unimpaired gall-bladder function, and small or medium-sized radiolucent stones. Radiological monitoring is required. Side-effects include diarrhoea, pruritus and minor hepatic abnormalities. Recurrence is common.

Drugs that modify appetite

Anorectic drugs

The commonest form of malnutrition in western society is obesity. Obesity is a killer disease and is preventable, since the obese are fat because they eat too much for their energy needs. Cure is ostensibly simple – they must eat less. In practice, however, treatment is much more difficult. Naturally a calorie-controlled diet and adequate but sensible amounts of exercise are the essentials of treatment. Unfortunately, the results of treating patients at weight-reduction clinics are disappointing – many patients default at an early stage, there is a high relapse rate, and only a few individuals achieve permanent weight loss. There has accordingly been a great deal of interest in the possibility of altering appetite pharmacologically in order to help the patient to reduce his or her calorie intake. Unfortunately, the causes of obesity are not well understood. There is conflicting evidence concerning the relative roles of overeating, lack of exercise and individual variation in the utilization of food energy. One hypothesis is that lean people do not become obese when they overeat because their tissues preferentially liberate heat (particularly from brown fat). Despite this uncertainty, there is no doubt that starvation leads to weight loss. Therefore, research into drugs for the treatment of obesity has concentrated on finding substances that inhibit appetite.

Social conditioning plays only a minor role in signalling normal satiety, but learned behaviour is probably important in determining the frequency of eating and whether food is taken between major meals. Stretch receptors in the stomach are stimulated by distention, but the main factors that terminate eating are humoral. Bombesin and somatostatin are two candidates for humoral satiety factors released by the stomach. The most important satiety factor released from the gastrointestinal tract beyond the stomach is cholecystokinin (CCK). A small peptide fragment of this (CCK-8) has been synthesized, and has been found to cause humans to reduce their food intake, possibly by acting on the appetite/satiety centre in the hypothalamus, but this agent is not in clinical use.

Amphetamine was first shown to be anorectic in humans in 1938, and since that time a number of congeners have been employed for this purpose. The site of action of these compounds appears to be in the hypothalamus, where they increase noradrenaline and dopamine levels by causing transmitter release and blocking reuptake. Cardiovascular effects are frequently observed with amphetamines, a dose-related increase in heart rate and blood pressure being the most common effect. **Phentermine** is licensed as a short-term appetite suppressant. It has abuse potential and may cause mood disturbance, tachycardia and hypertension. It has rarely been associated with primary pulmonary hypertension. **Dexfenfluramine** and **fenfluramine**, which are both associated with pulmonary hypertension, have been withdrawn following reports of valvular heart disease associated with their use.

Fluoxetine has shown useful activity in patients with bulimia.

In 1994 the gene for obesity (OB) in the mouse was identified. The OB gene encodes the protein leptin, which is produced only in fat cells and is secreted into the blood. The human homologue of the OB gene has now been identified. Leptin is thought to be a blood-borne signal from the adipose tissue that informs the brain about the size of the fat mass. Much more research is required to determine its exact role in neuroendocrine reproductive haematopoietic and metabolic control pathways, as well as its exact effects on body weight and energy expenditure. In the future, modulation of leptin activity may provide a method of treating obesity.

Orlistat, which inhibits gastrointestinal lipase enzymes, reduces fat absorption and is licensed for up to 2 years' use to treat obesity in combination with a weight management programme including a mildly hypocaloric diet. If no effect (minimum of 5% weight loss) is seen within 12 weeks it should be stopped. Systemic absorption is minimal. The main adverse effects are oily spotting from the rectum, flatus with discharge, faecal urgency and oily faeces. Although there is less absorption of the fat-soluble vitamins (vitamins A, D, E and K) and of β-carotene, this does not appear to cause pathological vitamin deficiency, and vitamin supplementation is not routinely indicated.

Bulk agents

Substances such as methylcellulose and guar gum acting as bulking agents in the diet are ineffective. A high-fibre diet may help weight loss, provided that total caloric intake is reduced, and is desirable for other reasons as well.

Miscellaneous

Diuretics cause a transient loss of weight through fluid loss, and their use for such an effect is to be deplored. Myxoedema is associated with weight gain. Thyroxine has been used to increase the basic metabolic rate and reduce weight in euthyroid obese patients. This is both dangerous and irrational.

Appetite stimulation

This is often difficult, as patients with a poor appetite may have a debilitating systemic illness or an underlying psychiatric disorder. Drugs that inhibit serotonin (5HT) receptors, (e.g. cyproheptadine, pizotifen) increase appetite and cause weight gain. Weight gain occurs during treatment with various other drugs, including chlorpromazine (but not other phenothiazines or butyrophenones), amitriptyline, lithium, corticosteroids and ACTH, and the oral contraceptive pill. Corticosteroids may help to improve appetite in terminally ill patients, but in general these effects are not therapeutically useful, and in fact rather the reverse is true.

Further reading

1997: Symposium: gastrointestinal disorders, *Prescriber's Journal* **37** (No. 4).

Liang TJ. 1998: Combination therapy for hepatitis C infection. *New England Journal of Medicine* **339**, 1549–50.

Reidenburg M. 1998: Drugs and the liver. *British Journal of Clinical Pharmacology* **46**, 351–9.

1998: Why and how should adults lose weight? *Drugs and Therapeutics Bulletin* **36** (No. 12).

CHAPTER THIRTY-FOUR

VITAMINS *and* OTHER NUTRIENTS

- Introduction
- General physiology of vitamins
- Vitamin A (retinoic acid) and its derivatives
- Vitamin B_1 (thiamine)
- Vitamin B_2 (riboflavine)
- Vitamin B_3 (niacin, nicotinic acid and nicotinamide)
- Vitamin B_6 (pyridoxine)
- Pantothenic acid
- Biotin
- Vitamin C (ascorbic acid)
- Vitamin E (tocopherol)
- Essential fatty acids
- Trace elements

INTRODUCTION

Vitamins were first recognized by a group of clinical syndromes relating to deficiency states (e.g. scurvy, beriberi). They are nutrients that are essential for normal cellular function (health), but are required in much smaller quantities than the aliments (carbohydrates, fats and proteins). Vitamins are essential cofactors to or components of enzymes that are integral in the intermediary metabolism of the aliments and for many other biochemical and cellular processes.

GENERAL PHYSIOLOGY OF VITAMINS

Humans are incapable of synthesizing adequate amounts of vitamins. Vitamin deficiency usually results from either inadequate dietary intake, increased demand (e.g pregnancy or growth) or impaired absorption (e.g malabsorption syndromes such as Crohn's disease or cystic fibrosis). Vitamin deficiencies are rarely diagnosed in the UK, but their true incidence is unknown and may be under-recognized, particularly in elderly people and certain ethnic groups.

Recently the concept has emerged that dietary supplements with various vitamins might decrease the incidence of a variety of diseases, including cancer and atheroma. Several large prospective controlled clinical trials have investigated these hypotheses, but to date evidence of clear clinical benefit is lacking. Not all vitamins are harmless when taken in excess (this is particularly true of vitamins A and D), and therefore in general vitamins should only be prescribed for the prevention or treatment of vitamin deficiency.

Vitamins fall into two categories:

1. *water soluble* – vitamin B complex (including pantothenic acid and biotin), vitamin C, vitamin B_{12} and folate;
2. *fat soluble* – vitamins A, D, E and K. Essential fatty acids are also fat-soluble nutrients which were not classed as vitamins due to historical accident.

Vitamin B_{12} and folate are discussed in Chapter 48, vitamin D in Chapter 38 and vitamin K in Chapter 29. In addition to its use in the treatment and prevention of folate deficiency anaemia, there is also interest in the use of folate supplementation to reduce neural-tube defects (see Chapter 9) and to decrease plasma homocysteine concentration, which has recently been recognized as an independent risk factor for ischaemic heart disease.

Key points

Major categories of vitamins

- Originally identified by characteristic deficiency states (now uncommon in developed countries).
- Water-soluble vitamins include the vitamin B complex and vitamin C.
- Fat-soluble vitamins include vitamins A, D, E and K.
- The vitamin B complex includes vitamins B_1 (thiamine), B_2 (riboflavin), B_3 (nicotinic acid), B_6 (pyridoxine), B_{12}, cobalamin, folate, pantothenic acid and biotin.

VITAMIN A (RETINOIC ACID) AND ITS DERIVATIVES

PHYSIOLOGY

This vitamin exists in several forms that are interconverted. Retinol (vitamin A_1) is a primary alcohol and is present in the tissues of animals and marine fishes; 3-dehydroretinol (vitamin A_2) is present in freshwater fishes; retinoic acid shares some but not all of the actions of retinol; retinol ethers and esters also show retinol-type activity. The plant pigment carotene is provitamin A and is readily converted into the vitamin in the body. Vitamin A has many physiological functions. It is essential for the integrity of epithelial cells, it stabilizes membranes, it is an essential component of the visual pigment rhodopsin, and it is required for skeletal and soft tissue growth. It is a cofactor in mucopolysaccharide synthesis, sulphate activation, hydroxysteroid dehydrogenation, cholesterol synthesis and microsomal drug-metabolizing enzyme function. There is accumulating evidence that vitamin A inhibits tumour growth. The normal adult daily requirement is about 2500–3000 IU, but for nursing mothers it is estimated to be 4000 IU. Vitamin A deficiency retards growth and development, and causes night blindness, keratomalacia, dry eyes and keratinization, and drying of the skin. Dietary sources rich in vitamin A include eggs, fish liver oil, liver, milk and vegetables.

USE

Vitamin A is used to prevent and treat deficiency states. Dietary supplementation with halibut liver oil capsules BP (containing vitamin A, 4000–5250 IU, and vitamin D, 450 IU) is used to prevent vitamin A deficiency. The doses used in clinical deficiency of vitamin A of the order of 5000 IU/kg daily. Although a single large intramuscular injection of retinol palmitate has been used in severe malnutrition, this should be followed by oral therapy. In vulnerable and malnourished communities intramuscular doses may be given to children 6-monthly. Regular dietary or parenteral supplementation of vitamin A may be necessary in patients with steatorrhoea (e.g. cystic fibrosis).

ADVERSE EFFECTS

Long-term ingestion of more than double the recommended daily intake of vitamin A can lead to toxicity and chronic hypervitaminosis A.

Chronic toxicity includes the following:

1. anorexia and vomiting;
2. itching and dry skin;
3. raised intracranial pressure (benign intracranial hypertension), irritability and headache;
4. tender hyperostoses in the skull and long bones;
5. hepatotoxicity;
6. congenital abnormalities.

Acute poisoning causes the following:

1. headache, vomiting and papilloedema;
2. desquamation.

PHARMACOKINETICS

Gastrointestinal absorption of retinol via a saturable active transport process is very efficient. Vitamin A absorption is impaired in patients with steatorrhoea, and under these circumstances water-miscible preparations of vitamin A can be administered. Carotene is converted to vitamin A by first-pass metabolism in the intestine. Esterified retinol reaches peak plasma concentrations 4 h after ingestion. About 100 μg/g is stored in the parenchymal and Kupffer cells of the liver. Vitamin E enhances vitamin A storage. Retinol is partly conjugated to a glucuronide and undergoes enterohepatic circulation. Retinol released from the liver is bound to the retinol-binding protein in the plasma. The normal plasma concentration of vitamin A is 30–70 μg/100 mL. When a vitamin A-deficient diet is taken, plasma concentrations are maintained for several months until the hepatic stores have been depleted. Clinical evidence of vitamin A deficiency appears when the plasma concentration falls below 20 μg/100 mL.

CONTRAINDICATIONS

Excess vitamin A during pregnancy causes birth defects (closely related compounds are involved in controlling morphogenesis in the fetus). Therefore pregnant women should not take vitamin A supplements, and should perhaps also avoid liver in their diet.

DERIVATIVES OF VITAMIN A (RETINOIDS)

Retinoids and the skin

Vitamin A derivatives such as etretinate and isotretinoin are discussed in Chapter 50.

Retinoids and cancer

Retinoids have powerful effects on cell differentiation and proliferation, and can inhibit or retard malignant transformation of cells *in vitro*. In animals they can prevent the action of carcinogens, and there is limited epidemiological evidence that retinoid status is a determinant of the risk of developing cancer. Clinical trials of retinoid therapy (e.g. β-carotene supplementation) as primary and secondary prevention of cancer have as yet yielded no evidence of clinical benefit, and in one large Scandinavian study β-carotene was associated with an *increased* incidence of malignancy. Retinoids, either alone (e.g. in acute promyelocytic leukemia) or in combination with established anti-cancer drugs (e.g. anthracyclines) are also being investigated as therapy for cancer (see Chapter 47).

VITAMIN B$_1$ (THIAMINE)

PHYSIOLOGY

All plant and animal cells require thiamine (in the form of thiamine pyrophosphate) for carbohydrate metabolism, as it is a coenzyme for decarboxylases and transketolases. Thiamine deficiency leads to the various manifestations of beriberi, including peripheral neuropathy and cardiac failure. Increased carbohydrate utilization requires increased intake because thiamine is consumed during carbohydrate metabolism. It is therefore useful to express thiamine needs in relation to the calorie intake. Diets associated with beriberi contain less than 0.3 mg thiamine/1000 kcal. If the diet provides more than this, *the excess is excreted in the urine*. Thus the recommended daily intake of 0.4 mg/1000 kcal provides a considerable safety margin. The body possesses little ability to store thiamine, and if the vitamin is withdrawn completely from the diet, beriberi develops within a few weeks.

Acute thiamine deficiency is precipitated by a carbohydrate load in patients who have been on a marginally deficient diet. This is especially important in alcoholics, and thiamine replacement should precede intravenous dextrose in alcoholic patients with a depressed conscious level. Failure to do this has historically been associated with worsening encephalopathy and permanent sequelae (e.g. Korsakoff's psychosis). Thiamine is found in many plant and animal foods (e.g. yeast and pork).

USE

Thiamine is used in the treatment of beriberi and other states of thiamine deficiency, or in their prevention. Such conditions include alcoholic neuritis, Wernicke's encephalopathy and the neuritis of pregnancy, as well as chronic diarrhoeal states and after intestinal resection. The parenteral route of administration is used in confused patients, and up to 30 mg is injected intramuscularly or by slow (10 min) IV injection 8-hourly. Once the deficiency state has been corrected the oral route (initially 5 mg daily) is preferred, unless gastrointestinal disease interferes with ingestion or absorption of the vitamin.

ADVERSE EFFECTS

Anaphylactoid reactions following parenteral thiamine delivery have been reported, so parenteral administration should be restricted to situations where it is essential.

PHARMACOKINETICS

Absorption of thiamine following intramuscular injection is rapid and complete. Thiamine is absorbed through the mucosa of the upper part of the small intestine by both active and passive mechanisms, and surplus intake is excreted unchanged in the urine.

VITAMIN B_2 (RIBOFLAVINE)

PHYSIOLOGY

Riboflavine is present in significant amounts in yeast, green vegetables, liver, eggs and milk, and is converted in the body into two essential coenzymes, namely flavine mononucleotide and flavine adenine dinucleotide. These are co-enzymes for proteins in the mitochondrial–respiratory electron transport chain, and a variety of important flavoproteins (e.g. nitric oxide synthase) are involved in electron transport. The minimum daily requirement is about 0.3 mg/1000 kcal. Riboflavine deficiency is common in developing countries, and also occurs sporadically among the poor and in alcoholics in the UK. Angular stomatitis and a sore tongue are early symptoms, and are followed by seborrhoeic dermatitis, itching and burning of the eyes with photophobia and corneal vascularization. Late findings include neuropathy and mild anaemia.

USE

Riboflavine, 5–20 mg orally daily, is prescribed for the prevention or treatment of deficiency.

PHARMACOKINETICS

Riboflavine is well absorbed from the small intestine (but absorption is impaired in liver disease) and from intramuscular sites. Very little is stored in tissues, and excess appears unchanged in the urine. On an average UK diet only about 10% is excreted in the urine.

VITAMIN B_3 (NIACIN, NICOTINIC ACID AND NICOTINAMIDE)

PHYSIOLOGY

Niacin is found in yeast, rice, liver and other meats. Its vital metabolic role is as a component of nicotinamide adenine dinucleotide (NAD) and nicotinamide adenine dinucleotide phosphate (NADP). Niacin can be generated in the body in small amounts from tryptophan, 60 mg of the amino acid yielding 1 mg of niacin. Deficiency causes pellagra, the clinical manifestations of which include dementia, dermatitis and diarrhoea. The pellagra-preventing properties of a diet are expressed as 'niacin equivalents' consisting of niacin itself together with tryptophan. Pellagra may develop on diets containing less than 5.0 mg niacin equivalents/1000 kcal. The recommended dietary intake is 6.6 niacin equivalents/1000 kcal.

USES

1 Niacin is used to treat and prevent pellagra. The oral dose is 50 mg up to three times daily. If oral treatment is not possible, intravenous injections of 25 mg are given two or three times daily.
2 Nicotinic acid (or nicotinic acid analogues, e.g. acipomox) in pharmacological doses is of limited use for treatment of hyperlipidaemia (see Chapter 26), but such use is limited by flushing.

ADVERSE EFFECTS

In replacement therapy for pellagra, adverse effects are uncommon. High doses (as used for hyperlipidaemia) causes the following:

1 vasodilatation due to prostaglandin D_2 – this can be reduced by premedication with aspirin;
2 nausea, vomiting and itching;
3 hyperglycaemia;
4 exacerbation of hyperuricaemia.

PHARMACOKINETICS

Both niacin and nicotinamide are well absorbed via the intestine and are distributed widely to all tissues. When the usual dietary amounts are administered, a high proportion is excreted as N-methyl nicotinamide and other metabolites. When increased doses are administered, a higher proportion is excreted unchanged in the urine.

VITAMIN B_6 (PYRIDOXINE)

PHYSIOLOGY

Vitamin B_6 occurs naturally in three forms, namely pyridoxine, pyridoxal and pyridoxamine. All three forms are converted in the body into pyridoxal phosphate, which is an essential cofactor in several metabolic reactions, including decarboxylation, transamination and other steps in amino acid metabolism. Pyridoxine is present in wheatgerm, yeast, bran, rice and liver. Deficiency causes glossitis, seborrhoea, fits, peripheral neuropathy and sideroblastic anaemia. Isoniazid prevents the activation of pyridoxal to pyridoxal phosphate by inhibiting the enzyme pyridoxal kinase, and slow acetylators of isoniazid are at increased risk of developing peripheral neuropathy for this reason (see Chapter 43). The minimum daily requirement is 1.25 mg/day/100 g of dietary protein.

USE

Pyridoxine hydrochloride, 10 mg/day, may be given to patients who are receiving long-term therapy with isoniazid to prevent peripheral neuropathy, and in deficiency states. In sideroblastic anaemias up to 100–400 mg of pyridoxine are given daily. Pyridoxine is also used to treat certain uncommon inborn errors of metabolism, including primary hyperoxaluria. Large doses are sometimes used to treat premenstrual syndrome, and there is a lobby of enthusiasts for this, despite a paucity of evidence.

ADVERSE EFFECTS

There have been reports of ataxia and sensory neuropathy following megadoses (2 g daily) of pyridoxine for more than 2 months.

PANTOTHENIC ACID

Pantothenic acid is present in many meats and vegetables. Its major role in cellular biochemistry is as an essential constituent of coenzyme A and acyl carrier proteins. Coenzyme A is a cofactor in a number of enzymic processes involved in two-carbon transfer. This is vital in gluconeogenesis, oxidative carbohydrate metabolism, fatty acid degradation and synthesis of steroid hormones and porphyrins. The daily requirement is 10–15 mg/day, and deficiency is uncommon, but patients with hepatic disease and alcoholics may develop symptoms of limb paraesthesiae and muscle weakness if they become deficient.

BIOTIN

Biotin is found in yeast, eggs and dairy products, and the intestinal microflora provides another source. The major biological role of biotin is as a coenzyme in β-carboxylation and deamination processes that require the fixation of carbon dioxide. The daily requirement is 0.3–0.5 mg/day, and deficiency states may occur in patients on long-term parenteral nutrition. Symptoms of biotin deficiency include lassitude, anorexia, gastrointestinal upsets and dermatitis. Deficiency is treated with 5–10 mg/day administered orally.

VITAMIN C (ASCORBIC ACID)

PHYSIOLOGY

Ascorbic acid is present in large quantities in citrus fruits, tomatoes and green vegetables. Vitamin C is essential to humans, monkeys and guinea pigs which, unlike other mammals, cannot synthesize it from glucose. Dietary lack of vitamin C causes scurvy, which is characterized by bleeding gums and perifollicular purpura. Ascorbic acid is involved in several metabolic processes, including collagen biosynthesis, steroid metabolism, functioning of the mitochondrial electron transport chain, activation of folic acid and the cytochrome P_{450} drug-metabolizing enzyme system. It is a potent water-soluble anti-oxidant. The nutritional status of vitamin C can be assessed by measuring the intracellular leucocyte concentration, but this is not routinely available. Daily intakes of 40–100 mg of vitamin C give whole blood concentrations of 34–68 μmol/L when the tissues are saturated. A daily intake of 10–15 mg results in approximately 50% tissue saturation.

USES

1 Ascorbic acid is used in the prophylaxis and treatment of scurvy. (Perhaps the first recorded clinical trial involved the distribution of citrus fruit to some, but not all, British naval vessels and observation of the incidence of scurvy. The admiralty were impressed, and British sailors were subsequently provided with limes – whence the term 'limeys'.) Normal dietary requirements are less than 70 mg daily, but this may double in the presence of infection. Daily ingestion of 120 mg meets the highest requirements in non-scorbutic individuals. In cases of fully developed scurvy, the dose is 1 g daily.

2 Ascorbic acid increases the absorption of orally administered iron.
3 The reducing properties of ascorbate may be used in the treatment of methaemoglobinaemia.
4 In scorbutic patients wound healing is delayed, and this is restored to normal by administration of ascorbic acid.

ADVERSE EFFECTS

Ascorbic acid is non-toxic in low doses. However, administration of 4 g daily raises the urinary excretion of oxalate by 12 mg, and a daily intake of 9 g results in a 68-mg increase in oxalate excretion. Large doses of vitamin C taken chronically have resulted in calcium oxalate urolithiasis. There is theoretical concern that high doses of vitamin C (in common with other anti-oxidants) can have pro-oxidant actions.

PHARMACOKINETICS

Ascorbic acid is well absorbed following oral administration, and its sodium salt may be given by intramuscular or intravenous injection. Ascorbic acid is mainly metabolized by oxidation to oxalic acid. Normally about 40% of urinary oxalate is derived from ascorbic acid. When the body stores of ascorbic acid are saturated, some ingested ascorbic acid is excreted in the urine unchanged.

VITAMIN E (TOCOPHEROL)

Vitamin E is found in many foods, including nuts, wheatgerm and bananas. Deficiency in animals causes abortion and degeneration of the germinal epithelium of the testes. No defined deficiency syndrome exists in humans, but low vitamin E intake is associated with anaemia in premature and malnourished infants. Vitamin E protects erythrocytes against haemolysis, and is a fat-soluble anti-oxidant and detoxifies free radicals. Free radicals cause membrane and epithelial injury and have been implicated in the pathophysiology of numerous diseases, including cancer and atheroma, and epidemiological evidence suggests that reduced intake is associated with increased atherogenesis (see Chapter 26). A clinical trial based in Cambridge suggested that supplementation of vitamin E in patients with established ischaemic heart disease reduces non-fatal myocardial infarction. However, the study was too small to detect an effect on mortality (which was, if anything, higher in the treated group), and larger studies are awaited. Despite the paucity of knowledge of its

Key points

Vitamin deficiency and disease

- In general, vitamin deficiencies are due to poor diet or malabsorption.
- Vitamin B deficiencies do not often occur in isolation.
- Vitamin A deficiency – night blindness.
- Vitamin B_1 (thiamine) deficiency – beriberi (neuropathy – paralysis, muscle wasting and cardiac failure).
- Vitamin B_3 (niacin) deficiency – pellagra (dermatitis, dementia and diarrhoea).
- Vitamin B_{12} and/or folate deficiency – megaloblastic anaemia.
- Vitamin C deficiency – scurvy (perifollicular petechiae, gingivitis and swollen joints).

Key points

Population groups at high risk for vitamin deficiency

- Infants.
- Pregnant women.
- Elderly people, especially the elderly with chronic disease.
- Alcoholics and drug abusers.
- Vegans and undernourished populations.
- Patients taking long-term anticonvulsants.
- Patients with malabsorption syndromes.

Key points

Vitamin toxicities

- Vitamin A – gastrointestinal upsets, headache (raised intracranial pressure), desquamation, hepatotoxicity and teratogenicity.
- Nicotinic acid – flushing, vasodilatation and hepatotoxicity.
- Vitamin B_6 (pyridoxine) – case reports of ataxia and sensory neuropathy.
- Vitamin C – hyperoxaluria and oxalate stones.
- Vitamin D – hypercalcaemia.

functions, vitamin E is widely consumed as part of the multiple vitamin therapies taken by some enthusiasts, and is apparently harmless.

Essential fatty acids

Several naturally occurring unsaturated fatty acids are essential dietary components. Linoleic and linolenic acids occur in vegetable oils and nuts, arachidonic acid occurs in meat, and longer-chain fatty acids (eicosapentanoic acid and docosahexanoic acid) are found in cold-water oily fish. Humans can synthesize arachidonic acid (C20:4) from shorter-chain (C18:2) essential fatty acids by chain elongation and desaturation. Arachidonic acid is present in the lipid component of cell membranes throughout the body. It is esterified on the 2′ position of glycerol in membrane phospholipids, and is liberated by phospholipases when cells are injured or otherwise stimulated. Such free arachidonic acid is the precursor of the 2–series of prostaglandins, thromboxanes and the 4–series of leukotrienes, and so is important in many mediator functions, including inflammatory and haemostatic processes. Deficiency states have been described in patients receiving long-term parenteral nutrition, and are prevented by the use of lipid emulsions.

Table 34.1: Trace element deficiencies and treatment

Element	Clinical features of deficiency	Biochemical activity	Normal serum/tissue concentration	Replacement therapy dose	Other comments
Copper	Osteoporosis, costochondral cartilage cupping and anaemia/leukopenia Menke's syndrome in children	Major enzyme dysfunction (e.g. cytochrome oxidase)	Plasma copper does not reflect tissue copper status well (12–26 μmol/L) Reduced red cell superoxide dismutase activity is a better indicator	Safe daily copper intake in adults is 1–3 mg copper/day maximum doses of copper sulphate 0.1 mg/kg/day)	Premature babies are predisposed to copper deficiency, as copper stores are built up in late pregnancy
Molybdenum	Symptoms of gout	Purine metabolism	Urine molybdenum 0.26–2.6 μmol/24 h		
Selenium	Myopathies, especially cardiomyopathy with heart failure	Protects against oxidation stresses, at active site of glutathione peroxidase	Plasma selenium = 0.3–0.6 μmol/L Red cell glutathione peroxidase activity is a surlogate measured for selenium stores	45–75 μg/day	Margin between replacement therapy and toxic dose is very narrow
Zinc	Skin rash (acrodermatitis enteropathica), hair thinning, diarrhoea, mental apathy and impaired T-cell function	At the active site of glutathione peroxidase and protects against oxidant stresses	Serum zinc 5 6–25 μmol/L	Adult daily requirement is 12–15 mg/day. Replacement therapy can be as much as 135 mg/day	Adverse effects of zinc include dyspepsia and abdominal pain

Case history

A 24-year-old woman was diagnosed as epileptic and was started on phenytoin. Many months later she complained of fatigue. Her haemoglobin was 8.6 g/dL, and mean corpuscular volume (MCV) was 103 fL.

Question

What additonal investigations would you undertake? What is the most likely diagnosis and how should you treat this patient?

Answer

This young woman has a macrocytic anaemia. After checking her vitamin B_{12} and folate levels, you find that the serum folate is low, with a normal B_{12}. This confirms your suspicion of phenytoin-induced folate deficiency, as a dietary assessment shows an apparently adequate intake, and there is no clinical evidence of other causes of malabsorption. Phenytoin commonly causes folate deficiency, impairing the absorption of dietary folate by inducing gastrointestinal enzymes involved in its catabolism. Treatment should consist of daily oral folate supplementation, keeping her on the phenytoin (as this has controlled her epilepsy), and further monitoring of her haematological status for response. During follow-up she should also be monitored for possible development of osteomalacia (suggested by proximal myopathy with low serum phosphate and calcium and raised alkaline phosphatase), as phenytoin also induces the metabolic inactivation of vitamin D.

TRACE ELEMENTS

A total of 14 nutritionally essential trace elements are recognized, namely fluorine, silicon, vanadium, chromium, manganese, iron, cobalt, nickel, copper, zinc, selenium, tin and iodine. These are required in the human body at $<0.01\%$ of body weight. Most of them are highly reactive chemically, and one or more of these elements is present at the active site of over 50% of the enzymes in humans, and they help to catalyse or inhibit chemical reactions. They are present in small but adequate amounts in a normal diet, but evidence is accumulating that in addition to iron, cobalt (see Chapter 48) and iodine (see Chapter 37), zinc, copper, selenium and molybdenum deficiencies can contribute to disease. Trace element deficiencies are most commonly due to inadequate intake or to intestinal disease reducing absorption.

The treatment of some major trace element deficiencies is summarized in Table 34.1.

FURTHER READING

Bender DA. 1992: *Nutritional biochemistry of the vitamins*. Cambridge: Cambridge University Press.

Charleux J-L. 1996: Beta-carotene, vitamin C and vitamin E: the protective micronutrients. *Nutrition Reviews* **54**, S109–14.

Fitzgerald FT, Tierney LM. 1984: Trace metals and human disease. *Advances in Internal Medicine* **30**, 337–58.

van Poppel G, van den Berg H. 1997: Vitamins and cancer. *Cancer Letters* **114**, 195–202.

PART VII

FLUIDS AND ELECTROLYTES

CHAPTER THIRTY-FIVE

DRUGS *and the* RENAL *and* GENITO-URINARY SYSTEMS: FLUID *and* ELECTROLYTE DISORDERS

- Volume overload (salt and water excess)
- Diuretics
- Overhydration
- Volume depletion
- Disordered potassium ion balance
- Drugs that alter urine pH
- Drugs that affect the bladder and genito-urinary system

VOLUME OVERLOAD (SALT AND WATER EXCESS)

Volume overload is usually caused by an excess of sodium chloride with accompanying water. Effective treatment is directed at the underlying cause (e.g. heart failure or renal failure), in addition to measures directed toward improving volume status *per se*. These include reducing salt intake and increasing its elimination by the use of diuretics. Limiting water intake is seldom useful in patients with volume overload, although modest limitation is of value in patients with ascites due to advanced liver disease.

Diuretics increase urine production and Na^+ excretion. They are among the most widely prescribed drugs, and are of central importance in managing hypertension (see Chapter 27) as well as the many diseases associated with oedema and volume overload, including heart failure (see Chapter 30), cirrhosis, renal failure and nephrotic syndrome. In all of these disorders it is important to assess the distribution of salt and water excess in different body compartments – a patient with gross peripheral oedema and ascites due to cirrhosis may none the less have a relatively contracted blood volume. Glomerular filtrate derives from plasma, so diuretic treatment primarily reduces plasma volume. It takes time for tissue fluid to re-equilibrate after an acute change in blood volume caused by a diuretic. Consequently, attempts to produce a vigorous diuresis are inappropriate in some oedematous states, and may lead to cardiovascular collapse and prerenal renal failure. The principles of using diuretics in the management of hypertension and heart failure are described in other chapters, but before considering individual classes of diuretic drugs in more detail, it is appropriate to describe briefly the management of nephrotic syndrome and cirrhosis of the liver. In both of these conditions there is hypoalbuminaemia, which affects the kinetics of several drugs through its effects on protein binding (see Chapter 7) and, paradoxically, an apparently inadequate intravascular volume in the face of fluid overload in the body as a whole. This results in an increased risk of nephrotoxicity from several common drugs, particularly non-steroidal anti-inflammatory drugs (NSAIDs). Consequently, particular caution is needed when prescribing and monitoring the effects of therapy for intercurrent problems in such patients.

Nephrotic syndrome

The primary problem in nephrotic syndrome is loss of the barrier function of glomerular membranes with leakage of plasma albumin into the urine. The oncotic pressure exerted by the plasma falls because of the resulting hypoalbuminaemia, and water passes from the circulation into the tissue spaces, producing oedema. The fall in effective blood volume stimulates the renin–angiotensin–aldosterone system, causing sodium retention. Depending on the nature of the glomerular pathology, it may be possible to reduce albumin loss with corticosteroid or other immunosuppressive drugs. However, in nephrotic syndrome caused by many types of glomerular pathology, treatment is only symptomatic. Diuretics are of only limited value, but diet is important. Individuals vary in their ability to compensate for increased urinary protein loss by increased hepatic synthesis of albumin. Salt intake should be restricted, and a high protein intake should be established in patients with an adequate glomerular filtration rate.

Cirrhosis of the liver

Fluid retention in cirrhosis of the liver usually takes the form of ascites, the localization of the fluid being due to portal hypertension leading to loss of fluid from the portal system, although dependent oedema also occurs. Other important factors are the low concentration of albumin in the plasma (caused by failure of synthesis by the diseased liver) and hyperaldosteronism (due to activation of volume receptors and reduced hepatic aldosterone catabolism). Cirrhosis is an irreversible pathological state, and no current medical therapy is effective in improving the damaged hepatic architecture. Transplantation may be appropriate in cases where the underlying pathology (most commonly alcoholism) is judged to have been cured or (as in some rare inherited metabolic disorders) will not recur in the donor liver. Nevertheless, symptomatic treatment is all that is available for most patients.

Diet is especially important. Protein is restricted because of the risk of precipitating hepatic encephalopathy. The protein that is consumed should be of high quality to provide an adequate supply of essential amino acids. High energy is desirable to minimize catabolism of body protein, and is provided by supplementary carbohydrate. Salt restriction and moderate water restriction are essential. Frequent accurate weighing is the best way of monitoring progress with regard to volume status. Diuretics should be used with particular care in this situation, as excessively rapid diuresis may precipitate renal failure, as explained above. A loss of approximately 0.5 kg daily is ideal.

Because of aldosterone excess, thiazides or loop diuretics cause especially marked potassium depletion and alkalosis in these patients, in whom these disturbances are more important than in patients with other diseases (e.g. hypertension) as they may precipitate hepatic encephalopathy by altering amino acid metabolism and increasing renal ammonia production. **Amiloride** or **spironolactone** can be used in this setting (see below), but if these drugs are not adequate, more powerful diuretics may be given with potassium supplements while monitoring plasma potassium levels. Salt-free albumin (25–50 g/day intravenously given slowly) increases the response to diuretics in cirrhotic patients by causing extracellular fluid to redistribute from tissue spaces to plasma, but it is rapidly metabolized, so its effects are short-lived, and it is also expensive.

Diuretics

Diuretics cause natriuresis, and are therefore used to treat patients with volume overload. As well as uses related to their natriuretic effect, some diuretics have a distict therapeutic niche because of specific actions within the kidney (e.g. the use of **frusemide** to treat hypercalcaemia, or the use of thiazide diuretics to treat nephrogenic diabetes insipidus) or elsewhere in the body (e.g. the use of

acetazolamide to treat glaucoma, or the use of **mannitol** to treat cerebral oedema).

THIAZIDES

See also Chapter 27.

USES

Thiazide diuretics in common clinical use include **bendrofluazide** and **hydrochlorothiazide**. **Metolazone**, which has a long duration of action, is used in the treatment of resistant oedema in combination with a loop diuretic (see below). Except for some differences in duration of action and potency per unit weight (rather than in maximum effect achievable at the top of the dose–response curve), there is little to choose between them. Thiazides are usually taken orally in the morning, and produce a mild to moderate diuresis throughout the day. Diuresis starts after about 2 h and lasts for 8–20 h depending on the drug. Thiazides are used in:

1 *hypertension* – this is currently the main indication for thiazide diuretics, and their clinical use for this indication is more extensively discussed in Chapter 27;
2 *cardiac failure* – thiazides are seldom potent enough to treat heart failure, although they are sometimes useful when it is very mild;
3 *resistant oedema* – thiazides, despite having only mild effects when used alone, may be extremely effective in treating resistant oedema when combined with a loop diuretic;
4 *prevention of stones* – thiazides reduce urinary calcium excretion and thus help to prevent urinary stone formation in patients with idiopathic hypercalciuria. Regular treatment with a thiazide together with maintenance of a high urine output (> 2.5 L/day) approximately halves the rate of recurrence in such patients;
5 *diabetes insipidus* – paradoxically, thiazides reduce urinary volume in diabetes insipidus by preventing the formation of hypotonic fluid in the distal tubule; they are therefore sometimes used to treat nephrogenic diabetes insipidus.

Thiazides are also sometimes prescribed for premenstrual oedema. However, this may worsen cyclical oedema and lead to diuretic abuse, and should be avoided.

MECHANISM OF ACTION

Originally discovered by modification of the sulphonamide structure of inhibitors of carbonic anhydrase, thiazides have a weak inhibitory effect on this enzyme. Their main effect is to decrease sodium chloride reabsorption in the early part of the distal convoluted tubule, thus increasing excretion of sodium, chloride and water. Only about 8% of filtered sodium is reabsorbed by this mechanism, limiting the potency of these drugs. Thiazides also relax vascular smooth muscle by indirect mechanisms that are not understood. This may contribute to their therapeutic effect in hypertension.

PHARMACOKINETICS

Thiazides are given orally. The duration of action of individual agents depends on their water solubility and protein binding. They are highly tissue and plasma protein bound, and gain access to their renal site of action via the proximal tubular non-selective organic-acid secretory mechanism. They are also metabolized to a variable extent.

ADVERSE EFFECTS AND CONTRAINDICATIONS

1 *Impotence* is common, dose related and (provided it is indeed drug related) reversible.
2 *Impairment of glucose tolerance* limits their use in patients with non-insulin-dependent diabetes mellitus. After 6 years of continuous thiazide therapy, up to 10% of hypertensive patients develop a frankly diabetic glucose tolerance curve, and the risk increases with age and obesity. The effect is dose related and usually reversible. Where glucose intolerance that occurs during treatment with a thiazide persists after treatment is discontinued, this is probably due to the independent onset of non-insulin-dependent diabetes.
3 *Hyperuricaemia* contraindicates the use of thiazides in patients with a history of gout. Competition with uric acid at the non-specific acid secretion site in the proximal tubule results in uric acid retention which, combined with a decreased extracellular fluid volume, causes a rise in plasma uric acid concentration.
4 *Hyponatraemia* may be severe, especially in elderly people.
5 *Hypokalaemia* and *hypomagnesaemia* are common during treatment with thiazide diuretics, but are seldom clinically important unless there is

increased risk of arrhythmia (e.g. during concurrent treatment with digoxin).

6 *Allergy* (including non-thrombocytopenic purpura and photosensitivity) and blood dyscrasias (including thrombocytopenia) occur rarely during treatment with thiazide diuretics.

DRUG INTERACTIONS

Thiazide diuretics can be usefully combined with various other drugs when treating patients with moderate or severe hypertension, including β-adrenoceptor antagonists, converting-enzyme inhibitors and α_1-adrenoceptor antagonists. Thiazides (and other diuretics) reduce the excretion of lithium, so a reduced dose of lithium carbonate is needed if these drugs are coadministered.

LOOP DIURETICS

USES

The main clinical use of loop diuretics is in the treatment of heart failure, and this is described more fully in Chapter 30. Several loop diuretics are marketed, including frusemide and **bumetanide**. In the absence of idiosyncratic or other adverse effects, frusemide is the standard agent. Frusemide can be given by slow intravenous injection (not more than 4 mg/min) in initial doses of 20–80 mg to patients with pulmonary oedema caused by acute left ventricular failure, in whom it may produce dramatic symptomatic relief within a few minutes. It is also given orally to patients with chronic congestive heart failure (usual dose 20–80 mg daily). Diuresis begins about 30 min after oral dosage, and lasts for about 6 h.

Frusemide is sometimes administered by continuous infusion (4–16 mg/h) in refractory oedema. An alternative is to combine a loop diuretic with other diuretics that act at different sites in the nephron including potassium-sparing distally acting drugs (e.g. amiloride) and thiazides (e.g. metolazone).

Frusemide is useful in patients with chronic renal failure who are suffering from fluid overload and/or hypertension. Unlike thiazides, which are ineffective in patients with a glomerular filtration rate (GFR) less than 25 mL/min, frusemide can produce some diuresis despite a low GFR when large doses (e.g. 0.25–2.0 g daily) are used. In patients with incipient acute renal failure, frusemide in doses of 250–500 mg intravenously sometimes produces diuresis, and may prevent the development of established failure, although this is difficult to prove.

Loop diuretics increase urinary calcium excretion (in contrast to thiazides, which reduce it), and the hypercalciuric effect of frusemide can be exploited in the treatment of hypercalcaemia when it is given following volume replacement with physiological saline.

MECHANISM OF ACTION

Loop diuretics are the most potent diuretics currently available. They have steep dose–response curves and much higher maximum effects than thiazide or other diuretics, being capable of increasing fractional sodium excretion (i.e. the fraction of sodium filtered at the glomerulus appearing in the urine) to as much as 35%. They act from within the tubular fluid to inhibit a transport mechanism in the thick ascending limb of the loop of Henlé which transports Na^+ and K^+ together with $2Cl^-$ ions from the lumen ('Na^+ K^+ $2Cl^-$ cotransport').

PHARMACOKINETICS

Frusemide is rapidly and extensively absorbed from the gut. It is 95% bound to plasma protein, and elimination is mainly via the kidneys, both filtration and proximal tubular secretion being involved. It is not reabsorbed substantially from the luminal fluid. Approximately two-thirds of water reabsorption occurs iso-osmotically in the proximal convoluted tubule, so frusemide and other loop diuretics are substantially concentrated before they reach their site of action in the thick ascending limb. This accounts for their selectivity for the renal Na^+ K^+ $2Cl^-$ cotransport mechanism, as opposed to Na^+ K^+ $2Cl^-$ cotransport at other sites, such as the inner ear. The luminal site of action of these drugs also contributes to the resistance to their effect in patients with nephrotic syndrome, in whom heavy proteinuria results in substantial protein binding within the lumen. After intravenous injection, 77% of a dose of frusemide is excreted in the urine within 4 h, most of the remainder being metabolized or excreted in the faeces. The plasma $t_{\frac{1}{2}}$ is 1.5–3.5 h. In renal failure the $t_{\frac{1}{2}}$ is prolonged to 10 h or more. In these circumstances, non-renal clearance increases and may account for up to 98% of total elimination.

ADVERSE EFFECTS

These include the following:

1 *acute renal failure* – loop diuretics in high dose cause massive diuresis, the urine flow rate increasing to up to 35% of GFR or 2.5 L/h! This causes a profound decrease in blood and extracellular fluid volume. The normal blood volume in an adult is approximately 5 L. Acute hypovolaemia can precipitate pre-renal renal failure, especially in elderly or debilitated patients. Those receiving other potentially nephrotoxic drugs, such as gentamicin, non-steroidal anti-inflammatory drugs or angiotensin-converting enzyme (ACE) inhibitors are especially at risk. Loop diuretics may also precipitate acute urinary retention in men with pre-existing prostate disease;
2 *hyperuricaemia* and *gout*;
3 *hypokalaemia* – inhibition of K^+ reabsorption in the loop of Henlé as well as increased delivery of Na^+ to the distal nephron (where it can be exchanged for K^+) results in increased urinary potassium loss, and some degree of hypokalaemia is common, although as with thiazide-induced hypokalaemia this is often clinically unimportant in the absence of additional risk factors for arrhythmia, such as digoxin treatment. Digoxin is now less commonly used in the treatment of heart failure than previously, whereas the early use of converting-enzyme inhibitors (which increase the plasma potassium concentration) is widely accepted, so the uncritical and excessive use of combination preparations (such as Frumil™ and Burinex-A™) is to be deplored;
4 *hypomagnesaemia* – magnesium clearance is increased and loop diuretics can cause hypomagnesaemia. Alcoholism and a diet low in magnesium are exacerbating factors. Magnesium and potassium metabolism are linked, and correction of potassium deficiency is impeded by coexisting magnesium deficiency. The most important clinical features of magnesium deficiency are increased cardiac excitability with ventricular arrhythmias and refractory atrial fibrillation. Digoxin toxicity is increased. Other symptoms are depression and muscle weakness;
5 *carbohydrate intolerance* may occur, but is less of a problem than with thiazide diuretics;
6 *ototoxicity* with hearing loss is associated with excessive peak plasma concentrations caused by too rapid intravenous injection. It may be related to inhibition of Na^+ K^+ $2Cl^-$ cotransport, which is involved in the formation of endolymph and is usually reversible. However, this is probably not the full story, since irreversible hearing loss has been caused by **ethacrynic acid** (another loop diuretic, now seldom used). Loop diuretics potentiate the ototoxic effects of aminoglycoside antibiotics;
7 *metabolic alkalosis* – the increased water and chloride excretion caused by loop diuretics results in contraction alkalosis, i.e. the extracellular fluid volume contracts with an increase in plasma bicarbonate concentration. This is seldom of clinical importance, although it can be a problem in patients with heart failure caused by chronic lung disease (cor pulmonale) in whom plasma bicarbonate levels are high in compensation for respiratory acidosis;
8 idiosyncratic *blood dyscrasias* occur rarely.

DRUG INTERACTIONS

Loop diuretics increase the nephrotoxicity of cephaloridine. More recently introduced cephalosporins are less nephrotoxic than cephaloridine, and less likely to interact in this way with loop diuretics. Renal prostaglandins, including PGE_2 and PGI_2, are natriuretic, and non-steroidal anti-inflammatory drugs such as indomethacin inhibit prostaglandin biosynthesis and oppose the diuretic effect of loop diuretics, as well as inhibiting their secretion into the tubule by competition for the transport mechanism. As with the thiazides, lithium reabsorption is reduced by loop diuretics, and the dose of lithium carbonate often needs to be reduced.

POTASSIUM-SPARING DIURETICS

Natriuresis caused by diuretics is usually accompanied by increased excretion of potassium, as described above. However, some diuretics inhibit distal Na^+/K^+ exchange, thereby causing potassium retention at the same time as mild natriuresis. These are not potent diuretics, but have been aggressively marketed in combination with thiazide or loop diuretics which have long outlived their patent lives when prescribed as single agents. The commercial implications of this have been substantial, but the clinical benefits are less certain. That is not to say that these drugs lack a valuable niche in therapeutics when used appropriately. They fall into two categories:

1 competitive antagonists of aldosterone (of which only one, spironolactone, is widely used;
2 Na^+/K^+ exchange antagonists that do not compete with aldosterone, of which there are two, namely amiloride and triamterene.

Spironolactone

Aldosterone promotes sodium retention and potassium loss by increasing the amount of sodium exchanged for potassium in the distal tubule. Spironolactone is structurally related to aldosterone and competes with it at receptors in the distal tubule. It increases sodium and water excretion and conserves potassium in patients with elevated circulating aldosterone concentrations. Hyperaldosteronism plays a key part in Conn's syndrome (primary hyperaldosteronism) and in ascites and fluid overload caused by cirrhosis (secondary hyperaldosteronism). The use of spironolactone has been limited to these situations, because it is poorly tolerated. It causes gynaecomastia and breast tenderness in men and menstrual irregularity in women, probably because it is structurally related to oestrogens. It causes tumours in rodents. However, it has recently been shown to improve longevity in patients with heart failure, and its use, for this indication, is likely to increase dramatically.

Amiloride

Amiloride is a non-competitive antagonist of aldosterone in the distal nephron. Its effect on sodium transport at this site is responsible for its therapeutic action, although at higher concentrations than are encountered therapeutically it also has other actions on sodium transport, including inhibition of Na^+/H^+ and Na^+/Ca^{2+} exchange. It is most commonly used in combination with frusemide (co-amilofruse), in which setting it should be restricted to patients with heart failure who develop clinically significant hypokalaemia when treated with a loop diuretic as sole agent, or with a thiazide (co-amilozide) for hypertension. Such combinations often cause hyponatraemia. Only 20% of the drug is absorbed after oral administration. It is not given intravenously because it can cause severe hypotension when administered by this route, possibly via histamine liberation. It is not metabolized, and is excreted unchanged by the kidneys. The plasma $t_{\frac{1}{2}}$ is 6 h, but its action following a 10–20 mg dose lasts for approximately 24 h.

ADVERSE EFFECTS AND DRUG INTERACTIONS

The main adverse effect is potassium retention leading to hyperkalaemia. Plasma potassium and creatinine levels should be monitored carefully, as the indications for which diuretics are used (including heart failure and hypertension) are important causes of progressive renal impairment, especially in the elderly, and life-threatening hyperkalaemia can occur in patients who are treated with potassium-sparing drugs in whom renal impairment supervenes. Diabetics are especially prone to hyperkalaemia because of hyporeninaemic hypoaldosteronism. Patients who are taking potassium supplements or ACE inhibitors (which increase plasma potassium levels by inhibiting angiotensin II-stimulated aldosterone secretion) or NSAIDs (which block PGI_2-induced renin release) are especially at risk.

Triamterene

This is a substituted pteridine with only weak natriuretic properties, the maximum fractional excretion of sodium that it causes being less than 2% of the filtered load. It inhibits Na^+/K^+ exchange in the distal tubule, but not by aldosterone antagonism. It can be used (like amiloride) in conjunction with thiazides or loop diuretics to potentiate their diuretic effect and prevent hypokalaemia. In combination with a thiazide (co-triamterzide) it was used in elderly patients in the European Working Party on Hypertension in the Elderly study, which demonstrated a beneficial effect of treatment in reducing the occurrence of myocardial infarction. Absorption after oral administration is rapid (the drug is not used parenterally). It is rapidly metabolized, 90% circulating as metabolites, and both the drug and its metabolites appear in the urine and bile. The plasma $t_{\frac{1}{2}}$ is 1.5–2 h. Diuresis starts within 2 h of administration and is complete within 8–10 h. Considerations with regard to adverse effects are similar to those for amiloride.

Carbonic anhydrase inhibitors

USE AND MECHANISM OF ACTION

The main carbonic anhydrase inhibitor is **acetazolamide**, a sulphonamide which is a non-competitive enzyme inhibitor. **Dorzolamide** is a topical carbonic anhydrase inhibitor for use in glaucoma (see Chapter 51). Carbonic anhydrase plays an important part in bicarbonate reabsorption from the proximal tubule. Consequently, acetazolamide inhibits reabsorption of sodium bicarbonate, resulting in an alkaline diuresis with loss of sodium and bicarbonate in the urine. Urinary alkalinization with acetazolamide has been used in the treatment of children with cysteine stones due to cysteinuria as cysteine is more soluble at alkaline than at acid pH. In the past it was suggested that urinary alkalinization with acetazolamide could also be used to increase salicylate elimination in cases of aspirin overdose. However, although salicylate elimination is indeed increased in an alkaline urine (see Chapter 53), the effects of acetazolamide on acid–base status (see below) are such as to increase salicylate toxicity by favouring its entry across the blood–brain barrier. Bicarbonate administration and not acetazolamide is therefore recommended for treating appropriately selected cases of salicylate overdose.

As a consequence of increased urinary elimination of bicarbonate during acetazolamide treatment, the plasma bicarbonate concentration falls without accumulation of any unmeasured anions, giving a normal anion gap metabolic acidosis, as in renal tubular acidosis. The reduction in plasma bicarbonate leads to a reduced filtered load of this ion, so less bicarbonate is available for reabsorption from proximal tubular fluid. The diuretic effect of acetazolamide is therefore self-limiting. Its metabolic effect is exploited in the *prevention of mountain sickness*, since it permits rapid acclimatization to altitude (which entails renal compensation for respiratory alkalosis caused by hyperventilation) by facilitating bicarbonate excretion.

More importantly than its diuretic effect, acetazolamide inhibits carbonic anhydrase in the eye and thereby decreases the rate of secretion of the aqueous humour in the anterior chamber and lowers intra-ocular pressure. *Treatment of glaucoma* is currently the major use of acetazolamide. In acute closed-angle, glaucoma 250 mg is given intravenously, followed by 250 mg four times daily. In open-angle glaucoma, 125 mg is given three times daily. In the lower-dose range acetazolamide can be given for long periods, and fortunately the change in acid–base status does not interfere with its action on aqueous humour formation.

Carbonic anhydrase is also present in the brain, and acetazolamide has *anticonvulsant* properties. Its use as an anticonvulsant is limited to a few specific situations (e.g. infantile spasms). Carbonic anhydrase in the choroid plexus participates in the formation of cerebrospinal fluid, and acetazolamide is sometimes used in the management of *benign intracranial hypertension*.

PHARMACOKINETICS

Acetazolamide is well absorbed from the intestine. It is renally excreted and has a plasma $t_{\frac{1}{2}}$ of about 3 h. However, its effect on the kidney lasts for about 6 h, and sustained-release tablets allow twice daily dosing.

ADVERSE EFFECTS

Adverse effects are common with large doses of acetazolamide, and relate both to its metabolic effects and to its sulphonamide structure. Large doses cause paraesthesiae, fatigue and dyspepsia. Prolonged use predisposes to renal stone formation due to reduced urinary citrate (citrate increases the solubility of calcium in the urine). As with other sulphonamides, hypersensitivity reactions and blood dyscrasias occur.

Osmotic diuretics

USE AND MECHANISM OF ACTION

Osmotic diuretics undergo glomerular filtration but are poorly reabsorbed from the renal tubular fluid. Their main diuretic action is exerted on the proximal tubule. This section of the tubule is freely permeable to water, and under normal circumstances sodium is actively reabsorbed accompanied by an isosmotic quantity of water. The presence of a substantial quantity of a poorly absorbable solute opposes this, because as water is reabsorbed the concentration and hence the osmotic activity of the solute increases. Osmotic diuretics (e.g. mannitol) also interfere with the establishment of the medullary osmotic gradient which is necessary for the formation of a concentrated urine. Mannitol is poorly absorbed from the intestine and is given intravenously as a 10% or 20% solution (25–50 g dose). It is not metabolized, but is filtered by the renal glomeruli and is not reabsorbed from the tubules.

Unlike other diuretics, osmotic diuretics increase the plasma volume (by increasing the entry of water to the circulation as a result of increasing intravascular osmolarity), so they are unsuitable for the treatment of most causes of oedema, especially cardiac failure. It is possible that, if used early in the course of incipient acute renal failure, osmotic diuretics may stave off the occurrence of acute tubular necrosis by increasing tubular fluid flow and reducing the accretion of material that would otherwise plug the tubules. Indeed, it has been suggested that the rarity of acute tubular necrosis in diabetic ketoacidosis is a consequence of the osmotic diuresis caused by heavy glycosuria. If mannitol is used in patients with incipient acute renal failure, intensive monitoring is needed to avoid precipitating pulmonary oedema secondary to the osmotic load if renal function in fact deteriorates. Low-dose dopamine (see Chapter 30) causes diuresis by selectively dilating renal vasculature, and is commonly used in this situation. Osmotic diuretics are mainly used for reasons unconnected with their ability to cause diuresis. Because they do not enter cells or some anatomical areas, such as the eye and brain, they cause water to leave cells down the osmotic gradient. This 'dehydrating' action is used in two circumstances:

1 *reduction of intra-ocular pressure* pre-operatively in closed-angle glaucoma – urea, 1.5 g/kg intra-

Key points

Salt overload and diuretics

- Several diseases are associated with excess salt and water, including:
  heart failure;
  renal failure;
  nephrotic syndrome;
  cirrhosis.
- Treatment involves restriction of dietary salt, and administration of diuretics to increase salt excretion.
- The main classes of diuretics are:
  thiazides (e.g. bendrofluazide);
  loop diuretics (e.g. frusemide);
  K^+-sparing diuretics (e.g. spironolactone, amiloride).
- In addition to treating salt/water overload, diuretics are also used in:
  systemic hypertension;
  glaucoma (carbonic anhydrase inhibitors);
  acute reduction of intracranial or intra-ocular pressure (osmotic diuretics);
  hypercalcaemia (frusemide);
  nephrogenic diabetes insipidus (thiazides).

Key points

Diuretics

Diuretics are classed by their site of action.

- Thiazides (e.g. bendrofluazide) inhibit Na^+/Cl^- reabsorption in the early distal convoluted tubule; they produce a modest diuresis and are used in particular in hypertension.
- Loop diuretics (e.g. frusemide) inhibit $Na^+/K^+/2Cl^-$ cotransport in the thick ascending limb of Henlé's loop. They cause a large effect and are used especially in heart failure and oedematous states.
- Potassium-sparing diuretics inhibit Na^+/K^+ exchange in the collecting duct either by competing with aldosterone (spironolactone), or non-competitively (e.g. amiloride, triamterene). They cause little diuresis, but are sometimes combined with thiazide or loop diuretics to prevent hypokalaemia.
- Carbonic anhydrase inhibitors (e.g. acetazolamide) inhibit HCO_3^- reabsorption in the proximal tubule. They are weak diuretics, cause metabolic acidosis, and are used to treat glaucoma rather than for their action on the kidney.
- Osmotic diuretics (e.g. mannitol) are used in patients with incipient acute renal failure, and acutely to lower intra-ocular or intracranial pressure.

venously, or glycerol, 1.5 g/kg orally, are used for this purpose as alternatives to mannitol;

2 *emergency reduction of intracranial pressure* in conditions such as brain tumour.

OVERHYDRATION

Overhydration without excess salt is much less common than salt and water overload, but occurs when antidiuretic hormone (ADH) is secreted inappropriately (e.g. by a neoplasm or following head injury or neurosurgery), giving rise to the syndrome of inappropriate secretion of ADH (SIADH). This is sometimes caused by drugs, notably the anticonvulsant carbamazepine, which stimulates ADH release from the posterior pituitary, and sulphonylureas, which potentiate its action on the renal collecting ducts. Antidiuretic hormone secretion results in a concentrated urine, while continued drinking (as a result of dietary habit) leads to progressive dilution of the plasma, which becomes hypo-osmolar and hyponatraemic. The plasma volume is slightly increased and urinary sodium loss continues. Some causes of SIADH resolve spontaneously (e.g. some cases of head injury), whereas others may improve after specific treatment of the underlying cause (e.g. following chemotherapy for small-cell carcinoma of the bronchus). Hyponatraemia that has arisen gradually can be corrected gradually by *restricting fluid intake*. This does not cause thirst (because the plasma is hypo-osmolar), but may not be well tolerated because of habit. Rapid correction of hyponatraemia to levels greater than 125 mmol/L is potentially harmful and is associated with severe central nervous system damage, including central pontine myelinolysis, with resultant devastating loss of brainstem function, sometimes with cortical function preserved (so-called 'locked-in syndrome').

Demeclocycline inhibits adenylyl cyclase and renders the collecting ducts insensitive to ADH (thereby producing a form of nephrogenic diabetes insipidus). It has been used to treat SIADH. In common with other tetracyclines, it increases plasma urea levels and can produce deterioration of renal function and increased loss of sodium in the urine. Electrolytes and renal function should therefore be monitored during treatment.

VOLUME DEPLETION

PRINCIPLES OF FLUID REPLACEMENT

Volume depletion is seldom treated with drugs. Even in situations such as Addisonian crisis, where ultimately the definitive treatment is replacement with glucocorticoid and mineralocorticoid hormones, emergency treatment pivots on replacement of what is depleted, i.e. salt and water in the form of adequate volumes of isotonic (physiologically 'normal', i.e. 140 mM) sodium chloride solution (see Chapter 39). The same is true when treating diabetic ketoacidosis, where the critical life-saving intervention is the rapid infusion of large volumes of isotonic saline at the same time as giving low doses of insulin by intravenous infusion (see p. 421–2). In patients with hypovolaemia due to acute and rapid blood loss, the appropriate fluid with which to replace is blood. Whole blood is now not always available because blood transfusion centres frequently separate plasma as a source of clotting factors. Consequently, a combination of 'packed' red cells with isotonic saline may be appropriate. In some situations, particularly when hypoalbuminaemia and oedema coexist with acute blood volume depletion, infusion of solutions of high-molecular-weight colloid (e.g. dextran or gelatin) may be preferable to low-molecular-weight readily diffusible crystalloid (e.g. isotonic saline). Anaphylactoid reactions are an unusual but severe adverse effect of such treatment. As mentioned above, *human serum albumin* is a seemingly logical but expensive alternative to artificial colloid solutions when there is hypoalbuminaemia. Its beneficial effect is short-lived.

DIABETES INSIPIDUS AND VASOPRESSIN

'Pure' water deprivation (i.e. true dehydration) is much less common than loss of salt and water (i.e. desalination). Plasma osmolality rapidly increases if fluid intake is inadequate, to make up insensible losses. This causes thirst, which leads to drinking and restoration of plasma osmolality, and to secretion of antidiuretic hormone (ADH, arginine vasopressin) by the posterior pituitary, which results in the formation of a small volume of concentrated urine. Vasopressin acts at the cellular level by combining with specific receptors coupled to G-proteins. The most physiologically important actions of vasopressin, including its antidiuretic and vasodilator effects and its ability to release factor VIII and von Willebrand factor, are mediated by V_2-receptors which are coupled to adenylyl cyclase. V_1-receptors activate the phosphatidyl inositol signalling system in vascular smooth muscle, mobilizing cytoplasmic calcium and causing intense vasoconstriction. V_{1a} receptors are also present in the liver, kidney and brain causing glycogenolysis, stimulating prostaglandin synthesis and inhibiting renin release, and influencing central functions such as memory, cerebrospinal fluid formation and the central control of blood pressure. V_{1b}-receptors in the anterior pituitary stimulate the release of corticotropin.

Vasopressin renders the collecting ducts permeable to water. Consequently, water leaves the collecting ducts passively down its osmotic gradient from tubular fluid (which is hypotonic at the beginning of the distal tubule) into the highly concentrated papillary interstitium. This process results in the formation of a small volume of highly concentrated urine under the influence of vasopressin. These homeostatic mechanisms fail when a patient is denied oral fluid, usually because of surgery ('nil by mouth'). Fluid must then be administered parenterally if dehydration with increased plasma sodium ion concentration is to be prevented. Pure water must not be given intravenously because this would cause haemolysis. Instead, an isotonic (5%) solution of glucose is used in these circumstances, as the glucose is rapidly metabolized to carbon dioxide, leaving water unaccompanied by solute. Surgical patients also lose salt, but unless they have been vomiting or losing electrolyte-rich fluid from the gastrointestinal tract via a drain or fistula, salt is lost at a lower rate than the loss of water. Consequently, post-operative patients are often given two or three volumes of 5% glucose for every volume of isotonic saline, modified if necessary depending on the results of serial serum electrolyte determinations.

Diabetes insipidus is an uncommon disorder in which either the secretion of ADH is deficient ('central' diabetes insipidus which can follow neurosurgery or head injury or complicate diseases such as sarcoid that can infiltrate the posterior pituitary), or in which the sensitivity of the collecting ducts to ADH is deficient ('nephrogenic' diabetes insipidus). Nephrogenic diabetes insipidus is sometimes drug induced, lithium being a common cause. If so, use of an alternative treatment may be possible. Severe nephrogenic diabetes insipidus is a rare X-linked disease caused by a mutation in the V_2-receptor gene. In such cases exogenous vasopressin or DDAVP is ineffective. Paradoxically, *thiazide diuretics* can reduce polyuria in nephrogenic diabetes insipidus, and are combined with mild salt restriction.

Dehydration is not invariably a problem in diabetes insipidus, because increasing plasma osmolality stimulates thirst. The consequent polydipsia prevents dehydration and hypernatraemia. However, patients with diabetes insipidus are at greatly increased risk of dehydration if they become unconscious for any reason (e.g. anaesthesia for an intercurrent surgical problem).

Polydipsia and polyuria in central diabetes insipidus can be prevented by vasopressin. However, ADH is not well absorbed across mucous membranes, so treatment necessitates the inconvenience of repeated injections. Currently, the usual treatment is therefore with a stable analogue, namely desamino-D-arginine vasopressin (DDAVP, desmopressin). This is sufficiently well absorbed through the nasal mucosa for it to be administered intranasally (adult dose 10–40 μg daily, given as one or two doses). Furthermore, it is selective for V_2-receptors, which are responsible for the effects of vasopressin on collecting ducts, and it lacks the pressor effect of arginine vasopressin which is mediated by V_1-receptors on vascular smooth muscle cells in resistance arterioles.

Desmopressin is also used for *nocturnal enuresis* (20–40 μg intranasally at bedtime in children over the age of 7 years). Caution is needed when it is used for this indication in adults who may have coexisting cardiovascular disease. (Children over 5 years old with regular enuresis may be helped by training using an enuresis alarm.) Desmopressin is used intravenously in patients with *von Willebrand's disease* before undergoing elective surgery, because it increases circulating von Willebrand factor and also increases factor VIII in patients with *mild/moderate haemophilia*.

Key points

Volume depletion

- Volume depletion can be caused by loss of blood or other body fluids (e.g. vomiting, diarrhoea, surgical fistulas).
- Replacement should be with appropriate volumes of blood or crystalloid.
- Excessive renal loss of salt (e.g. Addison's disease) or water (e.g. diabetes insipidus) can be due to renal or endocrine disorders and requires appropriate treatment (e.g. fludrocortisone in Addison's disease, desmopressin in central diabetes insipidus).

Disordered potassium ion balance

Hypokalaemia

Hypokalaemia commonly accompanies loss of fluid from the gastrointestinal tract (e.g. vomiting or diarrhoea), or loss of potassium ions into the urine due to diuretic therapy. Hypokalaemia in untreated patients with hypertension is suggestive of mineralocorticoid excess (e.g. Conn's syndrome, liquorice abuse). Barter's syndrome is a rare cause of severe hypokalaemia that should be considered in normotensive children who are not vomiting. Severe hypokalaemia causes symptoms of fatigue and nocturia (because of loss of renal concentrating ability), and can cause arrhythmias. Mild degrees of hypokalaemia (often associated with diuretic use) are generally well tolerated and of little clinical importance. Patients at risk of developing more serious hypokalaemia include the following:

1 those receiving large doses of diuretics, especially combinations of loop diuretics and thiazides;
2 patients receiving other drugs that cause increased potassium loss (e.g. systemic steroids or chronic laxative treatment);
3 those with a low potassium intake, notably poor and/or elderly people;
4 patients with diseases associated with high circulating aldosterone concentrations, particularly those with cirrhosis (in whom hypokalaemia may precipitate hepatic encephalopathy), as well as those with nephrotic syndrome and severe cardiac failure. Relatively mild potassium depletion exacerbates the toxicity of digoxin, incurring the risk of serious arrhythmias.

Against this background a practical approach is as follows.

1 Potassium replacement is not usually required in hypertensive patients on small doses of diuretics and taking a full mixed diet. Marked hypokalaemia (< 3.0 mmol/L) raises the possibility of Conn's syndrome, and needs attention. If this has been excluded, and replacement with food with a high potassium content (fruit and vegetables) is ineffective, use of a *combined thiazide/K^+-retaining diuretic* (e.g. triamterzide, coamilozide) should be considered. These drugs should be avoided if possible in situations where an angiotensin-converting enzyme inhibitor is likely to be needed because of the risk of hyperkalaemia. *Effervescent potassium supplements* are unpalatable, but contain larger amounts of potassium (e.g. 14 mmol per tablet) than conventional slow-release potassium preparations (approximately 7 mmol per tablet, formulated in a wax matrix). Slow-release preparations are usually inadequate (see below) unless impractically large numbers of tablets are prescribed, and carry the risk of causing gastrointestinal injury if held up within the gastrointestinal tract (e.g. in the oesophagus from an enlarged left atrium pressing backwards on the oesophagus in patients with mitral stenosis). Effervescent potassium tastes less unpleasant if it is dissolved in fruit juice. Intravenous replacement with KCl is dangerous, but is important (with appropriate monitoring) in emergency situations such as diabetic ketoacidosis.
2 The plasma potassium ion concentration should be monitored in patients with *congestive cardiac failure, cirrhosis* or *nephrotic syndrome*.
3 Patients treated with digoxin should receive a K^+-retaining diuretic or K^+ supplements if there is clinically significant hypokalaemia.
4 Patients who require diuretics and who develop cardiac arrhythmias and/or have recently had a myocardial infarct should have

relatively aggressive potassium replacement, together with consideration of magnesium supplementation.

5 Patients with other risk factors should be monitored and given replacements as required.

POTASSIUM REPLACEMENT

There are two ways to increase plasma potassium levels, namely by potassium supplements or by use of potassium-sparing diuretics.

Potassium supplements

To be effective, 30–50 mmol potassium daily is required. Combined diuretic and potassium tablets are inadequate, as they contain only 7–8 mmol. Potassium salts may be given orally as either an effervescent or slow-release preparation. Diet can be supplemented by foods with a high potassium content, such as fruit and vegetables. Intravenous potassium is usually given in the form of potassium chloride, and is used either to maintain body potassium levels in patients receiving intravenous feeding, or to restore potassium levels in severely depleted patients (e.g. those with diabetic ketoacidosis). The main danger associated with intravenous potassium is hyperkalaemia, which can cause any type of arrhythmia, including cardiac arrest. Potassium chloride caused 12 adverse effects per 100 exposures in the Boston Collaborative Drug Surveillance Program, and had the dubious distinction of the highest frequency of fatal adverse reactions of any drug. Potassium chloride solution is infused at a maximum rate of 10 mmol/h unless there is severe depletion, when 20 mmol/h can be given with electrocardiographic monitoring. The dose should not usually exceed 120 mmol/24 h unless there is severe depletion. Particular care is needed if there is impaired renal function. Potassium chloride for intravenous replacement should be diluted with saline or glucose in the bag before infusion. Potassium chloride should not be combined with blood, mannitol, amino acids or lipids.

Potassium-sparing diuretics

An alternative to potassium supplementation is to combine a thiazide or loop diuretic with a potassium-retaining diuretic (see p. 403–4). Potassium-retaining diuretics are better tolerated than potassium supplements, but are not without risk (especially of hyperkalaemia if renal impairment supervenes and/or other potassium-retaining drugs such as ACE inhibitors are prescribed).

HYPERKALAEMIA

Hyperkalaemia in untreated patients suggests the possibility of renal failure or of mineralocorticoid deficiency (e.g. Addison's disease, hyporeninaemic hypoaldosteronism). Most commonly, however, it is caused by drugs. Hyperkalaemia can develop either with potassium supplements or with potassium-sparing diuretics (still more so in patients treated with both!). Hyperkalaemia is particularly likely to occur in patients with impaired renal function, in the elderly (in whom renal impairment may be unrecognized because the plasma creatinine concentration is normal) and in patients receiving ACE inhibitors, K^+ supplements or non-steroidal anti-inflammatory drugs.

Key points

Disordered K^+ metabolism

- Hypokalaemia is caused by urinary or gastrointestinal K^+ loss in excess of dietary intake, or alternatively by a shift of K^+ into cells without a reduction of total body K^+. Diuretic (loop or thiazide) use is a common cause. Endocrine causes include Conn's and Barter's syndromes. β_2-agonists shift K^+ into cells.
- Mild hypokalaemia is often unimportant, but severe hypokalaemia can cause dysrhythmias. Hypokalaemia increases digoxin toxicity.
- Emergency treatment (e.g. in diabetic ketoacidosis) involves intravenous replacement, which requires close monitoring (including ECG).
- Foods rich in K^+ include fruit and vegetables. Oral K^+ preparations are unpalatable and not very effective.
- K^+-retaining diuretics (e.g. amiloride) are used to prevent hypokalaemia. They predispose to hyperkalaemia, especially in patients with impaired renal function or with concomitant use of K^+ supplements, ACE inhibitors or NSAIDs.

TREATMENT

The effects of an abnormal intracellular/extracellular K^+ ratio may be counteracted by the following measures.

1 *Calcium gluconate* is potentially life-saving in patients with arrhythmias caused by hyperkalaemia (see p. 322). A total of 10–30 mL of a 10% solution is given intravenously over 5 min with ECG monitoring. Calcium ions decrease membrane excitability. Emergency measures to reduce hyperkalaemia must be instituted without delay.
2 *Glucose and insulin* shift extracellular potassium into cells. A total of 200–500 mL of 10% glucose is given intravenously over 30 min accompanied by 10 units of soluble insulin.
3 *Sodium bicarbonate*, 100–150 mmol, given intravenously also shifts K^+ into cells.
4 The above measures may buy a brief period of time that can be used to *mobilize emergency dialysis*.
5 *Ion-exchange resin* made of sodium polystyrene sulphonate exchanges sodium for potassium ions in the gut lumen. It is given as a retention enema (30 g) or by mouth (15 g three or four times daily). It removes potassium from the body rather than altering its distribution. This effect usually begins about 1 h after administration. The sodium ions exchanged for potassium may lead to sodium overload. A calcium resin is available to avoid this problem. Ion-exchange resins are useful for preventing hyperkalaemia in patients with chronic renal failure. The main adverse effect when resins are given chronically in this way is constipation, which can be avoided if the resins are suspended in a solution of sorbitol.

> **Key points**
>
> Drugs and plasma potassium
>
> - *Hypokalaemia* predisposes to digoxin toxicity and to *torsardes de pointes* caused by drugs that prolong the QT interval (e.g. amiodarone). Mild degrees of hypokalaemia associated with thiazide or loop diuretics are common, and are seldom harmful *per se*.
> - Where hypokalaemia is clinically important it can be corrected and/or prevented with K^+ supplements or more conveniently with K^+-retaining diuretics. However, these predispose to hyperkalaemia.
> - *Hyperkalaemia* can cause arrhythmias that are often fatal. Converting-enzyme inhibitors predispose to hyperkalaemia, especially when there is renal impairment.
> - Emergency treatment of broad complex tachycardia caused by hyperkalaemia includes IV calcium gluconate.
> - Glucose and insulin IV cause redistribution of potassium into cells.
> - Sodium bicarbonate IV can cause redistribution of potassium into cells in exchange for hydrogen ions.
> - Haemodialysis is frequently indicated.
> - Ion-exchange resins administered by mouth may be useful.

DRUGS THAT ALTER URINE pH

ACIDIFICATION

Ammonium chloride given orally results in urinary acidification. Ammonium ions are converted to urea in the liver, with the release of hydrogen ions. This produces a metabolic acidosis to which the kidney responds by excreting acidic urine. There is increased excretion of chloride ions, together with balancing cations and water, which results in a transient diuresis. Ascorbic acid (vitamin C) is excreted in the urine, which it acidifies if given in sufficiently large doses (> 2 g). It is safer than ammonium chloride.

USE

Ammonium chloride can be used diagnostically in the investigation of renal tubular acidosis, to determine the ability of the kidney to form acidic urine. It is a gastric irritant and is given (dose 8–12 g) as enteric-coated tablets. The elimination of some basic drugs (e.g. morphine and amphetamine) is enhanced by acidification of the urine.

ADVERSE EFFECTS

Ammonium chloride causes nausea, vomiting and abdominal pain. It should not be given in hepatic failure, as it can precipitate encephalopathy, and it exacerbates the acidosis of renal failure.

Alkalinization

Sodium bicarbonate causes urinary alkalinization, but if given by mouth it reacts with hydrochloric acid in the stomach to produce carbon dioxide, so it is poorly tolerated and not very effective. Instead, a citric acid/potassium citrate mixture can be used, as citrate is absorbed from the gut and metabolized via the tricarboxylic acid cycle with generation of bicarbonate. The usual dose is 3–6 g every 4–6 h until the urine pH is > 7. Potassium must be avoided in renal failure, as retention of potassium ions may cause hyperkalaemia.

Use

Alkalinization of the urine is used to give symptomatic relief for the dysuria of cystitis, and to prevent the formation of uric acid stones, especially in patients who are about to undergo cancer chemotherapy. The use of forced alkaline diuresis to increase urinary excretion of salicylate following overdose is discussed in Chapter 53.

Drugs that affect the bladder and genito-urinary system

Drugs for urological pain

The acute pain of ureteric colic may be relieved by morphine or pethidine. Diclofenac (a non-steroidal anti-inflammatory drug) compares favourably with the opiates in the treatment of ureteric colic if used parenterally. It is given intramuscularly in a dose of 75 mg, which is repeated after 30 min if necessary.

Drugs to increase bladder activity

Drugs that increase bladder activity are sometimes used to treat patients with chronic retention of urine. These should never be used in the presence of severe obstruction, and are never used to treat acute urinary retention, which is managed by catheterization. Muscarinic agonists (e.g. bethanechol, carbachol) stimulate the detrusor muscle and are occasionally used in patients with chronic retention due to peripheral neurological damage rather than to obstruction. Anticholinesterases (e.g. distigmine) are used similarly for their parasympathomimetic action.

Drugs to decrease bladder activity

Increased frequency of micturition is often a symptom of infection. When infection is absent, unstable detrusor contractions may be responsible, the consequences ranging in severity from trivial inconvenience to urge incontinence that severely impairs quality of life. Drug treatment is usually disappointing. Antimuscarinic drugs such as **oxybutinin** and **propantheline** are not very effective and have a high incidence of antimuscarinic side-effects (e.g. dry mouth, dry eyes, blurred vision, constipation, confusion). Tricyclic antidepressants (e.g. amitryptyline, imipramine) are sometimes useful, perhaps in part because of their antimuscarinic effects. They are also used in nocturnal enuresis, but are less effective than desmopressin (see p. 469).

Drugs for prostatic obstruction

Prostatic obstruction is usually managed surgically. Symptoms of benign prostatic hypertrophy may be improved by a 5α-reductase inhibitor (e.g. finasteride, p. 461) or by an α_1-adrenoceptor antagonist (e.g. doxazosin, p. 271). **Tamsolusin**, a recently licensed α_1-adrenoceptor antagonist said to be selective for the α_{1A}-adrenoceptor subtype that is present in prostatic smooth muscle, may produce less postural hypotension than other α_1-adrenoceptor antagonists. Hormonal manipulation with anti-androgens and analogues of luteinizing hormone-releasing hormone (LHRH) is valuable in patients with prostatic cancer (see Chapter 47).

Drugs for impotence

Erectile failure has numerous organic as well as psychological causes. Replacement therapy with **testosterone** given intramuscularly as an oily injection or, more recently, by skin patch, is effec-

Case history

A 35-year-old woman has proteinuria (3 g/24 h) and progressive renal impairment (current serum creatinine 220 (μmol/L) in the setting of insulin-dependent diabetes mellitus. In addition to insulin, she takes captopril regularly and buys ibuprofen over the counter to take as needed for migraine. She develops progressive oedema which does not respond to oral frusemide in increasing doses of up to 250 mg/day. Amiloride (10 mg daily) is added without benefit, and metolazone (5 mg daily) is started. She loses 3 kg over the next 3 days. One week later she is admitted to hospital having collapsed at home. She is conscious but severely ill. Her blood pressure is 90/60 mmHg, heart rate is 86 beats/min and regular, and she has residual peripheral oedema, but the jugular venous pressure is not raised. Serum urea is 55 mmol/L, creatinine is 350 μmol/L, K^+ is 6.8 mmol/L, glucose is 5.6 mmol/L and albumin is 3.0 g/dL. Urinalysis shows 4+ protein. An ECG shows tall peaked T-waves and broad QRS complexes.

Question

Decide whether each of the following statements is true or false.

(a) Insulin should be withheld until the patient's metabolic state has improved.
(b) Metolazone should be stopped.
(c) The frusemide dose should be increased in view of the persistent oedema.
(d) Ibuprofen could have contributed to the hyperkalaemia.
(e) Captopril should be withheld.

Answer

(a) False.
(b) True.
(c) False.
(d) True.
(e) True.

Comment

Although highly effective in causing diuresis in patients with resistant oedema, combination diuretic treatment with loop, K^+-sparing and thiazide diuretics can cause acute prerenal renal failure with a disproportionate increase in serum urea compared to creatinine. Resistance to frusemide may be related to the combination of reduced GFR plus albuminuria. The combination of an NSAID, captopril and amiloride is extremely dangerous, especially in diabetics, and will have contributed to the severe hyperkalaemia. The NSAID may also have led to reduced glomerular filtration. Glucose with insulin would be appropriate to lower the plasma K^+.

tive in cases associated with proven androgen deficiency. Drug treatment of other causes of impotence is generally disappointing, but several promising agents are currently being developed. Intracavernosal injection of vasodilators (initially under specialist medical supervision) can be effective. **Prostaglandin E_1** is licensed for this indication. Adverse effects are related to the route of administration (e.g. haematoma, fibrosis) as well as to local (e.g. persistent erection necessitating emergency aspiration of the corpora cavernosa) and systemic (e.g. hypotension, headache, flushing and syncope) drug actions. Nitric oxide is involved in erectile function both as a vascular endothelium-derived mediator and as a non-adrenergic non-cholinergic neurotransmitter. This has led to the development of Type V

Case history

A 73-year-old man has a long history of hypertension and of osteoarthritis. Three months ago he had a myocardial infarction, since when he has been progressively oedematous and dyspnoeic, initially only on exertion but more recently also on lying flat. He continues to take coamilozide for his hypertension and naproxone for his osteoarthritis. The blood pressure is 164/94 mmHg and there are signs of fluid overload with generalised oedema and markedly elevated jugular venous pressure. Serum creatinine is 138 μmol/L and K^+ is 5.0 mmol/L. Why would it be hazardous to commence frusemide in addition to his present treatment? What alternative strategy could be considered?

Comment

The patient may go into prerenal renal failure with the addition of the loop diuretic to the two more distal diuretics he is already taking in the coamilozide combination. The NSAID he is taking makes this more likely, and also makes it more probable that his serum potassium level (which is already high) will become dangerously elevated. It would be appropriate to consider hospital admission, stopping naproxen (perhaps substituting paracetamol for pain if necessary), stopping the coamilozide, and cautiously instituting a converting-enzyme inhibitor (which could improve his prognosis from his heart failure as described in Chapter 30) followed by introduction of frusemide with close monitoring of blood pressure, signs of fluid overload and serum creatinine and potassium levels over the next few days.

phosphodiesterase inhibitors as oral agents to meet erectile dysfunction. Sildenafil (Viagra™) is the first of these to be introduced (see page 461). It is taken by mouth approximately 30 min before sexual activity. Adverse effects include flushing and headache, and it must not be given with organic nitrates since it potentiates their action. It is more effective and better tolerated that intracavernosal injections. Despite the anxiety regarding its cost, it is actually less expensive (currently approximately £8/dose) than intracavernosal PGE_1.

FURTHER READING

Brater DC. 1998: Drug therapy: diuretics. *New England Journal of Medicine* **339**, 387–95.

Clark BA, Brown RS. 1995: Potassium homeostasis and hyperkalemic syndromes. *Endocrinology and Metabolism Clinics of North America* **24**, 573–91.

Cohn JN. 1996: The management of chronic heart failure. *New England Journal of Medicine* **335**, 490–8.

Epstein M. 1995: Renal sodium retention in liver disease. *Hospital Practice* **30**, 33–7 and 41–2.

Greger R, Heidland A. 1998: Action and clinical use of diuretics. In Davison AM, Cameron JS, Grünfeld J-P (eds), *Oxford textbook of clinical nephrology*, 2nd edn. Oxford: Oxford University Press, 2679–706.

Hoes AW, Grobbee DE, Peet TM, Lubsen J. 1994: Do non-potassium-sparing diuretics increase the risk of sudden cardiac death in hypertensive patients? Recent evidence. *Drugs* **47**, 711–33.

Kaplan NM. 1996: Diuretics: cornerstone of antihypertensive therapy. *American Journal of Cardiology* **77**, 3B–5B.

Saggar-Malik AK, Cappuccio FP. 1993: Potassium supplements and potassium-sparing diuretics. A review and guide to appropriate use. *Drugs* **46**, 986–1008.

PART VIII

THE ENDOCRINE SYSTEM

CHAPTER THIRTY-SIX

DIABETES MELLITUS

- Pathophysiology
- Principles of management
- Diet in diabetes mellitus
- Drugs used to treat diabetes mellitus

PATHOPHYSIOLOGY

Insulin is the most important hormone of the endocrine pancreas. It is secreted by the β-cells of the islets of Langerhans. It is an anabolic hormone and controls the metabolic disposition of all three major aliments (carbohydrate, fats and amino acids). Insulin is synthesized as a precursor (pro-insulin) which is shortened by proteolysis in the Golgi complex of β-cells to a double-chained molecule consisting of an α-chain connected to a β-chain (insulin). The inactive connecting C-peptide and insulin are co-secreted in equimolar proportions together with a small proportion ($<10\%$ in normal healthy subjects, higher in type 2, non-insulin-dependent diabetics) of pro-insulin. C-peptide is a useful index of endogenous insulin secretion, as its plasma concentration is low or absent in patients with true insulin-dependent diabetes. Conversely, its plasma concentration is very high in patients with functional insulinomas, but is not elevated in patients with hypoglycaemia as a result of surreptitious self-injection with insulin. Its measurement, together with insulin, can therefore be helpful diagnostically.

Diabetes mellitus (defined by a fasting blood glucose level of >7 mmol/L or, by some authorities, an abnormal glucose tolerance test) is caused by an absolute or relative lack of insulin. Insulin secretion is triggered by many stimuli, including carbohydrate (glucose) and some amino acids. Inhibitors of insulin secretion include insulin itself, somatostatin, adrenaline and other α-adrenergic agonists, β-adrenoceptor antagonists and diazoxide (a K^+-channel agonist used in the past to treat hypertensive emergencies). The control of insulin secretion is now well understood. The problem is the linkage between insulin secretion and variable metabolic demand. The membrane potential in pancreatic β-cells is controlled by adenosine triphosphate (ATP)-sensitive potassium channels. Following a meal, blood glucose levels increase, cytoplasmic ATP in β-cells increases, and this metabolic signal turns off the potassium channels, hence depolarizing these cells and activating voltage-sensitive calcium channels. The resulting influx of calcium ions causes secretion of the insulin-containing vesicles as well as increased synthesis of new hormone.

In type 1, insulin-dependent diabetes mellitus (IDDM, or 'juvenile-onset' diabetes) there is an absolute deficiency of insulin, and unless insulin treatment is given the patient will ultimately develop diabetic ketoacidosis. Such patients are usually (but not invariably) young and non-obese at presentation. There is an inherited predisposition to the disease, with a 10-fold increase in first-degree relatives of an index case, and a strong positive association with particular human leucocyte antigen (HLA) types and a negative ('protective') association with others. However, twin studies have shown that genetically predisposed individuals must also be exposed to an environmental factor in order to express this tendency (concordance in identical twins is somewhat less than 50%). Viruses (including Coxsackie and Echo viruses) are one such environmental factor, and may cause direct damage to islet cells which results in exposure of antigens and initiation of an autoallergic process that is then self-perpetuating and which, after a variable period, eventually results in destruction of the islets. More than 90% of the islets have to be destroyed before the individual becomes frankly diabetic.

By contrast, in type 2 diabetes mellitus, previously known as non-insulin-dependent diabetes (NIDDM) or 'maturity-onset' diabetes, there is a relative lack of insulin secretion coupled with marked resistance to its action. The circulating concentration of immunoreactive insulin measured by standard assays (which do not discriminate well between insulin and pro-insulin) may be normal or even increased, but more discriminating assays indicate that there is an increase in pro-insulin, and that the true insulin concentration is reduced. Such patients are usually (although not invariably) middle-aged or elderly at presentation, and are usually obese. Twin studies show that concordance of this form of diabetes in identical twins is nearly 100%. Type 2 diabetes is not associated with diabetic ketoacidosis, although it can be complicated by non-ketotic hyperosmolar coma or, rarely (in association with treatment with metformin), with lactic acidosis. In both types of diabetes mellitus the increased concentration of glucose in the circulating blood gives rise to osmotic effects:

1 diuresis (*polyuria*) with consequent volume reduction and thirst, leading to *polydipsia*;
2 altered refraction due to the altered refractive index of a sugary solution in the aqueous humour and lens leads to blurred vision (or occasionally and paradoxically to improved vision, in individuals in whom the change in refraction is fortuitously beneficial).

In addition, glycosuria predisposes to *Candida* infection, especially in women. The loss of calories in the urine is coupled with inability to store energy in glycogen or fat, or to lay down protein in muscle, and weight loss with loss of fat and muscle ('amyotrophy') is common in uncontrolled diabetics.

Both types of diabetes mellitus are complicated by both microvascular and macrovascular complications. Microvascular complications include *retinopathy*, which consists of background retinopathy (dot and blot haemorrhages and hard exudates which do not of themselves threaten vision), and proliferative retinopathy, in which new vessels form, probably because of growth factors secreted in ischaemic areas of the retina, and can bleed and cause blindness. Cataracts are also more common in diabetics, perhaps because of the accumulation of sorbitol in the lens. A similar explanation may be important in diabetic *neuropathy*, which typically causes a stocking distribution of loss of sensation (especially to vibration sense) with associated painful paraesthesiae. Microangiopathy of the vasa nervorum and glycosylation of membrane proteins are additional pathophysiological factors. The other form of microvascular complication of special importance is glomerulopathy. Only approximately one-third of diabetic patients ultimately develop diabetic nephropathy, which leads to renal failure, and it is not known what factors render certain individuals susceptible to this complication. Microalbuminuria is prognostically useful, as it is a forerunner of overt diabetic *nephropathy*. There is evidence that an inherited abnormality of red-blood-cell cation transport detected as an increased rate of Na^+/Li^+ ion countertransport predicts individuals who are predisposed to develop this complication, but this is a research rather than routine investigation.

Macrovascular disease is the result of *accelerated atheroma*, and results in an increased incidence of myocardial infarction, peripheral vascular disease (manifested as claudication and amputation) and stroke. The pathophysiological connection between diabetes mellitus and atheroma is not fully understood, but factors of probable relevance include a strong association (pointed out by Reaven) between diabetes and obesity, hypertension and hyperlipidaemia (especially hypertriglyceridaemia).

PRINCIPLES OF MANAGEMENT

It is important to define ambitious but realistic goals for each patient. In the case of young type 1 patients there is good evidence that improved diabetic control reduces the incidence of microvascular complications. It is well worth trying hard to minimize the metabolic derangement associated with diabetes mellitus in order to reduce the development of such complications. Education and support are essential to motivate the patient to learn how to adjust their insulin dose to optimize control. This can only be achieved by the patient performing blood glucose monitoring at home and learning to adjust their insulin dose accordingly. The treatment regimen must be individualized, and usually requires either twice daily or four times daily subcutaneous injections. Follow-up must include structured care with regular screening for evidence of microvascular disease. This is especially important in the case of proliferative retinopathy (and also of maculopathy), because prophylactic laser therapy in patients with early disease has been shown (in controlled trials in which therapy was only given to one eye) to reduce the incidence of blindness caused by proliferative retinopathy.

By contrast, striving for tight control of blood sugar in type 2 patients is only appropriate in selected cases. Evidence that tight control reduces macrovascular complications is less convincing than in type 1 patients, perhaps because metabolic abnormality may precede diagnosis by many years, and therefore much damage will already have been done before treatment is started. In older type 2 patients (aged > 65 years) treatment should aim to minimize symptoms of polyuria, polydipsia or recurrent candidal infection, and to avoid the patient slipping into non-ketotic hyperosmolar coma. Aggressive therapy of the elderly increases the risk of hypoglycaemia and has no proven clinical benefit. In contrast, aggressive treatment of *hypertension* in Type 2 diabetics is of substantial benefit.

Maintenance of glucose levels as close as possible to normal throughout the day without producing hypoglycaemia or severely restricting the patient's life is achieved by:

1 diet;
2 diet plus insulin;
3 diet plus oral hypoglycaemic drugs.

By maintaining blood glucose levels below 8 mmol/L and limiting glycosuria to less than 20 g daily, polyuria, polydipsia, dehydration and weight loss can usually be avoided. Glycosylated haemoglobin (HbA_{1c}) provides a convenient integrated measure of blood glucose over the life of the red cell (120 days) and should be < 7%. In older diabetics, even these modest goals may not be achieved without considerable sacrifice and difficulty for the patient, and it may be necessary to accept some glycosuria and moderate hyperglycaemia.

There are many possible reasons for failure to obtain good control, and the following possibilities should be considered:

1 failure to adhere to diet;
2 infection (e.g. urinary tract infection, tonsillitis, pneumonia);
3 chronic renal failure provoking hypoglycaemic reactions;
4 violent/erratic exercise;
5 insulin resistance;
6 pregnancy;
7 drugs (e.g. corticosteroids, thiazide diuretics);
8 coexisting endocrine disorders (e.g. thyrotoxicosis, Cushing's syndrome);
9 alcohol.

DIET IN DIABETES MELLITUS

The aim for patients with either type 1 or type 2 diabetes is to achieve and maintain ideal body weight. If the patient is obese, calorie intake should be restricted so that weight is gradually (at a rate of not more than 1 kg/week) lost. The emphasis is on providing a healthy diet identical to that recommended for other individuals to reduce the risk of developing atheromatous disease. This means a diet high in vegetable fibre (fruit and fresh vegetables) and low in saturated fat and refined sugar. A relative increase in polyunsaturated or monounsaturated fat is appropriate. Excessive protein intake is undesirable, especially in the setting of potentially progressive renal impairment. Tissue insensitivity to insulin in type 2 patients is associated with reduced numbers of insulin receptors on the surface of fat and muscle cells. Weight loss (by caloric restriction) and increased exercise result in an increase in the number of insulin receptors, and hence in greater insulin sensitivity and a fall in blood glucose levels.

The diet for patients with type 1 diabetes must match caloric intake with insulin injections. Healthy people show considerable latitude in the timing and caloric value of individual meals, but patients who rely on injected insulin must time their food intake accordingly. A common way to distribute daily calories is to give 2/7th at each of three meals and the remaining 1/7th at bedtime. This approach may need modification for individual patients. The carbohydrate content of a healthy diabetic diet approximates to that of normal individuals, i.e. 45–55% of total calories. Simple sugars should be restricted because they are rapidly absorbed, causing postprandial hyperglycaemia, and they should be replaced by polysaccharides (complex sugars) that are broken down to simple sugars by digestion and absorbed more slowly. A fibre-rich diet reduces peak plasma glucose levels after meals and reduces the dose of insulin required. Pulses such as beans and lentils flatten the glucose absorption curve. Protein calories should constitute around 20% of total intake. Protein sources containing little fat (e.g. low-fat milk, poultry, fish and vegetable proteins) should be recommended to reduce atheromatous disease. Saturated fat and cholesterol intake should be minimized. There is no place for commercially promoted 'special diabetic foods', which are expensive and also often high in fat and calories at the expense of complex carbohydrate.

DRUGS USED TO TREAT DIABETES MELLITUS

Insulin

USE

Insulin is indicated in all patients with type 1 diabetes mellitus (although it is not strictly necessary during the early 'honeymoon' period before islet cell destruction is complete) and in some patients with type 2 diabetes mellitus. Insulin is usually administered by subcutaneous injection. Many insulin preparations are available that differ in their pharmacokinetics of absorption and thus in their duration of action. Insulin can be extracted from either ox or pig pancreas, but such animal insulins have now been almost entirely replaced by recombinant human insulin. The main advantage of human insulin is that production by bacterial culture can be standardized. In addition, there are rather fewer allergic side-effects, although this advantage is modest. The effective dose of human insulin is usually rather less than that of animal insulins because of the lack of blocking antibodies. Consequently, some patients have become hypoglycaemic when switched from an animal insulin to the same number of units of human insulin. Awareness of hypoglycaemia and counter-regulatory hormone release tends to diminish as diabetic patients age, and initially there was concern that human insulin might differ qualitatively from animal insulins in causing less awareness of hypoglycaemia. Double-blind crossover comparisons of human and animal insulins in which hypoglycaemia was deliberately induced under controlled conditions have not borne out these fears, and there is no difference between the symptoms of hypoglycaemia caused by human and animal insulins.

Soluble insulin is the only preparation suitable for intravenous use. It is administered intravenously in diabetic emergencies, and is also given subcutaneously before meals in chronic management. If the effect wanes before the next dose is due, a longer-acting insulin with a later onset, such as isophane insulin, can be added. Formulations of human insulins are available in various ratios of short-acting and longer-lasting forms (e.g. 30:70, commonly used twice daily). Some of these are marketed in prefilled injection devices ('pens') which are extremely convenient for patients. Injections are often given twice daily so that insulin reaches its peak activity at 3–4 p.m. and 3–4 a.m. The small dose of soluble insulin controls hyperglycaemia just after the injection. The main danger is of a hypoglycaemic reaction in the early hours of the morning. When starting a diabetic on a two-dose regime it is therefore helpful to divide the daily dose into two-thirds to be given before breakfast and one-third to be given before the evening meal. If the patient is engaged in strenuous physical work, the morning dose of insulin is reduced somewhat to prevent exercise-induced hypoglycaemia. The dose is determined by monitoring the blood sugar level when insulin is expected to be maximally active. If this is done, it is usually possible to increase the dose to improve hyperglycaemia without causing hypoglycaemia at other times.

Diabetics with absolute insulin deficiency must be treated with exogenous insulin. Insulin is also required for symptomatic maturity-onset diabetics in whom diet and/or oral hypoglycaemic drugs fail. Approximately one-third of type 2 patients require insulin treatment within 15 years of diagnosis. Unfortunately, insulin makes weight loss considerably more difficult because of the appetite-stimulating effect of lowering blood sugar, but the anabolic effects of insulin are valuable in some wasted patients, especially those with diabetic amyotrophy. Insulin is needed in acute diabetic emergencies such as ketoacidosis, during pregnancy, peri-operatively and in severe intercurrent disease (infections, myocardial infarction, burns, etc.).

Insulin requirements are increased by up to one-third by intercurrent viral infection, and patients must be instructed to intensify home blood sugar monitoring when they have a cold or other infection (even if they are eating less than usual) and increase the insulin dose if necessary. The dose will subsequently need to be reduced when the infection has cleared. Vomiting often causes patients incorrectly to stop injecting insulin (for fear of hypoglycaemia), and this may result in ketoacidosis.

Patients who are having elective surgery should be admitted to hospital 48 h before operation and, if they are on long-acting insulins, should be changed to a regime of three times daily soluble insulin. Patients who are receiving oral hypoglycaemic agents should be switched to insulin if they have proved difficult to control with oral agents. During surgery it is easiest to infuse 1–3 units of soluble insulin hourly together with a glucose infusion. The infusion rates are adjusted to produce a blood glucose concentration of 6–8 mmol/L. This is continued until oral feeding and intermittent subcutaneous injections of soluble insulin can be resumed. A similar regime is suitable for emergency operations, but more frequent measurements of blood glucose are required. Patients with very mild diabetes can be managed without insulin, but the blood glucose must be regularly checked during the post-operative period.

KETOACIDOSIS

The metabolic changes in ketoacidosis resemble those of starvation since, despite the increased concentrations of glucose and ketones in the plasma, these substrates are not available to the metabolizing enzymes within cells ('starving amidst plenty'). Increased glycogenolysis and gluconeogenesis in the liver result in hyperglycaemia, which in turn leads to osmotic diuresis, electrolyte depletion and desalination. A total body deficit of potassium ions is inevitable since, in the face of acidosis and an osmotic diuresis, conservation of potassium is even less efficient than that of sodium. However, the plasma potassium concentration can be increased due to a shift from the intracellular to the extracellular compartment, so large amounts of potassium chloride should not be administered empirically until blood results are available and the urine output is established. Increased breakdown of muscle releases glucogenic amino acids that are taken up by the liver and converted to glucose. Fat is mobilized from adipose tissue, releasing glycerol (which is converted to glucose by the liver) and free fatty acids that are metabolized by β-oxidation to acetyl coenzyme A (CoA). In the absence of glucose breakdown, acetyl CoA is converted to acetoacetate with a consequent excessive production of ketone bodies (acetone, acetoacetate and β-hydroxybutyrate). Increased release of ketogenic amino acids from proteolysis also contributes to the formation of ketone bodies. These are buffered by plasma bicarbonate, leading to a fall in bicarbonate concentration (metabolic acidosis) and compensatory hyperventilation ('Küssmaul' breathing). Hyperglycaemia gives rise to an osmotic diuresis with loss of electrolytes and water. There are therefore a number of abnormalities that require correction.

Desalination and potassium deficit A generous volume of physiological saline (0.9%), given intravenously, is crucial in order to restore extracellular fluid volume. An approximate guide is 1.5–2 L over the first 2 h, 2 L over the next 4 h and 2 L over the next 6 h. Monitoring of central venous pressure and urine output (following bladder catheterization) is a useful guide to the rate of volume replacement. When blood glucose levels fall below 17 mmol/L, 5% glucose is given in place of saline. Potassium must be replaced, and if the urinary output is satisfactory and the plasma potassium concentration is low, 20 mmol/h can be given, the rate of replacement being judged by frequent measurements of plasma potassium concentration and ECG monitoring.

Hyperglycaemia Intravenous insulin is infused at a rate of up to 0.1 unit/kg/h with a syringe pump until ketosis resolves (judged by blood pH, serum bicarbonate and blood ketones) and until the blood glucose is below 15 mmol/L. If ketones have not cleared at this blood glucose level, the infusion is slowed to 0.05 units/kg/h and 4 g of glucose/unit of insulin added to prevent hypoglycaemia, thus allowing continuation of the insulin until metabolic normality is restored. Intramuscular injection, although less satisfactory than intravenous infusion, is an acceptable alternative route of administration when facilities for intravenous infusion are not available, using a 10-unit starting dose followed by 5 units hourly depending on blood glucose levels. Subcutaneous injections are absorbed slowly, particularly in shocked patients, and should not be used in this situation.

Metabolic acidosis This usually resolves with adequate treatment with saline and insulin. Bicarbonate treatment to reverse the extracellular acidosis is controversial, and may paradoxically worsen intracellular and cerebrospinal fluid acidosis. We do not advocate its routine use. If the arterial pH is <7.0 the patient should be managed on the intensive-care unit if possible, and may need inotropic support.

Other measures These include aspiration of the stomach, as gastric stasis is common and inhalation of vomit can be fatal, and treatment of the precipitating cause of coma (e.g. antibiotics for bacterial infection).

HYPEROSMOLAR NON-KETOTIC COMA

Less insulin is required in this situation, as the blood pH is normal and insulin sensitivity is retained. Fluid loss is restored using physiological saline (there is sometimes a place for half-strength, 0.45% saline), and large amounts of intravenous potassium are often required. Magnesium deficiency is common, contributes to the difficulty of correcting the potassium deficit, and should be treated. There is a case for prophylactic heparin, as venous thrombosis is common.

MECHANISM OF ACTION

Insulin acts via receptors that are transmembrane glycoproteins which recycle between the plasma membrane and an intracellular pool. Each receptor has two insulin-binding sites, but occupancy of one results in a marked reduction in the affinity of the other. Insulin is internalized with the receptor and passed to lysosomes, leaving the receptor to be recycled to the plasma membrane. Receptor occupancy results in:

1 activation of insulin-dependent glucose transport processes (in adipose tissue and muscle) via a transporter known as 'Glut-4';
2 inhibition of adenylyl cyclase-dependent metabolism (lipolysis, proteolysis, glycogenolysis);
3 intracellular accumulation of potassium and phosphate, which is linked to glucose transport in some tissues.

Secondary effects include increased cellular amino acid uptake, increased DNA and RNA synthesis and increased oxidative phosphorylation.

ADVERSE REACTIONS

1 Hypoglycaemia is the most important complication of insulin treatment. It is treated with an intravenous injection of 50% glucose in unconscious patients, but sugar may be given orally in those with milder symptoms. **Glucagon** (1 mg given intramuscularly, repeated after a few minutes if necessary) is useful if the patient is unconscious and intravenous access is not available (e.g. to ambulance personnel during transfer to hospital, or to a partner or family member at home). Patients usually regain consciousness within 5 min and must then be given a sweet drink.
2 Insulin-induced post-hypoglycaemic hyperglycaemia (Somogyi effect) occurs when the patient develops mild hypoglycaemia which induces an overshoot of regulatory mechanisms (adrenaline, growth hormone, corticosteroids, glucagon) that elevate blood sugar. This sometimes occurs during twice daily insulin therapy when nocturnal hypoglycaemia coincides with the peak effect of intermediate-acting insulin. The situation is easily misinterpreted as requiring increased insulin, thus producing further hypoglycaemia.

3 There may be local or systemic allergic reactions to insulin, with itching, redness and swelling at the injection site.

4 Lipodystrophy is the disappearance of subcutaneous fat at or near injection sites. Atrophy is now less common due to better education regarding rotation of injection sites and wider use of pure insulins. Fatty tumours occur if repeated injections are made at the same site. Injections should therefore be made in unexposed areas.

5 Insulin resistance, defined arbitrarily as a daily requirement of more than 200 units, due to antibodies, is relatively unusual. Changing the patient to a highly purified insulin preparation is often successful. A small dose should be used initially to avoid hypoglycaemia.

PHARMACOKINETICS

Insulin is broken down in the gut and by the liver, and is given by injection. The $t_{\frac{1}{2}}$ is 3–5 min. It is metabolized to inactive α and β peptide chains largely by hepatic insulinase (insulin glutathione transhydrogenase), which breaks the disulphide bridges between α and β chains. Insulin from the pancreas is mainly released into the portal circulation and passes to the liver, where up to 60% is degraded before reaching the systemic circulation (presystemic metabolism). There is no evidence that diabetes ever results from increased hepatic destruction of insulin, but in cirrhosis the liver fails to inactivate insulin, thus predisposing to hypoglycaemia.

ORAL HYPOGLYCAEMIC DRUGS

Oral hypoglycaemic drugs are useful only as adjuncts to (and not in place of) continued dietary restraint. They should be prescribed only if an adequate trial of diet alone for at least 1 month has been unsuccessful. They fall into two major groups:

1 sulphonylureas;
2 biguanides.

Most type 2 patients initially achieve satisfactory control with diet either alone or combined with one of these agents. The small proportion who cannot be controlled with drugs at this stage (primary failure) require insulin. Subsequent failure after initially adequate control (secondary failure) occurs in about one-third of patients after 15 years.

The results of the University Group Diabetes Program (UGDP) performed in the USA and published in the 1970s have contributed to the controversy surrounding the use of these drugs. The objectives of this study were to evaluate the efficacy of treatment in the prevention of vascular complications by a long-term multicentre trial. After 8 years of follow-up there was excess cardiovascular mortality in patients treated with oral hypoglycaemic drugs. The results of this large study were generally ignored in the UK. Perhaps the most significant message is the importance of diet and the futility of putting exclusive faith in oral agents beyond their ability to improve symptoms such as polyuria.

Sulphonylureas

USE

These drugs (e.g. tolbutamide, chlorpropamide, glibenclamide, gliclazide) are used for type 2 diabetics who have not responded to diet alone and who show no tendency to ketosis. They improve symptoms of polyuria and polydipsia, but have not been shown to reduce vascular complications or increase longevity (see above), and they stimulate appetite, thus making weight loss more difficult to achieve. **Chlorpropamide** is associated with a higher incidence of adverse effects (especially hypoglycaemia, due to its long half-life, as well as flushing with alcohol; see below) than other drugs of this class, and is now largely obsolete. **Tolbutamide** and **gliclazide** are shorter-acting than **glibenclamide**, so there is less risk of hypoglycaemia, and for this reason they are preferred in the elderly. Glibenclamide is given once daily with breakfast, the usual starting dose being 2.5 or 5 mg increasing according to response to a maximum of 15 mg daily. Tolbutamide is started at a dose of 250 mg twice daily increasing to a maximum of 1 g twice daily according to response. Gliclazide is usually started as a single daily dose of 40 mg increasing to a maximum single dose of 160 mg with breakfast. The dose can be further increased if necessary to a maximum of 160 mg twice daily.

Glibenclamide 5mg OD. ↑ TDS
Gliclazide 40mg OD ↑ 160mg OD
Tolbutamide 250 mg OD ↑ 1gm

MECHANISM OF ACTION

The hypoglycaemic effect of these drugs depends on the presence of functioning β-cells and *in vitro* they stimulate insulin release from isolated islets of Langerhans. Sulphonylureas, like glucose, depolarize β-cells and release insulin. They do this by blocking ATP-dependent potassium channels in the cell membrane, thereby causing depolarization even when ATP levels in the cell are low. Depolarization causes entry of Ca^{2+} ions and insulin secretion. Consequently, acute administration results in a fall in blood sugar accompanied by a rise in plasma insulin. Thus even in normal subjects these drugs produce hypoglycaemia. Sulphonylureas differ in their effects on water excretion. Chlorpropamide has been employed as an antidiuretic agent in the treatment of patients with diabetes insipidus who have some residual antidiuretic hormone (see Chapter 35). Unsurprisingly, therefore, it can cause dilutional hyponatraemia. It probably acts both by stimulating antidiuretic hormone release and by potentiating its action on the kidney. Tolbutamide has similar but less marked activity, whereas glibenclamide is mildly diuretic.

ADVERSE EFFECTS

Hypoglycaemia from sulphonylureas can cause coma and irreversible neurological damage. Chlorpropamide, the longest acting agent, was responsible for many cases and also causes flushing in susceptible individuals when alcohol is consumed. Tolbutamide and other sulphonylureas are associated with adverse reactions in about 3% of patients, chiefly allergic skin reactions (ranging from mild maculopapular to severe generalized photosensitivity reactions occurring from within the first 6 months to up to 2 years of treatment), drug fever, gastrointestinal upsets, transient jaundice (usually cholestatic) and haematopoietic changes, including thrombocytopenia, neutropenia and pancytopenia. Serious effects other than hypoglycaemia are uncommon.

PHARMACOKINETICS

Sulphonylureas are all well absorbed from the gastrointestinal tract without presystemic metabolism, and the chief differences between them lie in their relative potencies and rates of elimination. Glibenclamide is almost completely metabolized by the liver. Glibenclamide is converted to weakly active metabolites before being excreted in the bile and urine. The activity of these metabolites is only clinically important in patients with renal failure, in whom they accumulate and can cause hypoglycaemia. The plasma $t_{\frac{1}{2}}$ in the later phases of elimination after oral administration is 6–12 h, but it has a more prolonged duration of action that may persist for over 16 h, presumably due to a delay in its elimination from pancreatic islet tissue, although tissue accumulation with repeated dosing has not been demonstrated. Tolbutamide is converted in the liver to inactive metabolites which are excreted in the urine. The $t_{\frac{1}{2}}$ shows considerable inter-individual variability, but is usually 4–8 h. Gliclazide is extensively metabolized, although up to 20% is excreted unchanged in the urine. The plasma $t_{\frac{1}{2}}$ ranges from 6 to 14 h (mean 10 h).

DRUG INTERACTIONS

Useful interactions include the concurrent use of sulphonylurea and metformin to achieve glycaemic control in patients who remain symptomatic on either agent alone. Oral hypoglycaemic drugs are, as a group, prone to producing adverse effects due to interaction with other drugs. Monoamine oxidase inhibitors potentiate the activity of sulphonylureas by an unknown mechanism. Several drugs (e.g. corticosteroids, thiazide diuretics) antagonize the hypoglycaemic effects of sulphonylureas by virtue of their actions on insulin release or sensitivity.

Biguanides: metformin

USES

Metformin is used in non-insulin-dependent diabetics without a tendency to ketosis in whom dietary carbohydrate restriction has not controlled hyperglycaemia and who remain symptomatic. Its main use is in the overweight patient, because its anorectic effect aids weight reduction. Metformin also exerts a useful additive effect in patients who are uncontrolled by sulphonylureas alone. The usual dose is 500 mg every 8 h, or 850 mg twice daily with or after meals. The usual maximum daily dose is 2 g (occasionally up to 3 g). It must not be used in patients at risk of lactic acidosis, and is contraindicated in the following conditions:

1 renal failure (it is eliminated in the urine, see below);
2 alcoholics;
3 cirrhosis;
4 chronic lung disease (because of hypoxia);
5 cardiac failure (because of poor tissue perfusion);
6 mitochondrial myopathy;
7 acute myocardial infarction and other serious intercurrent illness (insulin should be substituted).

Metformin should be withdrawn and insulin substituted before major elective surgery. Plasma creatinine and liver function tests should be monitored before and during its use.

MECHANISM OF ACTION

The mechanism whereby biguanides produce hypoglycaemia remains uncertain, but is quite different from that of the sulphonylureas. They do not cause hypoglycaemia and are effective in pancreatectomized animals. The effects of metformin include:

1 reduced glucose absorption from the gut;
2 facilitation of glucose entry into tissues by a non-insulin-responsive mechanism;
3 inhibition of gluconeogenesis in the liver;
4 suppression of oxidative glucose metabolism and enhanced anaerobic glycolysis.

ADVERSE EFFECTS

Metformin causes nausea, a metallic taste, anorexia, vomiting and intermittent diarrhoea. The symptoms are worst when treatment is first started, and about 3% of patients cannot tolerate even small doses because of these effects. Lactic acidosis, which has a mortality in excess of 60%, is uncommon provided that the above contraindications are respected. It presents with the features of a metabolic acidosis (drowsiness or coma, abdominal pain, vomiting and hyperventilation), often with shock. Treatment is by reversal of hypoxia and circulatory collapse and peritoneal or haemodialysis to alleviate sodium overloading and remove the drug. Phenformin (withdrawn in the UK) was more frequently associated with this problem than metformin. Absorption of vitamin B_{12} is reduced by metformin, but this is seldom clinically important.

PHARMACOKINETICS

Oral absorption of metformin is 50–60%; it is eliminated unchanged by renal excretion, clearance being greater than the glomerular filtration rate because of active secretion into the tubular fluid. Metformin accumulates in patients with renal impairment. The plasma $t_{\frac{1}{2}}$ ranges from 1.5 to 4.5 h, but its duration of action is considerably longer, permitting twice daily dosing.

DRUG INTERACTIONS

Sulphonylureas are additive with metformin. Alcohol predisposes to metformin-related lactic acidosis.

Key points

Type I diabetes mellitus and insulin

- Type I (insulin-dependent) diabetes mellitus is caused by degeneration of β-cells in the islets of Langerhans leading to an absolute deficiency of insulin.
- Without insulin treatment such patients are prone to diabetic ketoacidosis (DKA).
- Even with insulin treatment, such patients are susceptible to microvascular complications of retinopathy, nephropathy and neuropathy, and also to accelerated atherosclerotic (macrovascular) disease leading to myocardial infarction, stroke and gangrene.
- Management includes a healthy diet low in saturated fat (see Chapter 26), high in complex carbohydrates and with the energy spread throughout the day.
- Regular subcutaneous injections of recombinant human insulin are required indefinitely. Mixtures of soluble and longer-acting insulins are used and are given using special insulin 'pens' at least twice daily. Regular self-monitoring of blood glucose levels throughout the day with individual adjustment of the insulin dose is essential to achieve good metabolic control, which reduces the risk of complications.
- DKA is treated with large volumes of intravenous physiological saline, intravenous soluble insulin and replacement of potassium and, if necessary, magnesium.

Key points

Type 2 diabetes mellitus and oral hypoglycaemic agents

- Type 2 (non-insulin-dependent) diabetes mellitus is caused by relative deficiency of insulin in the face of impaired insulin sensitivity. Such patients are usually obese.
- About one-third of such patients finally require insulin treatment. This is especially important when they are losing muscle mass.
- The dietary goal is to achieve ideal body weight by consuming an energy-restricted healthy diet low in saturated fat (see Chapter 26).
- Oral hypoglycaemic drugs are useful in some patients as an adjunct to diet.
- Metformin, a biguanide, lowers blood glucose levels and encourages weight loss by causing anorexia. Diarrhoea is a common adverse effect. It is contraindicated in patients with renal impairment, heart failure, obstructive pulmonary disease or mitochondrial myopathies because of the risk of lactic acidosis, a rare but life-theatening complication.
- Acarbose, an α-glucosidase inhibitor, delays the absorption of starch and sucrose. It flattens the rise in plasma glucose following a meal, and may improve control when added to diet with or without other drugs. However, it can cause bloating, flatulence and diarrhoea associated with carbohydrate malabsorption.
- Sulphonylureas (e.g. tolbutamide) release insulin from β-cells by closing ATP-sensitive K^+ channels, thereby depolarizing the cell membrane. They are well tolerated and improve blood glucose at least initially, but stimulate appetite, thereby promoting weight gain. They differ from one another in their kinetics, the longer-acting drugs being particular likely to cause hypoglycaemia which can be severe, especially in the elderly.

Acarbose

Acarbose is used in type 2 diabetes mellitus in patients who are inadequately controlled on diet alone or diet and other oral hypoglycaemic agents. Acarbose is a reversible competitive inhibitor of intestinal α-glucoside hydrolases, and delays the absorption of starch and sucrose but does not affect the absorption of ingested glucose. The postprandial glycaemic rise after a meal containing complex carbohydrates is reduced and its peak is delayed. Fermentation of unabsorbed carbohydrate in the intestine leads to increased gas formation which results in flatulence, abdominal distension and occasionally diarrhoea. As with any change in a diabetic's medication, diet or activities, the blood glucose must be monitored. Further experience is required before the precise role of acarbose in the management of diabetes mellitus can be defined.

Case history

A 56-year-old woman with a positive family history of diabetes presents with polyuria, polydipsia, blurred vision and recurrent attacks of vaginal thrush. She is overweight at 92 kg, her fasting blood sugar is 12 mmol/L and haemoglobin A_{1C} is elevated at 10.6%. She is treated with glibenclamide once daily in addition to antifungal treatment for the thrush. Initially her symptoms improve considerably and she feels generally much better, but after 9 months the polyuria and polydipsia recur and her weight has increased to 102 kg.

Comment

Treatment with a sulphonylurea without attention to diet is doomed to failure. This patient needs to be motivated to take dietary advice, restricting her energy intake and reducing her risk of atherosclerosis.

Further reading

American Diabetes Association. 1993: Implications of the diabetes control and complications trial. *Diabetes* **42**, 1555–8.

Barnett AH, Owens DR. 1997: Insulin analogues. *Lancet* **349**, 47–51.

deFronzo RA, Goodman AM. Efficacy of metformin in patients with non-insulin-dependent diabetes mellitus. *New England Journal of Medicine* **333**, 541–9 (see also accompanying editorial on metformin by O.B. Crofford, pp. 588–9).

Gerich JE. 1989: Oral hypoglycemic agents. *New England Journal of Medicine* **321**, 1231–45.

Pickup JC, Williams J (eds) 1997: *Textbook of diabetes*, 2nd edn. Oxford: Blackwell Science.

Williams G. 1994: Management of non-insulin-dependent diabetes mellitus. *Lancet* **343**, 95–100.

Oral hypoglycaemics –

(A) Glibenclamide is largely excreted unchanged in urine.

(B) All display mild diuretic activity

(C) metformin ↓ intestinal glucose absorption

(D) chlorpropamide is a potent liver enzyme metabolising inducer

(E) sulphonylureas directly inhibit gluconeogenesis

CHAPTER THIRTY-SEVEN

THYROID

- Introduction
- Pathophysiology and principles of treatment
- Iodine
- Thyroxine and tri-iodothyronine
- Antithyroid drugs
- Special situations

INTRODUCTION

The thyroid secretes thyroxine (T_4) and tri-iodothyronine (T_3) as well as calcitonin, which is discussed in Chapter 38. The release of T_3 and T_4 is controlled by the pituitary hormone thyrotrophin (thyroid-stimulating hormone, TSH), which is the most important physiological regulator of thyroid function. It binds to receptors on thyroid follicular cells and activates adenylyl cyclase, resulting in increased cyclic 3′,5′-adenosine monophosphate (cAMP) formation. This stimulates iodine trapping, iodothyronine synthesis and release of thyroid hormones. TSH is secreted by basophil cells in the adenohypophysis. It consists of two conjoined polypeptide chains. The α-chain is identical to the α-chain of luteinizing hormone (LH) and follicle-stimulating hormone (FSH), and the β-chain confers specificity for the thyroid TSH receptor. Secretion of TSH by the anterior pituitary is stimulated by the hypothalamic peptide thyrotrophin-releasing hormone (TRH), which is a tripeptide (Glu-His-Pro). Circulating T_4 and, to a lesser extent, T_3 produce negative-feedback inhibition of TSH at pituitary and hypothalamic levels.

Drug treatment is highly effective in correcting under- or over-activity of the thyroid gland. Diagnosis of abnormal thyroid function and monitoring of therapy have been greatly facilitated by accurate and sensitive tests of TSH, because the serum TSH level accurately reflects thyroid state, whereas the interpretation of serum concentrations of T_3 and T_4 is complicated by very extensive and somewhat variable protein binding. Negative feedback of biologically active thyroid hormones ensures that when there is primary failure of the thyroid gland, serum TSH is elevated, whereas when there is overactivity of the gland, serum TSH is depressed. Hypothyroidism caused by hypopituitarism is relatively uncommon, and is associated with depressed sex hormone and adrenal cortical function. Hyperthyroidism secondary to excessive TSH is extremely rare.

PATHOPHYSIOLOGY AND PRINCIPLES OF TREATMENT

Thyroid disease is more common in women than in men, and is manifested either as goitre or as under- or over-activity of the gland (with or without goitre). *Hypothyroidism* is common, especially in the elderly. It is usually caused by autoimmune destruction of the gland, and if untreated it causes the clinical picture of myxoedema. Treatment is by lifelong replacement with thyroxine.

Hyperthyroidism is also common, and again autoimmune processes are commonly implicated. Treatment options include the following:

1 anti-thyroid drugs;
2 radioactive iodine;
3 surgery.

Antithyroid drugs enable a euthyroid state to be maintained until the disease remits or definitive treatment with radioiodine or surgery is undertaken. Radioactive iodine is well tolerated and free of surgical complications such as laryngeal nerve damage, whereas surgery is most appropriate when there are mechanical problems such as tracheal compression.

In older patients the commonest cause of hyperthyroidism is *multinodular toxic goitre*. In young women it is usually caused by autoimmune disease, an immunoglobulin being formed that binds to and stimulates the TSH receptor, thereby promoting synthesis and release of T_3 and T_4 independent of TSH. This results in a smooth vascular goitre and often in deposition of mucopolysaccharide in several tissues, most notably in the extrinsic eye muscles, which become thickened and cause proptosis. This clinical picture is known as *Graves' disease*. Graves' disease has a remitting/relapsing course, and often finally leads to hypothyroidism. Other aetiologies of hyperthyroidism include acute viral or autoimmune thyroiditis (which usually resolve spontaneously), iatrogenic iodine excess (e.g. thyroid storm following iodine-containing contrast media, and hyperthyroidism in patients treated with amiodarone; see Chapter 31), and acute postpartum hyperthyroidism.

IODINE

The thyroid gland selectively concentrates iodine from plasma. Dietary iodide normally amounts to 100–200 μg/day and is absorbed from the stomach and small intestine by an active process. Following uptake into the thyroid gland, iodide is oxidized to iodine, from which a series of iodinated tyrosine compounds including T_3 and T_4 are made. Iodine is used to treat simple non-toxic goitre due to iodine deficiency. Potassium iodide (3 mg daily po) prevents further enlargement of the gland, but seldom actually shrinks it. Iodized salt is used to prevent this type of endemic goitre in areas where the diet is iodine deficient, according to a defined World Health Organization (WHO) policy.

Pre-operative treatment with Lugol's iodine solution (an aqueous solution of iodine and potassium iodide) in combination with carbimazole or propylthiouracil is used to reduce the vascularity of the gland and inhibit thyroid hormone release. This action of iodine in inhibiting thyroid hormone release is only maintained for 1–2 weeks, after which thyroid hormone release is markedly *increased* if the cause of the hyperthyroidism has not been dealt with.

THYROXINE AND TRI-IODOTHYRONINE

USE

L-Thyroxine is used in the treatment of uncomplicated hypothyroidism, the dose being individualized according to serum TSH. The usual starting dose for an adult is 50 μg daily (25 μg in patients with ischaemic heart disease), increasing the dose by 50 μg (25 μg in patients with ischaemic heart disease) every 4 weeks until the patient has responded clinically and the TSH level has fallen to within the normal range. The optimal maintenance dose is usually 100–200 μg L-thyroxine daily. Excessive dosage or too rapid an increase in dose may precipitate cardiac complications, particularly in patients with overt ischaemic heart disease. If angina pectoris limits the dose of thyroxine, the addition of a beta-blocker (e.g. atenolol) will allow further increments in thyroxine dosage. Long-term overdosage is undesirable, and causes osteoporosis as well as predisposing to cardiac arrhythmias.

Congenital hypothyroidism ('cretinism') is treated similarly, and thyroxine must be given as early as possible. In the UK, the adoption of the Guthrie test has greatly facilitated the early detection of hypothyroidism.

The rapid action of T_3 is useful in treating myxoedema coma. It is given in doses of up to 100 μg 12-hourly intramuscularly, and at the same time maintenance therapy is commenced with thyroxine 50 μg given orally (or, if necessary, by a gastric tube). Hypothyroidism sometimes coexists with Addison's disease, and hydrocortisone is also given empirically to patients with myxoedema coma. Apart from primary thyroid hypofunction, hypothyroidism may result from hypopituitarism. This is also treated with oral thyroxine in the usual doses. Corticosteroid replacement must be started first, otherwise acute adrenal insufficiency will be precipitated.

MECHANISM OF ACTION

Thyroxine is a prohormone. After entering cells it is converted to T_3, which binds to receptor protein which interacts with DNA in the cell nucleus and causes the synthesis of new messenger RNA and hence of new proteins. The main actions of thyroid hormones are as follows:

1 stimulation of metabolism – raised basal metabolic rate;
2 promotion of normal growth and maturation, particularly of the central nervous system and skeleton;
3 sensitization to the effects of catecholamines.

ADVERSE EFFECTS

The adverse effects of the thyroid hormones relate to their physiological functions. Rapid increases in thyroxine dose in hypothyroidism can lead to sudden death due to ventricular fibrillation. Angina, myocardial infarction, tachycardia and congestive cardiac failure can also be precipitated. Diarrhoea is a common symptom of excessive thyroxine. Tremor, restlessness, heat intolerance and other features of hyperthyroidism are dose-dependent toxic effects of these hormones.

PHARMACOKINETICS

Thyroid hormones are absorbed from the gut. The effects of T_4 are not usually detectable before 24 h, and maximum activity is not attained for many days during regular daily dosing. T_3 produces effects within 6 h and peak activity is reached within 24 h. It is therefore often preferred for the urgent treatment of myxoedema coma. The $t_{\frac{1}{2}}$ of T_4 is 6–7 days in euthyroid individuals, but may be much longer than this in hypothyroidism, and that for T_3 is 2 days or less. It is therefore unnecessary to administer thyroid hormone more frequently than once a day.

The liver conjugates thyroid hormones, which undergo enterohepatic recirculation.

> **Key points**
>
> Iodine and thyroid hormones
>
> - Iodized salt is used to prevent endemic goitre in regions where the diet is iodine-deficient. Lugol's iodine (a solution of iodine in aqueous potassium iodide) is also used pre-operatively to reduce the vascularity of the thyroid.
> - Thyroxine (T_4) is used as a physiological replacement in patients who are hypothyroid. It is converted in the tissues to the more active tri-iodothyronine (T_3).
> - T_3 has a shorter elimination half-life than T_4, and is therefore used for emergency treatment of myxoedema coma (often with glucocorticoids because of the possibility of coexisting hypoadrenalism).

ANTITHYROID DRUGS

Carbimazole

USE

Carbimazole is used to treat hyperthyroidism. Patients are warned (see below) to report any evidence of infection (especially sore throat) immediately, and some centres use written advice leaflets and consent forms to highlight the importance of this. A single daily dose of 30–60 mg in adults (15 mg in children) is used until the patient is euthyroid, usually within 4–6 weeks. The dose of carbimazole is then reduced to a maintenance regime of 5–15 mg daily. Treatment is maintained for 1–2 years and the drug is then gradually withdrawn. If relapse occurs during drug withdrawal, the dose is again raised until clinical improvement is restored. If dosage adjustment proves difficult, smoother control may be obtained by giving thyroxine, 100 μg daily, together with a blocking dose of carbimazole, 60 mg daily.

MECHANISM OF ACTION

Carbimazole is hydrolysed to methimazole in plasma, and it is not possible to demonstrate the presence of carbimazole in the thyroid, although methimazole is present. Thus carbimazole acts by way of its active metabolite methimazole, which serves as a substrate for peroxidase and is itself iodinated and degraded within the thyroid, thus diverting oxidized iodine away from thyroglobulin and thereby decreasing thyroid hormone biosynthesis. Methimazole is concentrated by cells with a peroxidase system (salivary gland, neutrophils and macrophage/monocytes, in addition to thyroid follicular cells). It has an immunosuppressive action within the thyroid, and interferes with the generation of oxygen radicals by macrophages, thereby interfering with the presentation of antigen to lymphocytes. Methimazole also directly inhibits the synthesis of T_3 and T_4 by interfering with tyrosine iodination and the coupling of iodotyrosines, but does not affect hormone secretion. Thus hormone release decreases after a latent period, during which time the thyroid becomes depleted of hormone.

ADVERSE EFFECTS

Carbimazole is usually well tolerated, although pruritus and rashes are fairly common. These usually respond to switching to propylthiouracil as an alternative agent. Neutropenia is a rare but potentially fatal adverse effect. If the patient reports *sore throat* or other evidence of infection, an *urgent white cell count must be obtained*, and the drug should be stopped if there is neutropenia.Nausea and hair loss occasionally occur. Drug fever, leukopenia and arthralgia are rare. The use of carbimazole during pregnancy has rarely been associated with aplasia cutis in the newborn.

PHARMACOKINETICS

Carbimazole is rapidly absorbed after oral administration and hydrolysed to its active metabolite methimazole, which is concentrated in the thyroid within minutes of administration. Methimazole has an apparent volume of distribution equivalent to body water, and the $t_{\frac{1}{2}}$ varies according to thyroid status, being approximately 7, 9 and 14 h in hyperthyroid, euthyroid and hypothyroid patients, respectively. It is metabolized in the liver and thyroid.

Propylthiouracil

USE

Propylthiouracil has similar actions, uses and toxic effects to carbimazole, but has an additional action in inhibiting the peripheral conversion of T_4 to the more active T_3. As with carbimazole, dangerous leukopenia may develop but is very rare. The initial total daily dose is 300–600 mg and the maintenance dose is 50–150 mg. The scheme of attaining a euthyroid state with a large dose of drug and then reducing the dose to maintain this is carried out as with carbimazole. Propylthiouracil is rapidly absorbed from the intestine. The plasma $t_{\frac{1}{2}}$ is short, but the duration of action within the thyroid is prolonged, and as with carbimazole propylthiouracil can be given once daily, although many endocrinologists still prefer to give the drug in three divided doses. It can be used (by specialists) in pregnancy (see below), and has some advantages over carbimazole in this setting.

Potassium perchlorate

Potassium perchlorate prevents the trapping and concentration of iodine in the thyroid. It can produce aplastic anaemia, and is no longer used in the UK.

β-Adrenoceptor antagonists

Beta-blockers improve the symptoms and signs of hyperthyroidism, including anxiety, sweating, tachycardia, tremor and hyperactive reflexes. They inhibit the conversion of T_4 to T_3 in the tissues. This is a general property of β-blockade and occurs irrespective of β-selectivity or intrinsic sympathomimetic activity. These drugs are useful:

1 while awaiting laboratory confirmation, if the diagnosis is in doubt;
2 during initiation of therapy with antithyroid drugs, during the latent period while the gland is becoming depleted of hormone;
3 before treatment with radio-iodine, because they do not interfere with the uptake of iodine by the gland;
4 in thyroid crisis;
5 with iodine, as a rapid preparation for surgery;
6 in neonatal hyperthyroidism due to thyroid-stimulating immunoglobulin from the mother – this remits within about 6 weeks as maternally-derived immunoglobulin is cleared by the infant.

Hyperthyroid patients treated with beta-blockers are not biochemically euthyroid, even if they appear clinically euthyroid, and thyroid crisis ('storm') can supervene if treatment is discontinued.

Radioactive iodine

Radioactive iodine is an effective oral treatment for thyrotoxicosis caused by Graves' disease or by toxic nodular goitre. It is safe, causes no discomfort to the patient and has largely replaced surgery except when there are mechanical problems such as tracheal compression. It is contraindicated in pregnancy. Dosing has been the subject of controversy. It is now standard practice in many units to give an ablative dose followed by replacement therapy with thyroxine, so late-onset undiagnosed hypothyroidism is avoided. The isotope usually employed is ^{131}I with a $t_{\frac{1}{2}}$ of 8 days. Thyroxine replacement is started after 4–6 weeks and continued for life. There is no increased incidence of leukemia, thyroid or other malignancy after therapeutic use of ^{131}I, but concern remains regarding its use in children or young women. However, the dose of radiation to the gonads is less than that in many radiological procedures (e.g. barium enema), and there is no evidence that therapeutic doses of radioactive iodine damage the germ cells or reduce fertility. It is contraindicated during pregnancy because it damages the fetus, causing congenital hypothyroidism and consequently possible mental retardation ('cretinism'). Patients are usually treated as out-patients during the first 10 days of the menstrual cycle and after a negative pregnancy test. Pregnancy should be avoided for at least 4 months and a woman should not breast-feed for at least 2 months after treatment. High-dose ^{131}I is used to treat patients with well-differentiated thyroid carcinoma to ablate residual tumour after surgery. Thyroxine is stopped at least 1 month before treatment to allow TSH levels to increase, thereby stimulating uptake of isotope by the gland. Patients are isolated in hospital for several days to protect potential contacts.

Key points

Antithyroid drugs

- Carbimazole works via its active metabolite, methimazole. This is concentrated in cells that contain peroxidase, including neutrophils as well as thyroid epithelium. It is iodinated in the thyroid, diverting iodine from the synthesis of T_3 and T_4 and depleting the gland of hormone. It does not inhibit secretion of pre-formed thyroid hormones, so there is a latent period before its effect is evident after starting treatment.
- Neutropenia is an uncommon but potentially fatal adverse effect. Patients who develop sore throat or other symptoms of infection need to report for an urgent white blood count. Pruritus and rash are more common but less severe.
- Propylthiouracil is similar in its effects and adverse effects to carbimazole/methimazole, but in addition it inhibits peripheral conversion of T_4 to the more active T_3, and is therefore preferred in thyroid storm.
- β-Adrenoceptor antagonists suppress manifestations of hyperthyroidism and are used when starting treatment with specific antithyroid drugs, and in treating thyroid storm (together with propylthiouracil and glucocorticoids, which also the suppress the conversion of T_4 to T_3).
- Radioactive iodine (^{131}I) is safe in non-pregnant adults, and has largely replaced surgery in the treatment of hyperthyroidism, except when there are mechanical complications such as tracheal obstruction. Replacement therapy with T_4 is required after functional ablation.

SPECIAL SITUATIONS

GRAVES' OPHTHALMOPATHY

Eye signs usually occur within 18 months of the onset of Graves' disease, and commonly resolve over 1–2 years irrespective of the state of the thyroid. Over-aggressive treatment of hyperthyroidism in patients with eye signs must be avoided because of a strong clinical impression that iatrogenic hypothyroidism can exacerbate eye disease. Periorbital oedema can be reduced by sleeping with the head of the bed elevated. Simple moisturizing eyedrops (e.g. hypromellose) may be useful. Five per cent **guanethidine** eyedrops may improve the appearance of the eyes, and diuretics are sometimes prescribed in the hope of reducing orbital oedema. *Tarsoroplasty* is indicated to prevent corneal abrasion in severe cases. Radiotherapy is useful in moderate Graves' ophthalmopathy, provided that this is not threatening vision. Severe and distressing exophthalmos warrants a trial of prednisolone 60 mg daily. Urgent *surgical decompression* of the orbit is required if medical treatment is not successful and visual acuity deteriorates due to optic nerve compression.

Thyroid crisis

Thyroid crisis is a severe, abrupt exacerbation of hyperthyroidism with hyperpyrexia, tachycardia, vomiting, dehydration, hyperkinesis and shock. It can arise post-operatively, following radioiodine therapy or with intercurrent infection. Rarely, it arises spontaneously in a previously undiagnosed or untreated patient. The mortality rate is substantial and urgent treatment is required with the following:

1. β-adrenoceptor antagonists, which control tachycardia and tremor (and antagonize conversion of T_4 to T_3);
2. intravenous saline for volume replacement;
3. cooling to combat hyperthermia;
4. propylthiouracil (e.g. 200 mg every 4 h by nasogastric tube) to reduce hormone synthesis and conversion of T_4 to T_3;
5. Lugol's iodine to reduce secretion of T_4;
6. glucocorticoids (which antagonize the conversion of T_4 to T_3);
7. fast atrial fibrillation can be especially difficult to treat because of resistance to digoxin – DC cardioversion may be needed.

Aspirin must be avoided, because salicylate displaces bound T_4 and T_3 and also because of its uncoupling effect on oxidative phosphorylation, which renders the metabolic state even more severe.

Pregnancy and breast-feeding

Radioactive iodine is absolutely contraindicated in pregnancy, and surgery should be avoided if possible. T_4 and T_3 do *not* cross the placenta adequately and, if a fetus is hypothyroid, this results in congenital hypothyroidism with mental retardation caused by maldevelopment of the central nervous system. Antithyroid drugs (carbimazole and propylthiouracil) cross the placenta and enter breast milk, and management of hyperthyroidism during pregnancy requires specialist expertise. Overtreatment with antithyroid drugs must be avoided. Blocking doses of antithyroid drugs with added T_4 must *never* be used in pregnancy, as the antithyroid drugs cross the placenta but T_4 does not, leading inevitably to a severely hypothyroid infant. Propylthiouracil may be somewhat less likely than carbimazole to produce effects in the infant, since it is more highly protein bound and is ionized at pH 7.4. This reduces its passage across the placenta and into milk. Minimal effective doses of propylthiouracil should be used during pregnancy and breast-feeding.

Case history

A 19-year-old Chinese woman develops secondary amenorrhoea followed by symptoms of palpitations, nervousness, heat intolerance and sweating. There is a strong family history of autoimmune disease. On examination she appears anxious and sweaty, her pulse is 120 beats/min regular, and there is a smooth goitre with a soft bruit. There is tremor of the outstretched fingers and lidlag is present. A pregnancy test is positive, and you send blood to the laboratory for standard investigations, including T_3 and T_4.

Comment

This young woman has the clinical picture of Graves' disease, which is common in this ethnic group. Management is complicated by the fact that she is probably pregnant, and specialist input will be essential. Treatment with a β-adrenoceptor antagonist and a low dose of an antithyroid drug should be considered. Radioactive iodine is absolutely contraindicated in pregnancy, and a high dose of antithyroid drug should be avoided because of the risk of causing congenital hypothyroidism, and consequent mental retardation, in the baby.

Further reading

Franklin JA. 1995: The management of hyperthyroidism. *New England Journal of Medicine* **330**, 1731–8.

Franklin JF, Sheppard M. 1992: Radioiodine for hyperthyroidism: perhaps the best option. *British Medical Journal* **305**, 728–9.

Larkins R. 1993: Treatment of Graves' ophthalmology. *Lancet* **342**, 941–2.

Lazarus JH. 1997: Hyperthyroidism. *Lancet* **349**, 339–43.

Lindsay RS. 1997: Hypothyroidism. *Lancet* **349**, 413–17.

CHAPTER THIRTY-EIGHT

CALCIUM METABOLISM

- Introduction
- Vitamin D
- Calcium
- Principles of treatment of hypercalcaemia
- Bisphosphonates
- Calcitonin

INTRODUCTION

Plasma calcium is maintained within a narrow physiological range by parathyroid hormone (PTH), vitamin D and calcitonin. Parathyroid hormone (PTH) is rapidly metabolized by the liver and kidney so that a heterogeneous mixture of inactive PTH fragments is present in plasma. The plasma calcium concentration is the major factor controlling PTH secretion, and a reduction in calcium concentration stimulates PTH release. Acute hypomagnesaemia elevates plasma PTH, but prolonged magnesium depletion impairs secretion. This may result from a requirement for magnesium ions by the parathyroid adenylyl cyclase, as PTH release by hypocalcaemia is mediated via cyclic adenosine monophosphate (cAMP). Parathyroid hormone raises plasma calcium concentration and lowers plasma phosphate concentration. Parathyroid hormone acts on kidney and bone, where its effects are mediated intracellularly by stimulation of tissue adenylyl cyclase increasing cAMP. Parathyroid hormone causes phosphaturia and increased renal tubular reabsorption of calcium, which in association with mobilization of calcium from bone, increases the plasma calcium concentration. The effects of parathyroid hormone on bone include stimulation of osteoclast activity, formation of new osteoclasts from progenitor cells and transient depression of osteoblast activity. Parathyroid hormone also plays a role in the regulation of vitamin D metabolism. Increased gut absorption of calcium previously attributed to PTH is in fact an indirect effect via increased production of 1,25-dihydroxycholecalciferol. Parathyroid hormone replacement has no place in the long-term management of hypoparathyroidism. Parathyroid hormone is administered as a single test dose (200 units intravenously) in the diagnosis of pseudohypoparathyroidism. In this condition there is end-organ resistance to the hormone, so plasma calcium does not rise and there is no increase in urinary phosphate or cyclic AMP excretion.

Several important metabolic diseases affect the bones, notably hyperparathyroidism (treatment of which is surgical), osteomalacia and rickets, Paget's disease and osteoporosis. Some of these diseases (e.g. osteomalacia) are associated with normal or low plasma calcium concentrations,

Key points

Pathophysiology of common metabolic bone disease

- Osteoporosis is characterized by reduced bone quantity (density).
- Paget's disease is characterized by excessive new bone formation and bone resorption.
- Osteomalacia is characterized by lack of bone mineralization.

some (e.g. hyperparathyroidism) are associated with hypercalcaemia, and some (e.g. osteoporosis) are associated with normal calcium concentrations. The therapy of several of these conditions will be discussed in this chapter.

VITAMIN D

The term 'vitamin D' is used to cover a range of related substances that share the ability to prevent or cure rickets. These include ergocalciferol (vitamin D_2), cholecalciferol (vitamin D_3), α-calcidol (1-α-hydroxycholecalciferol) and calcitriol (1,25-α-dihydrocholecalciferol). The metabolic pathway of vitamin D is summarized in Figure. 38.1. Vitamin D_3 is synthesized in skin by the action of ultraviolet light on 7-dehydrocholesterol, or absorbed from food in the upper gut. It is fat soluble, and thus bile is necessary for its absorption. Renal 1-α-hydroxylase is activated by PTH and inhibited by phosphate, thus controlling the amount of active 1,25-dihydroxycholecalciferol (1,25-DHCC) produced. This enzyme is also suppressed by 1,25-DHCC itself. 1,25-Dihydroxycholecalciferol is effectively a hormone in that it is synthesized in the kidney and acts on the intestine to increase formation of a calcium-binding protein which augments intestinal calcium absorption. Vitamin D itself is the biologically inactive precursor of 1,25-DHCC. Enzyme induction, particularly that due to anti-epileptic drugs, causes metabolic inactivation of calciferol resulting in osteomalacia and rickets. 1,25-Dihydroxycholecalciferol mobilizes calcium from bone, and presumably this provides calcium for synthesis of new bone mineral. Its action on the kidney is to stimulate calcium reabsorption, although this is a minor effect. The maximum antirachitic effect of cholecalciferol is delayed for several weeks, and plasma calcium levels similarly increase only slowly. Storage of vitamin D occurs, so the plasma $t_{\frac{1}{2}}$ does not determine the duration of its action, and a single large dose may be effective for several weeks.

USES

In the UK, dietary deficiency of vitamin D occurs where there is poverty and poor diet accentuated

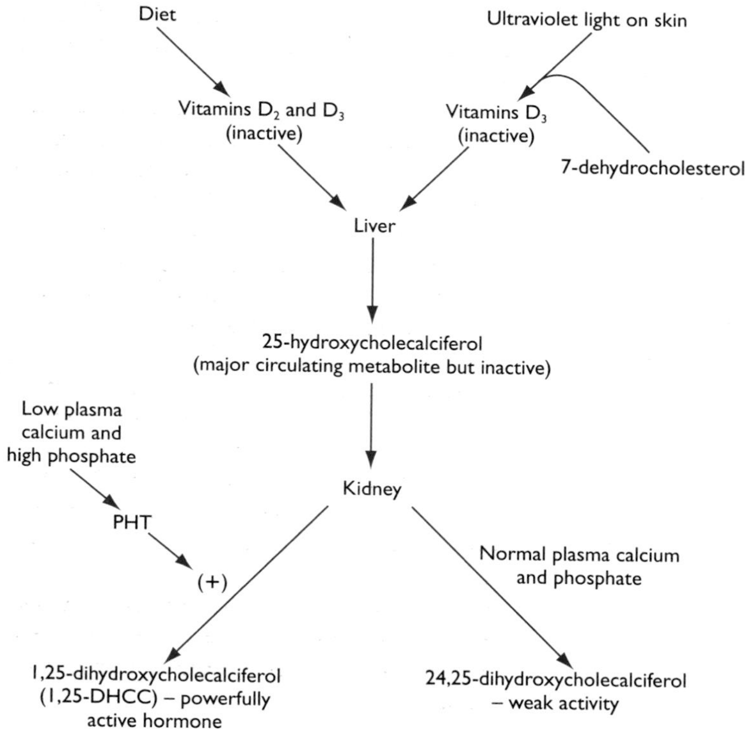

Figure 38.1: Metabolic pathway of vitamin D. PTH = parathormone.

by lack of sunlight, and is particularly common in Asian communities living in northern regions (chapatis and other unleavened breads also reduce the absorption of vitamin D), and in elderly people living alone. It results in rickets and osteomalacia. A daily dose of 10 μg of cholecalciferol is recommended in infants and children up to their seventh birthday, and 2.5 μg thereafter. Pregnant and lactating women should take about 20 μg daily. Several different vitamin D preparations are listed in the *British National Formulary*, which have different concentrations and uses.

1 Calcium and ergocalciferol tablets provide a physiological dose of vitamin D – ergocalciferol (vitamin D) 10 μg with 300 mg calcium lactate and 150 mg calcium phosphate. They are chewed or crushed before being taken, and are used in the prophylaxis and treatment of rickets and osteomalacia. The small dose of calcium (2.4 mmol) is unnecessary, but a preparation of vitamin D alone is not available.
2 Calciferol tablets, 250 μg or 1.25 mg, provide a pharmacological dose of vitamin D and are used for treatment of hypoparathyroidism and in cases of vitamin D-resistant rickets due to intestinal malabsorption or chronic liver disease.
3 1-α-Hydroxycholecalciferol (1-α-HCC). This metabolite is available for oral administration. It rapidly undergoes hepatic hydroxylation to 1,25-DHCC. It is used in:
   - renal rickets, where chronic renal failure leads to impaired 1,25-DHCC synthesis resulting in calcium malabsorption and hypocalcaemia with phosphate retention leading to secondary elevation of PTH levels. Bony changes of osteomalacia and hyperparathyroidism ensue. 1-α-Hydroxycholecalciferol is given in a dose of 1 μg daily (together with a phosphate-binding agent such as aluminum hydroxide);
   - hypoparathyroidism, which is usually treated with vitamin D in large doses, but the response is slow and unpredictable episodes of hypercalcaemia occur. This relative resistance to vitamin D is due to deficient 1,25-DHCC production secondary to PTH deficiency or hyperphosphataemia. 1-α-hydroxycholecalciferol, 1–2 μg, together with calcium supplements correct plasma calcium concentrations within a matter of days, and normocalcaemia may be maintained with smaller doses within a relatively narrow dosage range.
   - vitamin D-resistant rickets;
   - nutritional and malabsorptive rickets, which may also be treated with small doses (0.5–1 μg) of 1-α-HCC instead of conventional vitamin D.

The main adverse reaction is hypercalcaemia which can in turn cause renal failure, so regular plasma calcium and creatinine determinations (weekly initially) are essential. Hypercalcaemia is more likely to occur in patients with pre-existing renal dysfunction than in those with only osteomalacia. An advantage of using 1-α-HCC is that vitamin D intoxication is rapidly reversed when the drug is withdrawn, whereas reversal may take several weeks with the older vitamin D compounds.

Key points

Vitamin D and calcium metabolism

- Plasma calcium concentrations are tightly controlled by the balance of hypocalcaemic effects of calcitonin and hypercalcaemic effects of PTH and vitamin D and Ca^{2+} intake.
- Vitamin D is available in a number of forms, many of which are derived from each other by sequential metabolism in the skin, liver and kidney, and each of which has specific indications.
- The most potent and shortest-acting orally available vitamin D preparations are 1,25 dihydroxycholecalciferol, and 1-α-hydroxycholecalciferol. They are used in renal rickets or vitamin D resistant rickets.
- When patients are hypocalcaemic, calcium can be supplemented orally as calcium carbonate with or without various preparations of vitamin D. If urgent calcium replacement is required, a 10% solution of calcium lactate or gluconate (the former yielding more calcium) may be administered intravenously.
- Patients who are receiving vitamin D plus calcium should have periodic checks of their plasma Ca^{2+} concentrations, as the major adverse effect is hypercalcaemia.

4 Calcitriol (1,25-DHCC) is also available for the treatment of vitamin D-resistant rickets. Like 1-α-HCC it has a short biological half-life and less variable action than calciferol. Calcitriol is the treatment of choice for pseudohypoparathyroidism.

Prolonged or inappropriate use of these preparations will result in hypercalcaemia with calcium deposition in the tissues, particularly in the kidney, where it may cause irreversible renal failure.

CALCIUM

Calcium lactate or gluconate is used in conjunction with calciferol in the treatment of rickets and osteomalacia, and in hypocalcaemic tetany. Calcium chloride is also lifesaving in the emergency treatment of hyperkalaemia-induced cardiac arrhythmias (p. 322). If required intravenously, calcium gluconate injection BP (10% solution), 10–20 mL is given intravenously over 5–10 min every 2–4 h. It should not be given intramuscularly, at least to children, as it is painful and can cause tissue necrosis. Given intravenously its cardiac effects (which include bradycardia and ventricular arrhythmias) mimic and potentiate those of digoxin, and it should not be given to patients who are potentially digoxin toxic. The precise place of routine calcium supplements in the prevention and treatment of osteoporosis is not firmly established, but it is certainly justified to supplement the diet if intake is below 1 g of elemental calcium daily. Effervescent or chewable preparations of calcium carbonate are available, are easy to take, and can be taken with each meal, thereby delivering 200–300 mg into an acid-secreting stomach.

PRINCIPLES OF TREATMENT OF HYPERCALCAEMIA

Hypercalcaemia may be a life-threatening emergency and is produced by numerous pathological processes ranging from bony destruction by tumour to hyperparathyroidism. In patients with known disseminated untreatable malignancy, correction of hypercalcaemia may not always be in the patient's best interest. When treatment is indicated, it is important to use the time provided by whatever measure is effective in lowering plasma calcium to treat the underlying cause of the hypercalcaemia since the effect of other therapy is short-lived. Management can be divided into the general and specific.

GENERAL MANAGEMENT

This consists of the following measures:

1 maintenance of hydration with physiological saline, and avoidance of thiazide diuretics;
2 avoidance of excessive dietary vitamin D;
3 avoidance of immobilization.

SPECIFIC MANAGEMENT

Increasing calcium excretion

Physiologically normal saline is infused intravenously as rapidly as the patient's cardiovascular state permits. This restores blood volume and causes increased urinary elimination of calcium. Once extravascular volume has been restored, oral frusemide, 100 mg, further increases urinary calcium losses.

Decreasing bone resorption

The following measures are used:

1 biphosphonates (see below);
2 calcitonin (see below);
3 plicamycin (previously known as mithramycin) given intravenously in a dose of 15 μg/kg over 30 min on 4 successive days is often effective. It is a DNA intercalating agent and decreases osteoclast activity. Nausea and vomiting are common complications, and a bleeding disorder (endothelial damage, hepatic dysfunction and thrombocytopenia) and liver dysfunction occasionally occur.

Key points

Management of acute hypercalcaemia

- Avoid thiazides, vitamin D (milk), calcium and, if possible, immobilization.
- Vigorously replace fluid losses with intravenous 0.9% saline. Once replete, frusemide administration further increases urinary calcium loss.
- Give parenteral bisphosphonates (e.g. disodium etidronate or disodium pamidronate).
- Calcitonin lowers calcium levels more rapidly than bisphosphonates, and may be used concomitantly in severe cases.
- Plicamycin can be used in refractory cases
- Glucocorticosteroids should be given only for hypercalcaemia of sarcoidosis.

Glucocorticosteroids

Glucocorticosteroids are useful for treating the hypercalcaemia associated with sarcoidosis.

BISPHOSPHONATES

Bisphosphonates resemble pyrophosphate structurally, except that the two phosphorus atoms are linked by carbon rather than by oxygen. The P-C-P backbone structure renders such compounds very stable – no enzyme is known that degrades them – and allows for a number of analogues. These drugs have been used in the treatment of hypercalcaemia of malignancy, to reduce bone pain in patients with metastatic cancer, to prevent and reduce progression of osteoporosis, and in the treatment of Paget's disease.

Disodium etidronate

USES

Etidronate is active orally, and is indicated in Paget's disease and in hypercalcaemia of malignancy. Etidronate is combined with calcium carbonate to treat patients with established vertebral osteoporosis. In Paget's disease, etidronate is started at low dosage (5 mg/kg/day as a single dose) over 6 months when many patients achieve remission for 3–24 months; a further course may be given on relapse. Use for longer than 6 months at a time does not prolong remission. Higher doses (up to 20 mg/kg/day) should be used only if lower doses fail or if rapid control of disease is needed. Etidronate is effective when calcitonin has failed (and vice versa), and the two drugs may be used in conjunction. Bisphosphonates are indicated for treatment of Paget's patients with bone pain (which responds well), or if there is extensive involvement of the skull or spine with possible danger of irreversible neurological damage, or when a weight-bearing bone is involved or hypercalcaemia develops. Stress fractures in long bones contraindicate the use of etidronate, because of the reduction in new bone formation that it causes. In patients with hypercalcaemia, etidronate is given by intravenous infusion (7.5 mg/kg/day for 3 days) followed by 20 mg/kg by mouth daily for 30 days. It is not recommended for more than 3 months for this indication. To treat patients with severe vertebral osteoporosis, etidronate 400 mg/day is given by mouth for 14 days followed by calcium carbonate 1.25 g daily for 76 days. This 3–month cycle is then repeated and treatment is continued in this way for 3 years.

400 mg orally. OP x 2/52. $CaCO_3$ 1·25 gm x 76/7.

MECHANISM OF ACTION

Etidronate modifies the crystal growth of calcium hydroxyapatite by chemical adsorption to the crystal surface, and it binds to calcium phosphate. Etidronate also inhibits bone resorption and formation, primarily by inhibiting the osteoclast (the exact mechanism here remains undefined at present) and reduces accelerated bone turnover of Paget's disease, returning the histological bone pattern towards normal. Bisphosphonate inhibition of osteoclast activity takes about 48 h to manifest. Second- and third-generation bisphosphonates inhibit bone resorption similarly to etidronate, *but they do not inhibit bone mineralization* as etidronate does.

ADVERSE EFFECTS

Etidronate is well tolerated, and at low doses it has a low incidence of gastrointestinal disturbances (diarrhoea, nausea, abdominal bloating and pain, constipation, transient loss of taste). High doses can cause hyperphosphataemia, but this is probably harmless. Hypocalcaemia is usually mild and asymptomatic. A few patients with Paget's disease (approximately 5%) experience

Key points

Bisphosphonates and bone disease

- Used to treat malignant hypercalcaemia, bone pain from metastatic cancer, and Paget's disease, and to prevent and reduce the progression of osteoporosis.
- Inhibit bone resorption by osteoclasts; etidronate also inhibits mineralization with chronic use.
- Oral absorption is poor; short plasma $t_{\frac{1}{2}}$ and long $t_{\frac{1}{2}}$ in bone; renal clearance.
- Food and/or calcium-containing antacids further reduce gastrointestinal absorption of bisphosphonates.

The commonest side-effects are gastrointestinal disturbances (Note; with regard to oesophagitis and ulceration with alendronic acid, this drug must be taken with water and the patient must be able to stand for 30 min post-ingestion).

exacerbation of bone pain during treatment with high doses, and there is reduced healing of fractures.

PHARMACOKINETICS

Etidronate is given orally, but is poorly absorbed (1–5%). Food and antacids further reduce its absorption. It disappears from the blood extremely rapidly with a $t_{\frac{1}{2}}$ of 30–60 min, primarily moving into bone, where its effects persist. Within 24 h, approximately 50% of the absorbed dose is excreted unchanged in the urine, and the remainder is excreted over many weeks.

The uses and pharmacological properties of bisphosphonates are summarized in Table 38.1.

CALCITONIN

This hormone is a 32-amino-acid polypeptide secreted by thyroid parafollicular C-cells.

USES

Synthetic calcitonin (porcine, human and especially salmon) is used therapeutically to lower the plasma calcium concentration in some patients with hypercalcaemia, and in the treatment of pain and some of the neurological complications (e.g. deafness due to VIII nerve compression) of severe Paget's disease. Calcitonin is given by subcutaneous or intramuscular injection. Recently it has been found that sufficient absorption occurs across the nasal mucosa to enable this route to be employed clinically. This has opened up the possibility of widening its indications to include the prevention and/or treatment of osteoporosis in women at risk, especially those in whom oestrogen replacement is contraindicated. Calcitonin may induce antibody formation (salmon is less immunogenic than the porcine form), but this rarely interferes with treatment (as with insulin antibodies, pp. 420–23).

The two main indications for calcitonin treatment in patients with Paget's disease are hypercalcaemia and bone pain. Calcitonin use has been partly superseded by bisphosphonates in treating hypercalcaemia in this setting. Patients vary in their response, but pain relief usually occurs within 2 months of starting treatment (80 units 3 times weekly usually results in a fall in plasma calcium, phosphate and alkaline phosphatase with reduced urinary hydroxyproline excretion). In patients with nerve compression or severe pain, higher doses (e.g. 80–160 units daily for 3–6 months) may be used.

Hypercalcaemia due to malignancy, vitamin D intoxication, infantile hypercalcaemia or immobilization of patients with Paget's disease all respond to calcitonin. Doses of 4 units/kg/day are used, and in emergencies doses of 8 units/kg/6 h have been given subcutaneously or intramuscularly. Calcitonin is useful in the preparation of patients with severe hyperparathyroidism for surgery, but has no place in the long-term management of this condition. In postmenopausal osteoporosis it may be given (100 units daily subcutaneously or intramuscularly) with dietary calcium and vitamin D supplements if the diet contains inadequate amounts of these.

MECHANISM OF ACTION

Calcitonin produces its hypocalcaemic effects in a number of ways.

1 Its major effect is on bone, slowing osteoclastic resorption and reducing the release of calcium, phosphorus and hydroxyproline from bone. Calcitonin binds to cell-surface receptors which are linked via adenylyl cyclase, and it increases

Table 38.1: Uses and pharmacological properties of bisphosphonates

Drug	Formulation and dose	Oral bioavailability	Half-life	Toxicities	Other comments
First generation					
Etidronate	Oral and IV; for dosing	1–5 % (but variable)	30–60 min	Gastrointestinal upsets; hyperphosphataemia, hypocalcaemia	Used in Paget's disease, osteoporosis and malignant hypercalcaemia
Second generation					
Sodium clodronate	Oral dose 1.6–3.2 g daily in divided doses	1–10%	15–60 min	Gastrointestinal upsets, several cases of leukaemia reported in patients on the drug ? causality	Not widely used due to potentially sinister side-effects. Malignant hypercalcaemia and osteolytic bone metastases
Disodium pamidronate	IV Paget's 30–60 mg weekly for 6 weeks Maximum dose/cycle 360 mg Hypercalcaemia and osteolytic lesions and bone pain: 90 mg every 3–4 weeks	Not applicable	15–60 min	Gastrointestinal upsets; hyperphosphataemia hypocalcaemia	Used in Paget's disease, malignant hypercalcaemia
Third generation					
Alendronic acid	Oral dose: 10 mg once a day with water, stand for 30 min post injection and take before breakfast	1–10%	15–60 min	Gastrointestinal upsets, but notably severe oesophagitis and oesophageal ulceration if taken at night on an empty stomach; hyperphosphataemia, hypercalcaemia	Used in Paget;'s disease, post-menopausal osteoporosis. *Avoid use with NSAIDs*
Tiludronic acid	Oral dose: 400 mg single daily dose for 12 weeks; may be repeated after 6 months	1–10%	15–60 min	Gastrointestinal upsets; hyperphosphataemia, hypocalcaemia, skin reactions	Used in Paget's disease

Case history

A 52–year-old woman has had epilepsy since childhood, treated with phenytoin 300 mg/day and phenobarbitone 60 mg/day, and her fits have been well controlled. Since the loss of her job and the death of her husband she has become an alcoholic. At the age of 54 years she is seen by her local GP because of weakness in her legs, and difficulty in climbing stairs and getting out of her chair. She has no sensory symptoms in her limbs and no sphincter problems. Neurological examination of her legs is normal apart from signs of thigh and hip muscle weakness and slight wasting. Clinical investigations reveal that haemoglobin, white blood and platelets are normal, but her erythrocyte sedimentation rate is 30 mm/h, her blood glucose level is 5.4 mM, sodium is 136 mM, K is 4.6 mM, urea is 10 mM and creatinine is 100 μM. Liver function tests are all normal, except for an elevated alkaline phosphatase of 600 IU/L, and bilirubin is normal. A chest x-ray is normal. Further biochemical investigation reveals a plasma calcium concentration of 1.8 mM and a phosphate concentration of 0.6 mM.

Question

What is the likely cause of her metabolic disturbance and leg weakness, and how would you treat it ?

Answer

This patient has hypocalcaemia with hypophosphataemia and a raised alkaline phosphatase, but no renal dysfunction. This is the clinical picture of a patient with osteomalacia. The aetiology is secondary to her chronic anti-epileptic drug therapy. The mechanism of these effects is complex and relates to several actions of these drugs. Phenobarbitone and phenytoin are potent inducers of hepatic enzyme systems, including the enzymes involved in vitamin D metabolism, specifically metabolism of calciferol to 25'-hydroxycholecalciferol by the liver, and its further metabolism to inactive products. These drugs also impair the absorption of vitamin D from the gut. Treatment consists of giving the patient oral Ca^{2+} supplements together with low-dose 1-α-hydroxy vitamin D (0.5 μg per day), and continuing the anti-epileptic medications if necessary.

intracellular cAMP levels, thus inhibiting osteoclast activity. It also antagonizes the effects of parathormone on bone, thus causing a fall in plasma calcium and phosphate concentrations. The magnitude of the decrease in plasma calcium concentrations is greater during the initial states of high bone turnover (e.g. in Paget's disease or thyrotoxicosis). In normal adults the fall in plasma calcium concentrations are often unimpressive.

2 It promotes renal excretion of phosphate, calcium and sodium. This is less marked than its effect on bone.

3 It inhibits 1–α-hydroxylase and blocks the activation of vitamin D, reducing intestinal absorption of calcium.

ADVERSE EFFECTS

These include the following:

1 pain at the injection site;
2 nausea and diarrhoea;
3 facial flushing (20–30%).

FURTHER READING

Reichel H, Koeffler HP, Norman AW. 1989: The role of the vitamin D endocrine system in health and disease. *New England Journal of Medicine* **320**, 980–91.

Rosen CJ, Kessenich CR. 1996: Comparative clinical pharmacology and therapeutic use of bisphosphonates in metabolic bone disease. *Drugs* **51**, 537–51.

Stern PH. 1980: The D vitamins and bone. *Pharmacological Reviews* **32**, 47–80.

Watters J, Gerrand G, Dodwell D. 1996: The management of malignant hypercalcaemia. *Drugs*. **52**, 837–44.

CHAPTER THIRTY-NINE

ADRENAL HORMONES

- Adrenal cortex
- Adrenal medulla

ADRENAL CORTEX

The adrenal cortex secretes the following:

1 *glucocorticosteroids*, principally cortisol (hydrocortisone) and small amounts of corticosterone – the rate of secretion of cortisol shows diurnal variation. Normally the maximum concentration in the blood (170–720 nmol/L) occurs about 8.00 a.m. and the minimum concentration (< 220 nmol/L) around midnight.
2 *mineralocorticoids* – principally aldosterone and small amounts of desoxycorticosterone;
3 *androgens* (e.g. testosterone, androsterone) in relatively small amounts.

GLUCOCORTICOSTEROIDS

The actions of glucocorticosteroids and the effects of their over-secretion (Cushing's syndrome) and under-secretion (Addison's disease) are summarized in Table 39.1. Physiologically, glucocorticosteroids influence carbohydrate, protein and to a lesser extent lipid metabolism. Their increased secretion also plays a vital role in the human stress response. Glucocorticosteroids stimulate the mobilization of amino acids from skeletal muscle, bone and skin, promoting their transport to the liver where they are converted into glucose and stored as glycogen (gluconeogenesis). Fat mobilization by catecholamines is potentiated by glucocorticosteroids. The major therapeutic uses of the glucocorticosteroids exploit their powerful anti-inflammatory and immunosuppressive properties. They reduce circulating numbers of eosinophils, basophils and T-lymphocytes while increasing the number of circulating neutrophils. When potent steroids are applied topically to skin or mucous membranes they cause local vasoconstriction, and even when given systemically in massive doses (e.g. >1 g hydrocortisone) they can cause generalized vasoconstriction.

MECHANISM OF ACTION

After entering cells, glucocorticosteroids interact with a cytoplasmic glucocorticosteroid receptor causing its dissociation from a phosphorylated heat shock protein complex. This receptor–glucocorticosteroid complex is translocated to the nucleus, where it binds to certain areas of nuclear DNA known as glucocorticosteroid response elements (GREs) and acts as a transcription factor. This interaction brings about increases in the transcription of certain proteins (including the β_2 receptor, vasocortin-1, which reduces plasma exudation from blood vessels, lipocortin – which inhibits phospholipase A_2 reducing the formation of several other inflammatory mediators including eicosanoids of both the cyclo-oxygenase (e.g. prostaglandin E_2, thromboxane A_2) and lipoxygenase (e.g. leukotriene B_4) pathways – as

Table 39.1: Actions of cortisol and consequences of under- and over-secretion

	Actions	Deficiency	Excess
Carbohydrate, protein and fat metabolism	Enhances gluconeogenesis; antagonizes insulin; hyperglycaemia with or without diabetes mellitus; centripetal fat deposition; hypertriglyceridaemia; hypercholesterolaemia; decreased protein synthesis (e.g. diminished skin collagen)	Hypoglycaemia, loss of weight	Cushing's syndrome: weight gain, increase in trunk fat, moon face, skin striae, bruising, atrophy, wasting of limb muscles
Water and salt metabolism	Inhibits fluid shift from extracellular to intracellular compartment; antagonizes vasopressin action on kidney; increases vasopressin destruction and decreases its production. Sodium and water retention, potassium loss	Loss of weight, hypovolaemia, hyponatraemia	Oedema, thirst, polyuria; hypertension; muscular weakness
Haematological	Lowers lymphocyte and eosinophil counts; increases red blood cells, platelets and clotting tendency		Florid complexion and polycythemia
Alimentary	Increases production of gastric acid and pepsin	Anorexia and nausea	Dyspepsia; aggravation of peptic ulcer
Cardiovascular system	Sensitizes arterioles to catecholamines; enhances production of angiotensinogen Fall in high-density lipoprotein with increased total cholesterol	Hypotension, fainting	Hypertension, atherosclerosis
Skeletal	Decrease production of cartilage and osteoporosis; antivitamin D; increased renal loss of calcium; renal calculus formation		Backache due to osteoporosis, renal calculi, dwarfing in children (also anti-GH effect)
Nervous system	Altered neuronal excitability; inhibition of uptake of catecholamines		Depression and other psychiatric changes
Anti-inflammatory	Reduces formation of fluid and cellular exudate; fibrous tissue repair		Increased spread of and proneness to infections
Immunological	Large dose lyses lymphocytes and plasma cells (transient release of immunoglobulin)		Reduced lymphocyte mass, diminished immunoglobulin production
Feedback	Inhibits release of ACTH and MSH		Pigmentation of skin and mucosa

ACTH = adrenocorticotropic hormone, MSH = melanocyte-stimulating hormone, GH = growth hormone.

well as of platelet-activating factor (PAF). In addition, the glucocorticosteroid–receptor interacts with both NF κ B and AP-1 and inhibits them from enhancing transcription of many pro-inflammatory proteins (e.g. interleukin-1, interleukins 3–6, tumour necrosis factor-α, G-CSF, GM-CSF, nitric oxide synthase and adhesion molecules ICAM-1). Thus corticosteroids produce a profound but not immediate anti-inflammatory effect.

ADVERSE EFFECTS

The adverse effects of glucocorticosteroids tend to be common to all members of the group, and will be discussed prior to the uses of individual drugs.

Acute adrenal insufficiency rapid withdrawal after prolonged steroid administration can cause acute adrenal insufficiency, and gradual withdrawal is generally less hazardous. However, even in patients who have been successfully weaned from chronic treatment with corticosteroids, for 1–2 years afterwards a stressful situation (such as trauma, surgery, infection or an emotional crisis) may precipitate an acute adrenal crisis and necessitate the administration of large amounts of steroids, electrolytes, glucose and water. Suppression of the adrenal cortex is unusual if the daily dose of prednisolone is less than 5 mg or its equivalent. The rate at which patients can be weaned off their steroids depends on their underlying condition and also on the dose and duration of therapy. Provided that there is no exacerbation of disease, the daily dose may be reduced by 2.5–5.0 mg weekly down to a dose of 5 mg prednisolone per day. This is then reduced by 1 mg at a time depending on the symptoms and, if very prolonged therapy has been employed, plasma cortisol concentrations measured. These should reach 270 nmol/L in an early-morning sample before steroid treatment is finally discontinued. This may be followed by an adrenocorticotropic hormone (ACTH) stimulation test ('synacthen' test) to further establish adrenal function. After long-term steroid therapy has been discontinued the patient should continue to carry a steroid card for at least 1 year.

Intercurrent illness in patients receiving corticosteroids increases dose requirements and can precipitate acute adrenal failure. With moderate illness it is sufficient to double the dose of whichever steroid is normally being used. It is not usually necessary to give more than 40 mg prednisolone or its equivalent daily. In severely ill patients, particularly when vomiting or electrolyte loss is a problem, parenteral hydrocortisone hemisuccinate, 100 mg 6-hourly, is preferred.

Chronic administration of corticosteroids This leads to iatrogenic Cushing's syndrome (see Table 39.1). This usually only develops when exogenous glucocorticoid therapy is greater than physiological production (i.e. 7.5 mg prednisolone or more per day or its equivalent).

1. Cushingoid appearance.
2. Effects on inflammation – glucocorticosteroids decrease the inflammatory and immune responses, and resistance to infection is reduced. Symptoms and signs of acute infection are suppressed, but spread of infection is enhanced. Thus patients on steroids who develop an infection require vigorous treatment with the appropriate antibiotics. Steroids may increase susceptibility to opportunistic infections (e.g. *Mycbacterium* tuberculosis, fungi, *Pneumocystis carinii*, etc.).
3. Fluid and electrolyte imbalance – some salt and water retention is usual Potassium losses and hypokalaemia can be severe, especially when diuretics are used concomitantly.
4. Hypertension often accompanies glucocorticosteroid usage.
5. Diabetes mellitus (hyperglycaemia) may be precipitated or exacerbated by glucocorticosteroids, and may require the introduction or increased doses of insulin or oral hypoglycaemic drugs.
6. Osteoporosis is a major problem with long-term use, particularly with high dosage. Vertebral crush fractures are common and can occur even after short courses of high-dose glucocorticosteroids.
7. Peptic ulceration – a link between glucocorticosteroid therapy and peptic ulceration remains controversial, as there are few data as yet. Glucocorticosteroid therapy is probably weakly linked with peptic ulceration, but in addition it can mask the symptoms and signs of gastrointestinal perforation.

8 Mental changes – anxiety, elation, insomnia, depression and psychosis may develop. Special care is therefore required in patients with a history of mental illness.
9 Posterior subcapsular cataracts have both been reported with both systemic and high dose inhaled corticosteroids.
10 Proximal myopathy.
11 Linear growth – Prolonged use of pharmacological doses in childhood (e.g. in Still's disease) leads to stunting of growth, but this must be offset against the stunting effect of chronic disease itself (e.g. in chronic inflammatory bowel disease, growth improves as the disease is controlled with steroids).
12 Teratogenesis – animal studies show that glucocorticosteroids taken by the mother affect the fetus. The recent Committee on Safety of Medicines (CSM) experts panel review (1998) of pharmacological (supra-replacement) corticosteroid dosing in early pregnancy concluded that there was no evidence that corticosteroids increase the incidence of minor abnormalities such as cleft lip or palate in humans.
13 Aseptic necrosis of bone.

Hydrocortisone (cortisol)

USES

Hydrocortisone has predominantly glucocorticoid effects, but it also has significant mineralocorticoid activity (Table 39.2). At physiological concentrations it plays little if any part in controlling blood glucose, but it does cause hyperglycaemia (and can precipitate frank diabetes mellitus) when administered in pharmacological doses. This is caused by enhanced gluconeogenesis combined with reduced insulin sensitivity increasing overall insulin demand. Hydrocortisone is given (usually with fludrocortisone to replace mineralocorticoid) as replacement therapy in patients with adrenocortical insufficiency (due to autoimmune, tuberculous or other diseases producing adrenal cortex insufficiency). Clinically stable patients usually need 20 mg in the morning and 10 mg in the evening by mouth, but there is considerable interindividual variation, and plasma concentration profiling throughout the day is useful for individualizing doses. Stressful events (e.g. intercurrent surgery or infection) necessitate increased dosage, and emergency treatment of acute adrenal failure requires intravenous hydrocortisone succinate in

Table 39.2: Relative potencies of glucocorticosteroids and mineralocorticoids

Compound	Relative potency		Equivalent doses		
	Anti-inflammatory	Mineralocorticoid	For anti-inflammatory effect (mg)	Plasma half-life (h)	Effect duration (h)
Cortisol (hydrocortisone)	1	1	80	1.5–2	8–12
Cortisone	0.8	1	100	1.5–2	8–12
Deflazacort (prodrug) (active metabolite-21-desacetyl deflazacort)	3.5	–	24	1–2.5	8–24
Prednisolone and prednisone	4	0.8	20	3–4	12–36
Methylprednisolone	5	0.5	16	2–3	12–36
Triamcinolone	5	0	16	3	18–36
Dexamethasone	25–30	0	2	3–4	36–72
Betamethasone	25–30	0	2	4–5	36–72
Aldosterone	0	1000*	–	minutes	–
Fludrocortisone	10	500	–	0.5h	8–12

*Injected (other preparations administered as oral doses).

high doses (e.g. 100 mg 8-hourly) in addition to large volumes of 0.9% saline to correct hypovolaemia and glucose if the patient is hypoglycemic. Hydrocortisone is also used as replacement therapy in children with congenital adrenal hyperplasia due to 21-hydroxylase deficiency. This suppresses endogenous ACTH which otherwise stimulates over-production of adrenal androgens.

Intravenous hydrocortisone, 100–300 mg 6-hourly, is used to treat acute severe asthma (usually followed by oral prednisolone) or autoimmune inflammatory diseases (e.g. acute inflammatory bowel disease). Hydrocortisone acetate is an insoluble suspension which can be injected into joints or inflamed bursae (5–50 mg intra- or periarticularly) to provide a localized anti-inflammatory effect in rheumatoid or other seronegative arthritis. Many common skin diseases, including atopic eczema, improve with topical corticosteroid treatment, including hydrocortisone cream, which is relatively low in potency and hence of particular use on the face where more potent steroids are contraindicated (see pp. 611–13).

PHARMACOKINETICS

Hydrocortisone is rapidly absorbed from the gastrointestinal tract, but there is considerable inter-individual variation in bioavailability due to variable presystemic metabolism, mainly by cytochrome $P_{450\ 3A}$. It (and all other steroids) are metabolized in the liver (cytochrome $P_{450\ 3A4}$) and other tissues to tetrahydrometabolites that are conjugated with glucuronide before being excreted in the urine. The plasma $t_{\frac{1}{2}}$ is approximately 90 min, but the biological $t_{\frac{1}{2}}$ in terms of anti-inflammatory and other effects is 6–8 h.

Cortisone acetate

Cortisone acetate is a prodrug that is rapidly converted to hydrocortisone in the liver. Thus cortisone is unsuitable for topical use, but enterally it has been given as replacement therapy for patients with Addison's disease or congenital adrenal hyperplasia instead of hydrocortisone. However, it has little to commend it over hydrocortisone, its absorption from the intestine can be unreliable, and patients with liver disease may fail to convert it to the active metabolite, so its use is not recommended.

Key points

Glucocorticosteroids – pharmacodynamics and pharmacokinetics

- They have a potent anti-inflammatory action which takes 6–8 h to manifest after dosing.
- They act as positive transcription factors for proteins involved in inhibition of the production of inflammatory mediators (e.g. lipocortin), and they inhibit the action of transcription factors for pro-inflammatory cytokines.
- Mineralocorticoid effects decrease as the anti-inflammatory potency of synthetic glucocorticoids increases.
- Glucocorticosteroids have relatively short half-lives and are metabolized by hepatic cytochrome $P_{450\ 3A}$ to inactive metabolites.
- Their anti-inflammatory properties allow their wide use in disorders ranging from asthma to auto-immune rheumatological and pulmonary disease, and immunosuppression in transplant patients.

Key points

Glucocorticosteroids – major side-effects

- Feedback of adrenal suppression, reduced by once daily morning or alternate-day administration.
- After chronic therapy – slow dose reduction is needed, otherwise an adrenal crisis is likely to be precipitated.
- Acute side-effects include metabolic effects include (hyperglycaemia, hypokalemia) and insomnia, acute mood disturbances.
- Chronic side-effects include Cushingoid features (moon face, buffalo hump, etc.), hypertension, osteoporosis and proximal myopathy.
- Immunosuppression – susceptible to infection and opportunistic infections.
- Masked acute inflammation (e.g. perforated intra-abdominal viscus).
- Patients on chronic steroid treatment require a 'double-dose' increase for stresses such as infection or surgery.

PREDNISOLONE AND PREDNISONE

USES

Prednisolone and prednisone are analogues of hydrocortisone that are approximately 4–5 times as potent as the natural hormone with regard to anti-inflammatory metabolic actions, and involution of lymphoid tissue, but 0.8-fold as potent with regard to mineralocorticoid effects. Prednisone is almost completely converted into the biologically active form prednisolone, in the liver, and so is less preferable in patients with liver disease. There are no situations in which prednisone is preferred over its active metabolite, and the rest of this account refers to prednisolone alone.

Prednisolone can be used as replacement therapy in patients with adrenal insufficiency, but current practice is generally to use hydrocortisone (the natural hormone) for this indication. The anti-inflammatory effect of prednisolone can improve inflammatory symptoms of connective tissue and vasculitic diseases (p. 231), but whether this benefits the underlying course of the disease is often unclear, and if the drug is used for prolonged periods in high doses, the adverse Cushingoid effects are potentially appalling. Treatment must therefore be re-evaluated regularly, and if long-term use is deemed to be essential, the dose should be reduced to the lowest effective maintenance dose, if possible not more than 5 mg daily, given as a single dose first thing in the morning. Alternate-day dosing produces less suppression of the pituitary–adrenal axis, but not all diseases are adequately treated in this way (e.g. giant-cell arteritis). Prednisolone therapy is considered in progressive rheumatoid arthritis when other forms of treatment have failed, or as an interim measure while a slowly acting drug such as penicillamine or chloroquine has time to act. Intra-articular injection of 20 mg prednisolone or an equivalent dose of longer-acting steroid may be useful, but repeated use carries a substantial risk of damage to the joint cartilage. Low doses of prednisolone (5–10 mg daily) may be symptomatically useful in the short-term management of patients with severe articular symptoms from systemic lupus erythematosus, and larger doses (e.g. 60 mg daily) may be appropriate for limited periods in such patients with steroid-responsive forms of glomerulonephritis, or still larger doses (e.g. 150 mg daily) in those with active progression of central nervous system involvement.

Other diseases where prednisolone is effective are many, and they include the short-term and chronic treatment of severe asthma (pp. 347–8) and interstitial lung disease (e.g. intrinsic or extrinsic forms of fibrosing alveolitis, and some patients with sarcoidosis). Prednisolone is used in some forms of acute hepatitis (viral as well as alcoholic) and chronic active hepatitis, and acute and chronic inflammatory bowel disease (where formulations that are suitable for use include suppositories and enemas to minimize systemic effects) and minimal-change nephrotic syndrome. The immunosuppressant effect of prednisolone is further utilized in solid organ transplant patients, usually in combination with cyclosporin or azathioprine, in order to prevent rejection (Chapter 49). Benign haematological disorders for which prednisolone is indicated include autoimmune haemolytic anaemia and idiopathic thrombocytopenic purpura, and it is also very effective in treating certain haematological malignancies (e.g. lymphoma and Hodgkin's disease; see Chapter 47).

Dexamethasone

USES

Dexamethasone (9–α-fluoro-16–α-methyl prednisolone) is powerfully anti-inflammatory, but is reserved for a few distinct indications:

1 as a diagnostic agent in the investigation of suspected Cushing's syndrome (low- and high-dose dexamethasone suppression tests) *as it does not cross-react with endogenous cortisol* in conventional radioimmunoassays;
2 in the symptomatic treatment of cerebral oedema associated with primary or secondary brain tumours;
3 in the prevention of respiratory distress syndrome and intraventricular haemorrhage in premature neonates by administration to mothers at high risk of premature delivery;
4 in combination with anti-emetics such as metoclopramide or ondansetron to prevent and reduce vomiting in patients who are about to receive cytotoxic chemotherapy.

One other advantage of dexamethasone is that it is virtually devoid of mineralocorticoid activity, so it may be preferred to other agents when fluid retention is to be avoided. In therapeutic use, dexamethasone doses vary, but they range from 2–4 mg given three to four times a day. Alternatively, single daily doses of 10–20 mg may be used effectively. The pharmacological effects of the drug last for 36–72 h.

MINERALOCORTICOIDS

Aldosterone

Aldosterone is the main mineralocorticoid secreted by the adrenal cortex. It has no glucocorticoid activity, but is about 1000 times more active than hydrocortisone as a mineralocorticoid. Adrenocorticotrophic hormone (ACTH) has a minor stimulatory action on aldosterone production, but the main factors that control its release are plasma sodium, plasma potassium and angiotensin II. Pituitary failure, which results in a total absence of ACTH, allows aldosterone production by the zona glomerulosa to continue even though hydrocortisone is no longer released from the zona fasciculata.

Aldosterone acts on the distal nephron, binding intracellularly to the mineralocorticoid receptor which translocates to the nucleus and promotes the synthesis of proteins which cause Na^+/k^+ exchange, increasing intracellular sodium and causing urinary loss of potassium and hydrogen ions. The absence of aldosterone makes an important contribution to the clinical picture of Addison's disease due to adrenal cortical destruction, and results in sodium loss, potassium retention and a reduction in the volume of extracellular fluid. Primary hyperaldosteronism (Conn's syndrome) is due to either a tumour or hyperplasia of the zona glomerulosa of the adrenal cortex. Clinical features include nocturia, hypokalaemia, hypomagnesaemia, weakness, tetany, hypertension and sodium retention. Spironolactone competes with aldosterone for its receptors and is used as a potassium-sparing mild diuretic and to treat primary or secondary hyperaldosteronism (see Chapter 27). Aldosterone undergoes substantial presystemic metabolism in the gut and liver, and is therefore not used orally.

Key points

Mineralocorticoids

- Mineralocorticoids mimic aldosterone's effects on the distal nephron, causing sodium retention and k^+ and H^+ excretion.
- The synthetic mineralocorticoid fludrocortisone, which is effective orally, has 500 times more mineralocorticoid activity than hydrocortisone, and about half that of aldosterone.
- In patients with adrenal insufficiency who require mineralocorticoid replacement, fludrocortisone is used.
- Occasionally, fludrocortisone may be used in the treatment of severe postural hypotension.

Fludrocortisone

Fludrocortisone (9-α-fluorohydrocortisone) is a very potent synthetic mineralocorticoid, being approximately 500 times more powerful than hydrocortisone. It binds to the mineralocorticoid steroid receptor and mimics the action of aldosterone. It undergoes significant (90%) presystemic metabolism, but is active by mouth. The replacement therapy dose in adrenocortical insufficiency in adults is 50-300 μg/day. It is also sometimes used to treat patients with symptomatic postural hypotension.

ADRENAL MEDULLA

Epinephrine (adrenaline) is the main hormone produced by the adrenal medulla. It is usually used in emergency situations such as the management of acute anaphylactic shock (see Chapter 49) and other life-threatening disorders that require combined potent α-and β-agonist (mixed pressor) activity (e.g. bradycardic hypotension in a beta-blocker overdose, post-operative failure to come off cardiac bypass, coarsening of fine ventricular fibrillation in a cardiac arrest).

Key points

Adrenal cortex and medulla – pharmacology

- The adrenal cortex secretes three major hormones.
- Glucocorticosteroids, primarily in the form of hydrocortisone (cortisol), are secreted in a diurnal pattern from the zona fasciculata.
- Aldosterone controls sodium retention and K^+/H^+ ion excretion in the distal nephron, and is secreted from the zona glomerulosa.
- Small amounts of testosterone and androsterone are produced.
- The adrenal medulla secretes epinephrine (adrenaline) and norepinephrine (noradrenaline) in a ratio of about 9:1.

Case history

A 32-year-old man presents after collapsing in the street complaining of severe lower abdominal pain. His relevant past medical history is that for 10 years he has had chronic asthma, which is normally controlled with β_2-agonists, and inhaled beclomethasone 2000 μg/day. Initial assessment shows that he has peritonitis, and emergency laparotomy reveals a perforated appendix and associated peritonitis. His immediate post-operative state is stable, but approximately 12 h post-operatively he becomes hypotensive and oliguric. The hypotension does not respond well to intravenous dobutamine and dopamine and extending the spectrum of his antibiotics. By 16 h post-operatively he remains hypotensive on pressor agents (blood pressure 85/50 mmHg) and he becomes hypoglycaemic (blood glucose 2.5 mM). His other blood biochemistry shows Na^+ 124 mM, K^+ 5.2 mM and urea 15 mM.

Question

What is the diagnosis here, and how could you confirm it? What is the correct acute and further management of this patient?

Answer

In a chronic asthmatic patient who is receiving high-dose inhaled steroids (and may have received oral corticosteroids periodically) any severe stress (e.g. infection or surgery) could produce an acute adrenal insufficiency. In this case the development of refractory hypotension in a patient who is on antibiotics and pressors, and the subsequent hypoglycaemia, should alert one to the probability of adrenal insufficiency. This possibility is further supported by the low sodium, slightly increased potassium and elevated urea levels. This could be confirmed by sending plasma immediately for ACTH and cortisol estimation, although the results would not be available acutely.

The treatment consists of immediate administration of intravenous hydrocortisone, 100 mg, and intravenous glucose (50 mL of 50% dextrose). Hydrocortisone should then be given 8-hourly for 24–48 h together with intravenous 0.9% saline, 1 L every 3–6 h initially (to correct hypotension and sodium losses). Glucose should be carefully monitored further. With improvement the patient could then be given twice his normal dose of prednisolone (20–25 mg/day) or its parenteral equivalent for 5–7 days. This unfortunate clinical scenario could have been avoided if parenteral hydrocortisone (100 mg) was given preoperatively and every 8 h for the first 24 h post-operatively. His corticosteroids should be then continued at approximately twice their normal dose for the next 2–3 days post-operatively, before reverting to his normal dose (his clinical state permitting).

Further reading

Ansell BM. 1993: Overview of side-effects of corticosteroid therapy. *Clinical and Experimental Rheumatology* **9 (Suppl. 6)**, 19–20.

Barnes PJ, Adcock I. 1993: Anti-inflammatory actions of steroids: molecular mechanisms. *Trends in pharmacological Sciences* **14**, 436–41.

Schimmer BP, Parker KL. 1996: Adrenocorticotropic hormone; adrenocortical steroids and their synthetic analogs; inhibitors of the synthesis and actions of adrenocortical hormones. In Hardman JG, Limbird LE (eds), *The pharmacological basis of therapeutics*, 9th edn. New York: McGraw-Hill, 1457–91.

CHAPTER FORTY

REPRODUCTIVE ENDOCRINOLOGY

- Female reproductive endocrinology
- Male reproductive endocrinology

FEMALE REPRODUCTIVE ENDOCRINOLOGY

INTRODUCTION

Three main hormones are secreted by the ovary, namely oestradiol-17β, oestrone and progesterone. The ovary is also a source of androgens, although most androgen production in women is by the adrenal gland. Oestrogens are physiologically concerned with the development of secondary sex characteristics in the female, including breast development and female distribution of fat. Progesterone acts on the endometrium to render it receptive to the fertilized zygote and thus allow implantation to take place. It also causes the mid-cycle rise in basal body temperature. The pituitary gonadotrophins, follicle-stimulating hormone (FSH) and luteinizing hormone (LH) control ovarian steroid secretion. Oestrogens exert negative feedback control on both LH and FSH, whereas progesterone has less effect on gonadotrophin secretion. The hypothalamus secretes gonadotrophin-releasing hormone (GnRH), which stimulates the anterior pituitary to release LH or FSH. Follicle-stimulating hormone stimulates maturation of the ovarian follicle and release of oestrogens, whilst LH stimulates progesterone release from the corpus luteum, and in mid-cycle the sudden rise in LH causes ovulation.

Oestrogens

USES

1 They are used for oral contraception (see below).
2 Replacement hormone therapy at the menopause is effective in preventing menopausal symptoms of flushing and vaginal dryness. It also reduces osteoporosis, slowing or eliminating bone loss at all sites (including the vertebral bodies and femoral neck) in the early years following the menopause. Oestrogen replacement therapy also reduces the risk of cardiovascular disease (stroke and heart attack). There is an increased risk of endometrial cancer, so in women with a uterus a progestagen must be used in combination with the oestrogen during the latter part of the cycle, as this obviates the excess risk, albeit at the expense of side-effects from the progestagen. An effect of oestrogen replacement therapy on the risk of breast cancer has not been proven to date, but there is concern – based on the known biological features of breast cancer – that a small increase is likely, and present negative studies lack the statistical power to demonstrate an increase of a few per cent. Calendar packs of

oestrogen and progestagen are available and are convenient to use: 625 μg or 1.25 mg of conjugated oestrogen is given daily, with the addition of norgestrel, 150 μg, daily for 12 days from day 16 of the cycle. Transdermal patches are also available, but they are expensive and also about 15% of women develop local irritation due to the vehicle. There are theoretical advantages in a route of administration that avoids presenting the liver with a high concentration of oestrogen (e.g. there may be less effect on hepatic synthesis of coagulation factors and other proteins), but currently such patches are not justified for routine use, although they are useful for women who cannot tolerate an oral preparation.

3 Oestrogens are no longer used to suppress lactation, because of the risk of thrombo-embolism. **Bromocriptine** (see p. 168) is used instead.

4 Neoplastic disease – **stilboestrol** is less used for prostate cancer than in the past because of the risks of fluid retention and thrombosis, and because GnRH analogues (see p. 468–9) provide a safer and better tolerated alternative.

5 **Ethinylestradiol** is used under specialist supervision in the treatment of patients with hereditary haemorrhagic telangiectasia.

ADVERSE EFFECTS

Oestrogens commonly cause nausea and headaches. Gynaecomastia and impotence are predictable dose-dependent effects in men. Withdrawal uterine haemorrhage occurs 2–3 days after stopping oestrogen treatment. Salt and water retention with oedema, hypertension and exacerbation of heart failure can occur with pharmacological doses. The risk of thrombo-embolism is increased. Oestrogens are carcinogenic in some animals, and there is an increased incidence of endometrial carcinoma in women following uninterrupted treatment with exogenous oestrogen unopposed by progestagen. Some decades ago, treatment with stilboestrol during pregnancy was commonly employed in women with threatened miscarriage, without evidence of efficacy. An increased incidence of an otherwise extremely rare tumour, namely adenocarcinoma of the vagina, occurred in the daughters of those treated in this way during their teens and twenties (see Chapter 9).

PHARMACOKINETICS

Absorption of oestrogens via skin or mucous membranes is rapid. Synthetic derivatives such as ethinyl oestradiol and diethylstilboestrol are also well absorbed when given by mouth. The most potent natural oestrogen is oestradiol-17β. It is largely oxidized to oestrone and then hydrated to produce oestriol. These three oestrogens are metabolized in the liver and excreted as glucuronide and sulphate conjugates in the bile and urine. Estimation of urinary oestrogen excretion provides a measure of ovarian function. The synthetic oestrogen diethylstilboestrol is as potent as oestradiol, but has a longer action because it is metabolized more slowly. Ethinyl oestradiol is more potent still, and also has a prolonged action because of slow hepatic metabolism, the $t_{\frac{1}{2}}$ being about 25 h.

> **Key points**
>
> Main uses of oestrogen
>
> - Oral contraception
> - Replacement therapy

Oestrogen antagonists

Tamoxifen competes with oestrogen for its high-affinity receptors in target tissues, and it is of great value in the treatment of carcinoma of the breast (see Chapter 47). **Clomiphene** inhibits oestrogen binding to its receptors in the hypothalamus and anterior pituitary, thereby blocking feedback inhibition and increasing secretion of GnRH, FSH and LH. It is used as first-line treatment of infertility in anovulatory women, in a proportion of whom the increase in FSH and LH caused by clomiphene induces ovulation. However, there is an increased likelihood of multiple pregnancies.

Progesterone and progestagens

USES

Progestagens act on tissues primed by oestrogens, whose effects they modify. There are two main groups of progestagens, namely the naturally occurring hormone progesterone and its analogues, and the testosterone analogues such as norethisterone and norgestrel. The main therapeutic uses of progestagens are in the oral contraceptive (either alone or in combination with oestrogen, see below), in combination with oestrogen when this is used as hormone replacement therapy in women with an intact uterus (in order to prevent the increased risk of endometrial cancer caused by unopposed oestrogen action), for endometriosis and (with limited evidence of efficacy) in a variety of menstrual disorders (e.g. premenstrual tension, dysmenorrhoea and menorrhagia). Progestagens in common use include norethisterone, levonorgestrel (which is the active isomer of racemic norgestrel), desogestrel, norgestimate and gestodene, which are all derivatives of norgesterel. These differ considerably in potency (e.g. norgestimate is one-third to one-quarter as potent as gestodene). The newer progestagens (e.g. desogestrel, gestodene and norgestimate) produce good cycle control, gestodene being particularly effective, and have a less marked adverse effect on plasma lipids than the older progestagens. Recent studies have shown that oral contraceptives containing desogestrel and gestodene are associated with an increase of around twofold in the risk of venous thrombo-embolism compared to those containing other progestagens. Hence combined oral contraceptives (COCs) containing these progrestagens should not be used by women with risk factors for thrombo-embolic disease, and should only be used by women who are intolerant of other COCs and who are prepared to accept the extra risk.

MECHANISM OF ACTION

Progestagens act on cytoplasmic receptors and initiate new protein formation. Their main contraceptive effect is via an action on cervical mucus which renders it impenetrable to sperm. Nortestosterone derivatives are metabolized to a small extent to oestrogenic metabolites which may account for an additional anti-ovulatory effect in some women. In addition, a pseudodecidual (pseudopregnant) change in the endometrium discourages implantation. The pharmacological effects of large doses of progestagens include inhibition of uterine contractility, sodium retention and negative nitrogen balance.

ADVERSE AND METABOLIC EFFECTS

Progestagens cause or contribute to many of the symptoms of the contraceptive pill or hormone replacement therapy, including bloating with fluid retention and weight gain, acne, breast discomfort, altered libido, gastrointestinal and premenstrual symptoms. Testosterone-related progestagens (e.g. norethistrone) cause masculinization of a female fetus if used during pregnancy. Several of the earlier progestagens had adverse effects on lipid metabolism. Levonorgestrel if used continuously reduces the circulating concentrations of high-density lipoprotein (HDL) and is therefore no longer recommended when given in this way for women with risk factors for cardiovascular disease. Norethisterone has little effect on circulating lipoproteins, and desogestrel, gestodene and norgestimate cause small increases in HDL, although it is not known whether these potentially beneficial effects are clinically important.

Newer progestagens do not cause clinically important changes in blood glucose levels. Desogestrel, norgestimate and gestodene increase the serum concentrations of sex-hormone-binding globulin and reduce the free testosterone concentration. (These anti-androgenic effects can be clinically useful for reducing acne in adolescent females.)

PHARMACOKINETICS

Progesterone is subject to presystemic hepatic metabolism. It is more effective when injected intramuscularly or administered sublingually, and it is excreted in the urine as pregnanediol and pregnanelone. Norethisterone, a synthetic progestagen component of many oral contraceptives, is rapidly absorbed orally, is subject to little presystemic metabolism, and has a $t_{\frac{1}{2}}$ of 7.5–8 h.

The combined oral contraceptive (COC)

Since the original pilot trials in Puerto Rico proved that steroid oral contraception was feasible, this method has become the leading method of contraception world-wide. Nearly 50% of all women in their twenties in the UK use this form of contraception. It is the most consistently effective contraceptive method and allows sexual relations to proceed without interruption, but it lacks the advantage of protection against sexually transmitted disease that is afforded by condoms. The most commonly used oestrogen is **ethinyloestradiol** in a dose of 35 μg/day or less.

The main contraceptive action of the combined oral contraceptive is to suppress ovulation by interfering with gonadotrophin release by the pituitary via negative feedback on the hypothalamus. This prevents the mid-cycle rise in LH which triggers ovulation.

Progestagens currently used in combined oral contraceptives include **desogestrel**, **gestodene** and **norgestimate**. These 'third-generation' progestagens are only weak anti-oestrogens, have less androgenic activity than their predecessors (norethisterone, levonorgestrel and ethynodiol), and are associated with less disturbance of lipoprotein metabolism. However, desogestrel and gestadene have been associated with an increased risk of venous thrombo-embolism.

Endocrine effects of the combined oral contraceptive include the following:

1 prevention of the normal premenstrual rise and mid-cycle peaks of LH and FSH and of the rise in progesterone during the luteal phase;
2 increased hepatic synthesis of proteins, including thyroid-binding globulin, ceruloplasmin, transferrin, coagulation factors and renin substrate. Increased fibrinogen synthesis can raise the erythrocyte sedimentation rate;
3 reduced carbohydrate tolerance;
4 decreased albumin and haptoglobulin synthesis.

USE

The combined oestrogen–progestagen pill is taken daily for 21 consecutive days, the initial cycle being commenced on the first day of the menstrual cycle. Medication is either stopped for 7 days after the 3-week treatment or dummy tablets are taken, and withdrawal of oestrogen produces uterine bleeding some 2–3 days after the last active dose. The pill is restarted after 7 drug-free days and bleeding ceases. If a dose is forgotten the woman should take it as soon as she remembers, and the next tablet should be taken at the usual time. If she is more than 12 h late she should be advised to use additional contraception (e.g. a barrier method) for the next 7 days and, if this period extends beyond the current cycle, to start the next packet of pills immediately without a 7-day break and without taking dummy pills.

The combined contraceptive pill should be stopped 4 weeks before major elective surgery, because of the increased risk of venous thrombosis. Alternative contraception (e.g. a barrier method) should be used. Oral contraception can be restarted any time from 3–4 weeks after childbirth, but a progesterone-only preparation may be preferred by women who are breast-feeding because progestagen, unlike oestrogen, does not affect lactation.

> **Key point**
>
> Postcoital contraception
>
> Two doses each of ethinyloestradiol 100 μg and lenonorgestrel 500 μg given 12 h apart within 72 h of unprotected sexual intercourse.

Postcoital contraception (the 'morning-after' pill) consists of two doses each of ethinyloestradiol, 100 μg, and levonorgestrel, 500 μg, given 12 h apart within 72 h of unprotected intercourse. The failure rate of this method is 0–3%, but up to 50% of women experience nausea and vomiting (if one of the doses is vomited within 3 h of ingestion it should be repeated). A single dose of **mifepristone** (a progesterone antagonist), 600 mg, is highly effective as a postcoital contraceptive. The abortion statistics suggest that postcoital contraception is under-utilized in the UK.

ADVERSE EFFECTS

The overall acceptability of the combined pill is around 80%, and minor side-effects can often be controlled by a change in preparation. Users have an increased risk of venous thrombo-embolic disease, this risk being greatest in women over 35 years of age, especially if they smoke cigarettes and have used oral contraceptives for 5 years or more continuously. (This increased risk must not be confused with the decreased risk of stroke and myocardial infarction that is conferred by low doses of natural conjugated oestrogen given to menopausal women as hormone replacement.) The increased risk of thrombo-embolism made it desirable to reduce the oestrogen dose as much as possible. Deep vein thrombosis is uncommon with 35 μg or less of ethinyloestradiol, and lower doses or progestagen-only pills are appropriate in women at higher risk of thrombotic disease. Increased blood pressure is common with the pill, and is clinically significant in about 5% of patients. When medication is stopped, the blood pressure usually falls to normal levels. In normotensive non-smoking women without other risk factors for vascular disease, there is no upper age limit on using the combined oral contraceptive, but it is prudent to use the lowest effective dose of oestrogen, especially in women aged 35 years or over. Mesenteric artery thrombosis and small bowel ischaemia, and hepatic vein thrombosis and Budd–Chiari syndrome are rare but serious adverse events linked to the use of oral contraception. These cardiovascular adverse effects are related to oestrogen. Jaundice similar to that of pregnancy cholestasis can occur, usually in the first few cycles. Recovery is rapid on drug withdrawal. Oral contraceptives may affect migraine in the following ways:

1 precipitation of attacks in the previously unaffected;
2 exacerbation of previously existing migraine;
3 alteration of the pattern of attacks – in particular, focal neurological features may appear;
4 occasionally the incidence of attacks may decrease or they may even be abolished while the patient is on the pill.

Other important adverse effects include an increased incidence of gallstones. Early use of the pill for prolonged periods may increase the risk of breast cancer, although this remains uncertain, and there is no evidence of increased mortality from this cause in users of the contraceptive pill. There is an epidemiological association with increased risk of liver cancer, but a reduced risk of endometrial and ovarian cancer. The incidence of vascular adenoma is increased by the combined oral contraceptive, but it remains rare. There is a decreased incidence of benign breast lesions and functional ovarian cysts. Diabetes mellitus may be precipitated by the pill. Amenorrhoea after stopping combined oral contraception is not unusual (about 5% of cases) but is rarely prolonged, and although there may be temporary impairment of fertility, permanent sterility is very uncommon.

CONTRAINDICATIONS

Absolute contraindications include pregnancy, thrombo-embolism, multiple risk factors for arterial disease, ischaemic heart disease, severe hypertension, migraine with focal neurological symptoms, severe liver disease, porphyria, otosclerosis, breast or genital tract carcinoma, undiagnosed vaginal bleeding and breast-feeding. Relative contraindications include uncomplicated migraine, cholelithiasis, hypertension, hyperlipidaemia, diabetes mellitus, varicose veins, severe depression, long-term immobilization, sickle-cell disease and inflammatory bowel disease.

DRUG INTERACTIONS

1 Oral anticoagulants – oestrogens increase plasma levels of factor VII and reduce the efficacy of oral anticoagulants. This is not a contraindication to their continued use in patients to be started on warfarin (in whom pregnancy is highly undesirable, see Chapter 29), but it is a reason for increased frequency of monitoring of the international normalized ratio (INR) if oral contraception is started after a patient has been stabilized on warfarin.
2 Antihypertensive therapy is adversely affected by oral contraceptives, at least partly because of increased circulating renin substrate.

Enzyme inducers (e.g. rifampicin, carbamazepine, phenytoin and griseofulvin) decrease the plasma levels of contraceptive oestrogen, thus decreasing the effectiveness of the combined contraceptive pill. Breakthrough bleeding and/or unwanted pregnancy have been described. Oral contraceptive steroids undergo enterohepatic circulation, and conjugated steroid in the bile is broken down by bacteria in the gut to the parent

> **Key point**
>
> The main mechanism of action of the combined oral contraceptive is suppression of ovulation.

> **Key points**
>
> Combined oral contraception (COC) – adverse effects
>
> - Thrombo-embolic disease.
> - Increased blood pressure.
> - Jaundice.
> - Migraine – precipitates attacks or aggravates previously existing migraine.
> - Increased incidence of gallstones.
> - Associated with increased risk of liver cancer.

Key points

Combined oral contraceptive (COC) – absolute contraindications

- Pregnancy.
- Thrombo-embolism.
- Multiple risk factors for arterial disease.
- Ischaemic heart disease.
- Severe hypertension.
- Otosclerosis.
- Breast or genital carcinoma.
- Undiagnosed vaginal bleeding.
- Breast-feeding.
- Porphyria.

steroid and subsequently reabsorbed. Broad-spectrum antibiotics (e.g. ampicillin, tetracycline) alter colonic bacteria, increase faecal excretion of contraceptive oestrogen and decrease plasma concentrations, resulting in possible contraceptive failure. This does not appear to be a problem with progestagen-only pills.

Progestagen-only contraceptive

USE

Progestagen-only contraceptive pills (e.g. **norethisterone, norgestrel**) are associated with a high incidence of menstrual disturbances, but are useful if oestrogen-containing pills are poorly tolerated or contraindicated (e.g. in women with risk factors for vascular disease such as older smokers, diabetics, or those with valvular heart disease or migraine), or during breast-feeding. Contraceptive effectiveness is less than with the combined pill, as ovulation is suppressed in only approximately 40% of women, and the major contraceptive effect is on the cervical mucus and endometrium. This effect is maximal 3–4 h after ingestion and declines over the next 16–20 h, so the pill should be taken at the same time each day, preferably 3–4 h before the usual time of intercourse. Pregnancy rates are of the same order as those with the intrauterine contraceptive device or barrier methods (approximately 1.5–2 per 100 women per year, compared to 0.3 per 100 women per year for the combined preparation). Progestagen-only pills are taken continuously throughout the menstrual cycle, which is convenient for some patients.

Key points

Progestagen-only contraceptive (POP) – absolute contraindications

- Pregnancy.
- Undiagnosed vaginal bleeding.
- Severe arterial disease.
- Liver adenoma.
- Porphyria.

Depot progesterone injections are more effective than oral preparations. Aa single intramuscular injection of 150 mg **medroxyprogesterone acetate** provides contraception for 10 weeks with a failure rate of 0.25 per 100 women per year. It is mainly used as a temporary method (e.g. while waiting for vasectomy to become effective), but is occasionally indicated for long-term use in women for whom other methods are unacceptable. The side-effects are essentially similar to those of oral progestagen-only preparations. After 2 years of treatment up to 40% of women develop amenorrhoea and infertility, so that pregnancy is unlikely for 9–12 months after the last injection. Treatment with depot progestagen injections should not be undertaken without full counselling of the patient.

ADVERSE EFFECTS

There is no evidence of serious adverse effects associated with progestagen-only contraceptive pills, and the main problems are irregular menstrual bleeding (which can be heavy, but usually settles down after a few cycles), occasionally breast tenderness and uncommonly nausea, headache, appetite disturbance, weight changes and altered libido.

CONTRAINDICATIONS

These include pregnancy, undiagnosed vaginal bleeding, severe arterial disease, liver adenoma and porphyria.

Antiprogestagens

Mifepristone is a competitive antagonist of progesterone. It is used as a medical alternative to surgical termination of early pregnancy (currently up to 63 days' gestation, although it is also effective during the second trimester). The dose is 600 mg by mouth followed by **gemeprost** (a prostaglandin that ripens and softens the cervix), 1 mg, as a vaginal pessary unless abortion is already complete. Gemeprost can cause hypotension, so the blood pressure must be monitored for 6 h after the drug has been administered. The patient is followed up at 8–12 days, and surgical termination is essential if complete abortion has not occurred. Contraindications include ectopic pregnancy. Many women do not find this method as quick and trouble-free as they anticipated. Nevertheless, a large proportion of women who have had both surgical abortion and medical abortion by this method prefer the medical option.

HORMONE REPLACEMENT THERAPY (HRT)

Small doses of oestrogen have been shown to alleviate the vasomotor symptoms of the menopause, such as flushing, as well as menopausal vaginitis caused by oestrogen deficiency. In addition there is now reliable good evidence that giving small doses of oestrogen for several years, starting at around the time of the menopause, reduces the degree of post-menopausal osteoporosis as well as the incidence of stroke and myocardial infarction. However, there is an increased risk of endometrial carcinoma after several years of use which can be countered by progestagen. There is also possibly an increased risk of breast cancer.

For vaginal atrophy, oestrogen can be given as a local topical preparation for a few weeks at a time, repeated as necessary. However, the periods of treatment need to be limited, as again there is a risk of endometrial carcinoma. Vasomotor symptoms require systemic therapy, and this usually needs to be given for at least 1 year. In women with an intact uterus, progestagen needs to be added. Women undergoing an early natural or surgical menopause, i.e. before the age of 45 years, have a high risk of osteoporosis and have been shown to benefit from HRT given until at least the age of 50 years, and possibly for a further 10 years.

In women without a uterus, long-term HRT has been shown to be of benefit, and should be continued for about 10 years. However, in women with a uterus the need for prostagen may reduce the protective effect of low-dose oestrogen against myocardial infarction/stroke.

Although long-term HRT appears to be of benefit, chronic administration has to be viewed against the possible risk of breast carcinoma. Currently the analysis of pooled original data suggests that any excess risk of breast cancer disappears within 5 years of stopping HRT, and women who use HRT for a short period around the menopause have a very low excess risk. Approximately 45 in every 1000 women aged 50 years who are not using HRT will have breast cancer diagnosed over the next 20 years. This increases to two extra cases per 1000 women in those using HRT for 5 years, six extra cases per 1000 women in those using HRT for 10 years, and 12 extra cases per 1000 women in those using HRT for 15 years.

Recent studies have confirmed an increased risk of deep vein thrombosis and of pulmonary embolism in women taking hormone replacement therapy. However, the view is that the overall benefits of HRT outweigh the risk in women without predisposing factors for venous thrombo-embolism. In those with risk factors, the need for HRT should be reviewed and an individual risk–benefit assessment made.

In women with a uterus, oestrogen is given daily at a dose of either 625 µg or 1.25 mg with additional progestagen for the last 10 to 13 days of each 28-day cycle. Oestrogen is subject to first-pass metabolism via the oral route. Subcutaneous and transdermal routes of administration are available and may be suitable for certain women. However, subcutaneous implants can cause rebound vasomotor symptoms, as abnormally high plasma concentrations may occur.

Hormone replacement therapy does not provide contraception, and a woman is considered potentially fertile for 2 years after her last menstrual period if she is under 50 years of age, and for one year if she is over 50 years.

Women under 50 years without any of the risk factors for venous or arterial disease may use a low-oestrogen combined oral contraceptive pill to gain both relief of menopausal symptoms and contraception.

CONTRAINDICATIONS

Contraindications to HRT include pregnancy, oestrogen-dependent cancers, active thrombo-embolic disease, liver disease, undiagnosed vaginal bleeding and breast-feeding. Relative contraindications include migraine, history of breast nodules

Key points

HRT – indications

- Vasomotor symptoms.
- Vaginal atrophy and vaginitis.
- Osteoporosis prophylaxis.
- Cardiovascular prophylaxis.

Key points

HRT – absolute contraindications

- Pregnancy.
- Oestrogen-dependent cancers.
- Active thrombo-embolic disease.
- Liver disease.
- Undiagnosed vaginal bleeding.
- Breast-feeding.

and fibrocystic disease, pre-existing uterine fibroids, endometriosis, risk factors for thrombo-embolic disease and porphyria.

Although caution is recommended in certain other conditions, such as hypertension, cardiac or renal disease, diabetes, asthma, epilepsy, melanoma, otosclerosis and multiple sclerosis, there is unsatisfactory evidence to support this, and many women with these conditions may benefit from HRT.

SIDE-EFFECTS OF HRT

These include nausea and vomiting, weight changes, breast enlargement and tenderness, premenstrual-like syndrome, fluid retention, changes in liver function, depression and headache.

Oestrogens used in HRT include conjugated oestrogens, mestranol, oestrodiol, oestriol and oestropipate. Progesterones used in HRT include medroxyprogesterone, norgestrel, norethisterone, levonorgestrel and dydrogesterone.

Oxytocic drugs

Oxytocin

Oxytocin has relatively little antidiuretic activity, although large doses can cause fluid retention. It produces contractions of the smooth muscle of the fundus of the pregnant uterus at term, and of the mammary gland ducts. It is reflexly released from the pituitary following suckling, and also by emotional stimuli. Any role in the initiation of labour is not established. There is no known disease state of over- or under-production of oxytocin. Synthetic oxytocin is effective when administered by any parenteral route, and is usually given as a constant-rate intravenous infusion to initiate or augment labour, often following artificial rupture of membranes. A low dose is used to initiate treatment (e.g. 1 milliunit/min) titrated upwards if necessary. Oxytocin is also sometimes given as an intramuscular or intravenous bolus after delivery of the shoulders (usually with ergometrine, which acts more rapidly) to prevent or control postpartum haemorrhage. Like vasopressin, oxytocin has a short plasma $t_{\frac{1}{2}}$ (5–10 min), mainly because of tissue inactivation, but a small amount is excreted via the kidney.

SIDE-EFFECTS

The side-effects of oxytocin include uterine spasm, tetanic contractions, water intoxication and hyponatraemia, and uterine hyperstimulation.

Ergometrine

Ergometrine (an alkaloid derived from ergot, a fungus that infects rye) is a powerful oxytocic. The uterus is sensitive at all times, but especially so in late pregnancy. Ergometrine is used in the third stage of labour to decrease postpartum haemorrhage. It is given intramuscularly (200–500 μg: onset about 5 min, duration about 45 min), or intravenously in emergency (100–500 μg: onset within 1 min). It is often given with oxytocin (ergometrine, 500 μg, plus oxytocin, 5 IU), the actions of which it complements. Oxytocin produces slow contractions with full relaxations in between, whilst ergometrine produces faster contractions superimposed on a tonic persistent contraction (it is for this reason that ergometrine is unsuitable for induction of labour). If given intramuscularly, oxytocin acts within 1–2 min, although the contraction is brief, but ergometrine takes 5 min to act.

Ergometrine can cause hypertension, particularly in toxaemic patients, in whom it should be used with care, if at all.

Prostaglandins

Prostaglandins are naturally occurring lipid-derived mediators. They are 20–carbon unsaturated fatty acids containing a 5–carbon (cyclopentane) ring. Prostaglandins are involved in a wide range of physiological and pathological processes including inflammation (see Chapter 25) and haemostasis and thrombosis (see Chapter 29). Prostaglandin E_2 has a potent contractile action on the human uterus, and also softens and ripens the cervix. In addition, it has many other actions, including inhibition of acid secretion by the stomach, increased mucus secretion within the gastrointestinal tract, contraction of gastrointestinal smooth muscle, relaxation of vascular smooth muscle and increase in body temperature. Synthetic prostaglandin E_2 (dinoprostone) is used for the induction of late (second-trimester) therapeutic abortion, because the uterus is sensitive to its actions at this stage, whereas oxytocin only reliably causes uterine contraction later in pregnancy. Prostaglandin E_2 has also been used to induce or augment labour, but oxytocin is preferred for this, because it lacks the many side-effects of prostaglandin E_2 that relate to its actions on extra-uterine tissues. These include nausea, vomiting, diarrhoea, flushing, headache, hypotension and fever. Dinoprostone may be given by extra-amniotic instillation, or by vaginal tablets, 3 mg, which are dipped in water or saline before insertion, followed by a second dose 6–8 h later if necessary. Carboprost is used for postpartum haemorrhage in patients with an atonic uterus that is unresponsive to ergometrine and oxytocin.

Other specialized uses of prostaglandins in the perinatal period include the use of prostaglandin E_1 (alprostadil) in neonates with congenital heart defects that are 'ductus-dependent'. It preserves the patency of the ductus arteriosus until surgical correction is feasible. Conversely, in infants with inappropriately patent ductus arteriosus, indomethacin given intravenously can cause closure of the ductus by inhibiting the endogenous biosynthesis of prostaglandins involved in the preservation of ductal patency.

MALE REPRODUCTIVE ENDOCRINOLOGY

INTRODUCTION

The principal hormone of the testis is testosterone, which is secreted by the interstitial (Leydig) cells. Testosterone circulates in the blood while 95% bound to a plasma globulin. The plasma concentration is variable, but should exceed 10 nmol/L in adult males. Cells in target tissues convert testosterone into the more active androgen dihydrotestosterone by a 5-α-reductase enzyme. An inhibitor of this enzyme (finasteride) has recently been introduced for the treatment of benign prostatic hypertrophy. Both testosterone and dihydrotestosterone are inactivated in the liver. Androgens have a wide range of activities, the most important of which include actions on:

1 development of male secondary sex characteristics (including male distribution of body hair, breaking of the voice, enlargement of the penis, sebum secretion and male-pattern balding);
2 protein anabolic effects influencing growth, maturation of bone and muscle development;
3 spermatogenesis and seminal fluid formation.

Testicular function is controlled by the anterior pituitary.

1 Follicle-stimulating hormone acts on the seminiferous tubules and promotes spermatogenesis.
2 Luteinizing hormone stimulates testosterone production.

The release of FSH and LH by the pituitary is in turn mediated by the hypothalamus via gonadotrophin-releasing hormone.

ANDROGENS AND ANABOLIC STEROIDS

USES

Many cases of impotence are psychological in origin, in which case treatment with androgens is inappropriate. In impotent patients with low concentrations of circulating testosterone, replacement therapy improves secondary sex characteristics and may restore erectile function and libido, but it does not restore fertility. (Treatment of patients with hypogonadism secondary to hypothalamic or pituitary dysfunction who wish to become fertile includes gonadotrophins or pulsatile gonadotrophin-releasing hormone.) Replacement therapy is most reliably achieved by intramuscular injection of testosterone esters in oil, of which various preparations are available. They should usually be given at 2 to 3-week intervals to control symptoms. Alternatively, testosterone undecanoate or mesterolone can be taken by mouth; these drugs are formulated in oil, favouring lymphatic absorption from the gastrointestinal tract. The dose of mesterolone is 25 mg three or four times daily for the first few months, which may subsequently be reduced for maintenance according to the response. Delayed puberty due to gonadal deficiency (primary or secondary) or severe constitutional delay can be treated by testosterone esters or gonadotrophins. Care is needed because premature fusion of epiphyses may occur, resulting in short stature, and such treatment is best supervised by specialist clinics. Occasional patients with disseminated breast cancer derive considerable symptomatic benefit from androgen treatment.

Anabolic steroids (e.g. **nandrolone**, **stanozolol**, **danazol**) have proportionately greater anabolic and less virilizing effects than other androgens. They have generally been disappointing in therapeutics, and have been widely abused by athletes and body builders. Their legitimate uses are few, but include the treatment of some aplastic anaemias, the vascular manifestations of Behçet's disease and the prophylaxis of recurrent attacks of hereditary angioneurotic oedema. They dramatically reduce circulating concentrations of lipoprotein (a), which is a strong independent cardiovascular risk factor, but the biological meaning (if any) of this intriguing effect is unknown.

MECHANISM OF ACTION

Testosterone and dihydrotestosterone interact with cytoplasmic receptors in responsive cells that derepress DNA transcription, leading to synthesis of RNA and new proteins.

ADVERSE EFFECTS

Virilization in women and increased libido in men are predictable effects. In women, acne, growth of facial hair and deepening of the voice are common undesirable features produced by androgens. Other masculinizing effects and menstrual irregularities can also develop. In the male, excessive masculinization can result in frequent erections or priapism and aggressive behaviour. Young children may undergo premature fusion of epiphyses or other abnormal growth phenomena. Other adverse effects include jaundice, particularly of the cholestatic type, and because of this complication methyltestosterone is no longer prescribed. Azospermia occurs due to inhibition of gonadotrophin secretion. In patients treated for malignant disease with androgens, hypercalcaemia (which may be severe) is produced by an unknown mechanism. Salt and water retention is unusual with androgens compared to oestrogens. Oral testosterone preparations in oil cause various gastrointestinal symptoms including anorexia, vomiting, flatus, diarrhoea and oily stools.

PHARMACOKINETICS

Although testosterone is readily absorbed orally, considerable presystemic metabolism occurs in the liver. It can be administered sublingually, although this route is seldom used. Testosterone in oil is well absorbed from intramuscular injection sites, but is also rapidly metabolized. Esters of testosterone are much less polar and are more slowly released from oily depot injections and are used for their prolonged effect. Inactivation of testosterone takes place in the liver. The chief metabolites are androsterone and etiocholanolone, which are mainly excreted in the urine. About 6% of administered testosterone appears in the faeces having undergone enterohepatic circulation.

ANTI-ANDROGENS

Cyproterone

USES

Cyproterone acetate is used in men with inoperable prostatic carcinoma, before initiating treatment with gonadotrophin-releasing hormone analogues to prevent the flare of disease activity induced by the initial increase in sex hormone release. It has also been used to reduce sexual drive in cases of sexual deviation, and in children with precocious puberty. In women it has been used to treat hyperandrogenic effects (often seen in polycystic ovary disease), including acne, hirsutism and male-pattern baldness. Early fears raised by the occurrence of tumours in animal studies (pituitary and liver adenomas and mammary adenocarcinomas) have not been realized in humans, but the potentially adverse effects of cyproterone on HDL and LDL caution against long-term use, and the risk–benefit ratio should be considered carefully before embarking on treatment for relatively minor indications. The usual dose is 25–100 mg daily for 10 days of each cycle, and it is given with ethinyloestradiol to prevent pregnancy. Lower doses (2 mg/day) are used cyclically to suppress sebum production in combination with an oestrogen (ethinyloestradiol) when treating women with severe refractory acne.

MECHANISM OF ACTION

Cyproterone acts by competing with testosterone for its high-affinity receptors, thereby inhibiting prostatic growth, spermatogenesis and masculinization. It also has strong progestational activity and a very weak glucocorticoid effect.

ADVERSE EFFECTS

Side-effects include gynaecomastia in approximately 20% of patients (occasionally with benign nodules and galactorrhoea), inhibition of spermatogenesis (which usually returns to normal 6 months after cessation of treatment), and tiredness and lassitude (which can be so marked as to make driving dangerous).

FINASTERIDE

USE

Finasteride is a 5-α-reductase inhibitor used for benign prostatic hypertrophy. 5-α-Reductase metabolizes testosterone to the more potent 5-dihydrotestosterone. Previously the only alternative to surgery in this condition has been the use of an α-receptor antagonist (e.g. prazosin, doxazosin). Prostate-specific antigen should be measured before starting treatment with finasteride as there is concern that the diagnosis of prostate cancer might be delayed. The dose is 5 mg daily. Adverse effects include impotence and reduced libido.

DRUGS THAT AFFECT MALE SEXUAL PERFORMANCE

The complex interplay between physiological and psychological factors that determines sexual desire and performance makes it difficult to assess the influence of drugs on sexual function. In randomized placebo-controlled blinded studies a small but significant proportion of men who receive placebo discontinue their participation in the study because of the occurrence of impotence which they attribute to therapy. Drugs that affect the autonomic supply to the sex organs are not alone in interfering with sexual function. Indeed, bendrofluazide, a thiazide diuretic, caused significantly more impotence in the Medical Research Council (MRC) trial of mild hypertension than did propranolol, a β-receptor antagonist. Drugs that do interfere with autonomic function and can also cause erectile dysfunction include phenothiazines, butyrophenones and tricyclic antidepressants. Pelvic non-adrenergic non-cholinergic nerves are involved in erectile function, and utilize nitric oxide as their neurotransmitter. Nitric oxide release from endothelium in the corpus cavernosum is also believed to be abnormal in some cases of organic impotence, including that caused by diabetes mellitus. Replacement therapy with nitrates is currently being explored. Some cases of organic erectile failure (including some diabetics) can be successfully treated with intracavernosal injections of **papaverine**, a vascular smooth muscle relaxant, the starting dose being 7.5 mg, increasing if necessary to 30–60 mg. **Phentolamine**, an α-adrenoceptor antagonist, can be added in a dose of 0.25–1.25 mg if the response is not adequate. Intracavernosal and more recently urethral prostaglandlin E_1 alpostadil have also been licensed for this indication. Adverse effects consist of local changes due to the injection, including haematoma, priapism (which may necessitate emergency decompression by aspiration and metaraminol injection), fibrotic changes resembling Peyronie's disease, and systemic effects including hypotension and syncope. The initial doses must be given under close supervision.

Sildenafil, an oral selective phosphodiesterase inhibitor (PDE5), was marketed in the UK in 1998 for the treatment of erectile dysfunction. The NHS funding for the treatment has been very controversial. The drug itself prolongs cyclic guanosine monophosphate (vasodilator) activity, enhancing the erectile response to sexual stimulation. Peak plasma concentrations occur 30–120 min after an oral dose and are delayed by food. The drug is metabolized by cytochrome P_{3A4} and hence plasma concentrations may be increased by concomitant cimetidine and erythromycin. Unwanted effects include hypotension, particularly if the patient is on nitrate (in which case it is contraindicated), headache, flushing and dyspepsia and transient visual disturbances. Since the drug was marketed, sudden death and stroke have both been reported following its use.

The idea that aphrodisiac drugs exist that increase libido is probably a myth, although there is a market for such agents. The use of cocaine, amphetamine or yohimbine as sexual stimulants, as well as more traditional mixtures, has its devotees, but their medical use in the treatment of impotence is disappointing. Cannabis enjoys a reputation for enhancing sexual enjoyment and desire. The reason for this is unclear, but it may be due to a general release of inhibition. Continual smoking of cannabis increases prolactin secretion and lowers male serum testosterone levels. A few cases of reduced libido and impotence in males and females are associated with idiopathic hyper-

Case history

A 26-year-old woman consults you in your GP surgery regarding advice about starting the combined oral contraceptive pill.

Question

Outline your management of this patient.

Answer

It is very important to take a careful history in order to exclude any risk factors which would contraindicate the combined oral contraceptive, such as a past history of thrombo-embolic disease or risk factors for thrombo-embolic disease. In addition, it is important to ascertain whether the patient is a smoker and when she last had a cervical smear. It is important to exclude a history of migraine and to check her blood pressure.

The combined oral contraceptive is probably an appropriate form of contraception in a woman of this age, who would possibly be highly fertile, as it is the most reliable form of contraception available, provided that there are no risk factors to contraindicate the combined oral contraceptive. There are many COCs on the market, and selection for this individual would be dependent on a balance of achieving good cycle control, and weighing the beneficial effects on plasma lipids offered by the newer progestagens such as desogestrel, gestadine and norgestimate against the recently reported twofold increased risk of venous thrombo-embolism noted with desogestrel and gestadine. In a woman of this age the beneficial effects on plasma lipids are probably of minor importance, and in view of the increased risk of venous thrombo-embolism it would probably be appropriate to choose a pill containing norethisterone, levonorgestrel or norgestimate. The majority of women achieve good cycle control with combined oral contraceptives containing oestrogen at a dose of about 30–35 μg; pills containing the higher dose of oestrogen would only be required if the individual was on long-term enzyme-inducing therapy (e.g. rifampicin) or anticonvulsant medication.

Case history

A 50-year-old woman consults you about her symptoms of flushing and vaginal discomfort. She is a thin lady who is a smoker.

Question

Outline the therapy most likely to be of benefit, including the reasons for this.

Answer

This woman is probably menopausal and is suffering the consequences of the vasomotor effects of the menopause as well as vaginal dryness. The vaginal dryness could be treated locally with short periods of treatment with topical oestrogens. However, in view of her other symptoms, a better option would be to start her on hormone replacement therapy. If she still has an intact uterus then it is important to give both oestrogen and cyclical progestagen to protect the endometrium from hyperplasia. Depending on preference, life-style and the likelihood of compliance, either oral therapy or patches may be appropriate. In this woman, who has risk factors for osteoporosis such as smoking and thinness, it may be of benefit to continue the hormone replacement therapy for a period of at least 5 years and possibly longer, although it is important to exercise caution with regard to her risk for breast cancer.

prolactinaemia, and in such cases bromocriptine, 5–10 mg/day, may restore potency. Androgens play a role in both male and female arousal, but their use is not appropriate except in patients with reduced circulating concentrations of testosterone.

Further reading

Khaw KT. 1998: Hormone replacement therapy again. Risk–benefit relation differs between populations and individuals. *British Medical Journal* 316, 1842–4.

McKenna MJ. 1996: Risk of venous thrombosis with hormone replacement therapy. *Lancet* **348**, 1668.

McKinney K. 1996: Use of hormone replacement therapy. Evidence of risk of breast cancer associated with hormone replacement therapy is still inconclusive. *British Medical Journal* **313**, 686.

Marshall T. 1996: Hormone replacement therapy for all? Women must choose for themselves. *British Medical Journal* **313**, 1205.

Price EH, Little HK, Grant ECG. 1997: Women need to be warned about the dangers of hormone replacement therapy. *British Medical Journal* **314**, 376–7.

THE PITUITARY HORMONES *and* RELATED DRUGS

- Anterior pituitary hormones and related drugs
- Posterior pituitary hormones

ANTERIOR PITUITARY HORMONES AND RELATED DRUGS

Growth hormone (somatotropin)

Somatotropin (or growth hormone, GH) is a protein of molecular weight 27 000 daltons, that consists of 191 amino acids. Secretion from acidophil cells in the anterior pituitary is pulsatile with diurnal variation, being maximal during sleep, and is much greater during growth than in older individuals. Secretion is stimulated by hypoglycaemia, fasting and stress, and by agonists at dopamine, serotonin and at α-and β-adrenoreceptors. The serotoninergic pathway is involved in the stimulation of somatotropin release during slow-wave sleep. Secretion is inhibited by eating glucose and protein, and by administration of corticosteroids or oestrogens. The hypothalamus controls GH secretion from the pituitary by secreting a GH-releasing hormone, *somatorelin*-GHRH, and a GH-release-inhibiting hormone, *somatostatin*, which is also synthesized in D-cells of the islets of Langerhans in the pancreas. Somatostatin, a tetradecapeptide, has been synthesized commercially. It inhibits secretion of insulin, glucagon and gastrin as well as that of GH. Somatotropin is an anabolic hormone that promotes protein synthesis and is synergistic with insulin, causing amino acid uptake by cells. Its effect on skeletal growth is mediated by *somatomedin* (a small peptide synthesized in the liver, secretion of which depends on somatotropin).

Somatotropin is used to treat children with dwarfism due to isolated growth hormone deficiency or deficiency due to hypothalamic or pituitary disease. This is often difficult to diagnose, and requires accurate sequential measurements of height together with biochemical measurements of somatotropin during pharmacological (e.g. insulin, clonidine, glucagon, arginine or L-dopa) or physiological (e.g. sleep, exercise) stimulation. Somatotropin treatment also increases height in children with Turner's syndrome. Somatotropin derived from pooled human pituitary glands (obtained from a national programme that involved harvesting cadaver glands) was associated with transmission of Jakob–Creutzfeldt disease. It has been replaced by recombinant human somatotropin made in bacterial systems. Injections should start early before puberty in order to optimize linear growth, and should continue until growth ceases. The optimal dose is not yet defined, but 0.1 mg/kg/day subcutaneously has been recommended, and this should probably be increased during puberty. Its use in children with growth hormone deficiency after epiphyseal fusion is currently being investigated. Replacement therapy with gonadotrophin or sex hormones is delayed until maximum growth has been achieved. The availability of unlimited supplies of pure and safe human growth hormone produced by recombinant technology has stimulated considerable research into potential new indications, including its use in adults with hypopituitarism, and as an anabolic hormone in osteoporosis, major trauma, muscle wasting in the elderly, and heart failure.

Somatotropin over-secretion causes gigantism (in prepubertal children) or acromegaly (when over-secretion begins after puberty). This is usually associated with a functional adenoma of the acidophil cells of the adenohypophysis, and treatment is by neurosurgery and radiotherapy. The place of medical treatment is as an adjunct to this when surgery has not effected a cure, and while awaiting the effect of radiotherapy, which can be delayed by up to 10 years. The visual fields and size of the pituitary fossa must be assessed repeatedly in order to detect further growth of the tumour during such treatment. A drug that selectively inhibits somatotropin secretion and is entirely satisfactory for clinical use has yet to be found.

Somatostatin lowers somatropin levels in acromegalics, but has to be given by continuous intravenous infusion and also inhibits many gastrointestinal hormones. **Octreotide** is a long-acting analogue of somatostatin which lowers somatotropin levels. It is given subcutaneously three times a day, but recently a longer acting preparation for administration by deep intramuscular injection every 2 weeks has become available. Its other uses and pharmacology are discussed below. **Bromocriptine** suppresses somatotropin in a minority of patients with acromegaly (approximately 15–20% of cases are responsive), as well as suppressing prolactin secretion, and is an alternative to octreotide.

Octreotide

USES

Octreotide is a synthetic octapeptide analogue of somatostatin which inhibits peptide release from endocrine-secreting tumours of the pituitary or gastrointestinal tract. It is used to treat patients with symptoms caused by the release of pharmacologically active substances from gastro-enteropancreatic tumours, including patients with carcinoid syndrome, insulinoma, VIPoma or glucagonoma. It reduces the secretion of mediators such as serotonin, vasoactive intestinal peptide (VIP) and glucagon from such tumours, thereby reducing symptoms of flushing, diarrhoea or skin rash, but it does not reduce the size of the tumour. It is more effective than bromocriptine in lowering somatotropin levels in patients with acromegaly, but it is not generally an acceptable alternative to surgery. It is less convenient to use than bromocriptine because it must be administered parenterally. It is also effective in patients with TSH-secreting basophil tumours of the adenohypophesis causing thyrotoxicosis (an extremely rare cause of hyperthyroidism). It reduces portal pressure in portal hypertension, and is effective in the acute therapy of bleeding oesophageal varices. It is also used to reduce ileostomy diarrhoea and the diarrhoea associated with cryptosporidiosis in AIDS patients. The usual starting dose is 50 μg twice daily subcutaneously, increased gradually according to response to a maximum of 200 μg three times daily. Gastrointestinal side-effects are minimized if octreotide is given between meals. Clinical development of longer-acting analogue of octreotide is currently in progress, and a long- acting (slow-release) octreotide formulation in poly (alkyl cyanoacrylate) nanocapsules – a biodegradable polymer – became available recently.

ADVERSE EFFECTS

These include the following:

1 mainly gastrointestinal upsets, including anorexia, nausea, vomiting, abdominal pain, diarrhoea and steatorrhoea;
2 impaired glucose tolerance by reducing insulin secretion;
3 increased incidence of gallstones and/or biliary sludge after only a few months of treatment, especially at higher doses. Ultrasound evaluation of the gall-bladder is recommended before starting treatment.

PHARMACOKINETICS

Octreotide is extensively metabolized hepatically, little of the agent being excreted unchanged in the urine. The plasma $t_{\frac{1}{2}}$ of octreotide is 90–120 min (compared to 2-3 min for somatostatin). Its effects in suppressing hormone secretion last up to 8 h, allowing dosing two to three times daily.

Bromocriptine

USES

1 Suppression of lactation – bromocriptine is effective, but should *not* be used routinely.
2 Hyperprolactinaemia – this is an important cause of secondary hypogonadism in men and women. It accounts for about 10% of cases of secondary amenorrhoea. Milder degrees of hyperprolactinaemia may present as infertility with normal menstruation. Galactorrhoea occurs in only 30% of these patients. Isolated galactorrhoea is seldom due to hyperprolactinaemia. In men hyperprolactinaemia most commonly presents late with symptoms related to the underlying pituitary tumour, although a history of impotence with or without decreased volume of seminal ejaculate is often obtained on direct enquiry. Galactorrhoea and gynaecomastia are uncommon. The influence of prolactin on gonadal function is complex and incompletely understood, but bromocriptine is often successful in the treatment of impaired sexual function with hyperprolactinaemia. The dose required is usually 2.5–7.5 mg twice daily. Pituitary lactotroph adenomas usually (and often quite dramatically) decrease in size during treatment with bromocriptine. Visual fields are measured and the pituitary is imaged at diagnosis, and if a macroadenoma is present they are repeated during treatment. Fertility and cyclical ovarian function are usually restored rapidly. Fetal malformation has not been reported. Nevertheless, if pregnancy occurs the drug should be stopped during the first trimester (it can be restarted later in pregnancy if necessary). Bromocriptine does not cause multiple ovulation (as occurs with gonadotrophins and clomiphene). If a pituitary tumour (usually a lactotroph adenoma) is the cause of hyperprolactinaemia, the tumour may enlarge during pregnancy, necessitating restarting of bromocriptine treatment or surgical intervention. Thus visual fields should be carefully measured during bromocriptine therapy for infertility.
3 Hyperprolactinaemia may also be associated with hypothyroidism and with many drugs, including cannabis, antipsychotic drugs and oestrogens. In hypothyroidism, thyroid replacement therapy corrects hyperprolactinaemia. Drug therapy (especially phenothiazines, butyrophenones, metoclopramide, oral contraceptives and methyldopa) may produce galactorrhoea, which usually ceases when the drug is stopped. If the condition persists, a pituitary tumour should be excluded and bromocriptine treatment considered.
4 Acromegaly – bromocriptine is often tried in patients with persistently raised GH levels following surgery and radiotherapy.
5 Parkinson's disease (see Chapter. 20).

ADVERSE EFFECTS

With low doses of bromocriptine (2.5–12.5 mg daily) the only toxic effects commonly encountered are constipation and nausea. Postural hypotension occurs with initial doses of bromocriptine, which is therefore started at a low dose (2.5 mg) last thing at night and the dose is then increased gradually (by 2.5 mg every 3 days) to the required level. High doses (over 20 mg daily) cause nasal congestion, dry mouth, metallic taste, vascular spasm, cramps in the legs, dystonic reactions, visual hallucinations and cardiac arrhythmias.

MECHANISM OF ACTION

Bromocriptine is a semi-synthetic ergot derivative with dopamine D_2- receptor agonist properties. In addition, it has actions on 5-hydroxytryptamine receptors ($5HT_{1A}$, $5HT_2$) and adrenoreceptors. Bromocriptine stimulates inhibitory dopamine receptors in the anterior pituitary, thus inhibiting prolactin secretion. In normal subjects it produces a small increase in somatotropin secretion, but in acromegalics it suppresses somatotropin release, accounting for its clinical usefulness in this disorder.

PHARMACOKINETICS

Bromocriptine is administered orally, and 90% is absorbed via the small intestine. It is metabolized in the liver, and excretion is predominantly via the bile. The bromocriptine terminal elimination $t_{\frac{1}{2}}$ is 6–8 h. Raised prolactin and somatotropin levels fall within a few hours of starting treatment, but the duration of this effect appears to vary with the original level of the circulating hormone.

Key points

Growth hormone (GH, somatotropin)

- Recombinant GH is used to treat short stature due to:
  - GH deficiency;
  - Turner's syndrome.
- GH secretion is controlled physiologically by:
  - somatorelin (stimulates GH secretion);
  - somatostatin (inhibits GH secretion).
- Somatostatin is secreted by D-cells in the islets of Langerhans as well as centrally, and inhibits the secretion of many gut hormones in addition to GH.
- Octreotide is a somatostatin analogue used:
  - in acromegalics with persistent raised GH despite surgery/radiotherapy;
  - in functional neuroendocrine tumours (e.g. carcinoid, VIPomas, glucagonomas);
  - to reduce portal pressure in variceal bleeding (unlicensed indication).
- Bromocriptine (a dopamine agonist) inhibits secretion of GH in 10–20% of pituitary adenomas.
- Cabergoline (a long-acting dopamine agonist) is as effective as but better tolerated than bromocriptine.

Other dopamine agonists

Cabergoline is an orally available ergoline derivative, that is a potent, long-acting D_2 agonist. It is at least as effective and better tolerated than bromocriptine when used in the medical therapy of *acromegaly* or *hyperprolactinaemia*. Patients are started on 0.5 mg weekly or 0.25 mg twice weekly and the dose is increased by 0.5 mg/week every month until an optimal response in GH or prolactin is achieved. Absorption from the gastrointestinal tract is good, and cabergoline is extensively hepatically metabolized with only 10–20% of the parent drug appearing in the urine. It has a terminal elimination $t_{\frac{1}{2}}$ of 60–100 h. Dose adjustment for age, food or hepatic or renal insufficiency is not generally required. The side-effect profile is similar to that of bromocriptine, although the incidence of adverse effects may be lower. **Quinagolide** is an alternative that may be better tolerated than bromocriptine.

Gonadotrophins

The human pituitary gland secretes follicle-stimulating hormone (FSH) and luteinizing hormone (LH). Follicle-stimulating hormone is a glycoprotein (molecular weight 30 000) which in females controls development of the primary ovarian follicle, stimulates granulosa cell proliferation and increases oestrogen production, while in males it increases spermatogenesis. Luteinizing hormone is also a glycoprotein (molecular weight 30 000) which induces ovulation, stimulates thecal oestrogen production and initiates and maintains the corpus luteum in females. In males, LH stimulates androgen synthesis by Leydig cells, and thus has a role in the maturation of spermatocytes and the development of secondary sex characteristics.

Human menopausal urinary gonadotrophin (HMG), human chorionic gonadotrophin (HCG) and synthetic LH and recombinant FSH (follitropin α and β) are all commercially available. They are used to induce ovulation in anovulatory women with secondary ovarian failure in whom treatment with **clomiphene** has failed. Treatment must be supervised by specialists experienced in the use of gonadotrophins, and be carefully monitored with repeated pelvic ultrasound scans to avoid ovarian hyperstimulation and multiple pregnancies. Gonadotrophins are also effective in the treatment of oligospermia due to secondary testicular failure. They are, of course, ineffective in primary gonadal failure.

Clomiphene

USES

Clomiphene (see also Chapter 40) is used to treat anovulatory infertility. The main problem is multiple ovulation (resulting in multiple births). It has replaced partial or wedge resection of the ovary in treating infertility caused by polycystic ovary syndrome, but must be used with caution in this condition because of the risk of increasing the size of the cysts. For this indication it is given as a course of 50 mg daily for 5 days starting on the second to fifth day of a cycle (or on any day in amenorrhoeic women). A second course of 100 mg/day for 5 days can be tried if this is not effective. Three courses constitute an adequate therapeutic trial.

MECHANISM OF ACTION

Clomiphene is an antioestrogen which blocks oestrogen receptors in the hypothalamus. Thus feedback inhibition by oestrogen is blocked and gonadotropin (FSH/LH) secretion is stimulated.

ADVERSE EFFECTS

These include multiple pregnancy, visual disturbance, hot flushes, gastrointestinal symptoms, breast tenderness, weight gain, rashes, acute psychotic reactions and alopecia.

Danazol and gestrinone

USES

Danazol (see also Chapter 40) is used to treat endometriosis, and has also been used in the treatment of menorrhagia and gynaecomastia. It is also effective in preventing attacks of angioedema in some patients with hereditary angioneurotic odema. It is given starting on the first day of the menstrual cycle in a dose of 100 mg four times a day, adjusted according to response up to 200 mg four times daily, usually for 6 months. It is contraindicated in pregnancy and during breast-feeding. **Gestrinone** (2.5 mg orally twice weekly) is an alternative to danazol for endometriosis.

MECHANISM OF ACTION

Danazol inhibits gonadotropin secretion, and it combines androgenic activity with antioestrogen and antiprogestagen effects.

ADVERSE EFFECTS

Danazol causes fluid retention and hence weight gain. Nausea and effects related to its androgenic action including acne, hirsutism, deepening of the voice, male-pattern balding, cholestatic jaundice and, rarely, clitoral hypertrophy, can occur. Benign intracranial hypertension, neutropenia and thrombocytopenia have also been reported. It adversely affects serum lipids and glucose sensitivity, and its long-term use should be avoided if possible.

Gonadorelin analogues

Gonadorelin (gonadotrophin-releasing hormone, GnRH) is the FSH/LH-releasing factor produced in the hypothalamus. It may be used in a single intravenous dose to assess anterior pituitary reserve. Analogues of GnRH (Table 41.1) such as **goserelin**, **buserelin** and **leuprorelin** are also used to treat endometriosis, female infertility (see Chapter 40), prostate cancer and advanced breast

Table 41.1: GnRH analogues

Drug	Dose and route	Use and additional comments
Goserelin	3.6 mg subcutaneous injection (usually into anterior abdominal wall) every 28 days	Used to treat endometriosis, prostate cancer and advanced breast cancer
Leuprorelin	3.75 mg subcutaneous or intramuscular injection every 28 days	Used to treat endometriosis and prostate cancer
Buserelin	150-μg metered-dose nasal spray in each nostril (300 μg) tds	Used to treat endometriosis. Its use in prostate cancer requires intramuscular therapy with 500 μg tds for 1 week, then continuing on intranasal doses of 300 μg six times a day. *Specialist use only* for pituitary desensitization before induction of ovulation prior to IVF
Naferelin	200-μg metered-dose nasal spray taken twice daily	Used to treat endometriosis. *Specialist use only* for pituitary desensitization before induction of ovulation prior to IVF
Triptorelin	3 mg by intramuscular injection every 28 days	Used to treat endometriosis and prostate cancer

cancer (see Chapter 47). Buserelin is given intranasally (300 μg three times daily), and goserelin is usually given by subcutaneous injection/implant into the anterior abdominal wall (3.6 mg once monthly). In benign conditions use should be limited to a maximum period of 6 months because reduced oestrogen levels lead to reduced bone density in the long term. One rational strategy that can be used to avoid this for indications such as endometriosis is to combine a GnRH analogue with a small dose of oestrogen replacement.

MECHANISM OF ACTION

GnRH analogues initially stimulate the release of FSH/LH, but then down-regulate this response (usually after 2 weeks) and thereby reduce pituitary stimulation of male or female gonads, effectively leading to medical orchidectomy/ovariectomy (a state of hypopituitary hypogonadism) and permitting the avoidance of surgical orchidectomy/ovariectomy.

ADVERSE EFFECTS

Menopausal symptoms of hot flushes, vaginal dryness, reduced libido and reduced breast size are common, in addition to local symptoms caused by irritation of the nasal mucosa. Reduced oestrogen secretion causes a decrease in trabecular bone density, so long-term use of GnRH is not recommended for benign disease.

> **Key points**
>
> Gonadotrophins and GnRH analogues
>
> - FSH and LH are secreted in pulses and stimulate gonadal steroid synthesis.
> - GnRH analogues initially stimulate and then after 2 weeks down-regulate the release of FSH and LH.
> - GnRH analogues (e.g. goserelin, buserelin) are used in the treatment of :
>   - endometriosis;
>   - female infertility (highly specialized);
>   - prostate cancer;
>   - advanced breast cancer.
> - Side-effects of GnRH analogues include:
>   - menopausal symptoms;
>   - reduced bone density (by reducing oestrogen secretion).

PHARMACOKINETICS

All gonadorelin analogues are peptides, and thus they have to be given parenterally. Goserelin may be given as intravenous pulses to mimic the physiological release of GnRH. Depot preparations are available to suppress FSH/LH release (see above). GnRH analogues are cleared by a combination of hepatic metabolism and renal excretion. The plasma $t_{\frac{1}{2}}$ ranges from 80 min for buserelin to 4–5 h for goserelin.

Adrenocorticotrophic hormone

Adrenocorticotrophic hormone (ACTH) is no longer commercially available in the UK. A synthetic analogue of ACTH containing only the first 24 amino acids is available as tetracosactrin. This possesses full biological activity, the remaining 15 amino acids of ACTH being species specific and associated with antigenic activity. The $t_{\frac{1}{2}}$ of tetracosactrin (15 min) is slightly longer than that of ACTH, but otherwise its properties are identical. Tetracosactrin is used as a diagnostic test in the evaluation of patients in whom Addison's disease (adrenal insufficiency) is suspected. A single intravenous or intramuscular dose of 250 μg is administered, followed by venous blood sampling for plasma cortisol determination. There is a small but real risk of anaphylaxis.

POSTERIOR PITUITARY HORMONES

Vasopressin (antidiuretic hormone, ADH) and *oxytocin* are related octapeptide hormones synthesized in the supra-optic and paraventricular hypothalamic nuclei and transported along nerve fibres to the posterior lobe of the pituitary gland-for storage and subsequent release (neurosecretion). Vasopressin and desmopressin (DDAVP) are discussed in Chapter 36 in relation to diabetes insipidus. The use of oxytocin for induction of labour is described in Chapter 40.

Key points

Physiology of the pituitary

Anterior pituitary

Secretes:

- growth hormone (GH);
- follicle-stimulating hormone (FSH);
- luteinizing hormone (LH);
- adrenocorticotrophic hormone (ACTH);
- prolactin;
- thyroid-stimulating hormone (TSH).

Is controlled by:

- hypothalamic hormones (stimulatory/inhibitory);
- feedback inhibition.

Posterior pituitary

Related octapeptides, synthesized in the hypothalamus and released by neurosecretion:

1 Vasopressin (ADH):
   - increases blood pressure
   - causes renal water retention.
2 Oxytocin:
   - stimulates uterine contractions;
   - used in obstretrics (for induction of labour).

FURTHER READING

Chanson P Timsit J, Harris AG. 1993: Clinical pharmacokinetics of octreotide. Therapeutic applications in patients with pituitary tumours. *Clinical Pharmacokineics* **25**, 375–391.

Harris AG. 1994: Somatostatin and somatostatin analogues: pharmacokinetics and pharmacodynamic effects. *Gut* **35** (**Suppl.3**) S1–4.

Loy RA. 1994: The pharmacology and potential applications of GnRH antagonists. *Current Opinion in Obstetrics and Gynecology* **6**, 262–268.

Case history

A 64-year-old man was investigated for worsening chronic back pain and was found to have osteosclerotic bony metastases from prostate carcinoma. Analgesia with adequate doses of NSAIDs successfully controlled his bone pain, and he was started on GnRH analogue therapy with goserelin given subcutaneously, 3.6 mg per month. After 1 week his pain was worse, especially at night, without evidence of spinal compression.

Question

What is the likely cause of the deterioration in his symptoms, and how would you treat him ?

Answer

The most likely cause of his symptoms worsening in the first week of GnRH analogue therapy is the 'tumour flare reaction'. GnRH analogues increase secretion of FSH/LH for 1–2 weeks, causing an initial increase in testosterone. They subsequently produce down-regulation, leading to *decreased* secretion of FSH/LH and hence *decreased* testosterone levels. In patients with metastatic prostate cancer it is essential to initiate GnRH analogue therapy only after several weeks of treatment with an androgen receptor antagonist such as cyproterone acetate, flutamide or bicalutamide. The use of anti-androgens prevents the 'tumour flare'. Thus this patient should be given adequate analgesia and an androgen receptor antagonist (e.g. oral flutamide, 250 mg tds) started at once. Goserelin can then be re-started in several weeks' time.

PART IX

SELECTIVE TOXICITY

CHAPTER FORTY-TWO

ANTIBACTERIAL DRUGS

- Principles of antibacterial chemotherapy
- Bacterial resistance
- Drug combinations
- Prophylactic use of antibacterial drugs
- Commonly prescribed antibacterial drugs

PRINCIPLES OF ANTIBACTERIAL CHEMOTHERAPY

Bacteria are a common cause of disease but have beneficial as well as harmful effects. For example, the gastrointestinal bacterial flora of the healthy human assists in preventing colonization by pathogens. The widespread use of antibacterial drugs has led to the appearance of multiresistant bacteria which are now a significant cause of morbidity and mortality in the UK. Consequently, antibacterial therapy should not be used indiscriminately.

A distinction is conventionally drawn between bactericidal drugs that kill bacteria and bacteriostatic drugs that prevent their reproduction, elimination depending on host defence (Table 42.1). This difference is relative, as bacteriostatic drugs are often bactericidal at high concentrations and in the presence of host defence mechanisms. In clinical practice the distinction is seldom important unless the body's defence mechanisms are depressed. Antibacterial drugs can be further classified into four main groups according to their mechanism of action (Table 42.1).

The choice of an appropriate antibacterial drug depends on the following factors:

1. *diagnosis of infection* – this is usually made on the basis of history and clinical examination supported by appropriate investigations (e.g. chest X-ray, lumbar puncture and bacteriological culture and sensitivities). The site and severity of infection are important factors. The clinical features sometimes necessitate initiating drug treatment before bacteriological results are available (e.g. if the patient is hypotensive or shocked, or if there is neutropenia), and hence the initial drug choice is based on knowledge of likely causative bacteria in a particular clinical setting (e.g. cellulitis

Key points

Choice of antibacterial therapy

1. If practicable, take specimens for microbiological analyses before starting antibacterial therapy.
2. Consider the severity of the illness.
3. Consider the likely pathogen(s).
4. Consider patient factors, particularly allergies and potential drug interactions (see text).
5. Select the most appropriate route of administration.
6. Monitor the response and alter the therapy and route of administration as appropriate.
7. Some drugs require routine plasma concentration monitoring (e.g. aminoglycosides).
8. For most bacterial infections other than those involving bone, joint or heart valve tissue, 5 days of treatment are sufficient.

Table 42.1: Classification of antibacterial agents

Bactericidal	Bacteriostatic	Mechanism of action	Antibacterial agent
Penicillins	Erythromycin	Inhibition of cell wall synthesis	Penicillins
Cephalosporins	Tetracyclines		Cephalosporins
Aminoglycosides	Chloramphenicol		Monobactams
Co-trimoxazole	Sulphonamides		Vancomycin
	Trimethoprim	Inhibition of DNA gyrase	Quinolones
		Inhibition of RNA polymerase	Rifampicin
		Inhibition of protein synthesis	Aminoglycosides
			Tetracyclines
			Erythromycin
			Chloramphenicol
		Inhibition of folic acid metabolism	Trimethoprim
			Sulphonamides

is usually the result of streptococcal or staphylococcal infection). An up-to-date knowledge of prevalent organisms and their sensitivities can be invaluable in settings such as oncology wards where patients are undergoing cancer chemotherapy;

2 *patient factors* – these include age, sex (pregnant, lactating), weight, allergies, genetic factors, renal and hepatic function, immune status and concurrent medication that may cause drug interactions;

3 *drug factors* – these include antibacterial spectrum, pharmacokinetics, adverse effects, drug interactions, route of administration, convenience and cost.

The dose and route of administration also depend on the infection (e.g. anatomical site, severity) and patient factors (e.g. age, weight, renal function). In addition, the dose may be guided by plasma concentration measurements of drugs with a narrow therapeutic index (e.g. aminoglycosides). The duration of therapy depends on the nature of the infection and response to treatment.

Table 42.2 outlines the recommended initial treatments for common bacterial infections.

Close liaison with the local microbiology laboratory not only provides the physician with information on local prevalence of organisms and sensitivities, but also allows feedback on the quality of diagnostic specimens.

The MIC is often quoted by laboratories and in promotional literature. It is the *minimal inhibitory concentration* of a particular agent below which bacterial growth is not prevented. Although the MIC provides useful information for comparing the susceptibility of organisms to antibacterial drugs, it is an *in-vitro* test in a homogenous culture system, whilst *in vivo* the concentration at the site of infection may be considerably lower than the plasma concentration which one might predict to be bactericidal (e.g. drug penetration and concentration in an abscess cavity are very low).

BACTERIAL RESISTANCE

The resistance of bacterial populations to antimicrobial agents is constantly changing and can become a serious clinical problem, particularly if the resistant strain supplants the sensitive one, thus rendering a previously useful drug inactive. Although most multiresistant bacteria have developed in hospitalized patients, the majority of antimicrobial prescribing in the UK takes place in primary care. Resistant community pathogens are also increasing. Recommendations from a recent report of the Standing Medical Advisory Committee included a national campaign to improve understanding of the appropriate use and dangers of inappropriate use of antimicrobial drugs by health professionals and the public. In

Table 42.2: Summary of antibacterial therapy: all treatments are oral and for adults unless otherwise stated

Clinical conditions	Likely causative organism(s)	Suggested treatment
Bone and joint infections		
Acute osteomyelitis and septic arthritis	*Staphylococcus aureus*	Several weeks of treatment necessary. IV treatment rarely required for more than 3 days. Initially IV flucloxacillin *plus* oral sodium fusidate followed by oral flucloxacillin *For penicillin-allergic patients*: Initially IV erythromycin *plus* oral sodium fusidate, then erythromycin and oral sodium fusidate *or* clindamycin IV/oral
Wound, soft tissue, skin and superficial infections		
Erysipelas	*Streptococcus pyogenes*	Benzylpenicillin followed by phenoxymethyl penicillin *For penicillin-allergic patients*: Erythromycin
Cellulitis	*Staphylococcus aureus* and/or *Streptococcus pyogenes*	Phenoxymethyl penicillin and fluxcloxacillin or co-amoxiclav *If severe parenteral*: benzylpenicillin and flucloxacillin or co-amoxiclav *For penicillin-allergic patients*: erythromycin
Impetigo and other skin sepsis	*Staphylococcus aureus* and/or *Streptococcus pyogenes*	Flucloxacillin *For penicillin-allergic patients*: erythromycin
Wound infection after clean surgery	Usually *Staphylococcus aureus*	Flucloxacillin
Wound infection after contaminated surgery	Many possibilites depending on the prophylactic agents	Seek advice from microbiology laboratory
Human bites	Upper respiratory tract aerobes and anaerobes	Co-amoxiclav
Animal bites	Various	Co-amoxiclav
Bacterial meningitis		
Bacterial meningitis	Before smear/culture results are known	All patients should be treated until sensitivity known with ceftriaxone* IV
	N. meningitidis	Benzylpenicillin *or* ceftriaxone*
	Streptococcus pneumoniae	Benzylpenicillin
	H. influenzae	Ceftriaxone* IV
Oropharangeal infections		
Acute ulcerative gingivitis	Anaerobes	Metronidazole
Periodontitis	Anaerobes	Metronidazole
Dental abscesses	Mixed oral flora including anaerobes	Treat by surgical drainage (e.g. extraction). If surgical drainage is delayed, give phenoxymethlpenicillin *plus* metronidazole
Sialadentitis (suppurative-parotitis)	*Stapylococcus aureus*	Flucloxacillin

* Cefotaxime is an alternative to ceftriaxone

Table 42.2: continued

Clinical conditions	Likely causative organism(s)	Suggested treatment
Gastrointestinal infections and enteric fever		
Gastroenteritis	*Salmonella*	Ciprofloxacin
1 Acute diarrhoea (untreated)	*Shigella*	
2 Stool result available and still symptomatic	*Campylobacter*	Erythromycin or ciprofloxacin
3 Treating carriage (e.g. in food industry)	*Salmonella*	Ciprofloxacin orally
Enteric fever	*Salmonella typhi* *Salmonella paratyphi A,B*	Ciprofloxacin orally
Pseudomembranous colitis (antibiotic associated)	Toxin of *Clostridium difficile*	Stop other antibiotics Metronidazole *plus* brewer's yeast *In severe infections*: vancomycin (extremely expensive)
Acute biliary sepsis	Coliforms *Enterococci* Sometimes anaerobes	Cefuroxime *plus* gentamicin initially in severely septic patients. Metronidazole
Respiratory tract infections		
β-Haemolytic streptococcus Lancefield Group A will be referred to as *Streptococcus pyogenes*		
Pharyngitis	Virus	Most infections are viral and require symtomatic treatment only
Tonsillitis	*Streptococcus pyogenes* (occasionally resistant to erythromycin)	Phenoxymethylpenicillin or amoxycillin Avoid amoxycillin in young adults where glandular fever is a possible diagnosis *For penicillin-allergic patients*: erythromycin
Acute otitis media Sinusitis	*Streptococcus pyogenes* *H. influenzae* *Streptococcus pneumoniae*	amoxycillin If penicillin allergic: erythromycin Doxycycline is an alternative in sinusitis
Chronic bronchitis		
For guidelines for chronic obstructive pulmonary disease (COPD) see Chapter 32		
Patients with acute asthma		Usually there is no acute bacterial infection and treatment with an antibiotic is not needed
Acute exacerbation in patients with COPD	*H. influenzae* *M. catarrhalis* *Streptococcus pneumoniae*	First choice is oral amoxycillin *Penicillin-allergic patients or those with impared renal function*: doxycycline or ciprofloxacin
Patients with bronchiectasis	*H. influenzae* *M. catarrhalis* *Streptococcus pneumoniae* *Pseudomonas aeroginosa*	Seek advice from respiratory physicians Sputum culture is essential

Pneumonia		
Community-acquired presumptive pneumococcus (i.e. lobar) and not severely ill	*Streptococcus pneumoniae*	Amoxycillin *If penicillin-allergic*: erythromycin
Community acquired pneumonia, severely ill	*Streptococcus pneumoniae* *Mycoplasma* *Legionella* *Staphylococcus aureus* Many other possibilities	Initially erythromycin 1 g IV 6-hourly *plus* cefuroxime 1.5 g IV 8-hourly until pathogen is known. flucloxacillin if Staphylococcus is suspected
Pneumonia in the immunosuppressed	Wide variety of organisms including Gram-negative organisms, anaerobes and fungi	Microbiological diagnosis is essential
Hospital-acquired pneumonia	Many pathogens possible	Broad-spectrum cephalosporin (e.g. ceftazidime) or antipseudomonal penicillin (e.g. azlocillin) and aminoglycoside (e.g. gentamicin) Microbiological diagnosis is essential
Genito-urinary infections		
In hospital a urine specimen should be sent for microscopy and culture before treatment. If there is likely to be a delay in delivery, refrigerate the sample.		
Urinary tract infection in women	*E. coli* *Staphylococcus saprophyticus*	Cefadroxil or norfloxacin
In pregnancy		Prompt treatment is required to prevent progression to acute pyelonephritis. Oral cefadroxil should be given. Avoid trimethoprim, quinolones and tetracycline
Acute pyelonephritis	*E. coli*	The severely ill may need parenteral therapy with a broad-spectrum antibiotic such as cefuroxime. An oral 4-quinolone may be appropriate. Seek advice from microbiology laboratory. Requires treatment for 2 weeks
Urinary tract infection in men	*E. coli*	Often related to urological abnormality (e.g. prostate) and may require further investigation. Trimethoprim or a 4-quinolone is usually effective for urinary tract infection/prostatitis. The latter requires prolonged treatment and consultation with urologist/microbiology laboratory

Table 42.2: continued

Clinical conditions	Likely causative organism(s)	Suggested treatment
Catheter-associated urinary tract infection	Variety of organisms, usually multiply resistant	Seldom requires treatment unless instrumentation or catheter change in proven urinary tract infection. A single IV or IM dose of gentamicin, according to sensitivity, should be given before the procedure Avoid treating bacteria just because they have been isolated unless the patient is symptomatic Remove the catheter if possible and repeat the sample
Urethritis	*Neisseria gonorrhoeae*	Refer to genito-urinary medicine department. Amoxycillin and probenecid are usually effective. For penicillin-allergic patients: spectinomycin or a quinolone are alternatives
	Chlamydia	Uncomplicated infections: Doxycycline or erythromycin
Syphilis	*Treponema pallidum*	Procaine penicillin for 10–21 days *For penicillin-allergic patients*: tetracycline, doxycline or erythromycin for 14–21 days
Cardiovascular system		
Endocarditis	Many	See *British National Formulary*/local guidelines
	Penicillin-sensitive streptococci (e.g. *Streptococcus viridans*)	Benzylpenicillin (vancomycin if penicillin-allergic) and low-dose gentamicin

addition to emphasizing the value of prescribing guidelines, the report identified areas which could have an immediate effect on the volume of antimicrobials prescribed:

1 no prescribing of antibiotics for coughs and colds or viral sore throats;
2 limit prescribing for uncomplicated cystitis to 3 days for otherwise fit women; and
3 limit prescribing of antibiotics over the telephone to exceptional cases.

Antimicrobial resistance is particularly common in intensive-care units and transplant units where the use of antimicrobial agents is frequent and the patients may be immunocompromised.

The evolution of drug resistance arises by either of two processes:

1 selection of naturally resistant strains (which have arisen by spontaneous mutation) that exist within the bacterial population by elimination of the sensitive strain by therapy or environmental contamination. Thus the incidence of drug resistance is related to the prescription of that drug. The hospital environment with intensive and widespread use of broad-spectrum antibacterials is particularly likely to promote the selection of resistant organisms;
2 transfer of resistance between organisms can occur by transfer of naked DNA (transforma-

Key points

The prescriber can minimize bacterial resistance by:

1 avoiding unnecessary prescription of antimicrobial drugs – this requires education not only of health professionals but also of the general public;
2 use of an adequate dose for an appropriate length of time;
3 restriction of certain drugs (e.g. amikacin) for specific clinical and bacteriological indications;
4 use of drug combinations in selected circumstances (especially tuberculosis; see Chapter 43).

tion), by conjugation with direct cell-to-cell transfer of extrachromosomal DNA (plasmids), or by passage of the information by bacteriophage (transduction). In this way transfer of genetic information concerning drug resistance (frequently to a group of several antibiotics simultaneously) may occur between species.

Mechanisms of drug resistance can be broadly divided into three groups:

1 inactivation of the antimicrobial agent either by disruption of its chemical structure (e.g. penicillinase) or by addition of a modifying group that inactivates the drug (e.g. chloramphenicol, inactivated by acetylation);
2 restriction of entry of the drug into the bacterium by altered permeability (e.g. sulphonamides, tetracycline);
3 modification of the bacterial target – this may take the form of an enzyme with reduced affinity for an inhibitor (e.g. sulphonamide), or an altered organelle with reduced drug-binding properties (e.g. erythromycin and bacterial ribosomes).

Key points

Antibacterial resistance in the UK.

- Methicillin-resistant *Staphylococcus aureus* (MRSA) is a major problem in the UK.
- **Vancomycin** and **teicoplanin** were the mainstay of treatment of MRSA, but some *Staphylococcus aureus* isolates are now displaying resistance to these agents.
- The prevalance of resistant pneumococci has increased from 0.3% in 1989 to 7.5% in 1997.
- Enterococci are a particular problem in immunocompromised patients. They are intrinsically resistant to quinolones and cephalosporins. Resistant strains of Gram-negative bacteria such as *E.coli*, *Klebsiella* and *Proteus* are also a particular problem in the immunocompromised patient.

Key points

Hazards of inappropriate antibacterial drug use

- Development of resistant organisms.
- Superinfections, (e.g. broad-spectrum antibiotics leading to *Clostridium difficile* superinfection with subsequent life-threatening pseudomembranous colitis).
- Adverse drug effects.
- Obscuring the correct diagnosis.
- Cost.

It should be remembered that the commonest cause of pyrexia is a viral infection, and that antibiotics not uncommonly cause fever as an adverse effect.

DRUG COMBINATIONS

Most infections can be treated with a single agent. However, there are four main situations in which more than one antibacterial drug is prescribed concurrently:

1 to achieve broad antimicrobial activity in critically ill patients with an undefined infection (e.g. aminoglycoside plus a penicillin to treat septicaemia);
2 to treat mixed bacterial infections (e.g. following perforation of the bowel) in cases where no single agent would affect all of the bacteria present;
3 to prevent the emergence of resistance (e.g. in treating tuberculosis; see Chapter 43);
4 to achieve an additive or synergistic effect (e.g. use of co-trimoxazole in the treatment of *Pneumocystis carinii* pneumonia).

Prophylactic use of antibacterial drugs

There are a limited number of occasions when it is appropriate to use antibacterial drugs prophylactically. Wherever possible a suitable specific narrow-spectrum drug should be used. A summary of the common indications and drugs used for prophylactic therapy is given in Table 42.3.

Antibiotic prophylaxis of infective endocarditis

The guidelines shown in Figure 42.1 are based on the Working Party Report of the British Society for Antimicrobial Chemotherapy.

In addition to prophylactic antibiotics, the use of chlorhexidine 0.2% mouthwash 5 min before the procedure may be a useful supplementary measure.

Key points

Prevention of post-splenectomy infection

Beware *Streptococcus pneumoniae*, *Haemophilus influenzae*, *Neisseria meningitis*, malaria.

- Explain the risk to the patient – provide a warning card.
- Vaccinations (pneumovax, influenza vaccine, HIB vaccine, with or without meningococcal vaccine) but should not be given during chemotherapy/immunosuppressant therapy.
- Antibiotic prophylaxis – phenoxymethyl penicillin or erythromycin up to 15 years of age, then give a supply of amoxycillin or erythromycin to start if there is febrile illness, and seek medical advice.
- Malarial prophylaxis – travel.

Patients at risk

Patients at risk are those with congenital or acquired cardiac defects causing turbulent flow from high to

Table 42.3: Prophylactic antibiotics in medicine

Indications	Common pathogen	Recommendation
Neutropenic patients		Check local guidelines
Meningococcal disease: (very close contacts only)	*Meningitidis*	Ciprofloaxacin as a single dose (unlicensed indication) *or* rifampicin twice daily for 2 days (patient should be counselled on side-effects and interactions) Pregnant contacts can be given Ceftriaxone IM as a single dose (unlicensed indication)
Prevention of secondary case of diphtheria	*Diphtheriae*	Erythromycin
Sickle-cell disease or splenectomy patients	*Streptococcus pneumoniae* *Meningitidis influenzae*	Warning card should be given to all patients Note: check pneumococcal vaccination status
Recurrent cystitis	*Staphylococcus saprophyticus, coli*	Single dose at night of trimethoprin *or* nitrofurantoin *or* cranberry juice, 200–300 mL
Tetanus-prone wound	Prevention of tetanus and secondary infection	Immunized patients should have a booster dose of toxoid (unless this has already been given in the last 10 years). Extensive or dirty wounds will require human tetanus immunoglobulin (HTIG) plus antibiotics as below Non-immunized patients should have human tetanus immunoglobulin (HTIG) and a course of absorbed tetanus toxoid *plus* phenoxymethylpenicillin or amoxycillin for 5 days (in the event of delay or sepsis) *Penicillin-allergic patients*: erythromycin for 5 days

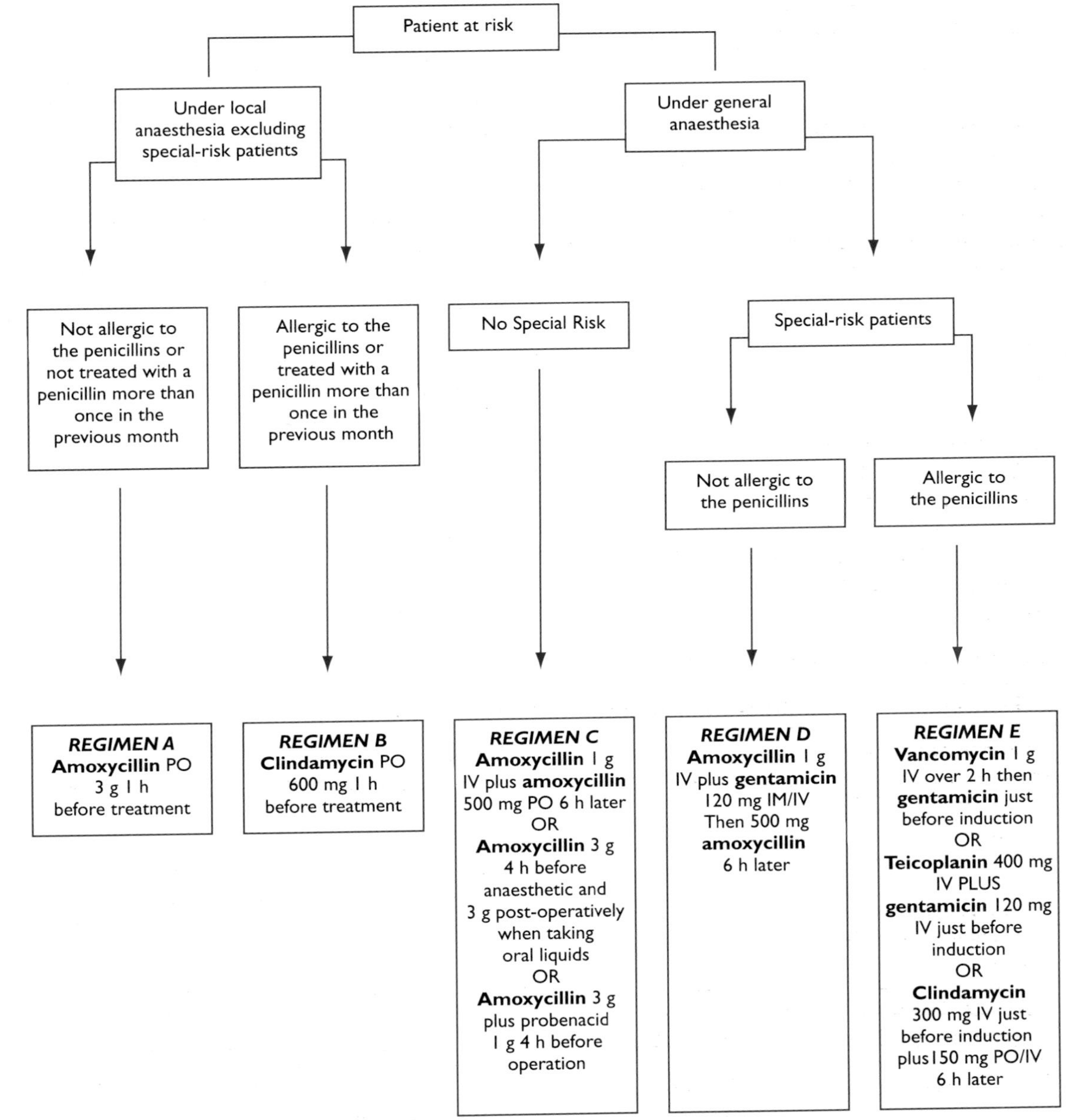

Figure 42.1 British Society for Antimicrobial Chemotherapy guidelines on antibiotic prophylactic regimens recommended for dental treatment. These guidelines are based on the Working Party Report of the British Society for Antimicrobial Chemotherapy (published in *Lancet* 1990: **i**, 88–9 and revised in *Lancet* 1992: **339,** 1292–3 and again in *Journal of Antimicrobial Chemotherapy* 1993: **31**, 437–53).

low pressure chambers, (e.g. small ventricular septal defect (VSD), but not atrial septal defect (ASD)), those with prosthetic heart valves, pacemakers or prosthetic joint replacements, those with a past history of infective endocarditis, drug addicts and alcoholics. Patients with a history of coronary thrombosis or cardiac surgery of the coronary artery graft type do not normally require cover.

Procedures to be covered

DENTAL TREATMENT

With regard to dental extractions, deep scaling and periodontal surgery, plan the dental treatment carefully in order to reduce the need for antibiotic cover. A patient at risk should normally be advised to have dubious teeth extracted, and to maintain meticulous dental hygiene. As much treatment as possible is performed under the same antibiotic cover.

OTHER PROCEDURES

See Table 42.4 and Figure 42.1.

- Oral amoxycillin should be given under supervision 1 h before the procedure and 6 h after the procedure, unless otherwise stated.
- Give IM and IV antibiotics immediately before the procedure (vancomycin should be infused over 100 min and followed by gentamicin. IV teicoplanin or clindamycin should be given at the time of induction of anaesthesia or 30 min before the dental procedure).
- Oral clindamycin should be given as a single dose 1 h before the procedure.
- IV clindamycin should be given in 50 mL of 0.9% sodium chloride or 5% dextrose and administered over 10 min.

SPECIAL-RISK PATIENTS

Special-risk patients include the following:

1 those who need a general anaesthetic and have received a penicillin more than once in the previous month, or who have a prosthetic valve or are allergic to penicillin;
2 all patients who have previously had endocarditis. Warning/information cards are available from most microbiology departments for patients who are at risk.

PROPHYLACTIC PRE-OPERATIVE ANTIBIOTICS

General principles

1 Prophylaxis should be used in cases where the procedure commonly leads to infection, or if infection, although rare, would be expected to have devastating results.
2 The antimicrobial agent should be bactericidal and directed against the likely pathogen.
3 The aim is to provide high plasma and tissue concentrations of an appropriate drug at the time of bacterial contamination. Intramuscular injections can usually be given with the premedication or intravenous injections at the time of induction. The duration of treatment should be short – usually not more than 48 h. Many problems in this area arise because of failure to discontinue 'prophylactic' antibiotics, a mistake that is easily made by a busy junior house-surgeon who does not want to take responsibility for changing a prescription for a patient who is apparently doing well post-operatively. Local hospital drug and therapeutics committees can help considerably by

Table 42.4: British Society for Antimicrobial Chemotherapy recommendations for other procedures

Procedure	Valve	Regimen (as in diagram for dental treatment)
Genito-urinary instrumentation	Native valve or prosthetic valve	No penicillin allergy: regimen D Penicillin allergy: regimen E
Obstetric/gynaecological procedures (including intrauterine device insertion)	Prosthetic valves only	As above
Gastrointestinal endoscopy, barium enema	Prosthetic valves only	As above
Tonsillectomy/adenoidectomy	Native valve	No penicillin allergy: regimen C Penicillin allergy: regimen E
	Prosthetic valve	No penicillin allergy: regimen D Penicillin allergy: regimen E

instituting sensible guidelines on the duration of prophylactic antibiotics.

4 Change to oral therapy as soon as possible post-operatively.
5 Administer metronidazole rectally whenever possible, instead of using the more expensive intravenous formulation, which is no more effective.

Table 42.5 summarizes the use of antibacterial drugs pre-operatively.

COMMONLY PRESCRIBED ANTIBACTERIAL DRUGS

β-LACTAM ANTIBIOTICS

This group is so named because each member contains a β-lactam ring. This can be broken down by β-lactamase enzymes produced by bacteria, notably by many strains of *Staphylococcus* and by

Table 42.5: Prophylactic pre-operative antibiotics

Indications	Common pathogens	Recommendation
1 Dirty/contaminated surgery	Anaerobes Coliforms	Cefuroxime IV at induction followed by 2 × IV doses at 8 and 16 h post-operatively *plus* metronidazole IV at induction and 2 doses at 8 and 16 h post-operatively
Elective colorectal surgery Head and neck surgery Upper gastrointestinal surgery Vaginal hysterectomy Caesarian section	Anaerobes	Note: *post-operative doses* are given at 8 and 16 h after operation
Suspected acute appendicitis	Non-sporing anaerobes Coliforms	Metronidazole suppositories (4 h before surgery) and cefuroxime IV at induction
2 Orthopaedic implants Vascular prosthetic surgery	*Staphylococcus aureus* Coliforms Coagulase-negative staphylococci	Cefuroxime IV at induction followed by 2 × IV doses at 8 and 16 h post-operatively
Cardiac surgery	*Staphylococcus aureus* Coliforms Coagulase-negative staphylococci	Cefuroxime IV for three doses
3 Urological procedure where there is bacteriuria (e.g. cystopy)	Coliforms *P. aeruginosa*	To prevent bacteraemia, gentamicin as a single IV dose
4 Transurethral resection of the prostate	Coliforms *P. aeruginosa*	Gentamicin IV single dose *after* procedure *plus* norfloxacin PO twice daily for 3 days (*Note*: norfloxacin is not licensed for this indication)
5 Transrectal biopsy	Anaerobes Coliforms	Gentamicin IV *plus* metronidazole PR as single doses before procedure *or* cefuroxime IV and metronidazole PR followed by norfloxacin PO twice daily for 3 days (*Note*: norfloxacin is not licensed for this indication
6 ERCP	Coliforms Enterococci	Amoxycillin orally/IV and gentamicin IV both for 3 doses only
7 CSF leak	Many possibilities	Prophylactic antibiotic not recommended. Monitor closely for signs and symptoms of meningitis

Key points

β-Lactam antibiotics

Penicillins	Comment
■ Benzylpenicillin	Narrow spectrum, parenteral only
■ Phenoxymethylpencillin	Oral
■ Flucloxacillin	β-Lactamase-resitant
■ Amoxycillin/ampicillin	Extended range
■ Co-amoxiclav	Extended range and β-lactamase resistant
■ Piperacillin	Anti-*Pseudomonas*
■ **Cephalosporins**	10% cross-sensitivity
■ Cefadroxil	Oral
■ Cefuroxime	Broad spectrum and lactamase resistant
■ Ceftriaxone/cefotaxime	Severe sepsis, penetrates blood–brain barrier well, greater activity against Gram-negative pathogens, less activity against *Staphylococcus aureus*
■ **Carbapenems**	
■ Imipenem (and cilastatin)	Very broad spectrum, imipenem is partially inactivated in the kidney by enzymatic activity; cilastatin, a specific enzyme inhibitor, blocks its renal metabolism
■ **Monobactams**	
■ Aztreonam	Narrow spectrum, Gram-negative aerobic bacteria

Haemophilus influenzae, which are thereby resistant. β-Lactam antibiotics kill bacteria by inhibiting bacterial cell wall synthesis. Penicillins are excreted in the urine. Probenecid blocks the renal tubular excretion of penicillin. This interaction may be used therapeutically to produce higher and more prolonged blood concentrations of penicillin. Antibiotics in this group include the penicillins, monobactams, carbapenems and cephalosporins.

Penicillins

USE

Benzylpenicillin (penicillin G) is the drug of choice for streptococcal, pneumococcal, gonococcal and meningococcal infections, and also for anthrax, diphtheria, gas gangrene, leptospirosis, syphilis, tetanus, yaws, and the treatment of Lyme disease in children. Benzylpenicillin is inactivated by gastric acid.

ADVERSE EFFECTS

1. Anaphylaxis can occur (1 in 100 000 injections); therefore always enquire about previous reactions before administration.
2. Skin rashes, usually morbilliform, occur in 3–5% of patients, and are rarely severe, but Stevens–Johnson syndrome can occur.
3. Serum sickness – type III hypersensitivity.
4. In renal failure, accumulation of the drug can rarely cause encephalopathy and fits, haemolytic anaemia and thrombocytopenia.

The main shortcomings of benzylpenicillin are as follows:

1. It is acid labile and so must be given parenterally (inactivated in gastric acid).
2. It has a short half-life, so frequent injections are required.
3. Development of resistant β-lactamase-producing strains can occur.
4. It has a narrow antibacterial spectrum.

Two preparations with similar antibacterial spectra are used to overcome the problems of acid lability/frequent injection:

1. *procaine penicillin* – this complex releases penicillin slowly from an intramuscular site, so a twice daily dosage only is required. **Bicillin**® is

a combination of benzyl penicillin and procaine penicillin for intramuscular administration.

2 *phenoxymethylpenicillin* – this is acid stable and so is effective when given orally (40–60% absorption). Although it is useful for mild infections, blood concentrations are variable, so it is not used in serious infections or with poorly sensitive bacteria. Tablets are given on an empty stomach to improve absorption.

β-LACTAMASE-RESISTANT PENICILLIN

Flucloxacillin was developed to overcome β-lactamase-producing strains. It has a similar antibacterial spectrum to benzylpenicillin, but is less potent. However, the lactam ring is not exposed and it is effective against β-lactamase-producing organisms. It is used for the treatment of staphylococcal infections (90% of hospital staphylococci are resistant to benzylpenicillin, and 5–10% are resistant to flucloxacillin).

EXTENDED-RANGE PENICILLINS

Ampicillin/amoxycillin

USES

These have a similar antibacterial spectrum to benzylpenicillin, but are also effective against most strains of *Haemophilus influenzae, E. coli, Streptococcus faecalis* and *Salmonella*. They are used for a variety of chest infections (e.g. bronchitis, pneumonia), otitis media, urinary tract infections, biliary infections and the prevention of bacterial endocarditis (amoxycillin). Amoxycillin is somewhat more potent than ampicillin, penetrates tissues better, and is given three rather than four times daily. Both are susceptible to β-lactamases.

ADVERSE EFFECTS

Rashes are common, and may appear after dosing has stopped. There is an especially high incidence in patients with infectious mononucleosis or lymphatic leukaemia.

PHARMACOKINETICS

The half-life of each drug is about 1.5 h, and they are predominantly renally excreted.

Co-fluampicil

Co-fluampicil is a mixture of equal parts by mass of flucloxacillin and ampicillin. It is indicated in mixed infections involving β-lactamase-producing *Staphylococcus*. It may be administered by the oral, intramuscular or intravenous route, and should be given four times daily.

Co-amoxiclav

Co-amoxiclav is a combination of amoxycillin and clavulanic acid, a β-lactamase inhibitor. In addition to those bacteria that are susceptible to amoxycillin, most *Staphylococcus aureus*, 50% of *E. coli*, some *Haemophilus influenzae* strains and many *Bacteroides* and *Klebsiella* species are susceptible to co-amoxiclav. Adverse effects are similar to those of amoxycillin, but abdominal discomfort is more common.

Antipseudomonal penicillins

Regular penicillins are not effective against *Pseudomonas*. This is not usually a problem, as these organisms seldom cause disease in otherwise healthy people. However, they are important in neutropenic patients (e.g. those undergoing cancer chemotherapy) and in patients with cystic fibrosis. Penicillins with activity against *Pseudomonas* have been developed, and are particularly useful in these circumstances. These include **piperacillin**, **azlocillin** and **ticarcillin**, which is combined with clavulanic acid

USES

These expensive intravenous penicillins are not used routinely. Their efficacy against Gram-positive organisms is variable and poor. They are useful against Gram-negative infections, particularly with *Pseudomonas*, and they are also effective against many anaerobes. These drugs have a synergistic effect when combined with aminoglycosides in *Pseudomonas* septicaemias. **Timentin**® is a combination of ticarcillin and clavulanic acid (a β-lactamase inhibitor) designed to overcome the problem of β-lactamase formation by *Pseudomonas*. **Tazocin**® is a combination of pipercillin and the β-lactamase inhibitor tazobactam.

ADVERSE EFFECTS

These drugs have a fairly broad spectrum of activity and predispose to superinfection. Rashes, sodium overload and thrombocytopenia or non-thrombocytopenic platelet dysfunction occur.

PHARMACOKINETICS

Absorption of these drugs from the gut is inadequate in the life-threatening infections for which they are mainly indicated. They are given intravenously every 4–6 h. Their half-lives range from 1 to 1.5 h, and they are renally excreted.

CEPHALOSPORINS

This group of antibiotics is derived from a strain of micro-organism found near a sewage outlet in the Mediterranean off the coast of Sardinia.

First-generation cephalosporins

So-called first-generation cephalosporins (e.g. cephalexin, cefaclor, cefadroxil) are effective against *Streptococcus pyogenes* and *Streptococcus pneumoniae*, *E. coli* and some staphylococci. They have few *absolute* (i.e. uniquely advantageous) indications. Their pharmacology is similar to that of the penicillins, and they are principally renally eliminated.

Second- and third-generation cephalosporins

The efficacy of second- and third-generation cephalosporins has been increased to include *H. influenzae* and in some instances *Pseudomonas* and anaerobes. This has only been achieved with some loss of efficacy against Gram-positive organisms. β-Lactamase stability has been increased. Arguably the most generally useful member of the group is **cefuroxime**, which combines lactamase stability with activity against streptococci, staphylococci, *H. influenzae* and *E. coli*. It is given by injection 8-hourly (an oral preparation is also available). It is expensive, although when used against Gram-negative organisms that would otherwise necessitate use of an aminoglycoside, this cost is at least partly offset by savings from the lack of need for plasma concentration determinations.

Of the third-generation cephalosporins, **ceftazidime**, **ceftriaxone** and **cefotaxime** are useful in severe sepsis, especially because (unlike earlier cephalosporins) they penetrate the blood–brain barrier well and are effective in meningitis.

ADVERSE EFFECTS

About 10% of patients who are allergic to penicillins are also allergic to cephalosporins. Some first-generation cephalosporins are nephrotoxic, particularly if used with frusemide, aminoglycosides or other nephrotoxic agents. Some of the third-generation drugs are associated with bleeding due to increased prothrombin times, which is reversible with vitamin K.

MONOBACTAMS

Monobactams (e.g. **aztreonam**) contain a 5–monobactam ring and are resistant to β-lactamase degradation.

Aztreonam

USES

Aztreonam is primarily active against aerobic Gram-negative organisms, and is an alternative to an aminoglycoside. It is used in severe sepsis, often hospital acquired, especially infections of the respiratory, urinary, biliary, gastrointestinal and female genital tracts. It has a narrow spectrum of activity and cannot be used alone unless the organism's sensitivity to aztreonam is known.

MECHANISM OF ACTION

The 5–monobactam ring binds to bacterial wall transpeptidases and inhibits bacterial cell wall synthesis in a similar way to the penicillins.

ADVERSE EFFECTS

Rashes occur, but there appears to be no cross-allergenicity with penicillins.

PHARMACOKINETICS

Aztreonam is poorly absorbed after oral administration, so it is given parenterally. It is widely distributed to all body compartments, including the cerebrospinal fluid. Excretion is renal, and the usual half-life (1–2 h) is increased in renal failure.

Imipenem–cilastatin

USES

This antibacterial agent combines a carbapenem (thienamycin), imipenem, with cilastatin, which is an inhibitor of the enzyme dehydropeptidase I found in the brush border of the proximal renal tubule. This enzyme breaks down imipenem in the kidney. Imipenem has a very broad spectrum of activity against Gram-positive, Gram-negative and anaerobic organisms. It is β-lactamase stable, and is used for treating severe infections of the lung and abdomen, and in patients with septicaemia, where the source of the organism is unknown.

ADVERSE EFFECTS

Imipenem is generally well tolerated, but seizures, myoclonus, confusion, nausea and vomiting, hypersensitivity, positive Coombs' test, taste disturbances and thrombophlebitis have all been reported.

PHARMACOKINETICS

Imipenem is both renally filtered and metabolized in the kidney by dehydropeptidase I. This is inhibited by cilastin in the combination. The half-life of the drug is 1 h. It is given intravenously as an infusion in three or four divided daily doses.

AMINOGLYCOSIDES

USES

Aminoglycosides are highly polar, sugar-containing derivatives of bacterial proteins. They are all powerful bactericidal agents that are active against many Gram-negative organisms and some Gram-positive organisms, with activity against staphylococci and *Enterococcus faecalis*, but not (when used alone) against other streptococci. They synergize with penicillins in killing *Streptococcus faecalis* in endocarditis. Aminoglycosides are used in serious infections including septicaemia, sometimes alone but usually in combination with other antibiotics (penicillins or cephalosporins). **Gentamicin** is the most widely used, and has a broad spectrum, but is ineffective against anaerobes, many streptococci and pneumococci.

Netilmicin is similar to gentamicin but is probably less ototoxic, and is therefore preferred in patients in whom prolonged treatment is envisaged, especially those with hearing or visual impairment or with impaired renal function, including the elderly. **Tobramycin** is probably somewhat less nephrotoxic than gentamicin. Amikacin is more effective than gentamicin for pseudomonal infections, and is occasionally effective against organisms resistant to gentamicin. It is principally indicated in serious infections caused by Gram-negative bacilli that are resistant to gentamicin. Topical gentamicin and tobramycin eyedrops are used to treat eye infections.

MECHANISM OF ACTION

These drugs are transported into cells and block bacterial protein synthesis by binding to the 30S ribosome. They are bactericidal. A post-antibiotic effect on Gram-negative organisms has been demonstrated.

ADVERSE EFFECTS

These are important and are related to duration of therapy and trough plasma concentrations. They are more frequent in the elderly and in renal impairment. Therapeutic monitoring is performed by measuring plasma concentrations before dosing (trough) and at 'peak' levels (at an arbitary 1 h after dosing). Three times weekly therapeutic monitoring is adequate for most patients with normal renal function during maintenance, but if the patient is severely ill and if acute tubular necrosis is a clinical possibility, more frequent monitoring initially is essential. Eighth nerve damage – cochlear (deafness) and vestibular (dizziness, loss of balance, seen especially with streptomycin treatment for tuberculosis) – is potentially catastrophic and is often irreversible. Acute tubular necrosis and renal failure are usually reversible if diagnosed promptly and the drug stopped or the dose reduced. Hypersensitivity rashes occur in patients and in those drawing up the drug, but are uncommon. Bone-marrow suppression is rare. Exacerbation of myasthenia gravis is predictable in patients with this disease.

PHARMACOKINETICS

Aminoglycosides are poorly absorbed from the gut, and are given by intramuscular or intravenous injections. They are poorly protein bound (30%) and are excreted renally. The half-life is short, usually 2 h, but once daily administration is

> **Key points**
>
> Aminoglycosides
>
> - Active against many Gram-negative and some Gram-positive organisms. Generally used parenterally in serious infections, and occasionally used topically. *Note: they are not used orally.*
> - Adverse effects related to duration of therapy and trough concentrations:
>   eighth nerve damage, often irreversible;
>   renal damage, usually reversible.
> - *Note that elimination is renal.* Monitor plasma concentrations (e.g. gentamicin, netilmicin).

usually adequate. This presumably reflects a post-antibiotic effect whereby bacterial growth is inhibited following clearance of the drug. In patients with renal dysfunction, dose reduction and/or an increased dose interval is required. Cerebrospinal fluid (CSF) penetration is poor, and neurosurgeons sometimes insert a reservoir with direct access to a lateral ventricle in patients with Gram-negative meningitis that is resistant to other antibiotics that penetrate the CSF better (e.g. chloramphenicol).

DRUG INTERACTIONS

Aminoglycosides enhance neuromuscular blockade of non-depolarizing neuromuscular antagonists. Loop diuretics potentiate their nephrotoxicity and ototoxicity.

CHLORAMPHENICOL

USES

Chloramphenicol has a broad spectrum of activity and penetrates tissues exceptionally well. It is bacteriostatic, but is extremely effective against streptococci, staphylococci, *H.influenzae*, salmonellae and others. Uncommonly it causes aplastic anaemia, so its use is largely confined to *H. influenzae* epiglottitis, meningitis, typhoid fever and topical use as eyedrops.

It was previously used widely in chronic respiratory disease, and still has a role in patients with life-threatening pulmonary infections in whom other antibiotics are contraindicated or likely to be ineffective.

MECHANISM OF ACTION

Chloramphenicol inhibits bacterial ribosome function by inhibiting the 50S ribosomal peptidyl transferase, thereby preventing peptide elongation.

ADVERSE EFFECTS

These include the following:

1 *haematological effects* – dose-related erythroid suppression is common and predictable, but in addition aplastic anemia occurs unpredictably with an incidence of approximately 1:40 000. This is irreversible in 50% of cases. It is only extremely rarely, if ever, related to the use of topical eyedrops. It provides a strong reason for not using the drug for trivial infections, but should not preclude its use in life-threatening situations – fatal anaphylactic reactions have been reported.
2 *grey baby syndrome* – the grey colour is due to shock (hypotension and tissue hypoperfusion). Chloramphenicol accumulates in neonates (especially if premature) due to reduced glucuronidation in the immature liver. The syndrome usually occurs at plasma concentrations greater than 50 μg/mL.
3 *other effects* – chloramphenicol can also cause sore mouth, diarrhoea, encephalopathy and optic neuritis.

PHARMACOKINETICS

Chloramphenicol is well absorbed following oral administration, and can also be given by the intramuscular and intravenous routes. It is widely distributed and CSF penetration is excellent. It mainly undergoes hepatic glucuronidation. Its half-life is 6 h, but neonates this is prolonged due to the immaturity of the glucuronidation enzymes.

DRUG INTERACTIONS

Chloramphenicol inhibits the metabolism of alcohol, warfarin, phenytoin and theophylline. This can cause clinically important toxicity if effects and/or plasma concentrations of these drugs are not monitored closely and their dose modified accordingly.

MACROLIDES

Macrolide antibiotics (e.g. **erythromycin**, **clarithromycin**, **azithromycin** and **spiramycin**) have an antibacterial spectrum similar but not identical to that of penicillin. Distinctively, they are effective against several unusual organisms, including *Chlamydia*, *Legionella* and *Mycoplasma*. Most experience has been obtained with erythromycin. The characteristics of the drugs belonging to this group are compared in Table 42.6.

Erythromycin

USES

These include the treatment of respiratory infections (including *Mycoplasma pneumoniae*, psittacosis and Legionnaires' disease), whooping cough, *Campylobacter enteritis*, and non-specific urethritis. Erythromycin is a useful alternative to penicillin in penicillin-allergic patients (with the notable exception of meningitis, because it does not penetrate the CSF adequately). It is useful for skin infections such as low-grade cellulitis and infected acne, and is an acceptable drug for patients with an infective exacerbation of chronic bronchitis. It is most commonly administered by mouth four times daily, although when necessary it may be given by intravenous infusion.

MECHANISM OF ACTION

Macrolides bind to bacterial 50S ribosomes and inhibit the ribosomal translocation enzyme.

PHARMACOKINETICS

Erythromycin is well absorbed orally. Food delays its absorption but may reduce gastrointestinal side-effects. The drug is distributed adequately to most sites except the brain and CSF. It is inactivated by hepatic N-demethylation, less than 15% being eliminated unchanged in the urine.

ADVERSE EFFECTS

Erythromycin is a remarkably safe antibiotic, and may be used in pregnancy and in children. Nausea, vomiting, diarrhoea and abdominal cramps are the most common adverse effects reported, and may be related to direct pharmacological action on vasoactive intestinal peptide (VIP) receptors. Cholestatic jaundice has been reported following prolonged use. Intravenous administration frequently causes local pain and phlebitis.

DRUG INTERACTIONS

Erythromycin inhibits cytochrome P_{450} and causes accumulation of theophylline, warfarin and terfenadine. This can result in clinically important adverse effects.

Azithromycin and clarithromycin

These macrolides have somewhat different activities *in vitro* to erythromycin. Each of them has greater activity against *H.influenzae*. Azithromycin is less effective against Gram-positive bacteria than erythromycin but has a wider spectrum of activity against Gram-negative organisms. The long half-life of azithromycin is probably related to its extensive tissue penetration and subsequent slow release from peripheral compartments. A single dose of azithromycin is as effective as 7 days' of treatment with tetracycline in the management of non-specific urethritis due to *Chlamydia*.

Azithromycin and clarithromycin are approximately four times more expensive than erythromycin.

Table 42.6: Comparison of macrolides

	Erythromycin	Azithromycin	Clarithromycin
Experience	Extensive	Limited	Limited
Oral dose frequency	Usually qds	od	bd
$t_{\frac{1}{2}}$	1–1.5 h	40–60 h	Approximately 5 h
Intravenous preparation available	Yes	No	Yes
Adverse gastrointestinal effects	Common	Less common	Less common
Tissue penetration	Reasonable	Extremely high	High

Key points

Macrolides

Similar antibacterial spectrum to penicillins (useful in penicillin allergy, but not effective in meningitis); also useful against atypical organisms including *Chlamydia, Legionella, Campylobacter* and *Mycoplasma*. They inhibit cytochrome-P_{450}.

Antibiotic	Comments
■ Erythromycin	Safe, gastrointestinal disturbances, (phlebitis with IV administration), QDS regime
■ Clarithromycin	Twice daily regime
■ Azithromycin	Excellent tissue penetration; $t_{\frac{1}{2}}$ 50 h, once daily dose

Key points

Tetracyclines

- Broad spectrum, but resistance is a problem, second-line drugs for acute bacterial exacerbations of chronic bronchitis, also useful for atypical organisms e.g. *Chlamydia, Mycoplasma, Lyme disease*), and used in the treatment of acne.
- Adverse effects include nausea, diarrhoea, superinfections, worsening of renal impairment, and discoloration and damage of developing teeth and bones.
- Oxytetracycline – interaction with food, renal elimination.
- Doxycycline – no interaction with food, can be given once daily, and is not contraindicated in renal impairment.

TETRACYCLINES

USES

Tetracyclines (e.g. **tetracycline**, **chlortetracycline**, **oxytetracycline**, **doxycycline**, **minocycline**) are molecular modifications of a four-ringed nucleus (hence the name). They have a broad range of antibacterial activity covering both Gram-positive and Gram-negative organisms and, in addition organisms such as *Rickettsia*, *Chlamydia* and *Mycoplasma*. They are used in atypical pneumonias and chlamydial and rickettsial infections, and remain useful in treating exacerbations of chronic bronchitis. They are not used routinely for staphylococcal or streptococcal infections because of the development of resistance. Minocycline is used to eliminate carriage of *Neisseria meningitidis* from the nasopharynx. Tetracyclines are used in the long-term treatment of acne (see Chapter 50).

MECHANISM OF ACTION

Tetracyclines bind to the 30S subunit of bacterial ribosomes and prevent binding of the aminoacyl-tRNA to the ribosome acceptor site, thereby inhibiting protein synthesis.

ADVERSE EFFECTS

These include the following:

1. nausea and diarrhoea;
2. fungal superinfection, and pseudomembranous colitis due to *Clostridium difficile*;
3. worsening of prerenal and renal failure;
4. discoloration and damage of teeth and bones of the fetus if the mother takes tetracyclines after the fifth month of pregnancy, and of children;
5. minocycline causes reversible and dose-related ataxia.

PHARMACOKINETICS

Tetracyclines are well absorbed orally when fasting, but their absorption is reduced by food and antacids. They undergo elimination by both the liver and the kidney. The half-life varies with the different members of the group, ranging from 6 to 12 h. The shorter-acting drugs are given four times daily, and the longer acting ones once daily. Doxycycline is given once daily, can be taken with food, and is not contraindicated in renal impairment, but is more expensive than other members of this group.

DRUG INTERACTIONS

Tetracyclines chelate with calcium salts in the stomach, and their absorption is reduced by the presence of antacids or food.

SODIUM FUSIDATE

USES

Fusidic acid is a steroid derivative used for the treatment of staphylococcal infections, including strains which are penicillin resistant. It penetrates tissues (including bone) well. It is normally used in conjunction with flucloxacillin for serious staphylococcal infections. It is also available as eyedrops for the treatment of bacterial conjunctivitis.

MECHANISM OF ACTION

Fucidin inhibits bacterial protein synthesis.

ADVERSE EFFECTS

Adverse effects are rare, but include cholestatic jaundice.

PHARMACOKINETICS

Fucidin is administered either orally or intravenously. Its half-life is 4–6 h and it is excreted primarily via the liver.

VANCOMYCIN

USES AND ANTIBACTERIAL SPECTRUM

Vancomycin is valuable in the treatment of resistant infections due to *Staphylococcus pyogenes*. It is also rarely used to treat other infections, for example *Staphylococcus epidermidis* endocarditis), and is given orally for the treatment of pseudomembranous colitis caused by *Clostridium difficile*.

MECHANISM OF ACTION

Vancomycin inhibits bacterial cell wall synthesis.

ADVERSE EFFECTS

These include the following:

1 hearing loss;
2 venous thrombosis at infusion site;
3 'red man' syndrome due to cytokine/histamine release following excessively rapid intravenous administration;
4 hypersensitivity (rashes, etc.);
5 nephrotoxicity.

PHARMACOKINETICS

Vancomycin is not absorbed from the gut, and is usually given as an intravenous infusion. It is eliminated by the kidneys. Because of its concentration-related toxicity, the dose is adjusted according to the results of plasma concentration monitoring.

TEICOPLANIN

Teicoplanin has a longer duration of action but is otherwise similar to vancomycin.

METRONIDAZOLE (Flagyl).

USES

Metronidazole is a synthetic drug with high activity against anaerobic bacteria, including *C. welchii* and *Bacteroides fragilis*. It is also active against several medically important protozoa and parasites (see Chapter 46). It is used to treat trichomonal infections, amoebic dysentrey, giardiasis, gas gangrene, pseudomembranous colitis and various abdominal infections, lung abscesses and dental sepsis. It is widely used prophylactically before abdominal surgery.

Giardiasis
Amoebiasis
Trichomonal
Gas gangrene.
And surgery.

MECHANISM OF ACTION

Metronidazole binds to DNA and causes strand breakage. In addition, it acts as an electron acceptor for flavoproteins and ferredoxins.

ADVERSE EFFECTS

These includes the following:

1 nausea and vomiting;
2 peripheral neuropathy;
3 convulsions, headaches;
4 hepatitis.

PHARMACOKINETICS

Metronidazole is well absorbed after oral or rectal administration, but is too often administered by the relatively expensive intravenous route. The half-life is approximately 6 h. It is eliminated by a combination of hepatic metabolism and renal excretion. Dose reduction is required in renal impairment.

DRUG INTERACTIONS

Metronidazole interacts with alcohol because it inhibits aldehyde dehydrogenase and consequently causes a disulfiram-like reaction. It is a weak inhibitor of cytochrome P_{450}.

SULPHONAMIDES AND TRIMETHOPRIM

Sulphonamides and trimethoprim inhibit the production of folic acid at different sites of its synthetic pathway, and are synergistic *in vitro*. There is now widespread resistance to sulphonamides, and they have been largely replaced by more active and less toxic antibacterial agents. Sulphonamides (e.g. sulphadimidine) alone are occasionally used to treat urinary tract infections. The sulphamethoxazole—trimethoprim combination (co-trimoxazole) is effective in urinary tract infections, prostatitis, exacerbations of chronic bronchitis and invasive *Salmonella* infections, but with the exception of *Pneumocystis carinii* infections (when high doses are used), trimethoprim alone is generally preferred as it avoids sulphonamide side-effects whilst having similar efficacy *in vivo*.

SULPHONAMIDES

ADVERSE EFFECTS

Sulphonamides frequently cause unwanted side-effects including hypersensitivity reactions such as rashes, fever and serum sickness-like syndrome and Stevens–Johnson syndrome. The latter is much more common with long-acting preparations. Rarely, agranulocytosis, megaloblastic, aplastic or haemolytic anaemia and thrombocytopenia occur. Sulphonamides are oxidants and can precipitate haemolytic anaemia in glucose-6–phosphate dehydrogenase (G6PD)-deficient individuals.

PHARMACOKINETICS

Sulphonamides are generally well absorbed after oral administration and are widely distributed to the body compartments. Acetylation and glucuronidation are the most important metabolic pathways. Some of the older sulphonamides precipitate in acid urine. The half-life of sulphamethoxazole is 11 h and that of sulphadoxine is 120–200 h.

DRUG INTERACTIONS

Sulphonamides potentiate the action of sulphonylureas, oral anticoagulants, phenytoin and methotrexate due to inhibition of metabolism.

Trimethoprim

USES

Trimethoprim is a broad-spectrum antibacterial drug and has largely taken the place of co-trimoxazole in the treatment of urinary tract infections and acute and chronic bronchitis.

ADVERSE EFFECTS

Trimethoprim is generally well tolerated, but occasionally causes gastrointestinal disturbances, skin reactions and (rarely) bone-marrow depression.

PHARMACOKINETICS

Trimethoprim is well absorbed, highly lipid soluble and widely distributed in the body. At least 65% is eliminated unchanged in the urine. Trimethoprim competes for the same renal clearance pathway as creatinine.

ADVERSE EFFECTS

In addition to the side-effects associated with trimethoprim and sulphonamides, the high doses used in the management of *Pneumocystis* pneumonia in immunosuppressed patients cause vomiting (which can be improved by prophylactic anti-emetics), a higher incidence of serious skin reactions, hepatitis and thromobocytopenia.

QUINOLONES

Nalidixic acid has been available for over 20 years but its low activity, poor tissue distribution and adverse effects limited its use to a second- or third-line treatment for urinary tract infections. Changes to the basic quinolone structure, such as the addition of fluorine and a piperazine ring, have dramatically increased its antibacterial potency, particularly against *Pseudomonas aeruginosa*. Its oral bioavailability is good and thus the 4–fluoroquinolones offer an oral alternative to parenteral aminoglycosides and antipseudomonal penicillins for treatment of *Pseudomonas* urinary and chest infections. Although the 4–fluoroquinolones have a very broad spectrum of activity, all of those currently available have very limited activity against streptococci. Most experience has been obtained with **ciprofloxacin**, which has the additional advantage of being available for intravenous use. The quinolones inhibit bacterial DNA gyrase.

USES

Ciprofloxacin is used for respiratory (*but not pneumococcal*), urinary, gastrointestinal and genital infections, septicaemia and meningococcal meningitis contacts. In addition to *Pseudomonas*, it is particularly active against infection with *Salmonella*, *Shigella*, *Campylobacter*, *Neisseria* and *Chlamydia*. It is ineffective in most anaerobic infections. The licensed indications for the other quinolones are more limited. Nalidixic acid, **cinoxacin** and **norfloxacin** are effective in uncomplicated urinary tract infections. **Ofloxacin** is also used for lower respiratory tract infections, gonorrhoea, NSU and

Case history

A 70-year-old man with a history of chronic obstructive pulmonary disease visits his GP in December during a local 'flu' epidemic. He complains of worsening shortness of breath, productive cough, fever and malaise. On examination his sputum is viscous and green, his respiratory rate is 20 breaths/min at rest but, in addition to wheezes, bronchial breathing is audible over the right lower lobe. The GP prescribes amoxycillin which has been effective in previous exacerbations of chronic obstructive pulmonary disease in this patient. Twenty-four hours later the patient is brought to the local casualty department confused, cyanosed and with a respiratory rate of 30 breaths/min. His chest X-ray is consistent with lobar pneumonia.

Question

In addition to controlled oxygen and bronchodilators, which three antibacterial drugs would you prescribe and why?

Answer

This patient is seriously ill with community-acquired lobar pneumonia. The previously abnormal chest, the concurrent flu epidemic and the rapid deterioration suggest *Staphylococcus*, but *Streptococcus pneumoniae* and *Legionella* are also possible pathogens. The following antibacterial drugs should be prescribed:

- Flucloxacillin – Active against *Staphylococcus* and Gram-positive organisms
- Cefuroxime – broadspectrum and active against *Straphylococcus*;
- Erythromycin – active against *Legionella* and *Mycoplasma*, and also some *Staphylococcus* and Gram-positive bacteria.

Case history

While on holiday in Spain a 66-year-old man develops a cough, fevers and breathlessness at rest. He is told that his chest X-ray confirms that he has pneumonia. He is started on a 7-day course of oral antibiotics by a local physician and stays in his hotel for the remainder of his 10-day holiday. When he returns home he is reviewed by his own GP who notices that he looks pale and sallow and is still breathless on exertion but his chest examination no longer reveals any signs of pneumonia. A full blood count reveals a haemoglobin level of 6.7 g/dL (previously normal), normal white blood count and platelets, and a reticulocyte count of 4.1%.

Question

What other tests should you do, and what antibiotics would be most likely to cause this clinical senario?

Answer

The patient received a course of antibiotics for pneumonia and then developed what appears to be a haemolytic anaemia. This could be further confirmed by raised unconjugated bilirubin levels, and low haptoglobin levels, and observation of target cells and poikilocytosis on the blood film. *Mycoplasma* pneumonia should be excluded by performing Myco titres, as this can itself be complicated by a haemolytic anaemia. However, considering the drugs as the potential cause, it is important to define the patients, glucose-6-phosphate dehydrogenase status, and if he was deficient then to consider such agents as co-trimoxazole (containing a sulphamethoxazole and sulphonamide, the fluoroquinolones (e.g. ciprofloxacin or nitrofurantoin) or chloramphenicol, which can cause haemolytic anaemia in susceptible individuals. Note that chloramphenicol is more commonly prescribed in certain countries on the European mainland. Aplastic anaemia (not the picture in this patient) is a major concern with the use of systemic chloramphenicol. If the patient's glucose-6-phosphate dehyrogenase status is normal, then rarely the β-lactams (penicillins or early (first and second)-generation cephalosporins) or (less likely) rifampicin may cause an autoimmune haemolytic anaemia due to the production of antibodies to the antibiotic which binds to the red blood cells. This could be further confirmed by performing an Direct Coombs' test in which the patient's serum in the presence of red cells and the drug would cause red cell lysis. Management involves stopping the drug, giving folic acid and monitoring recovery of the haemoglobin. It should be noted in the patient's record that certain antibiotics led him to have a haemolytic anaemia.

Case history

A 20-year-old man presented to his GP during a flu epidemic complaining of a throbbing headache which was present when he woke up that morning. He had been studying hard and was anxious about his exams. Physical examination was normal and he was sent home with paracetamol and vitamins. He presented to casualty 12 h later with a worsening headache. Examination revealed a temperature of 39°C, blood pressure of 110/60 mmHg, neck stiffness and a purpuric rash on his arms and legs which did not blanch when pressure was applied.

Question

Which antibacterial drugs would you use, and why?

Answer

This young man has meningococcal meningitis and requires benzylpenicillin IV immediately.

REMEMBER : Treatment of bacterial meningitis must never be delayed.

cervicitis. **Grepafloxacin** and **levofloxacin** have more activity against pneumococci than ciprofloxacin. The indiscriminate use of these expensive agents is likely to lead to unnecessary bacterial resistance – the 4–fluoroquinolones have some unique attributes among antibacterial agents, and their widespread prescription when equally effective and safe agents are available is to be deplored.

ADVERSE EFFECTS

Ciprofloxacin is generally well tolerated, but should be avoided by epileptics (it rarely causes convulsions), children (it causes arthritis in growing animals) and individuals with glucose-6-phospate dehydrogenase deficiency. Anaphylaxis, nephritis, vasculitis, dizziness, hepatic and renal damage have all been reported. An excessively alkaline urine and dehydration can cause crystallization.

PHARMACOKINETICS

Approximately 80% of an oral dose of ciprofloxacin is systemically available. It is widely distributed entering all body compartments including the eye and the CSF. Ciprofloxacin is removed primarily by glomerular filtration and tubular secretion. The half-life is 4 h.

DRUG INTERACTIONS

Co-administration of ciprofloxacin and theophylline causes elevated blood theophylline concentrations due to inhibition of cytochrome P_{450}. As both drugs are epileptogenic, this interaction is particularly significant.

FURTHER READING

Antimicrobial resistance. *British Medical Journal*, 5 September 1998, editorial, article and papers.

CHAPTER FORTY-THREE

MYCOBACTERIAL INFECTIONS

- Introduction
- Principles of management of *Mycobacterium tuberculosis* infections
- First-line drugs in tuberculosis therapy
- Treatment of tuberculous meningitis
- Chemoprophylaxis
- Tuberculosis and the acquired immune deficiency syndrome (AIDS)
- Corticosteroids in tuberculosis therapy
- Second-line drugs and treatment of tuberculosis
- *Mycobacterium leprae* infection

INTRODUCTION

Tuberculosis ('consumption') was the commonest cause of death in Victorian England, but its prevalence fell with the great improvements in living standards that occurred during the twentieth century. However, the incidence of *Mycobacterium tuberculosis* infection world-wide (including economically developed countries such as the UK and USA) is once again increasing, particularly among immigrants and in human immunodeficiency virus (HIV)-related cases. Infection with *Mycobacterium tuberculosis* usually occurs in the lungs, but may affect any organ, especially the lymph nodes, gut, meninges, bone, adrenal glands or urogenital tract. Other atypical (non-tuberculous) mycobacterial infections are less common, but are occurring with increasing frequency in HIV-1 infected individuals. *Mycobacterium tuberculosis* is an intracellular organism and an obligate aerobe in keeping with its predilection for the well-ventilated apical segments of the lung.

PRINCIPLES OF MANAGEMENT OF MYCOBACTERIUM TUBERCULOSIS INFECTIONS

Successful treatment of *M. tuberculosis* requires initial combination therapy with at least three (and sometimes four) drugs. The use of several drugs means that one is less likely to encounter a bacterium that is resistant to all agents, and is therefore more likely to achieve a cure, with a low relapse rate (0–3 %). The development of resistance is also thereby minimized. Following several Medical Research Council (MRC) clinical trials in Hong Kong and East Africa, the British Thoracic Society now recommends standard therapy for pulmonary tuberculosis for 6 months (longer regimes were used previously). A combination of **isoniazid, rifampicin, pyrazinamide** and **ethambutol** (or streptomycin) is administered for the first 2 months, followed by rifampicin and isoniazid for a further 4 months. Ethambutol and/or streptomycin may be omitted in patients who are at relatively low risk of carrying bacilli resistant to isoniazid, which includes 99% of the UK-born population. However, the initial use of four drugs is advisable in immigrants from countries where bacterial resistance to isoniazid is more frequent, and in HIV patients. In such patients the initial use of three drugs might lead to a higher incidence of treatment failures, because *M. tuberculosis* would only be sensitive to rifampicin and pyrazinamide – not the most effective antituberculous combination. Initial four-drug combination therapy should also be used in all patients with non-tuberculous mycobacterial infection, which often involves organisms that are resistant to both isoniazid and pyrazinamide. Patients with open active tuberculosis are initially isolated on the ward to reduce the risk of spread, but may be considered non-infectious after 14 days of therapy. In cases where compliance with a daily regimen is a problem, the initial 2 months of triple or quadruple chemotherapy can be given on an intermittent supervised basis two or three times a week. At the end of the 2-month period the precise identification and sensitivities of the organism will be available. If they are fully sensitive, treatment will continue with daily or intermittent rifampicin and isoniazid for a further 4 months. After 6 months, treatment can usually be discontinued unless the sputum remains positive or the patient is immunocompromised or poorly compliant. If the initial drug sensitivities reveal isoniazid resistance, treatment with ethambutol plus rifampicin must be continued for a total of 12 months. The duration of chemotherapy will also need to be extended if either isoniazid, rifampicin or pyrazinamide has to be discontinued because of side-effects.

The usual drug doses for daily and intermittent treatment are shown in Table 43.1. The regimens described are applicable to patients infected with tubercle bacilli that are either fully sensitive or resistant to only isoniazid and/or streptomycin. The treatment of tuberculosis which is resistant to multiple drugs is more difficult, and regimens have to be individualized according to drug sensitivity.

Key points:

Mycobacterium tuberculosis infection

M. tuberculosis:

- is an obligate aerobe;
- grows slowly;
- has a great propensity to develop drug resistance.

FIRST-LINE DRUGS IN TUBERCULOSIS THERAPY

Isoniazid (isonicotinic acid hydrazide)-INH

USES

This is one of the most important agents for the treatment of tuberculosis. It is bactericidal only to *Mycobacterium tuberculosis*, with a minimal inhibitory concentration (MIC) of about 0.2

Table 43.1: Dose of commonly used antituberculous drugs (mg)

Drug	Daily dosing (mg) Weight <50 kg	Daily dosing (mg) Weight >50 kg	Twice weekly dosing (mg) Weight <50 kg	Twice weekly dosing (mg) Weight >50 kg	Three times weekly dosing (mg) Weight <50 kg	Three times weekly dosing (mg) Weight >50 kg
Isoniazid	300	300	15 mg/kg	15 mg/kg	15 mg/kg	15 mg/kg
Rifampicin‡	450	600	600	600–900	600	600–900
Pyrazinamide	1500	2000	3000	3500	2000	2500
Ethambutol	15 mg/kg	15 mg/kg	45 mg/kg	45 mg/kg	30 mg/kg	30 mg/kg
Streptomycin	750*	1000†	750*	1000†	750*	1000‡

* Reduced to 500 mg in patients aged 40–60 years.
† Reduced to 750 mg in patients aged 40–60 years.
‡ Rifampicin (another Rifamycin) is an alternative. Dose is 150–450 mg orally once a day. Dose reduced in renal failure.

μg/mL. In tuberculosis a daily dose of 5 mg/kg (Table 43.1) for adults and 6 mg/kg for children is usually employed. High doses are used in tuberculous meningitis, where an injectable preparation is available for patients who are unable to take oral drugs. Isoniazid is often given in combination with rifampicin or ethambutol. When using high-dose isoniazid (e.g. treating tuberculous meningitis) or in patients with special risk factors (e.g. diabetes, alcoholism) pyridoxine, 10–30 mg daily, is given to prevent peripheral neuropathy (see Chapter 34).

MECHANISM OF ACTION

Isoniazid acts only on growing bacteria, possibly by interference with the synthesis of mycolic acid, a constituent of the *M. tuberculosis* cell wall.

ADVERSE EFFECTS

Toxic effects are uncommon with the usual dose of 300 mg/day. Adverse effects include the following:

1. restlessness, insomnia and muscle twitching;
2. peripheral neuropathy, which is commoner in patients who are slow acetylators, and which may be prevented by administration of supplemental pyridoxine, 10–30 mg daily;
3. hepatitis, which is clinically significant in 1% of patients, and rarely progress to hepatic necrosis. It is possible that acetylisoniazid is responsible for this effect, since enzyme inducers such as rifampicin result in higher production of the acetyl metabolite in the liver, and are associated with increased toxicity;
4. drug-induced systemic lupus erythematosus;
5. Bone marrow suppression-anemia, agranulocytosis.

PHARMACOKINETICS

Isoniazid is readily absorbed from the gut, diffuses widely into the body tissues, including the cerebrospinal fluid (CSF) and penetrates into macrophages, being effective against intracellular tubercle bacilli. It undergoes genetically controlled polymorphic acetylation in the liver (see Chapter 14). The proportions of a given population that are characterized as fast or slow acetylators depend on the population's ethnic make-up, a high percentage of fast acetylators being found in Japanese and Eskimo populations, In European populations 40–45% are rapid acetylators. The $(t_{\frac{1}{2}})$ of isoniazid is less than 80 min in fast acetylators and more than 140 min in slow acetylators. Around 50–70% seventy per cent of a dose is excreted in the urine within 24 h as metabolite or free drug. Impaired renal function is not usually a problem, but abnormally high and potentially toxic concentrations of isoniazid may be reached in slow acetylators with renal impairment.

DRUG INTERACTIONS

Isoniazid undergoes some metabolism by hepatic cytochrome P_{450} and inhibits the metabolism of several anticonvulsants, including phenytoin and carbamazepine. This is clinically important, as it leads to anticonvulsant toxicity in some patients.

Rifampicin

USES

Rifampicin is a derivative of rifamycin, which is produced by *Streptomyces mediterranei*. Tubercle bacilli are inhibited at concentrations well below 0.5 μg/mL. Rifampicin is given as 450–600 mg once daily before meals (Table 43.1). It may also be used to treat nasopharyngeal meningococcal carriers (it is present in saliva, tears and nasal secretions), the dose being 600 mg twice daily for 2 days or 2400 mg once daily. Other uses include the treatment of Legionnaires' disease (600 mg daily by intravenous infusion).

MECHANISM OF ACTION

Rifampicin acts by inhibiting bacterial RNA polymerase (binding to its β-subunit) and, because of its high lipophilicity, it diffuses easily through cell membranes to kill intracellular bacteria.

ADVERSE EFFECTS

Large doses (as in intermittent therapy) of rifampicin produce toxic effects in about one-third of patients:

1. After a few hours influenza-like symptoms, flushing and rashes occur;
2. Abdominal pain;
3. Hepatotoxicity – hepatitis and cholestatic jaundice may occur. It is important to measure pre- and intra-treatment hepatic aminotransferases, particularly in patients at high risk of hepatitis (e.g. alcoholics). Serious liver damage is uncommon, but minor histological changes and rises

in aminotransferase activity are common, and in the absence of jaundice they are not an indication for stopping treatment;

4 Thrombocytopenia is rare;

5 Urine and tears become orange/pink in colour, which may be a useful guide to drug compliance.

Does not penetrate CSF well.

PHARMACOKINETICS

Absorption from the gut is almost complete, but is delayed by food. Peak plasma concentrations of about 10 μg/mL are reached 3 h after a single oral dose of 600 mg. The $t_{\frac{1}{2}}$ is 1–5 h. Around 85–90% of rifampicin is protein bound in plasma, but it penetrates well into most tissues, cavities and exudates. However, little rifampicin enters the brain and CSF. It is metabolized by deacetylation, and both the metabolite and parent compound are excreted in the bile and undergo prolonged enterohepatic circulation. Toxicity is increased by biliary obstruction or impaired liver function. Less than 10% appears unchanged in the urine, and thus dosing is unaffected by renal failure.

DRUG INTERACTIONS

Rifampicin markedly induces hepatic microsomal cytochrome P_{450} activity, thereby accelerating the metabolism of many commonly used drugs. Clinically important interactions due to reduced concentration and loss of effect are common, and include the following:

1 corticosteroids;
2 warfarin;
3 sex steroids (rendering oral contraception unreliable);
4 immunosuppressants (including cyclosporine, tacrolimus as well as corticosteroids, and leading to graft rejection);
5 oral hypoglycaemic drugs (e.g. tolbutamide);
6 anticonvulsants (phenytoin and carbamazepine);
7 Several antimicrobial drugs (including antibacterials, antivirals, antifungals and antiprotozoals).

In addition, clinically important interactions may occur after rifampicin is discontinued when the dose of a second drug (e.g. warfarin) has been increased during rifampicin therapy to compensate for the increased metabolism. If the effect of such a drug is not closely monitored in the weeks following cessation of rifampicin treatment and the dose reduced accordingly, serious problems (e.g. bleeding from warfarin) may ensue.

Ethambutol

This is the D-isomer of ethylenediiminodibutanol. It inhibits about 75% of strains of *Mycobacterium tuberculosis* at a concentration of 1 μg/mL. Other organisms are completely resistant. Resistance to ethambutol develops slowly, and the drug often inhibits strains that are resistant to isoniazid or streptomycin. The daily dose is 15–25 mg/kg (Table 43.1).

MECHANISM OF ACTION

The cellular mechanism of action of ethambutol is unclear. It inhibits bacterial cell wall synthesis and is bacteriostatic.

ADVERSE EFFECTS

These include the following:

1 retrobulbar neuritis with scotomata and loss of visual acuity occurs in 10% of patients on the higher dose. The first signs are loss of red-green perception. Prompt withdrawal of the drug may be followed by recovery. Testing of colour vision and visual fields should precede treatment, and the patient should be regularly examined for visual disturbances;
2 rashes, pruritus and joint pains;
3 nausea and abdominal pain;
4 confusion and hallucinations;
5 peripheral neuropathy.

PHARMACOKINETICS

Ethambutol is well absorbed (75–80%) from the intestine, and a single dose of 25 mg/kg gives a peak plasma concentration of 5 μg/mL at 2–4 h. The plasma $t_{\frac{1}{2}}$ is 5–6 h. The drug is concentrated in red cells, and this provides a depot for re-entry into plasma. About 80% is excreted unchanged in the urine. Ethambutol is contraindicated in renal failure.

Pyrazinamide

USES

This is a powerful drug which is well tolerated in an oral dose of 20–35 mg/kg/day (maximum 3.0 g/day; see Table 43.1). Because of its ability to kill bacteria in the acid intracellular environment of a macrophage, it exerts its main effects in the first 2–3 months of therapy. Pyrazinamide is most active against slowly or intermittently metabolizing organisms, but is inactive against atypical mycobacteria. Resistance to this drug develops quickly if it is used alone. Pyrazinamide should be avoided if there is a history of alcohol abuse, because of the occurrence of hepatitis (see below), and liver enzymes should be monitored.

MECHANISM OF ACTION

The enzyme pyrazinamidase in mycobacteria cleaves off the amide portion of the molecule, producing pyrazinoic acid which is bactericidal by a mechanism that is as yet unknown.

ADVERSE EFFECTS

These include the following:

1. facial flushing, rash and photosensitivity;
2. nausea, anorexia and vomiting;
3. hyperuricaemia – may precipitate gout;
4. hepatitis (in approximately 5–15% of patients);
5. sideroblastic anaemia (rare);
6. hypoglycaemia – secondary to increased glucose uptake by adipose tissue – is also uncommon.

PHARMACOKINETICS

Pyrazinamide is converted by an amidase in the liver to pyrazinoic acid, and this undergoes further metabolism to hydroxypyrazinoic acid by xanthine oxidase. Peak concentrations of the metabolites occur 6 h after oral administration. Pyrazinamide is almost completely absorbed and has $t_{\frac{1}{2}}$ of 11–24 h. Pyrazinamide and its metabolites are excreted via the kidney, and renal failure necessitates dose reduction. It crosses the blood–brain barrier to achieve therapeutic CSF concentrations almost equal to those in the plasma, and is therefore a drug of first choice in tuberculous meningitis.

Streptomycin

USE

This is an aminoglycoside antibiotic. It has a wide spectrum of antibacterial activity, but is primarily used to treat mycobacterial infections. It is only given parenterally (intramuscularly). Once daily dosing of 750–1000 mg is adequate. Therapeutic drug monitoring of trough plasma concentrations may be performed to minimize the risk of toxicity and allow dosage optimization.

MECHANISM OF ACTION

Like other aminoglycosides it is actively transported across the bacterial cell wall, and its antibacterial activity is due to specific binding to the P12 protein on the 30S subunit of the bacterial ribosome, which inhibits protein synthesis.

ADVERSE EFFECTS

These are the same as for other aminoglycosides (see Chapter 42). The main problems are eighth nerve toxicity (vestibulotoxicity more than deafness), nephrotoxicity and, less commonly, allergic reactions.

CONTRAINDICATIONS

Streptomycin is contraindicated in patients with eighth nerve dysfunction, in those who are pregnant, and in those with myasthenia gravis, as it has weak neuromuscular blocking activity.

PHARMACOKINETICS

Oral absorption is minimal, and therefore it is given intramuscularly. Streptomycin is mainly excreted via the kidney, and renal impairment requires dose adjustment. The $t_{\frac{1}{2}}$ of streptomycin is in the range 2–9 h. It crosses the blood–brain barrier when the meninges are inflamed.

PREPARATIONS CONTAINING COMBINED ANTI-TUBERCULOSIS- DRUGS

Several combination preparations of the first-line drugs are now available. They are helpful when patients are established on therapy, and the reduced number of tablets should aid compliance and importantly avoid monotherapy. Combined preparations available include Mynah (ethambutol and INH – in varying dosages), Rifinah and Rimactazid (containing rifampicin and INH) and Rifater (containing INH, 50 mg, rifampicin, 120 mg, and pyrazinamide, 300 mg).

THERAPEUTIC DRUG MONITORING IN TB THERAPY

In order to optimize therapy, reduce the development of resistance (and check compliance) certain authorities are undertaking therapeutic drug monitoring of anti-TB drugs in patients with multidrug resistant tuberculosis or in populations where there may be problems with drug absorption (e.g. HIV-positive patients).

Key points:

Mycobacterium Tuberculosis treatment

- Treatment is with multiple drugs to mimimize the development of resistance.
- Triple (pyrazinamide plus rifampicin plus INH) or quadruple (pyrazinamide plus rifampicin plus INH and ethambutol or streptomycin) therapy is given for the 2 first months.
- Two drugs (usually rifampicin and INH, depending on sensitivity) are given for a further 4 months, or longer if the patient is immunosuppressed.
- Formulations containing two (e.g. rifampicin/isoniazid) or three (e.g. rifampicin/isoniazid/pyrazinamide) drugs may improve compliance.
- Multi-drug-resistant *M. tuberculosis* requires four drugs initially, while awaiting sensitivity results.
- Drug combinations using second-line agents (e.g. ethionamide, cycloserine, capreomycin), based on sensitivities, are required to treat multi-drug-resistant *M. tuberculosis*. Such drugs are toxic, and treatment should be supervised by a clinician experienced in their use.

Treatment of tuberculous meningitis

Many of the problems involved in treating tuberculous meningitis arise from the poor penetration of most antimicrobials into the CSF. Pyrazinamide and isoniazid are the most useful drugs. They are highly effective and achieve concentrations in the CSF that are inhibitory to tubercle bacilli. Streptomycin penetrates well only when the meninges are inflamed, and is therefore only effective in the early stages of treatment. Ethambutol is also used with satisfactory penetration in the acute stage of the disease, particularly with higher dosage levels. Rifampicin penetrates poorly into the CSF, presumably because of the high protein-bound fraction in the plasma, and the concentration in the CSF only just reaches the minimum inhibitory concentration for tubercle bacilli.

The optimal regimen and duration for treating tuberculous meningeal infection have yet to be defined. The regimen of isoniazid, 10 mg/kg, with pyridoxine, 10 mg daily, rifampicin, 10mg/kg daily and pyrazinamide, 30 mg/kg daily, for 2 months followed by isoniazid and rifampicin continued for a further 10 months is effective. Streptomycin and ethambutol only penetrate the CSF well during the early stages when the meninges are inflamed. Corticosteroids are used in the initial stages of treatment of severe cases to reduce the risk of meningeal adhesions and obstructive hydrocephalus. Intrathecal drug administration is unnecessary.

Chemoprophylaxis

Contacts of patients with tuberculosis (especially children under 16 years of age who have not previously been innoculated with BCG) who have a positive reaction to tuberculin but no other evidence of disease should be considered for chemoprophylaxis. The usual regimen is isoniazid, 300 mg daily for 6 months, but with the increasing resistance of *M. tuberculosis* to isoniazid, combination therapy with rifampicin, 450–600 mg, and isoniazid, 300 mg/day for 3 months, is also used.

Tuberculosis and the acquired immune deficience syndrome (AIDS)

The immunocompromised state in HIV infection increases the difficulty of eradicating the tubercle bacillus. The absence of a normal immune defence necessitates prolonged courses of therapy. Treatment is continued either for 9 months, or for 6 months after the time of documented conversion to being culture negative, whichever is longer. Quadruple drug therapy should be used initially, because of increasing multi-drug resistance in this setting. Adverse drug reactions and interactions are commoner in HIV -positive patients, who must be carefully monitored.

Corticosteroids in tuberculosis therapy

Corticosteroids are seldom essential in tuberculosis therapy, the one absolute indication being adrenal failure (Addison's disease). (Tuberculous adrenal disease used to be the commonest cause of Addison's disease in the nineteenth century, and is again increasing.) However, corticosteroids may, be useful adjuncts to antituberculous therapy in several clinical situations, including the following:

1 resolution of large lymph nodes;
2 suppression of allergic drug reactions, including drug fever;
3 large pleural or pericardial effusions;
4 patients who are likely to die before chemotherapy can be effective;
5 tuberculous meningitis (to reduce the formation of meningeal adhesions).

The usual dose of corticosteroid should be doubled in patients who are receiving rifampicin (see above).

Second-line drugs and treatment of refractory tuberculosis

The commonest cause of *M. tuberculosis* treatment failure or relapse is non-compliance with therapy. The previous drug regimen used should be known and the current bacterial sensitivity defined. If the organisms are still sensitive to the original drugs, then more fully supervised and prolonged therapy with these drugs should be prescribed. Alternative drugs (which are toxic and difficult to use) are needed if bacterial resistance has arisen. Treatment should be supervised by a clinician who is experienced in their use. Organisms that are resistant to INH, rifampicin, pyrazinamide and ethambutol are now emerging, especially in the USA but also in the UK.

Several second-line antitiberculous drugs are listed in Table 43.2.

Mycobacterium leprae infection

This organism causes leprosy, an infection with two forms of clinical manifestations, namely lepromatoid (the organism being localized to skin or nerve) or lepromatous (a generalized bacteraemic

Table 43.2: Second-line antituberculous drugs, used mainly for drug-resistant TB

Drug	Childrens dose (mg/kg)	Adult dose (mg) Weight <50 kg	Weight >50 kg	Route	Major adverse effects
Ethionamide and Prothionamide	15–20	750	1000	Oral	Hepatitis, gastrointestinal and CNS disturbances, insomnia
PAS†	300	10–15 g	10–15 g	Oral	Gastrointestinal, rash, hepatitis
Thiacetazone	4	150	150	Oral	Gastrointestinal, rash, vertigo and conjunctivitis
			Divided doses		
Capreomycin*	1500	1 g	1 g	IM	Similar to streptomycin
Kanamycin*	15	0.5–1 g	0.5–1 g	IM	Similar to streptomycin
Cycloserine*	15	750	1000	Oral	Depression, fits and psychosis

* Adults only.
† PAS = *para*-aminosalicylic acid.

disease that effects many organs, analogous to miliary tuberculosis). The main drugs used in therapy are dapsone and rifampicin. **Dapsone** is 4,4′-diaminodiphenyl sulphone, and is given as 100 mg (1–2 mg/kg/day) once daily. Rifampicin is a more expensive alternative, and as resistance develops quickly it must be combined with a second agent. It is usually given as a single daily dose (450–600 mg orally). Other agents used in leprosy therapy are ethionamide, prothionamide and clofazimine. The advised World Health Organization (WHO) regimen for multibacillary leprosy is as follows:

1 rifampicin, 600 mg orally once monthly;
2 clofazimine, 50 mg daily unsupervised plus 300 mg supervised every 4 weeks (see Chapter 45).
3 dapsone, 100 mg daily unsupervised given for 24 months.

Dapsone

USES

Dapsone is a bacteriostatic sulphone. It has been the standard drug for treating all forms of leprosy, but irregular and inadequate duration of treatment as a single agent has produced resistance. Dapsone is used to treat dermatitis herpetiformis as well as leprosy, *Pneumocystis* and, combined with pyrimethamine, for malaria prophylaxis. It is administered orally, 100 mg once a day, for leprosy.

MECHANISM OF ACTION

Dapsone is a competitive inhibitor of dihydrofolate synthase, thereby blocking the production of dihydrofolic acid.

ADVERSE EFFECTS

These include the following:

1 anaemia and agranulocytosis;
2 gastrointestinal disturbances and (rarely) hepatitis;

Case history

A 27-year old Asian woman presents to her physician with a history of streaky haemoptysis and weight loss for the past 2 months. Clinical examination is reported as normal. Her chest X-ray shows patchy right upper lobe consolidation and her sputum is positive for acid-fast bacilli. After having obtained three sputum samples, she is started, while in hospital, on a four-drug regimen, pyrazinamide (800 mg/day), ethambutol (600 mg/day), isoniazid (300 mg/day) and rifampicin (450 mg/day). She is also given pyridoxine 10 mg daily (to reduce the likelihood of developing peripheral neuropathy secondary to INH). She tolerates the therapy well, without evidence of hepatic dysfunction, and her systemic symptoms improve. After 2 weeks on treatment she is discharged home. Three months later, when reviewed in the out-patient clinic, she has been off pyrazinamide and ethambutol for just over 1 month, and she complains of daily nausea and vomiting, and is found to be 8 weeks pregnant. She is taking the low-dose oestrogen contraceptive pill and is adamant that she has been meticulously compliant with all of her anti-TB medications and the contraceptive pill.

Question

What therapeutic problem has occurred here, and how can you explain the clinical situation? How could this outcome have been avoided?

Answer

Ethambutol, isoniazid, rifampicin and pyrazinamide are all potent inducers of hepatic cytochrome P_{450}. Over a period of several weeks they induce several cytochrome P_{450} isoenzymes, especially cytochrome $P_{450\ 3A4}$, such that the hepatic metabolism of oestrogen and progesterone are markedly enhanced, reducing their efficacy as contraceptives. Thus in this case, hepatic cytochrome P_{450} enzyme induction caused a failure of contraceptive efficacy and so the patient was 'unprotected' and became pregnant. The patient should continue on her anti-TB drug regimen, as there is no evidence that these agents are harmful to the developing fetus, except for streptomycin, which should never be given in pregnancy.

This outcome could have been prevented by advising the patient to double the usual dose of her oral contraceptives while taking anti-TB therapy, and to take additional contraceptive precautions - (e.g. barrier methods), or to abandon the pill altogether and use an alternative effective contraceptive measure (e.g. an intranterine contaceptive device) during her TB treatment.

3 allergy and rashes, including Stevens–Johnson syndrome'
4 peripheral neuropathy;
5 methaemoglobinaemia;
6 haemolytic anaemia, especially in glucose-6-phosphate dehydrogenase (G6PDH)-deficient patients in whom it is contraindicated.

PHARMACOKINETICS

Dapsone is well absorbed from the gastrointestinal tract (> 90%) and widely distributed. The $t_{\frac{1}{2}}$ is long (on average 27 h). It is extensively metabolized in the liver, partly by N-acetylation. There is some enterohepatic circulation, with only 10–20% of the parent drug being excreted in the urine.

DRUG INTERACTIONS

The metabolism of dapsone is increased by hepatic enzyme inducers (e.g. rifampicin) such that its $t_{\frac{1}{2}}$ is reduced to 12–15h.

FURTHER READING

Joint Tuberculosis Committee of the British Thoracic Society. 1990: Chemotherapy and management of tuberculosis in the UK. *Thorax* **45**, 403–8.

Joint Tuberculosis Committee of the British Thoracic Society. 1994: Control and prevention of tuberculosis in the UK. Code of practice. *Thorax* **49**,1193–2000.

Subcommittee of the Joint Tuberculosis Committee of the British Thoracic Society. 1992: Guidelines for the management of tuberculosis and HIV infections in the UK. *British Medical Journal* **304**, 1231–3.

CHAPTER FORTY-FOUR

FUNGAL *and* VIRAL INFECTIONS

- Antifungal drug therapy
- Antiviral drug therapy (excluding anti-HIV drugs)
- Interferons
- Immunoglobulins

ANTIFUNGAL DRUG THERAPY

INTRODUCTION

Fungi, like mammalian cells but unlike bacteria, are eukaryotic and possess nuclei, mitochondria and cell membranes. However, their membranes are unusual in containing distinctive sterols. The very success of antibacterial therapy has created ecological situations in which opportunistic fungal infections can flourish. In addition, potent immunosuppressive and cytotoxic therapies have produced patients with seriously impaired immune defences, in whom fungi that are non-pathogenic to healthy individuals become pathogenic and cause disease. Table 44.1 summarizes an approach to antifungal therapy in immunocompromised patients.

POLYENES

Amphotericin B

USES

Amphotericin is an antibiotic derived from *Streptomyces nodosus*, and is invaluable in treating life-threatening systemic fungal infections, but has considerable toxicity. The antifungal spectrum of **amphotericin B** is broad and includes *Candida* species (local and systemic infections), *Blastomyces dermatitidis* (which causes North American blastomycosis), *Histoplasma capsulatum* (which causes histoplasmosis), *Cryptococcus neoformans* (which causes cryptococcosis), *Coccidioides immitis* (which causes coccidioidomycosis) and *Sporotrichum schenckii* (which causes local and systemic sporotrichosis). *Aspergillus* species are also usually sensitive. Resistance is seldom acquired during treatment. Amphotericin is insoluble in water but can be complexed to bile salts to give an unstable colloid which can be administered intravenously. Several liposomal or lipid or colloidal complex amphotericin preparations have now been formulated, and they are less toxic (in particular less nephrotoxic) but more expensive than the standard formulation. They should be reserved for patients who experience unacceptable adverse effects from regular amphotericin. Amphotericin B is normally given as an intravenous infusion freshly prepared in 5% dextrose over 4–6 h. A 1-mg test dose is given at least 6 h before starting treatment. The initial dose is 5 mg daily in 500 mL of 5% dextrose which is increased daily by 5 mg up to a dose of 0.5–1 mg/kg daily and continued for 6–12 weeks. Treatment on alternate days at 1–1.5 mg/kg may reduce toxicity. Amphotericin may also be administered topically as lozenges (10 mg 3-hourly) or as a suspension for oral or oesophageal and gastrointestinal moniliasis, respectively. There is some evidence that effective

Table 44.1: Antifungal drug therapy in the immunocompromised host

Fungal infection	Drug therapy for superficial infection	Drug therapy for deep-seated infection
Candida	Nystatin – topical Clotrimazole – topical Miconazole – topical Fluconazole – oral	Amphotericin B with or without flucytosine Fluconazole – oral or IV Itraconazole or ketoconazole- oral
Aspergillus		Amphotericin B IV Itraconazole
Cryptococcus		Amphotericin B IV with or without flucytosine Fluconazole – oral or IV OR Itraconazole followed by chronic suppressive therapy with either fluconazole or itraconazole
Disseminated histoplasmosis		Itraconazole or Amphotericin B IV (or fluconazole)
Disseminated coccidiomycosis		Fluconazole or Amphotericin B IV (plus flucytosine) OR itraconazole
Blastomycosis		Itraconazole OR amphotericin B IV for severe infection

systemic therapy may be achieved by reduced doses and therefore lower toxicity if amphotericin is combined with 5–flucytosine. The dose of amphotericin should then be 0.3 mg/kg/day.

MECHANISM OF ACTION

Amphotericin is a polyene macrolide with a hydroxylated hydrophilic surface on one side of the molecule and an unsaturated conjugated lipophilic surface on the other. The lipophilic surface binds to sterols in fungal cell membranes and increases membrane permeability by creating a 'membrane pore' with a hydrophilic centre which causes leakage and loss of small molecules such as glucose and potassium ions. Amphotericin has a higher affinity for the ergosterol of fungal membranes than for the cholesterol of mammalian membranes, resulting in clinically useful selectivity.

ADVERSE EFFECTS

These include the following:

1 fever, chills, headache, nausea and vomiting, and hypotension during intravenous infusion. Pulse and temperature should be monitored every 30 min and the infusion can be halted if necessary;
2 nephrotoxicity is almost invariable and results from vasoconstriction, tubular damage leading to renal tubular acidosis and acute renal failure. Fortunately, most of these effects are reversible if they are detected early enough and the drug is discontinued or the dose reduced;
3 hypokalaemia and hypomagnesaemia;
4 normochromic normocytic anaemia due to temporary marrow suppression is common.

PHARMACOKINETICS

Amphotericin is poorly absorbed following oral administration, and therefore for systemic mycoses it must be given by intravenous infusion. Liposomal or lipid/micellar delivery systems yield adequate plasma concentrations with a lower incidence of systemic and nephrotoxicity. Amphotericin distributes very unevenly throughout the body – CSF concentrations are $\frac{1}{40}$ of the plasma concentration. Amphotericin B is over 90% protein bound, but is concentrated in the reticuloendothelial system. The $t_{\frac{1}{2}}$ is 18–24 hours. Only 5% is excreted in the urine and drug elimination is unaffected by renal failure.

Nystatin

Nystatin is another polyene antifungal antibiotic isolated from *Streptomyces* with an identical mode of action to amphotericin B, but its greater toxicity precludes systemic use. In general, nystatin has a broad antifungal spectrum, but Epidermophytes are not sensitive to it. Its indications are limited to cutaneous/mucocutaneous and intestinal infections, especially those caused by *Candida* species. Little or no nystatin is absorbed systemically from the oropharynx or gastrointestinal tract, and resistance to nystatin does not develop during therapy. Preparations of nystatin include tablets, pastilles, lozenges or suspension, given in doses of 100 000–500 000 units three times daily for oral or intestinal *Candida* infections. Patients may often prefer topical amphotericin B because nystatin has an intensely bitter taste. Cutaneous infections are treated with ointment, and vaginitis is treated by suppositories.

ADVERSE EFFECTS

Nystatin causes nausea and diarrhoea only when large doses are administered orally.

> **Key points**
>
> Polyene antifungal therapy
>
> - Wide spectrum of anti-fungal activity – fungicidal–makes 'pores' in fungal membranes.
> - Available for topical (nystatin and amphotericin) treatment of common mucocutaneous fungal infections.
> - Amphotericin is used intravenously for deep-seated and severe fungal infections (e.g. *Aspergillus* or histoplasmosis).
> - Intravenous amphotericin is toxic, causing fever, chills, hypotension during infusion, nephrotoxicity, electrolyte abnormalities and transient bone-marrow suppression.
> - Systemic toxicity of amphotericin is reduced by using the liposomal/lipid/micellar formulations.
> - Amphotericin combined with 5-flucytosine is used in severe infections and immunosuppressed patients.

AZOLES–IMIDAZOLES

Imidazole antifungal drugs are fungistatic at low concentrations and fungicidal at higher concentrations. They are used topically and are active against both dermatophytes and yeasts such as *Candida*. Some imidazoles are also used systemically, although they have limited efficacy and significant toxicity, limiting their systemic use. They act by interfering with the synthesis of an important component of fungal cell membranes, namely ergosterol. Imidazoles competitively inhibit lanosterol 14-α-demethylase (a fungal cytochrome-haem P_{450} enzyme), which is a major enzyme in the pathway that synthesizes ergosterol from squalene. Inhibition of this enzyme causes disruption of the acyl chains of phospholipids, increasing membrane fluidity and causing membrane leakage and dysfunction of membrane-bound enzymes such as adenosine triphosphatase (ATPase). The imidazoles have considerable specificity/affinity for the fungal cytochrome-haem P_{450} enzymes.

Ketoconazole

USES

Ketoconazole is used as oral or topical therapy for dermatophytic infections and some phycomycetes. It is active against systemic infection with *Candida*, *Blastomyces*, *Histoplasma capsulatum* and *Cryptococcus neoformans*. *Aspergillus* and *Mucor* species are resistant. It is given orally (200–400 mg once daily). Its systemic use has waned because of the relatively high incidence of hepatic and endocrine side-effects.

ADVERSE EFFECTS

These include the following:

1. nausea and vomiting, which can be reduced by giving the drug with food;
2. transient liver enzyme abnormalities occur in 5–10% of patients, but fulminant hepatic damage, jaundice and fever are rare;
3. gynaecomastia (by blocking testosterone synthesis);
4. impotence and azoospermia;
5. adrenal insufficiency (by inhibiting cortisol biosynthesis).

PHARMACOKINETICS

Ketoconazole is given orally and achieves maximum plasma concentrations within 1–2 h. It is approximately 90% protein bound and is relatively widely distributed in the tissues. However, cerebrospinal fluid concentrations are only 5% of those in the plasma. Ketoconazole is extensively metabolized by hydroxylation and oxidative N-dealkylation by the liver, and only 2–4% of the dose is found in the urine as parent drug. The mean elimination $t_{\frac{1}{2}}$ is 8 h.

DRUG INTERACTIONS

Azoles are involved in multiple drug–drug interactions, the most dangerous being due to their inhibition of cytochrome $P_{450\,3A4}$. Examples of common/dangerous interactions are given below, but the reader should also consult drug interaction texts as this list is *not* comprehensive:

1. Antacids, H_2-blockers and proton-pump inhibitors (e.g. omeprazole) reduce ketoconazole absorption.
2. Ketoconazole reduces the metabolism of cyclosporin, increasing its plasma concencration and thus its toxicity (e.g. nephrotoxicity).
3. Ketoconazole reduces warfarin metabolism, enhancing its anticoagulant effect.
4. Ketoconazole reduces the metabolism of antihistamines and cisapride enhancing their cardiotoxic (pro-arrhythmic) effects.
5. Ketoconazole reduces metabolism and increases the plasma concentrations of the statins (e.g. simvastatin), leading to a higher risk of myositis/rhabdomyolysis.
6. Rifampicin increases the metabolism of ketoconazole.
7. Ketoconazole should not be used with amphotericin B because it reduces its effectiveness.

The properties of other commonly used imidazoles are listed in Table 44.2.

AZOLES – TRIAZOLES

This group of drugs (e.g. fluconazole) is derived from the imidazoles, but they are nitroimidazoles and have a wider antifungal spectrum. Their mechanism of action is identical to that of the imidazoles (e.g. ketoconazole). However, fluconazole is more specific for this fungal cytochrome P_{450} enzyme and consequently less likely to cause adverse effects due to inhibition of human hepatic $P_{450\,3A4}$ or human steroid biosynthetic enzymes for testosterone or cortisol.

Fluconazole

Uses

Fluconazole is a potent and broad-spectrum antifungal agent. It is active against *Candida* species, *Cryptococcus neoformans* and *Histoplasma capsulatum*. However, *Cryptococcus cruseii* and *Aspergillus* species are resistant and resistant *Candida* species are now being isolated from AIDS patients. Fluconazole is used clinically to treat superficial *Candida* infections and oesophageal *Candida*, for the acute therapy of disseminated *Candida*, systemic therapy for blastomycosis and histoplasmosis, for dermatophytic fungal infections and for prophylaxis in neutropenic patients. It may be given orally or intravenously as a once daily dose. For superficial infections it is given as 50–100 mg/day. In systemic or meningitic infections 200–400 mg are required intravenously daily for 4–6 weeks, followed by a daily maintenance dose. For prophylaxis in cytotoxic immunosuppressed patients 50–100 mg are adequate.

ADVERSE EFFECTS

Unlike ketoconazole, fluconazole does not reduce the synthesis of testosterone or cortisol. Adverse effects include the following:

1. gastrointestinal upsets with nausea, abdominal distension, diarrhoea and flatulence;
2. skin rashes, including erythema multiforme;
3. hepatitis.

CONTRAINDICATIONS

Fluconazole is contraindicated in pregnancy because of fetal defects in rodents. Breast-milk concentrations are similar to those in plasma, and fluconazole should not be used in nursing mothers.

PHARMACOKINETICS

Fluconazole is rapidly absorbed after oral administration, with maximum plasma concentrations achieved within 1–2 h. Absorption is virtually complete, and is unaffected by food or gastric pH. There is no presystemic metabolism, and its mean elimination $t_{\frac{1}{2}}$ is 30 h. Fluconazole is 11% bound to plasma proteins and is widely distributed throughout the body. CSF concentrations reach 50–80% of those in the plasma. About 80% is excreted by the kidney, and thus dose reduction is

Table 44.2: Properties of other commonly used imidazoles (see also Chapter 50)

Drug*	Use	Standard dosing regimen	Side-effects	Pharmacokinetics	Other specific comments
Clotrimazole	Topical therapy for dermatophyte and for *Candida* infections	1% cream or powder applied twice daily	Local irritation	Poorly absorbed from gastrointestinal tract	Induces its own metabolism – not used systemically
Miconazole	Oral *Candida* Topical therapy for ringworm, *Candida* and pityriasis	Oral gel, 25 mg/mL; 10 mL in mouth 4 times daily 2% cream or powder applied twice daily	Nausea and vomiting, rashes Local irritation	Systemic absorption is very poor, undergoes extensive hepatic metabolism	
Tiaconazole	Topical treatment for nail infections with dermatophytes and yeasts	Apply 28% solution to nails and local skin twice daily for 6 months	Minor local irritation	Systemic absorption is negligible	

* Other drugs in this group that are used topically include butoconazole, econazole, fentionazole, isoconazole and sulconazole.

required in renal failure. Fluconazole is a weak inhibitor (compared to ketoconazole) of human hepatic cytochrome $P_{450\ 3A}$.

DRUG INTERACTIONS

Fluconazole reduces the metabolism of several drugs by inhibiting cytochrome $P_{450\ 3A}$, such drugs including cyclosporin, warfarin, diltiazem, benzodiazepines, the taxanes, etc. The plasma concentrations and toxicity of these drugs will increase during concomitant treatment with fluconazole. Rifampicin enhances the metabolism of fluconazole.

The properties of other clinically important triazoles are shown in Table 44.3.

> **Key points**
>
> Azole antifungal treatment
>
> - Relatively wide spectrum of antifungal activity, fungistatic, but fungicidal with higher concentrations.
> - Impairs ergosterol biosynthesis by inhibiting lanosterol 14-α-demethylase (fungal cytochrome enzyme).
> - Available as intravenous, oral and topical formulations.
> - Can be used as therapy for superficial (e.g. *Candida*) and serious deep-seated (e.g. *Cryptococcus*) fungal infections
> - Ketoconazole is hepatotoxic, but fluconazole is much less so.
> - Ketoconazole (imidazole) to a greater extent than fluconazole (triazole) inhibits human P_{450} enzymes (especially cytochrome $P_{450\ 3A}$), reduces human sex and adrenal steroid biosynthesis, and causes multiple drug interactions.

ALLYLAMINES

Terbinafine

Terbinafine is an allylamine and is fungicidal. It can be given orally and is used to treat ringworm (*Tinea pedis*, *T. cruris* or *T corporis*) or dermatophyte infections of the nails if oral therapy is considered appropriate. It is given as a 250-mg dose once daily for 2–6 weeks or longer in infections of the nailbed as an alternative to griseofulvin. It acts by inhibiting the enzyme squalene epoxidase, which is involved in fungal ergosterol biosynthesis. It interferes with human cytochrome P_{450}, but only to a limited extent (e.g. 10–15% increase in cyclosporin concentrations). It is well absorbed, strongly bound to plasma proteins and concentrated in the stratum corneum. It is eliminated by hepatic metabolism and the mean elimination $t_{\frac{1}{2}}$ is 17 h. Its major side-effects are nausea, abdominal discomfort, anorexia, diarrhoea and rashes (including urticaria). Dose reduction is needed in hepatic failure and if cimetidine is given concurrently. Rifampicin increases terbinafine metabolism, requiring a dose increase. **Naftifine**, another allylamine, will be available for topical administration.

OTHER ANTIFUNGAL AGENTS

Flucytosine (5–fluorocytosine)

USES

Flucytosine is used to treat systemic candidiasis and cryptococcosis, provided that the strain is sensitive. Its spectrum is relatively restricted to *Cryptococcus neoformans*, *Candida albicans* and some other *Candida* species, *Torulopsis* species and *Cladosporum* species. Even certain strains of these species are resistant (5–15%), and filamentous fungi, especially *Aspergillus*, are resistant. The optimal oral dose is 200 mg/kg/day every 6 h. For very ill patients an intravenous preparation is available. It is *only* used in combination therapy (e.g. with amphotericin B). Single agent and topical use is avoided due to the widespread and rapid emergence of resistant *Candida* species.

MECHANISM OF ACTION

Flucytosine enters the fungus by active transport. Its precise mode of action is unknown. It is deaminated to 5–fluorouracil (by the enzyme cytosine deaminase, which is only present in fungal cells), a known precursor of the antimetabolite 5-FdUMP that inhibits thymidylate synthetase, thereby impairing DNA synthesis.

ADVERSE EFFECTS

These include the following:

1 gastrointestinal upsets;
2 leukopenia;

Table 44.3: Clinical therapeutics of other triazole antifungal agents

Drug	Use	Standard dosing regimen	Side-effects	Pharmacokinetics	Other specific comments
Itraconazole	Systemic fungal infections not treatable by other antifungal agents	Oral dose 200 mg daily (or 200 mg twice daily if severe)	Gastrointestinal upsets, rashes, hepatitis	Orally 85% absorbed, first-pass effect, hepatic metabolism, 99% protein bound, $t_{\frac{1}{2}}$ is 20 h	Absorption is reduced by drugs that reduce gastric acid levels
	Dermatophyte infections, oral *Candida* and *Pityriasis versicolor*	Oral dose 100 mg daily	Does not cause endocrine disturbances like ketoconazole		Inhibits cytochrome $P_{450\ 3A4}$ drug interactions are fewer than with fluconazole Hepatic enzyme-inducers lower plasma concentrations
Voriconazole and several other new triazoles	Currently undergoing pre-clinical and early clinical development				

3 hepatitis may occur, so liver function tests should be monitored.

At plasma concentrations below 100 μg/mL there is little danger of toxicity. Depression of bone marrow and hepatotoxicity are associated with higher concentrations. Plasma concentration measurement is helpful in managing patients with impaired renal function.

PHARMACOKINETICS

Flucytosine is well absorbed from the gut, peak concentrations of 75–90 μg/mL being reached on a dose of 50 mg/kg 6-hourly. It penetrates adequately into the CSF, in contrast to amphotericin B, and consequently is particularly useful when combined with amphotericin to treat cryptococcal meningitis. It is excreted largely unchanged by glomerular filtration, less than 10% of the dose undergoing metabolism. The $t_{\frac{1}{2}}$ is 6 h, and is prolonged in renal failure.

DRUG INTERACTIONS

The effect of flucytosine is antagonized by concurrent administration of cytosine arabinoside. Amphotericin (and azoles) act additively or synergistically with flucytosine. Flucytosine should *only* be used in combination. These combinations are useful because amphotericin is more effective but also more toxic than flucytosine, which also penetrates the blood–brain barrier better than amphotericin. Concurrent use of amphotericin reduces the likelihood of resistance to flucytosine emerging during therapy.

Griseofulvin

USES

Griseofulvin was isolated from *Penicillium griseofulvium*. It is orally active, but its spectrum is limited to dermatophytes (ringworm fungi). It is concentrated in keratinized cells and is the drug of choice for treatment of childhood dermatophyte infections. It is given orally (0.5–1 g daily in two divided doses) with meals. Therapy is recommended for 6 weeks for skin infections, and for up to 12 months for nail infections.

MECHANISM OF ACTION

Griseofulvin is actively taken up by fungi. Its mode of action is obscure, but it binds to the microtubules that form the mitotic spindle, blocking polymerization of the microtubule. It also interferes with fungal DNA replication, resulting in distorted hyphal growth.

ADVERSE EFFECTS

These include the following:

1 headaches and mental dullness or inattention;
2 diarrhoea or nausea;
3 rashes and photosensitivity;
4 griseofulvin can precipitate attacks of acute intermittent porphyria and can cause drug-induced systemic lupus enythematosus.

PHARMACOKINETICS

Griseofulvin is almost insoluble in water and is formulated as micronized particles. Its absorption is facilitated by a fatty meal. The onset of action is slow due to its uptake into slow-growing keratinized structures prior to reaching the site of infection. The cell turnover time determines the efficacy of treatment, so palmar and plantar skin require at least 8 weeks of treatment, fingernails require 6 months and toenails up to 1 year for eradicative treatment. Griseofulvin is metabolized by the liver to inactive 6-demethylgriseofulvin, which is excreted in the urine. Less than 1% of free griseofulvin is renally excreted, so it can be used in normal doses in renal failure.

DRUG INTERACTIONS

Griseofulvin induces hepatic cytochrome P_{450} enzyme activity and consequently interacts with many drugs, reducing their therapeutic effect (e.g. it decreases the anticoagulant effect of warfarin). Other inducing agents (e.g. rifampicin, barbiturates) enhance griseofulvin metabolism.

ANTIVIRAL DRUG THERAPY (EXCLUDING ANTI-HIV DRUGS)

INTRODUCTION

Many viral illnesses are mild and/or self-limiting, but a few of them are inherently deadly (e.g. the now extinct smallpox and the global HIV-1 epidemic). Patients who are immunocompromised, especially by HIV-1 infection, are also at risk of serious illness from viruses that are seldom serious in otherwise healthy hosts. Antiviral drug therapy is therefore increasingly important, and is considered in this section apart from the specific anti-human immunodeficiency virus (HIV) drugs, which are considered separately in Chapter 45. Antiviral therapy is more difficult than antibacterial therapy because its therapeutic targets often involve human cellular processes or its enzymes involves targets which are not that different to the equivalent enzymes/structures in human cells.

1. Viral replication is essentially intracellular, so drugs must penetrate cells in order to be effective.
2. Viral replication, although under the control of the viral genome, involves the metabolic enzymes and processes of host cells.
3. Although viral replication begins almost immediately after the host cell has been penetrated, the clinical signs and symptoms of infection often appear after peak replication is over. Clinical manifestations often result from inflammatory and other processes mounted by the host in response to viral tissue damage.

There are several events in viral colonization which might prove susceptible as drug targets:

1. when the virus is outside cells it is susceptible to antibody attack, but it has proved difficult to find drugs that are non-toxic yet which can destroy viruses in this situation;
2. viral attachment to the cell surface probably involves a specific chemical reaction between the virus coat and the cell surface. Neuraminidase, an enzyme that destroys myxovirus receptors, including those on cell surfaces, has an effect on experimental infections in animals;
3. penetration of the cell membrane can be prevented (e.g. for influenza A amantadine, or neuraminidase inhibitors);
4. uncoating of the virus with release of viral nucleic acid intracellularly;
5. viral nucleic acid acts as a template for new strands of nucleic acid that in turn direct the production of new viral components utilizing the host cell's synthetic mechanisms. Most antiviral drugs in current use act at this stage of viral replication;
6. extracellular release of new viral particles.

NUCLEOSIDE ANALOGUES

ACYCLOVIR

USES

Acyclovir is a potent and selective inhibitor of herpes viruses (particularly herpes simplex). It is also effective against herpes zoster, but is much less active against cytomegalovirus (which also belongs to the group of herpes viruses). Acyclovir and its newer analogues make the continued use of idoxuridine obsolete.

1. Three per cent acyclovir ointment applied five times daily for up to 14 days accelerates healing in herpetic keratitis.
2. The efficacy of local application of acyclovir in genital and labial herpes simplex has been unimpressive. Despite its low bioavailability, 200 mg given orally five times daily accelerates healing in genital herpes. It is much less effective in secondary than in primary infection. It does not eliminate vaginal carriage, so Caesarean section is indicated to avoid neonatal herpes.
3. Treatment of shingles (herpes zoster) should be started within 72 h of the onset, and is useful for patients with severe pain, although it shortens the illness by only a short time and is expensive. Acyclovir, 800 mg five times daily, is given for 7 days.
4. In generalized herpes simplex or herpetic meningoencephalitis acyclovir can be given intravenously in doses of 5 mg/kg infused intravenously over 1 h three times daily for 5 days. The acyclovir dose in immunocompromised hosts with herpes simplex, shingles or herpes simplex encephalitis is 10 mg/kg IV three times daily for at least 10 days. A reduced dosage is required for patients with impaired renal function.

MECHANISM OF ACTION

Acyclovir is an acyclic analogue of guanosine. Its selective action results from metabolic activation to its monophosphate, solely in infected cells, by a specific thymidine kinase that is coded for by the virus but not by the host genome. Acyclovir monophosphate (is converted intracellularly to its di- and triphosphate (ACYC-TP). The viral DNA polymerase is inhibited competitively by ACYC-TP from synthesizing nascent viral DNA.

ADVERSE EFFECTS

These include the following:

1 a reversible rise in plasma urea and creatinine;
2 neurological disturbances;
3 rashes;
4 nausea and vomiting;
5 hepatitis.

CONTRAINDICATIONS

Acyclovir is relatively contraindicated in pregnancy as it is an analogue of guanosine and so potentially teratogenic in the first trimester.

PHARMACOKINETICS

The bioavailability of acyclovir in humans is only 20% after administration of 200 mg orally, and may be dose dependent. Acyclovir has a mean elimination $t_{\frac{1}{2}}$ of 3 h, and crosses the blood–brain barrier to give a CSF concentration that is approximately 50% of that in plasma. Plasma protein binding is approximately 20%. Clearance is largely renal and includes an element of tubular secretion; renal impairment requires dose/schedule adjustment.

DRUG INTERACTIONS

Probenecid prolongs the half-life of acyclovir by 20% by inhibiting renal tubular secretion.

Key points

Acyclovir and its analogues

- Acyclovir is an acyclic guanosine analogue, that is active against the herpes virus.
- These agents are initially phosphorylated by virally coded thymidine kinase and further phosphorylated to their triphosphate form, which inhibits the viral DNA polymerase.
- They are used to treat oral herpes simplex (topical), genital herpes simplex (oral therapy) and herpes encephalitis (intravenous therapy).
- Acyclovir has low oral bioavailability. Famciclovir (prodrug of penciclovir) and valaciclovir (an acyclovir prodrug) have much greater bioavailability than acyclovir.
- Side-effects are mild – increased creatinine levels, rashes, hepatitis and gastrointestinal disturbances.
- Viral resistance to acyclovir is developing.

Foscarnet (trisodium phosphonoformate)

USES

Foscarnet is active against several other important viruses, notably HIV-1 and all human herpes viruses, including acyclovir-resistant herpes viruses and cytomegalovirus (CMV). It is used to treat CMV infections (retinitis, pneumonitis, colitis and oesophagitis) and acyclovir-resistant herpes simplex virus (HSV) infections in immunocompetent and immunosuppressed hosts. Foscarnet is given as a loading dose of 30 mg/kg intravenously over 30 min followed by 60–90 mg/kg as a 1-h infusion 8-hourly. After 2–3 weeks of treatment, doses are reduced to 20–30 mg/kg/day. Dose reduction is required in patients with renal failure.

MECHANISM OF ACTION

Foscarnet is a nucleotide analogue that acts as a non-competitive inhibitor of viral DNA polymerase and inhibits the reverse transcriptase from several retroviruses. It is inactive against eukaryotic DNA polymerases at concentrations that inhibit viral DNA replication.

ADVERSE EFFECTS

These include the following:

1 nephrotoxicity, a problem that can be minimized by adequate hydration and dose reduction if the creatinine level rises; monitoring of renal function is mandatory;
2 central nervous system effects include irritability, anxiety and fits;
3 nausea, vomiting and headache;
4 thrombophlebitis;
5 hypocalcaemia and hypomagnaesemia;
6 hypoglycaemia (rare).

PHARMACOKINETICS

Foscarnet is poorly absorbed (2–5%) after oral administration. It does not undergo presystemic metabolism, is only 14–17% protein bound, and is widely distributed. Plasma concentrations decay in a triphasic manner, and the terminal $t_{\frac{1}{2}}$ is 18 h. Foscarnet is excreted renally by glomerular filtration and tubular excretion. Approximately 20% remains in the body bound in bone.

DRUG INTERACTIONS

The nephrotoxicity of foscarnet is potentiated in the presence of other nephrotoxins such as pentamidine, gentamicin, cyclosporin and amphotericin B. Administration with pentamidine can also cause marked hypocalcaemia.

Ganciclovir (dihydroxy-propoxymethylguanine DHPG)

USES

Ganciclovir, a guanine analogue, is used to treat sight-or life-threatening CMV infections (e.g. retinitis, pneumonitis, colitis and oesophagitis) in immunocompromised hosts. It also has potent activity against herpes viruses 1 and 2. It is administered at an induction dose of 5 mg/kg every 12 h for 14–21 days as an intravenous infusion over 1 h, followed by a maintenance dose of 6 mg/kg for 5 days every week or 5 mg/kg for 7 days a week continuously. Oral ganciclovir is now available for therapy despite its poor bioavailability, and is given as 500 mg every 4 h. Comparative studies have shown that oral treatment is slightly less effective than intravenous therapy in CMV retinitis in AIDS patients, but is easier for the patients and less expensive. Intravitreal ganciclovir implants are also effective in treating CMV retinitis.

MECHANISM OF ACTION

Ganciclovir is metabolized intracellularly to its monophosphate in herpes-infected cells by virally encoded thymidine kinase. It undergoes further phosphorylation by host kinases to its triphosphate anabolite which competitively inhibits the CMV (or HSV) DNA polymerase. If it is incorporated into nascent viral DNA, it causes chain termination. Ganciclovir is concentrated 10 times in infected cells compared to uninfected cells.

ADVERSE EFFECTS

These include the following:

1 neutropenia and bone-marrow suppression (thrombocytopenia and less often anaemia)–cell counts usually return to normal within 2–5 days of discontinuing the drug;
2 temporary or possibly permanent inhibition of spermatogenesis or oogenesis;
3 phlebitis and pain at the infusion site;
4 rashes and fever;
5 gastrointestinal upsets;
6 transient increases in liver enzymes and creatinine in underhydrated patients.

CONTRAINDICATIONS

Ganciclovir is contraindicated in pregnancy (it is teratogenic in animals) and in breast-feeding women.

PHARMACOKINETICS

Only 4–7.5% of an oral dose of ganciclovir is absorbed, indicating that intravenous administration is to be preferred. It is less than 2% protein bound and is widely distributed, with a mean elimination $t_{\frac{1}{2}}$ of 2–5 h. Ganciclovir is virtually totally excreted by the kidney, and dose reduction is needed in renal failure.

DRUG INTERACTIONS

Probenecid reduces renal clearance of ganciclovir. Antineoplastic drugs, co-trimoxazole and amphotericin B increase its toxic effects on rapidly dividing tissues including bone-marrow, skin and gut epithelium. Zidovudine should not be given concomitantly with ganciclovir because of the potentiation of bone marrow suppression.

The properties of some recently available acyclovir-like antiviral drugs are shown in Table 44.4.

Tribavirin (ribavirin)

USES

Tribavirin is active against a number of RNA and DNA (HSV-1 and HSV-2, influenza) viruses. Its main use is in the treatment of bronchiolitis secondary to respiratory syncytial virus infection in infants and children, although its efficacy is disputed. Administration for bronchiolitis is via aerosol inhalation or nebulizer of a solution of 20 mg/mL for 12–18 h (dose is 6 g daily) for between 3 days and a maximum of 7 days.

MECHANISM OF ACTION

Tribavirin is taken up into cells and phosphorylated to tribavirin 5′-monophosphate by adenosine kinase, and is then rapidly phosphorylated to its di- and triphosphates by other cellular kinases. Tribavirin 5′-triphosphate inhibits the guanylation reaction in the formation of the 5′ cap of

Table 44.4: Summary of the properties of recently available acyclovir-like antiviral agents and others

Drug*	Use	Standard dosing regimen	Side-effects	Pharmacokinetics	Other specific comments
Famciclovir	Herpes simplex virus (HSV) and recurrent genital HSV varicella zoster (VZV)	Orally 250 mg tds or 750 mg od in UK	See acyclovir	Prodrug of peniciclovir Bioavailability of penciclovir is 77% from famciclovir $t_{\frac{1}{2}}$ is 2.5 h Renal excretion	High bioavailability, prodrug of penciclovir Acyclovir-resistant isolates are cross-resistant
Penciclovir	Systemic therapy for HSV and VZV and hepatitis B virus Topical therapy for HSV	IV/topical IV 5 mg/kg/day for 8 days Topical 1% cream	See acyclovir Same as placebo for topical use	Bioavailability is very good. $t_{\frac{1}{2}}$ is 2.5 h Renal excretion (In renal failure $t_{\frac{1}{2}}$ = 18 h.) Intracellular triphosphate is longer-lasting (7–20 h) than acyclovir	High bioavailability. Viral DNA polymerase not as sensitive to Pen-TP Acyclovir-resistant isolates are cross-resistant
Valaciclovir	HSV infection but uncertainty about VZV and CMV in future	Oral dosing 500–2000 mg tds	L-valyl ester of acyclovir Haemolytic – uraemic /TTP syndrome in immunosuppressed individuals	Rapid absorption bioavailability is 54% Converted to acyclovir before phosphorylation	High bioavailability Acyclovir-resistant isolates are cross-resistant
Cidofovir	Intravenous therapy for HSV and CMV	Intravenous, once weekly for 2 weeks, then every two weeks 5 mg/kg/dose	See ganciclovir, but has been noted to cause renal failure	Plasma $t_{\frac{1}{2}}$ of parent is 2.6 h and of cidofovir diphosphate (active) is 17–30 h Cidofovir is renally excreted	CMV isolates resistant to ganciclovir are sensitive. Not to be used in patients with renal failure
Lobucavir	Analogue of ganciclovir. Systemic therapy for CMV	Oral dose to be determined – 20–200 mg bd	See ganciclovir	Oral bioavailability is 20–40%	Still undergoing clinical development

* Other new drugs in the antiviral arena undergoing future clinical development include sorivudine (nucleoside analogue for VZV) *n*-Docosanol (topical cream for recurrent herpes labialis) and ISIS 2922 (an antisense phosphorothioate oligonucleotide complementary to human CMV immediate-early mRNA, currently being investigated in AIDS patients).

mRNA and inhibits viral RNA methyltransferase. It has little or no effect on mammalian RNA methyltransferase.

ADVERSE EFFECTS

No systemic adverse effects of tribavirin have been reported following administration by aerosol or nebulizer. General adverse effects include the following:

1 worsening respiration and bacterial pneumonia;
2 pneumothorax;
3 teratogenic potential even with aerosol exposure in health care workers.

PHARMACOKINETICS

Following nebulized administration, negligible amounts of tribavirin are absorbed systemically.

Amantadine (or rimantidine)

Amantadine is effective in preventing the spread of influenza A, and it also has an unrelated action in Parkinson's disease (see Chapter 20). Its usefulness as an antiviral agent is limited to influenza A – it is inactive against influenza B and only weakly active on influenza C and rubella. These are all RNA viruses. Its mode of action is unknown. Prophylaxis with amantadine (100–200 mg daily) has an advantage over immunization in that the latter can be ineffective when a new antigenic variant arises in the community and spreads too rapidly for a killed virus vaccine to be prepared and administered. Prophylaxis by amantadine during an epidemic should be considered for persons at special risk, for (e.g. patients with severe cardiac or lung disease, or health-care personnel). Amantadine is less effective during periods of antigenic variation than during periods of relative antigenic stability. Treating established influenza infections with amantidine within 48 h yields some amelioration of headache and upper respiratory tract infection symptoms. The mean elimination $t_{\frac{1}{2}}$ is approximately 12 h, and clearance is via renal excretion. Thus dose reductions are needed when amantadine is given to patients with renal failure.

ADVERSE EFFECTS

These include the following:

1 dizziness, nervousness and headaches with short-term use;
2 livedo reticularis.

Zanamivir

This inhibitor of influenza virus neuraminidases has shown early promise in treating the symptoms of influenza A and B, if topical intranasal therapy is initiated early.

> **Key points**
>
> Antiviral therapy
>
> - Selective toxicity for viruses is more difficult to achieve than for fungi or bacteria.
> - Viruses survive and proliferate inside human cells and often use human cellular enzymes and processes to undertake part of their replicative process.
> - Certain viruses encode virus-specific enzymes that can be targeted (e.g. herpes virus and acyclovir; CMV virus and its DNA polymerase which is a target for ganciclovir).

INTERFERONS

Interferons are cytokines (mediators of cell growth and function). They are glycoproteins secreted by cells infected with viruses or foreign double-stranded DNA. They are non-antigenic, and are active against a wide range of viruses, but unfortunately they are relatively species specific. Thus it is necessary to produce human interferon to act on human cells. Interferon production is triggered not only by viruses but also by tumour cells or previously encountered foreign antigens. Certain interferons are also important in immune cell regulation.

Four main types of interferon, with different structures, derivation and properties, are recognized:

1 **interferon-α** – known previously as leukocyte or lymphoblastoid interferon. Subspecies of the human α gene produce variants designated by the addition of a number, e.g. interferon-α_2, or in the case of a mixture of proteins, by Nl, N2, etc. Two methods of commercial production

have been developed and these are indicated by *rbe* (produced from bacteria (*Escherichia coli*) genetically modified by recombinant DNA technology), and *lns* (produced from cultured lymphoblasts stimulated by Sendai virus). Interferon-α_2 may also differ in the amino acids at positions 23 and 24, and these are shown by the addition of a letter. Thus α-2a has lys–his at these sites whilst α-2b has arg–his. It is not yet clear whether these different molecules have different therapeutic properties;

2 **interferon-β** from fibroblasts;
3 **interferon-ω** with 60% homology to interferon-α, and not yet clinically available;
4 **interferon-γ** formerly called 'immune' interferon because it is produced by lymphocytes in response to antigens and mitogens.

Commercial production of interferon by cloning of human interferon genes into bacterial and yeast plasmids is now available, facilitating large-scale production.

USES

Interferon-α provides effective therapy for chronic hepatitis B and C infection (see Chapter 33), and is given three times a week by subcutaneous injection of 1–5 million units, for 6–12 months. Interferon-β has been shown to be of some benefit in patients with relapsing multiple sclerosis. Interferon-β_{2B} is used to treat condylomata acuminata by intralesional injection. All three interferons are used to treat hairy cell leukaemia. Interferon-α_{2a} and interferon-α_{2b} are used to treat Kaposi's sarcoma in AIDS patients, and interferon-α_{2b} is effective in recurrent or metastatic renal cell carcinoma (see Chapter 47). Recombinant interferon-γ_{1b} has been used for the treatment of chronic granulomatous disease, and is under investigation for the treatment of mesothelioma and carcinoma of the ovary. Interferon therapy is beneficial in chronic myelogenous leukaemia, multiple myeloma, refractory lymphoma and metastatic melanoma. Interferons are being investigated for the treatment of rheumatoid arthritis and mycosis fungoides, and as an additional component of standard chemotherapy combinations.

MECHANISM OF ACTION

Interferons bind to a common cell-membrane receptor, except interferon-γ, which binds to its own receptor. Following receptor binding, interferons produce a complex series of effects which follow a tyrosine phosphorylation cascade and lead to the activation of various signal transducers and activators of transcription proteins, the latter being transported to the nucleus where in combination with interferon stimulated gene factor-3 (ISGF-3) or GAF, they cause transcription of certain genes. Consequently, the quantities of a number of enzymes with antiviral activity are increased, namely 2′,5′ – oligoadenylate synthetase (which activates ribonuclease L, which preferentially cuts viral RNA) and protein kinase activity. The onset of these effects takes several hours, but may then persist for days even after plasma interferon concentrations have fallen to undetectable levels. Interferon also increases the presentation of viral antigens in infected cells, and up-regulates macrophage activation and T-cell and natural-killer-cell cytotoxicity, thereby increasing viral elimination. The interferon concentrations needed to produce their antiviral effects are lower than those required for their antiproliferative effects.

ADVERSE EFFECTS

These include the following:

1 fever, malaise, chills – an influenza-like syndrome, and neuropsychiatric symptoms similar to a postviral syndrome;
2 lymphocytopenia and thrombocytopenia are reversible, and tolerance may occur after a week or so;
3 anorexia and weight loss;
4 alopecia;
5 transient loss of higher cognitive functions, confusion, tremor and fits;
6 transient hypotension or cardiac arrhythmias;
7 hypothyroidism.

PHARMACOKINETICS

Most clinical experience has been gained with interferon-α, which has been given intravenously and intramuscularly, subcutaneously. Absorption of more than 80% of an intramuscular dose occurs and, following subcutaneous administration, peak plasma concentrations occur at 4–8 h and decline over 1–2 days. The mean elimination $t_{\frac{1}{2}}$ is 3–5 h. Polyethylene glycol (PEG)-conjugated interferons are being studied clinically because they have a protracted half-life and may be given less frequently. Bodily clearance of interferons is

Case history

A 45-year-old female insulin-dependent diabetic developed a severe oral *Candida* infection. She also had chronic oesophageal reflux exacerbated by gastroparesis, for which she took omeprazole and cisapride. She was started on itraconazole, 100 mg daily, and after a few days her oropharyngeal symptoms were improving. About 1 week into the treatment she was brought into a local hospital casualty unit with *torsades de pointes* (polymorphic ventricular tachycardia) that was difficult to treat initially, but which eventually responded to administration of intravenous magnesium and direct current (D/C) cardioversion. There was no evidence of an acute myocardial ischaemia/infarction on post reversion or subsequent ECGs, the patient's cardiac enzymes were not diagnostic of a myocardial infarction, and her electrolyte and magnesium levels measured immediately on admission were normal.

Question

What is the likely cause of this patient's life threatening arrhythmia and how could this have been avoided ?

Answer

In this case the recent prescription of itraconazole and the serious cardiac event while the patient was on this drug are temporally linked. It is widely known that all azoles can inhibit cytochrome $P_{450\ 3A4}$ which happens to be the enzyme responsible for metabolizing cisapride. Cisapride has recently been found (like terfenadine – now prescription only) to cause prolongation of the QT interval in humans in a concentration-dependent manner. Thus there is an increased likelihood of a patient developing ventricular tachycardia (VT) if the concentrations of cisapride are increased, as occurs when its metabolism is inhibited by a drug (e.g. itraconazole) that inhibits hepatic cytochrome $P_{450\ 3A4}$. This is exactly what happened here. Other common drugs whose concentrations increase (with an attendant increase in their toxicity) if prescribed concurrently with azoles (which should be avoided) are listed in the table below:

In this patient the problem could have been avoided by either stopping the cisapride prior to starting the azole or if cisapride was such a necessary component of therapy using a topical polyene such as amphotericin or nystatin lozenges to cure her oral *Candida*. Neither of these polyene anti-fungal agents inhibit $P_{450\ 3A4}$ mediated hepatic drug metabolism.

Table 44.5

Drug or drug class	Toxicity caused by reduced metabolism
Astemizole	*Torsades de pointes* (polymorphic ventricular tachycardia)
Cyclosporin (and Tacrolimus-FK 506)	Nephroxicity and seizures
Warfarin	Haemorrhage
HMG Co A reductase inhibitors (statins such as simvastatin)	Myositis and rhabdomyolysis
Calcium channel-blockers	Hypotension
Sildenafil citrate (Viagra)	Protracted hypotension

complex. Inactivation occurs in the liver, lung and kidney, but interferons are also excreted in the urine.

Key points

Non-HIV antiviral drugs

- Specific anti-CMV agents are ganciclovir and foscarnet.
- Both are active against acyclovir-resistant herpes viruses.
- Foscarnet is not absorbed orally, and ganciclovir is very poorly absorbed; both are renally excreted.
- Ganciclovir and foscarnet are best given intravenously.
- Ganciclovir (bone-marrow suppresion) and foscarnet (nephrotoxicity) are much more toxic than acyclovir.
- Interferon-α is effective against chronic hepatitis B and C.

IMMUNOGLOBULINS

Some pooled human immunoglobulins have high titres against specific viruses such as cytomegalovirus, hepatitis A, hepatitis B, varicella and measles. Immunoglobulin is given intramuscularly as near as possible to the time of exposure, and may be used prophylactically (see Chapter 49). Immunoglobulins administered parenterally reach peak serum concentrations in 4–6 days, which then decline with a $t_{\frac{1}{2}}$ of 20–30 days.

FURTHER READING

Albengeres E, Le Leouet H., Tillement JP. 1998: Systemic antifungal agents: drug interactions and clinical significance. *Drug Safety*; **18**, 83–97.

Alrabiah FA, Sacks SL. 1996: New antiherpes virus agents: their targets and therapeutic potential. *Drugs* **52**, 17–32.

Como JA, Dismukes WE.1994: Drug Therapy. Oral azole drugs as systemic antifungal therapy. *New England Journal of Medicine* **330**, 263–72.

Hayden FG, Osterhaus AD, Treanor JJ *et al*. 1998: FH *et al*. Efficacy and safety of the neuraminidase inhibitor zanamir in the treatment of influenza virus infections. *New England Journal of Medicine* **337**, 874–80.

CHAPTER FORTY-FIVE

HIV *and* AIDS

- Introduction
- Immunopathogenesis of HIV-1 infection
- Guidelines for treating HIV-seropositive individuals
- Anti-HIV drugs
- Opportunitic infections in HIV-1 seropositive patients
- *Mycobacterium tuberculosis* therapy in HIV patients
- *Mycobacterium avium-intracellulare* complex therapy
- Antifungal therapy
- Anti-herpes virus therapy

Introduction

By the end of 1994 approximately 23 000 cases of AIDS had been reported in the UK. World-wide, by the end of 1995 there were 6 million cases of AIDS reported and an estimated 20 million people infected with HIV-1. The World Health Organization estimates that by the year 2000 there will be 30 to 40 million people world-wide infected with HIV-1, more than 90% of whom will be in developing countries. These countries must take major public health measures to attempt to control the spread of HIV-1, otherwise this pandemic will exterminate considerable proportions of several generations of the human population.

Immunopathogenesis of HIV-1 infection

Following inoculation of a naive host with biological fluid (e.g. blood, blood products or sexual secretions) containing HIV-1, the virus adheres to cells expressing the CD4 and its coreceptor – CCR5 – the chemokine receptor (lymphocytes, macrophages and dendritic cells in the blood, lymphoid organs and central nervous system) and enters the cell, the viral envelope being absorbed into the host membrane. After uncoating, the viral genome is released into the host cell, where viral reverse transcriptase produces complementary DNA (cDNA), using the viral RNA as a template. This viral DNA is then integrated into the host genome by a viral integrase enzyme . Viral cDNA is then transcribed by the host, producing mes-

Key points

HIV-1 epidemiology and HIV life-cycle and dynamics

- World-wide, it has been estimated that there will be 30 to 40 million HIV-infected people by 2000 AD.
- Exposed individuals have CD4/CCR5-expressing cells invaded; HIV produces its own DNA (from RNA) which is incorporated into the host DNA, and this is then replicated.
- Infected T-cells have a half-life of 1.6 days.
- Plasma virions have a half-life of 0.24 days.
- The rate of production of HIV is 10.3×10^9 virions per day.
- The mean time period needed for HIV generation (time from release of virion into plasma until it infects another cell and causes release of a new generation of viruses) is 2.6 days.
- The HIV viral load is best assessed by measuring the number of copies of HIV RNA/mL of plasma.
- Plasma HIV RNA/ml is strongly correlated (inversely) with CD4 count and survival.

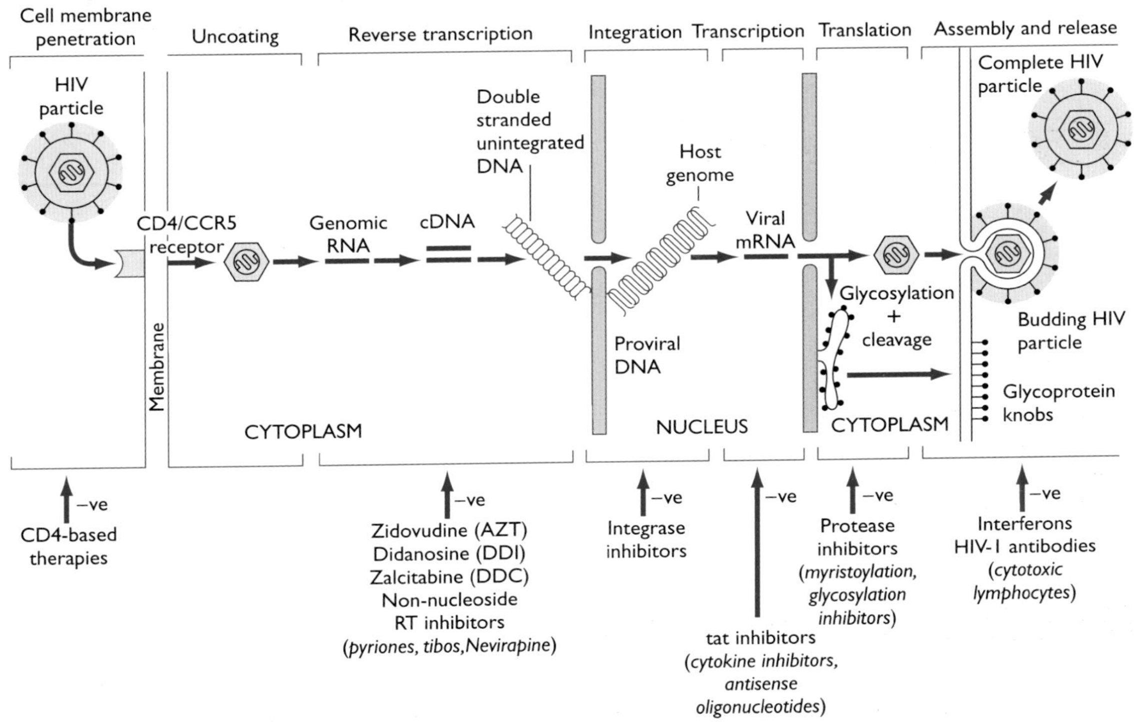

Figure 45.1: Life cycle of human immunodeficiency virus-1 (HIV-1) illustrating the actual and potential (in italics) sites of action of antiviral agents. RT = reverse transcriptase, cDNA = complementary DNA, mRNA = messenger RNA.

senger RNA (mRNA) which is translated into viral peptides. These peptides are then cleaved by the HIV protease to form the structural viral proteins that eventually make up the new infectious virion containing viral RNA. Figure 45.1 summarizes the HIV-1 life-cycle, and also shows the potential therapeutic targets which are enumerated below:

1 entry of virus into the cell via the CD4 and chemokine-R (CCR5) receptor combination;
2 the HIV-1 DNA polymerase (reverse transcriptase);
3 the integrase enzyme;
4 the transactivator of transcription (tat) protein that accelerates replication of viral RNA;
5 the HIV-1 protease.

Newly formed HIV-1 virions infect previously uninfected CD4/CCR5–positive cells and subsequently impair the host immune response by killing or inhibiting CD4/CCR5–positive cells, thus rendering the host immunosuppressed and consequently at high risk of infections by commensal and opportunistic organisms. The diagnosis of HIV-1 infection is based on enzyme-linked immunosorbent assay (ELISA) techniques that identify HIV-1 antibodies and/or structural proteins in blood (see Figure 45.2 for details of the structure of the virus). In patients who are infected with HIV-1, massive amounts of viral replication occur (10.3 × 10^9 virions per day) in the 4–8 weeks immediately post infection. By 8–12 weeks viral replication has started to fall, and within 6–12 months of infection viral replication has stabilized and a 'latent period' (which may last 5-12 years) of good health develops. During this latent period the viral load has fallen from its initial peak values, but remains stable at a plateau value (which if assessed by HIV RNA copy number/mL of plasma lies in the range 10^2–10^6). The HIV RNA copy number rises again prior to the development of AIDS. During the latent phase a dynamic equilibrium of HIV replication, T-cell infection and

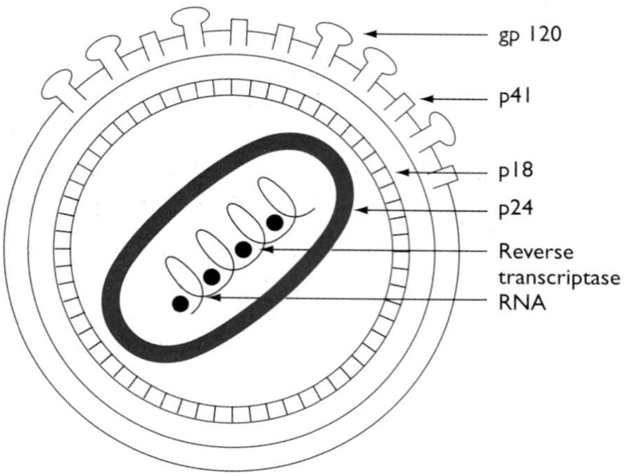

Figure 45.2: HIV structure consisting of membrane glycoprotein gp120 and peptide protein p41 plus an outer membrane of p18 and a nuclear membrane of p24 protein containing viral RNA and the reverse transcriptase enzyme.

subsequent destruction and new T-cell generation is occurring with a slow and inexorable decline in the number of CD4 cells. Only after the CD4 lymphocyte count has fallen to < 500 and certainly to below 200 × 10^6/L is the individual predisposed to opportunistic infections and certain malignancies (e.g. Kaposi's sarcoma and lymphoma). Ultimately it is these infections and malignancies that define the later stages of HIV-1 infection, which is known as the acquired immune deficiency syndrome (AIDS).

Guidelines for treating HIV-seropositive individuals

Most physicians would agree that recent clinical studies (the Delta study, the CAESAR study and the CPRCA study) have shown that combination drug antiretroviral therapy should be given to patients before substantial immunodeficiency ensues. The primary aim of treating patients with HIV infection is maximal suppression of HIV replication for as long as possible, which means improved survival time. With the advent of sensitive assays for determination of plasma HIV RNA and the development of novel, potent anti-HIV drugs, this objective becomes tenable. *The current standard of care for HIV patients is a three-drug combination of two nucleoside analogues plus a protease inhibitor with high anti-HIV potency* in vivo. These combinations were found to reduce the viral load to < 500 copies of HIV RNA/mL in 80% of subjects in clinical studies after 12 months. Not all patients will tolerate triple therapy due to toxicity and alternate double therapy (with two nucleoside, analogue in one nucleoside and one protease inhibitor, or some other two-drug combinations) may be used. This therapeutic area is in constant flux, and future therapeutic developments may well involve four (two protease inhibitors) or more drug combinations, or sequential changes in drug combinations. Clinical studies are already in progress to assess such strategies.

The recommended criteria for initiating anti-HIV therapy are as follows. First, all patients with HIV RNA above 5000 – 10 000 copies/mL of plasma are eligible. Secondly, consider treatment at all CD4 counts, but especially if CD4 is < 500 × 10^6/L or if there is a rapid decline in CD4 count of > 300 × 10^6/L over 12 months. Treatment may be deferred if CD4 counts are stable in the range 350–500 × 10^6/L and plasma HIV RNA is < 5000–10 000 copies/mL of plasma. Thirdly, all HIV seropositive patients with symptoms should receive treatment. *The recommended regimens for initial therapy are shown in Table 45.1 and are expected to reduce the HIV RNA copy number/mL of plasma by > 0.5 log by week 8 of therapy, and ultimately to undetectable levels, and to maintain this state. The plasma HIV RNA copy number is the accepted gold standard for assessing/monitoring the efficacy of therapy, and correlates inversely with the CD4 count.*

HIV-1–infected patients who develop infections with *Pneumocysis carinii* and who recover require secondary prophylaxis with oral co-trimoxazole (two tablets twice daily). AIDS patients with CD4 counts of < 200 may be considered for primary prophylaxis with co-trimoxazole. Patients who have recovered following oesophageal candidiasis or crytococcal meningitis require prophylactic therapy with fluconazole, 200 mg once daily. A number of other opportunistic infections in HIV-1–infected individuals once treated acutely also require maintenance prophylaxis.

Table 45.1: Combinations to be used as initial anti-HIV drug therapy*

Two nucleoside analogues + protease inhibitor	e.g. ZDV + ddl/ddC/ 3TC + Ind/Nel/Rit d4T + ddl/ddC/3 TC + Ind/ Nel/ Rit
Two nucleoside analogues + non-nucleoside reverse transcriptase inhibitor	e.g. ZDV + ddl/ddC/3TC + Del/ Nvp d4T + ddl ddC 3 TC + Del/Nvp

ZDV = zidovudine; ddl = dideoxyinosine; ddC = dideoxycytidine (Zalcitabine); 3-TC = 3-thiacytidine (Lamivudine); d4T = didehydrothymidine (Stavudine); Ind = indinavir; Nel = nelfinavir; Rit = ritonovir; Del = delaverdine; Nvp = nevirapine.
*Combinations always include either ZDV or d4T because they have better CSF penetration than other nucleoside analogues and combinations attempt to avoid overlapping toxicities, and to avoid using agents that are phosphorylated by the same enzymes (combinations of ZDV + d4T and 3-TC and ddC are avoided).

Key points

General guidelines for anti-HIV-1 therapy

- Treat before significant immunosuppression develops.
- Treatment criteria are HIV RNA copies if 5000–10 000/mL or more, or CD4 count (if < 500) or symptoms.
- Combination therapy is used – monotherapy is no longer acceptable.
- Standard of care therapy is two nucleoside analogue RT inhibitors plus one protease inhibitor.
- The standard therapy regimen is, for example, ZDV plus 3TC plus indinavir.
- If there is treatment failure or resistance, change at least two and preferably all three drugs being used.

ANTI-HIV DRUGS

NUCLEOSIDE ANALOGUE REVERSE TRANSCRIPTASE (RT) INHIBITORS

Of these agents, only **zidovudine** (ZDV) has been shown in clinical studies to reduce mortality in late-stage AIDS, and to reduce the incidence of opportunistic infections and possibly reduce the rate of progression of HIV-1 infection to AIDS. **Didanosine** (ddI) and **zalcitabine** (ddC) and the newer agents (d4T, 3-TC) in this class, when used in combination with ZDV, appear to reduce HIV-1 viral replication as indicated by surrogate markers, (e.g. the plasma HIV RNA load).

Zidovudine (ZDV, Azidothymidine-AZT)

This was originally synthesized as a nucleoside analogue in 1964, and was the first nucleoside analogue to be licensed for the treatment of HIV-1 infection. It is an analogue of thymidine in which the 3′-hydroxyl has been replaced by an azido (N_3) group.

USE

ZDV is only licensed for the treatment of HIV-1 infection. It is given orally as 200 mg three times daily (or 300 mg twice a day to improve compliance) to patients who have developed AIDS.

MECHANISM OF ACTION

The parent drug ZDV enters the cells by diffusion and undergoes anabolic phosphorylation first to its monophosphate (ZDV-MP), then to the diphosphate (ZDV-DP) (the rate-limiting step) and finally to the triphosphate (ZDV-TP). The intracellular $t_{\frac{1}{2}}$ of ZDV-TP is 2–3 h. ZDV-TP is a competitive inhibitor of the HIV-1 reverse transcriptase (RT) (competing with endogenous thymidine triphosphate) and when incorporated into nascent viral DNA it causes chain termination because the incoming nucleotide triphosphate cannot make a phosphate bond with the 3′ carbon which lacks a hydroxyl group (Figure 45.3). The human nuclear DNA polymerases are much less sensitive (by at least 100-fold) to inhibition by ZDV-TP, thus producing a selective effect on viral replication. This mechanism of action is common to all anti-HIV nucleoside analogues.

ADVERSE EFFECTS

These include the following:

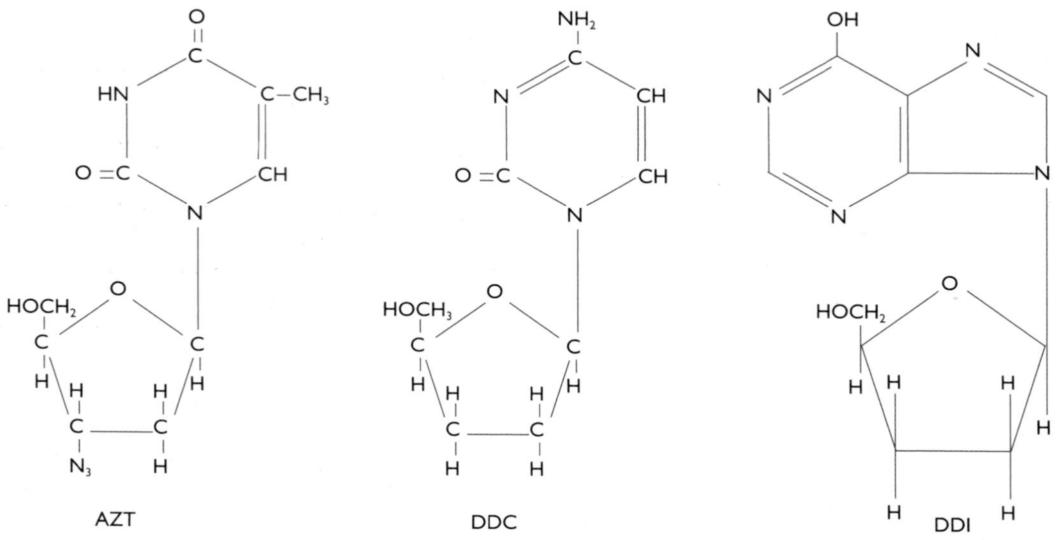

Figure 45.3: Molecular structures of AZT, DDC and DDI.

1 bone-marrow suppression causing anaemia with reticulocytopenia and granulocytopenia, which are dose dependent. This occurred in 15% of patients in the original studies with high-dose ZDV. At the currently recommended lower dose (200 mg three times daily or 300 mg bd) it occurs in only 1–2% of patients;
2 nausea and vomiting;
3 fatigue and headache;
4 melanonychia (blue-grey nail discoloration);
5 insomnia;
6 mitochondrial myopathy (uncommon) and (rarely) a lactic acidosis;
7 it is mutagenic and carcinogenic in animals. However, ZDV is used in HIV-positive pregnant women as it reduces HIV maternal–fetal transmission and thus fetal/neonatal HIV-1 infection, and has not been shown to be teratogenic if given to women after the first trimester.

PHARMACOKINETICS

Zidovudine is almost totally absorbed (>90%) from the gut. The plasma elimination $t_{\frac{1}{2}}$ is 1–2 h. It is widely distributed, achieving cerebrospinal fluid (CSF) concentrations that are 50% of those in plasma. The rate of plasma protein binding is 30–40%. About 25–40% of a dose undergoes presystemic metabolism in the liver. The major metabolite (80%) is the glucuronide, and approximately 20% of a dose appears unchanged in the urine. Plasma concentrations after a single oral dose of 100–300 mg achieve the concentration that inhibits 90% growth (IC_{90}) for cells acutely infected with HIV-1.

DRUG INTERACTIONS

The following list is not comprehensive, as only the commonest interactions are listed:

1 probenecid inhibits the glucuronidation and renal excretion of ZDV;
2 ZDV glucuronidation is reduced by atovaquone;

Key points

Anti-HIV drugs – nucleoside analogue reverse transcriptase inhibitors – ZDV

- Used in combinations to increase anti-HIV efficacy and reduce resistance.
- Zidovudine is phosphorylated intracellularly to ZDV-TP, which inhibits viral RT.
- Good oral absorption, penetration of CSF, hepatic metabolism and short half-life.
- Adverse effects include bone-marrow suppression and myopathy in the long term.
- Used in HIV-positive pregnant women, in whom it reduces transmission to the fetus/neonate by approximately 60%.
- Resistance develops slowly.

3 ZDV and rifamycins cause increased ZDV metabolism;
4 ZDV and antituberculous chemotherapy cause a high incidence of anaemia;
5 ganciclovir and ZDV combined therapy produces profound bone-marrow suppression;
6 clinical studies have confirmed the *in vitro* data that ZDV/ddI or ZDV/ddC or ZDV/3TC combinations are synergistic. Such combination therapy also reduces the development of resistance.

NON-NUCLEOSIDE ANALOGUE REVERSE TRANSCRIPTASE INHIBITORS

These drugs are now routinely used as part of the triple combination therapy schedules with the nucleoside analogue RT inhibitors (e.g. ZDV + 3–TC). The established agents in this group are **nevirapine** and **delavirdine**.

Nevirapine

Nevirapine is administered orally as 200 mg once a day for the first 7–14 days and then as 200 mg twice daily. This gradual increase in dose reduces the potential for it to cause skin rashes which can be dose limiting. Unfortunately, such gradual dose increases are not effective in the case of delavirdine. These agents cause a marked (> 50%) reduction in viral load during 8 weeks of therapy, and are synergistic with drugs such as ZDV. Another reason why they are used in combination anti-HIV therapy is that HIV rapidly develops resistance to them if they are used as monotherapy.

MECHANISM OF ACTION

Non-nucleoside agents such as nevirapine inhibit the HIV reverse transcriptase by binding to an allosteric site (i.e. not the substrate-binding site) and causing non-competitive enzyme inhibition, reducing the ability of the virus to produce viral DNA. Their anti-HIV action is synergistic *in vitro* when combined with nucleoside analogue reverse transcriptase inhibitors (ZDV, etc.).

ADVERSE EFFECTS

These include the following

1 skin rashes – often dose limiting;
2 hepatitis;

> **Key points**
>
> Anti-HIV drugs – Non-nucleoside analogue reverse transcriptase inhibitors
>
> - Used in combination, because of synergy with drugs such as ZDV.
> - Nevirapine and delavirdine are allosteric (non-competitive) inhibitors of HIV RT.
> - Oral absorption is good, hepatic metabolism by $P_{450\ 3A4}$, short-intermediate half-lives.
> - Adverse effects include skin rashes and drug interactions.
> - Resistance develops quickly.

3 drug–drug interactions–complex effects on other hepatically metabolized drugs (see below).

PHARMACOKINETICS

Nevirapine is well absorbed orally (> 90% bioavailability) with a $t_{\frac{1}{2}}$ of 25–30 hours. It is metabolized in the liver by cytochrome $P_{450\ 3A4}$, to desalkylnevirapine. Its pharmacokinetics are linear over the dose range that is used clinically. Less than 5% is found unchanged in the urine. It causes autoinduction of its own metabolism during the first 10–14 days of therapy, and it induces metabolism of drugs by hepatic glucuronyl transferase.

DRUG INTERACTIONS

Nevirapine induces hepatic cytochrome P_{450} and thus increases the clearance of agents such as the oral contraceptives or other HIV inhibitors. Other drugs metabolized by cytochrome $P_{450\ 3A4}$ and hepatic glucuronyl transferase (e.g. ZDV) may also be less effective due to increased metabolism.

ANTI-HIV PROTEASE INHIBITORS

USES

The curently available compounds in this class are **ritonavir**, **indinavir**, **nelfinavir**, and **saquinavir**. They cause the most rapid and dramatic reduction of HIV-1 replication *in vitro* and *in vivo* as measured by a fall of 100-to 1000-fold over 4–12 weeks in the number of HIV RNA copies/mL of plasma. Reductions in viral load were paralleled by increases in CD4 count (the mean increase was 100–150 × 10^6/L). The effect on HIV RNA as monotherapy is dose and concentration dependent. Resistance is becoming a problem, and this leads to cross-resistance between agents. Ritonavir is administered orally twice daily, but because it induces its own metabolism, it is started at 300 mg bd for 3 days, and then increased to 400 mg bd for 3 days, then 500 mg bd for 3 days and finally 600 mg bd, if tolerated. The regimens for the other agents in the group are shown in table 45.4. These drugs are used in combination therapy (not as monotherapy) (see Table 45.1).

MECHANISM OF ACTION

These agents prevent the HIV protease from cleaving the gag and gag–pol protein precursors encoded by the HIV genome in acutely and chronically infected cells, arresting maturation and thereby blocking the infectivity of nascent virions. These agents are active against isolates of HIV-1 and HIV-2. The protease enzyme is a dimer and has aspartyl-protease activity. Anti-HIV protease drugs contain a synthetic analogue structure of the phenylalanine–proline sequence of positions 167–168 of the gag–pol polyprotein. Thus they act as competitive inhibitors of the viral protease and inhibit maturation of viral particles to infectious virion. They have K_i values in the range 0.1–2 nM. These drugs are inactive or only weakly active against human aspartyl-proteases, with K_i values of at least 10 000 nM for renin and pepsin.

ADVERSE EFFECTS

These include the following:

1 nausea, vomiting and abdominal pain;
2 circumoral paraesthesia;
3 glucose intolerance, including insulin resistance and diabetes mellitus;
4 fatigue;
5 hypertriglyceridaemia;
6 fat redistribution – buffalo hump, increased abdominal girth;
7 multiple drug–drug interactions – complex effects on other hepatically metabolized drugs (see below).

PHARMACOKINETICS

Ritonavir is well absorbed orally, with 65–75% bioavailability, and peak plasma concentrations are achieved 2–4 h post dosing. Food increases absorption, and therefore the drug should be taken with meals. It is 98–99% protein bound with a $t_{\frac{1}{2}}$ of 3–5 h. It is metabolized in the liver by cytochrome $P_{450\ 3A4}$, and causes autoinduction of its own metabolism in the first 7–14 days of therapy. It also induces hepatic glucuronyl transferase activity. Ritonavir inhibits the metabolism of certain cytochrome $P_{450\ 3A4}$ substrates (and certain drugs metabolized by cytochrome $P_{450\ 2D6}$), and increases the metabolism of others. Therefore drug–drug interactions are complex.

DRUG INTERACTIONS

For a comprehensive list, a drug interaction text should be consulted

1 Most protease inhibitors are inhibitors of the hepatic cytochrome $P_{450\ 3A4}$ enzyme system, and this can lead to toxicity of a number of co-administered drugs often with severe adverse effects (e.g. midazolam, triazolam cause increased sedation, and astemizole, terfenadine, and cisapride cause ventricular tachycardia; both of these sets of combinations are contraindicated). Protease inhibitors inhibit the metabolism of rifabutin thereby potentiating the risk of rifabutin toxicity, and this combination is therefore also contraindicated.
2 Enzyme inducers (e.g. rifamycins – rifampin/rifabutin; or nevirapine) will enhance the metabolism of the protease inhibitors, making them less effective, producing subtherapeutic plasma concentrations and thus increasing the

> **Key points**
>
> Anti-HIV drugs – protease inhibitors
>
> - Used in combinations because of synergy with anti-HIV RT inhibitors and reduced resistance.
> - They inhibit HIV protease enzyme, and are the most potent and rapid blockers of HIV replication available.
> - Oral absorption is variable, hepatic metabolism is mainly by cytochrome $P_{450\ 3A4}$.
> - Side-effects: include gastrointestinal upsets, hyperglycaemia, fat redistribution and drug–drug interactions.
> - Ritonavir is not as well tolerated as other protease inhibitors because of its gastrointestinal effects.
> - HIV resistance to one agent usually means cross-resistance to others in the group.

Table 45.2: Properties of the other anti-HIV nucleoside analogue RT inhibitors

Anti-HIV nucleoside analogue	Standard oral dosing regimen*	Side-effects	Pharmacokinetics	Additional comments
Didanosine (ddI-dideoxyinosine	200 mg twice a day (< 60 kg 125 mg bd)	Peripheral neuropathy, pancreatitis, bone-marrow toxicity is rare. Gastrointestinal upsets and hyperuricaemia	Acid-labile absorption affected by pH – given as a buffered capsule. Plasma $t_{\frac{1}{2}}$ is 0.5–1.5 h Renal excretion (50%) and hepatic metabolism	Intracellular triphosphate anabolite ddA-TP has a $t_{\frac{1}{2}}$ of 24–40 h Didanosine decreases absorption of drugs requiring acid pH (e.g. keto- or itraconazole)
Zalcitabine (ddC-dideoxycytidine	0.75 mg every 8 h	Reversible sensori-motor neuropathy, pancreatitis, stomatitis, rashes; bone-marrow toxicity is rare	Well absorbed (85% bioavailability), plasma $t_{\frac{1}{2}}$ is 1–2 h Renal excretion (70%)	Intracellular triphosphate has $t_{\frac{1}{2}}$ of 2–3 h
Stavudine (d4T-didehydro-thymidine)	40 mg 12-hourly (patients < 60 kg take 30 mg bd)	Peripheral neuropathy	Well absorbed (86% bioavailability). T_{max} is 2 h; plasma $t_{\frac{1}{2}}$ is 1 h, rapidly cleared by renal (50%) and non-renal routes	Intracellular triphosphate has $t_{\frac{1}{2}}$ of 3–4 h *In vitro* data show antagonism with ZDV against HIV
Lamivudine (3TC; 2-deoxy-3-thiacytidine)	150 mg 12-hourly (patients < 50 kg, 2 mg/kg)	Well tolerated Uncommon gastrointestinal upsets, hair loss, myelosuppression, neuropathy	Well absorbed; $t_{\frac{1}{2}}$ of 3–6 h. Renal excretion (unchanged), requires dose reduction in renal impairment	Intracellular triphosphate has $t_{\frac{1}{2}}$ of 12 h Synergy *in vitro* with ZDV against HIV Co-trimoxazole reduces clearance by 40%
Zidovudine + lamivudine (Combivir)	1 tablet 12-hourly (the tablet contains ZDV, 300 mg, and 3TC, 150 mg)			
Others still in clinical development (e.g. Abacavir, slow-release ZDV)				

Table 45.3: Properties of the other anti-HIV non-nucleoside analogue RT inhibitors

Anti-HIV non-nucleoside analogues	Standard oral dosing regimen*	Side-effects	Pharmacokinetics	Additional comments
Delavirdine	400 mg 8-hourly (> 3 ounces of water)	Rashes and headaches	Well absorbed (85% bioavailable), non-linear pharmacokinetics $t_{\frac{1}{2}}$ of 4–6 h Hepatic metabolism by cytochrome $P_{450\ 3A4}$ (> 5%)	Inhibits cytochrome $P_{450\ 3A4}$ thus drug interactions occur Resistance develops if used as monotherapy (unchanged in urine)
Loviride				Still under phase II/III development
Others still in clinical devlopment (e.g. Efavirez, Atevirdine)				

* Adult doses.

likelihood of HIV resistance developing.

3 Several protease inhibitors reduce the metabolism of co-administered protease inhibitors, thereby increasing plasma concentrations and potentially leading to greater toxicity.

Changing anti-HIV therapy for treatment failure and/or resistance

A change in anti-HIV therapy may be required because of treatment failure, adverse effects, poor compliance, potential drug–drug interactions or current use of a suboptimal regimen. When changing regimens because of treatment failure, one should adopt the principle of changing all previous drugs, or at least two of them. Viral resistance to nucleoside and non-nucleoside analogue RT inhibitors and protease inhibitors may cause treatment failure. Reduced susceptibility of HIV-1 isolates to ZDV, ddI and ddC is spreading. Resistance to ZDV emerges more quickly and to a greater degree in the later stages of the disease. Progressive stepwise reductions in susceptibility of the HIV reverse transcripase (RT) correlate with the acquisition of mutations in the gene for the RT protein. There is only cross-resistance to other nucleosides with the 3′-azido side-chain, and therefore such isolates are currently still sensitive to ddI/ ddC/3TC. However, resistance to other nucleoside inhibitors has been documented in patients on long-term therapy with ddI or ddC. Alternative anti-retroviral therapy to initially used regimens for treatment failure/resistance is suggested in Table 45.5.

The future holds exciting therapeutic prospects for anti-HIV treatment. This includes more potent protease inhibitors, integrase enzyme inhibitors and the ongoing clinical search for an effective anti-HIV vaccine, one candidate is now going into phase II/III clinical trial in Thailand. Anti-HIV therapy has become a complex arena, and is only likely to increase further in its complexity. Thus it necessitates specialist supervision.

Table 45.4: Properties of available anti-HIV protease inhibitors

Protease non-nucleoside analogues	Standard oral dosing regimen*	Side-effects	Pharmacokinetics	Additional comments
Indinavir	800 mg every 8 h with water 1–2 h before meals	Renal stones (5–15%), gastrointestinal upsets fewer than with other PIs, hepatic dysfunction, hyperglycaemia, fat redistribution	Well absorbed (65% (bioavailable). T_{max} is 0.8–1.5 h, $t_{\frac{1}{2}}$ is 2 h 60–65% protein bound Hepatic metabolism	Does not induce cytochrome P_{450} but does inhibit it, especially cytochrome $P_{450\ 3A4}$ – drug interactions
Saquinavir (Invirovase – hard gel may be phased out in 1998. Fortavase – soft gel	600 or 1200 mg every 8 h, with or within 2 h of a meal	Gastrointestinal upsets, hepatitis hyperglycaemia, fat redistribution	Poorly absorbed (<4% bioavailability of hard gel Hepatic metabolism Improved absorption with soft gel preparation	Does not induce cytochrome P_{450}, but does inhibit it, it at the concentrations achieved clinically (cytochrome $P_{450\ 3A4}$)
Nelfinavir	750 mg every 8 h, with food	Gastrointestinal >20%, hyperglycaemia, fat redistribution, transaminitis	Well absorbed (20–80% bioavailable). T_{max} is 2–4 h, $t_{\frac{1}{2}}$ is 3.5–5 h 98% protein bound Hepatic metabolism	Does induce cytochrome P_{450} and does inhibit it, especially cytochrome $P_{450\ 3A4}$
Amprenavir	Capsules and oral solution 1200 mg every 12 h	Gastrointestinal upsets, Skin rashes, fat redistribution	Well absorbed T_{max} 1–2 h $t_{\frac{1}{2}} = 7–10$ h. Hepatic metabolism cytochrome $P_{450\ 3A4}$	Inhibits cytochrome $P_{450\ 3A4}$

* Adult doses.

Table 45.5: Examples of alternative anti-HIV drug therapy combinations

Initial treatment regimen	Alternate regimen
ZDV + ddI + Ind	d4T + 3-TC + Nel d4T + 3-TC + Nel Rit + Sqv + 3-TC
d4T + 3-TC + Ind	ZDV + ddI + Nel ZDV + ddI + Nvp Rit + Sqv + ZDV

ZDV= zidovudine; ddI = dideoxyinosine; ddC = dideoxycytidine (Zalcitabine); 3-TC = 3-thiacytidine (Lamivudine); d4T = didehydrothymidine (Stavudine); Ind = Indinavir; Nel = nelfinavir; Rit = ritonovir; Sqv = saquinivir. Del = delavirdine; Nvp = nevirapine.

OPPORTUNISTIC INFECTIONS IN HIV-1-SEROPOSITIVE PATIENTS

PNEUMOCYSTIS CARINII

In moderate to severe cases of *Pneumocystis carinii* pneumonia (PCP) where the arterial PO_2 is less than 60 mmHg, treatment consists not only of anti-*Pneumocystis* therapy but, in addition, involves the use of glucocorticosteroids. Prednisolone is given as 80 mg/day for 5 days, 40 mg/day for 5 days and 20 mg/day for 11 days. This has been shown to reduce the number of patients who require mechanical ventilation, and to improve survival.

Co-trimoxazole

High-dose co-trimoxazole (see Chapter 42) is first-line standard therapy for PCP in patients with HIV infection. It is given intravenously at the equivalent of 20 mg/kg/day trimethoprim in two divided doses for a total of 21 days. If the patient improves after 5–7 days, oral therapy may be substituted for the remainder of the course. The major adverse effects of this therapy are nausea and vomiting (which is reduced by the prior intravenous administration of an anti-emetic), rashes, hepatitis, bone-marrow suppression and hyperkalaemia. Treatment may have to be discontinued in 20–55% of cases because of side-effects, and one of the alternative therapies listed below substituted instead. After recovery from an episode of PCP, secondary prophylaxis with oral co-trimoxazole (one double strength tablet two or three times daily) is preferred to nebulized pentamidine, as it reduces the risk of extrapulmonary as well as pulmonary relapse. Dapsone, 100 mg orally once daily, is also effective for secondary prophylaxis.

Pentamidine

USES

This is an aromatic amidine and is supplied for parenteral use as **pentamidine isethionate**. It has activity against a range of pathogenic protozoa, including *Pneumocystis carinii*, African trypanosomiasis (*Trypanosoma rhodesiense* and *T. congolese*) and kala-azar (*Leishmania donovani*). It is effective in 70–80% of *Pneumocystis carinii* pneumonia (PCP) episodes, and is administered as a slow intravenous infusion over 2 h at 4 mg/kg/day for 21 days. Parenteral administration via the intramuscular route has been used, but sterile injection site abscesses commonly occur. Pentamidine has also been given via the nebulized route to treat PCP (4 mg/kg/day, up to 600 mg/day), but the recurrence rate is higher than with systemic therapy.

MECHANISM OF ACTION

Pentamidine has a number of actions on protozoan cells. It damages cellular DNA, especially extranuclear (mitochondrial) DNA, and prevents its replication. It also inhibits RNA polymerase and, at high concentrations, it damages mitochondria. Polyamine uptake into protozoa is also inhibited by pentamidine. *Pneumocystis carinii* is killed even in the non-replicating state.

ADVERSE EFFECTS

Nebulized route Cough and bronchospasm occur, but can be reduced by pre-administration of a nebulized β_2–agonist.

Intravenous route Adverse effects include the following:

1. hypotension and acidosis (due to cardiotoxicity) if given too rapidly;
2. dizziness and syncope;
3. hypoglycaemia due to toxicity to the pancreatic β-cells producing hyperinsulinaemia;
4. nephrotoxicity (rarely irreversible);
5. pancreatitis;
6. reversible neutropenia;
7. prolongation of the QTc interval.

Intramuscular route The above problems occur, together with pain at the injection site and sterile abscesses.

PHARMACOKINETICS

Pentamidine is not significantly absorbed after oral administration, and must be given parenterally. The half-life varies, but is approximately 6 h after the first intravenous dose. There is drug accumulation in tissue and plasma with repeated dosing. The major route of clearance from plasma is by tissue binding and uptake. Pentamidine has a large volume of distribution, but does not cross the blood–brain barrier well. The rate of renal excretion is low (<5%), so renal failure does not necessitate dose adjustment. There are no data on pentamidine metabolism in humans. Nebulized therapy yields lung concentrations that are at least as high (if not higher) than those achieved after intravenous infusion.

DRUG INTERACTIONS

Pentamidine inhibits human cholinesterase *in vitro*. This suggests potential interactions in enhancing the effect of suxamethonium and reducing that of competitive muscle relaxants, but it is not known whether this is of clinical importance.

Alternative regimens for treating PCP are summarized in Table 45.6.

Table 45.6: Alternative regimens for treating PCP

Alternative PCP treatment	Additional comments
Trimethoprim, 20 mg/kg/day in two divided doses plus dapsone, 100 mg daily	Oral therapy for 21 days, used in mild to moderate PCP Check glucose-6-phosphate dehydrogenase
Primaquine, 30 mg/day po and clindamycin, 900 mg tds IV for 11 days and 450 mg qds for 10 days	Therapy for 21 days, used in mild to moderate PCP Check glucose-6-phosphate dehydrogenase
Atovaquone (a hydroxynaphthoquinone), 750 mg qds for 21 days	Oral therapy used in mild to moderate PCP. Blocks protozoan mitochondrial electron transport chain and *de novo* pyrimidine synthesis. Side-effects include nausea, vomiting, rash and hepatitis

TOXOPLASMA GONDII

Pyrimethamine and sulphadiazine

USE

This combination is the first-line therapy for cerebral and tissue toxoplasmosis. **Pyrimethamine** is given as an oral loading dose of 100–200 mg, then 50–100 mg/day, together with oral (or intravenous) **sulphadiazine** as a dose of 10 mg/kg/day. Treatment should be continued for 4–6 weeks after clinical and neurological resolution, and for up to 6 months thereafter. Folinic acid is given prophylactically at 10–50 mg/day to reduce drug-induced bone-marrow suppression.

MECHANISM OF ACTION

Sulphadiazine acts as a competitive inhibitor of dihydrofolate synthase (competing with *p*-aminobenzoic acid) in folate synthesis. Pyrimethamine is a competitive inhibitor of dihydrofolate reductase, which converts dihydrofolate to tetrahydrofolate. Together they sequentially block the first two major steps in the synthesis of folate in the parasite. Their selective toxicity is due to their greater specificity as inhibitors of these enzymes in the protozoan than in humans. Humans obtain their dihydrofolate from dietary folate, thus circumventing the block of sulphadiazine, while adding folinic acid (which is not absorbed by these parasites) helps to reduce the effects of pyrimethamine on the bone marrow.

ADVERSE EFFECTS

The major toxic effects of the combination are as follows:

1. nausea and vomiting;
2. fever and rashes which may be life-threatening (Stevens–Johnson syndrome);
3. bone-marrow suppression, especially granulocytopenia;
4. hepatitis;
5. nephrotoxicity, including crystalluria and obstructive nephropathy.

PHARMACOKINETICS

Oral absorption of pyrimethamine is good (>90%). It undergoes extensive hepatic metabolism but approximately 20% is recovered unchanged in the urine. The plasma $t_{\frac{1}{2}}$ is long, ranging from 35 to 175 h. Because of its high lipid solubility it has a large volume of distribution, and achieves CSF concentrations that are 10–25% of those in plasma.

Sulphadiazine is rapidly and completely absorbed after oral administration. However, there is, substantial first-pass hepatic metabolism, the major metabolite being the acetyl derivative. The mean plasma $t_{\frac{1}{2}}$ is 10 h. Cerebrospinal fluid concentrations are 70% of those in plasma. Clearance is a combination of hepatic metabolism and renal excretion, with 50% of a dose being excreted in the urine, so dose reduction is needed in cases of renal failure.

DRUG INTERACTIONS

These are primarily due to the sulphadiazine (Chapter 42) and the combined bone-marrow suppressive effect of pyrimethamine with other antifolates.

An alternative anti-toxoplasmosis regimen consists of pyrimethamine in combination with clindamycin (at a dose of 900–1200 mg every 6–8 h), with folinic acid as above. Therapies which are still undergoing investigation for treatment of cerebral toxoplasmosis as salvage therapy include one of the newer macrolides (azithromycin, clarithromycin; see Chapter 42) and atovaquone.

Mycobacterium tuberculosis therapy in HIV patients

See also Chapter 43.

Bacille Calmette-Guérin vaccine should *not* be given to HIV-1 infected individuals as it is a live, albeit attenuated, strain. Quadruple therapy with isoniazid, 300 mg/day, plus rifampicin, 600 mg/day (450 mg for patients weighing less than 50 kg) and pyrazinamide, 20–30 mg/kg/day, plus either ethambutol (15–25 mg/kg/day) or streptomycin (0.75–1.0 g/day) is recommended. This regimen should be given orally for 2 months, and then rifampicin and isoniazid continued for 9 months or for 6 months after the sputum converts to negative for bacterial growth, whichever is longer. Isoniazid may be used as long-term chemoprophylaxis in patients after successful treatment. If there is isoniazid resistance and/or resistance to other drugs, then the regimen will need to be based on the sensitivities of the isolated organism. This may require therapy with second-line anti-TB drugs. Response rates in HIV patients are generally high (around 90%), provided that there is good compliance, with a relatively low recurrence rate (10%). The incidence of adverse effects from antituberculous therapy is high in these patients, and may necessitate a change in medication. *Mycobacterium tuberculosis* strains are becoming multi-drug resistant (to rifampicin, INAH, ethambutol and even pyrazinamide), and are present in this population, so *in vitro* sensitivity determinations are essential.

Mycobacterium avium-intracellulare complex therapy

This infection is a systemic multi-organ system infection in HIV-infected patients. It has not been convincingly shown to be communicable to other individuals as has *M. tuberculosis*, and the benefit of chronically treating this infection in HIV-infected individuals is now more clearly defined. Prophylactic treatment is best achieved with either clarithromycin (500 mg daily) or azithromycin. Both drugs have potent anti-*M. avium-intracellulare* complex (MAC) activity *in vitro*. The regimens used for treatment are three-or four-drug combination therapies because of the resistance patterns of the organism. One such successful regimen consists of rifabutin (600 mg/day), ethambutol (15 mg/kg/day) and clarithromycin (1000 mg bd). Other effective agents include rifampicin (600 mg/day), clofazimine (100 mg/day), ciprofloxacin (1500 mg/day) and amikacin (7.5–10.0 mg/kg/day – dosage determined by plasma concentrations) intravenously or intramuscularly. If a clinical response is produced (usually within 2–8 weeks), secondary prophylaxis (suppressive therapy) with oral drugs should be given for life.

Antifungal therapy

See Chapter 44 on antifungal and antiviral therapy.

Candida

For *Candida*, if the disease is confined locally then initial therapy with nystatin/amphotericin given topically is adequate. However, if the infection is more extensive, treatment should be with fluconazole, 50 mg daily for 1–2 weeks. Alternatives are itraconazole, 200 mg daily for 1–2 weeks, or even ketoconazole. Prophylaxis with fluconazole, 150 mg weekly, has been established.

Cryptococcus neoformans

First-line therapy is with amphotericin B given intravenously initially at 0.5–1 mg/kg/day (maximum 100 mg/day). The lower dose is used in combination with intravenous flucytosine. However, flucytosine often causes bone-marrow suppression in HIV-1–infected patients. Such combination therapy is preferred in severely ill patients. An effective alternative is fluconazole initially given as oral or intravenous therapy, 400 mg/day, reduced to 200–400 mg/day as maintenance therapy if the patient responds. Liposomal amphotericin B has reduced systemic toxicity and can be used in combination with fluconazole. Itraconazole, 200–400 mg daily, is an alternative and is also effective as prophylactic therapy.

Histoplasmosis

Treatment is with amphotericin B, 1 mg/kg daily intravenously for 6 weeks, or itraconazole, 400 mg daily for 6 weeks. Prophylactic maintenance therapy with itraconazole, 400 mg/day, is recommended.

Coccidiomycosis

Treatment is with amphotericin B, 0.5–1 mg/kg daily intravenously for 6 weeks, followed by itraconazole, 400 mg/day, as maintenance prophylaxis.

Case history

A 69-year-old man had a blood transfusion 12 years ago following surgery for a perforated gastric ulcer. He now complains of a history of fatigue for 18 months and recent weight loss of 5 lb. After thorough clinical assessment and investigation he was found to be HIV-positive. His HIV RNA was 150 000 copies/mL, and his CD4 count was 300×10^6/L on two occasions. He was started on ZDV (300 mg bd) and lamivudine (150 mg bd) given as the combination tablet 'Combivir' 1 tablet twice a day, and saquinivir, 600 mg tds (soft gel), taken with food. Two months later, he feels no better and despite his HIV isolate being sensitive to all agents in the regimen, his HIV RNA is 120 000 copies/mL. He was adamant that he was taking his medication and this was confirmed by his wife. His physician reduces his saquinavir dose to 400 mg bd and adds oral ritonavir, starting at 300 mg bd for 3 days and then increasing to 400 mg bd, which he tolerates well. When reviewed 4 weeks later he has put on weight and feels less tired, and his plasma HIV RNA is 30 000 copies/mL.

Question

Why did this patient show an initial poor response to therapy and then a rapid improvement in clinical symptoms and HIV RNA copy number?

Answer

This patient with late-stage HIV was appropriately started on a 'triple' combination therapy regimen consisting of two nucleoside analogue reverse transcriptase inhibitors (ZDV and 3TC) and a protease inhibitor. There are several possible reasons for a poor response, including poor compliance, viral resistance and inadequate drug treatment. In this case the most likely cause is the poor bioavailability (< 4% and somewhat variable) of the soft gel saquinavir, even with a fatty meal, resulting in inadequate plasma concentrations. The physician revised the patient's regimen, and added ritonavir to saquinavir as a second protease inhibitor. Subsequent follow-up showed the patient to be symptomatically better, with a significant further reduction in the HIV RNA copy number. The explanation for this effect is that the combination causes the systemic saquinavir AUC to be increased by at least 2000%, yielding more effective anti-HIV blood concentrations at a lower dose. In addition, saquinavir potentially increases the AUC of ritonavir, although the extent of this interaction has not yet been clearly defined. These effects on the bioavailability and metabolism of each of these protease inhibitors are thought to be primarily due to mutual inhibition of metabolism by the gastrointestinal and hepatic cytochrome $P_{450\ 3A4}$ isoenzyme. Recent data suggest that saquinavir is a P-glycoprotein substrate and that inhibition of the gastrointestinal P-glycoprotein drug efflux transporter may also contribute to ritonavir increasing the bioavailability of saquinavir in this complex but clinically beneficial drug–drug interaction. A further drug–drug interaction that needs to be considered in this quadruple combination regimen is ritonavir, which reduces the AUC of ZDV by approximately 25% by hepatic glucoronyl transferase enzyme induction, but in the above case this does not appear to have had a significant adverse clinical effect.

ANTI-HERPES VIRUS THERAPY

See also Chapter 44 on antifungal and antiviral therapy.

HERPES SIMPLEX VIRUS I

Acyclovir is used for treatment, and in some patients it has been given orally (200 mg twice daily) as maintenance prophylaxis against recurrence . Unfortunately, this has led to the development of acyclovir resistance of herpes virus isolates in many HIV patients. The newer acyclovir analogues (Famciclovir), which achieve higher blood concentrations of acyclovir or its equivalent are useful here, as are foscarnet or cidofovir.

CYTOMEGALOVIRUS (CMV) INFECTION

CMV infection may be multi-system or confined to the eyes, lungs, genito-urinary system or gastrointestinal tract. Successful therapeutic regimens consist of induction therapy with either ganciclovir or foscarnet, followed by a maintenance regimen. For ganciclovir and foscarnet dosing regimens, see Chapter 44. In the treatment of CMV retinitis, studies suggested that foscarnet was superior and allowed the continued use of ZDV with an improved survival time. This was perhaps due to its lack of bone-marrow suppressive effects, unlike ganciclovir, which together with ZDV causes profound marrow suppression. The tolerance of ganciclovir in AIDS patients is improved when it is used with G-CSF to minimize granulocytopenia. Innovations of drug delivery have also shown the efficacy of slow-release implants of ganciclovir (Ocusert) from a reservoir inserted into the vitreous humour in patients with retinal CMV infection.

FURTHER READING

Anonymous. 1998: Report of the NIH panel to define principles of therapy of HIV infection and guidelines for use of anti-retroviral agents in HIV-infected adults and adolescents. *Annals of Internal Medicine* **128,** 1079–100.

Barry M, Mulcahy F, Back DJ. 1998: Anti-retroviral therapy for patients with HIV disease. *British Journal of Clinical Pharmacology* **45,** 221–28.

BHIVA Co-ordinating Committee. 1997: British HIV Association guidelines for anti-retroviral treatment of HIV seropositive individuals. *Lancet*. **349,** 1086–92.

Collier AC, Coombs RW, Schoenfeld DA *et al*. 1996: Treatment of human immunodeficiency virus infection with saquinivir, zidovudine and zalcitabine. *New England Journal of Medicine* **334,** 1011–17.

Flexner C. 1998: Drug therapy: HIV protease inhibitors. *New England Journal of Medicine* **338,** 1281–92.

Moyle GJ, Gazzard BG, Cooper DA, Gatell J. 1998: Anti-retroviral therapy for HIV infection: a knowledge-based approach to drug selection and use. *Drugs* **55.** 383–404.

CHAPTER FORTY-SIX

MALARIA *and* OTHER PARASITIC INFECTIONS

- Malaria
- Trypanosomal infection
- Helminthic infection

MALARIA

Malaria is the commonest of the six major parasitic diseases defined by the World Health Organization. The global incidence is 200 million cases and 2 million deaths per annum. Malaria is endemic wherever there is a hospitable habitat for its vector, the anopheles mosquito, and this includes much of the world, especially equatorial regions. It is transmitted to humans in the saliva of a mosquito bite, and is caused by protozoan organisms of the genus *Plasmodium*, of which there are four species, namely *P.falciparum*, *P.vivax*, *P. ovale* and *P.malariae*. *P.falciparum is the most lethal form*. Most cases of acute malaria in the western world occur in patients who have contracted the disease in an endemic area and subsequently travelled. The speed of air travel and the appreciable incubation period of the disease have ensured that malaria is not uncommon even in areas where it is not endemic (e.g. general hospitals near international airports in the UK).

Antimalarial drugs are used for:

1 chemoprophylaxis;
2 treatment of acute malaria;
3 cure of chronic malaria.

Visitors to endemic areas must be warned about the risks of infection and advised that prophylactic drug therapy should be taken, *but that it is not 100% effective*. They should also be advised to wear long-sleeved clothing to cover extremities (especially in the evenings, when mosquitos feed) to use mosquito-repellent sprays, to sleep in properly screened rooms with mosquito nets (impregnated with pyrethroids) around the bed and/or to burn and vaporize synthetic pyrethroids during the night. In addition to antimalarial prophylactic drug therapy, travellers to remote areas should be advised to carry standby malarial drug therapy consisting of either halofantrine or quinine. Where there is doubt concerning the suitability of drug

Key points

The malaria parasite

- *Plasmodium falciparum* infection has the highest mortality, and causes cerebral malaria.
- *P. malariae*, *P. ovale* and *P.vivax* cause more benign disease.
- The hepatic forms of *P. ovale* and *P. vivax* cause relapses.
- Antimalarial drugs act at different stages of the malaria parasite's life-cycle.
- Resistance, especially of *P.falciparum*, to chloroquine, sulphadoxine–pyrimethamine and even mefloquine is an increasing problem world-wide

therapy for malaria prophylaxis or treatment, this should be discussed with the malaria reference laboratory at the London School of Hygiene and Tropical Medicine (tel 0171–387–4411 for treatment only and 0171–636–8636 for prophylaxis).

Figure 46.1 illustrates the *Plasmodium* life-cycle and the points of therapeutic drug attack.

MALARIA PROPHYLAXIS

All malaria prophylaxis is relative, and the agents are chosen mainly on the basis of the susceptibility patterns of the local *Plasmodium* species. The arylaminoalcohols (mefloquine), 4–aminoquinolines (chloroquine) and the antifolate agents (dapsone, pyrimethamine and proguanil) are the major prophylactic antimalarial agents. Prophylactic drug treatment *must start at least 1 week* (and preferably 2 weeks) before entering a malaria endemic region, and *must continue for 4 weeks afterwards*.

Chloroquine is only used as a prophylactic in regions where falciparum malaria is not chloroquine resistant; the dose is 300 mg weekly. Proguanil, 200 mg daily, or amodiaquine, 400 mg weekly, are alternatives. Suggested regimens for the prophylaxis of chloroquine-resistant falciparum malaria include the following:

1 mefloquine, 250 mg weekly;
2 chloroquine, 300 mg weekly plus proguanil, 200 mg daily;
3 maloprim (12.5 mg pyrimethamine plus 100 mg dapsone) plus chloroquine, 300 mg weekly.

Key points

Malaria prophylaxis

- All travellers to an endemic area should be made aware of the risks.
- Use appropriate measures to avoid mosquito bites (e.g. repellents, appropriate cover at night, mosquito nets).
- The choice of chemoprophylaxis regimen is dependent on the local strains and resistance pattern.
- Chemoprophylaxis must start before, and continue after, travel to and from an endemic area.
- Full compliance with the chemoprophylaxis regimen is necessary.
- Drug choice and doses may need to be altered in patients with renal or hepatic dysfunction.
- *Prophylaxis is not 100% effective.*

must start 1 week before and continue for 4 weeks afterwards. chloroquine 300 mg weekly. or/and proguanil. 200mg OD.

mefloquine 250mg weekly

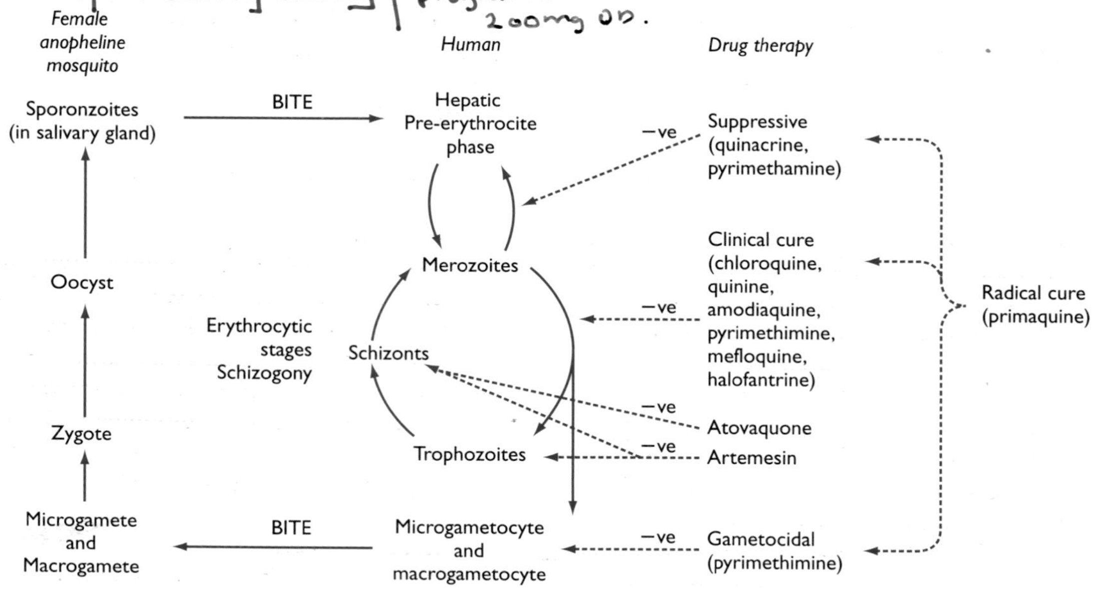

Figure 46.1: Malaria life cycle and type of drug treatment.

Prevention of malaria in pregnancy

This is a difficult problem owing to the theoretical risk to the fetus from antimalarial drugs. Folic acid (5 mg daily) supplements should be prescribed if pyrimethamine or proguanil are used, because the selectivity of these folate inhibitors for the malarial parasite may not be absolute. Maloprim (pyrimethamine combined with dapsone) is not used in the first trimester. Chloroquine and proguanil are believed to be the safest antimalarial drugs for use in pregnancy.

DRUG TREATMENT OF ACUTE MALARIA

The 4-aminoquinolines – (chloroquine and amodiaquine)

Chloroquine

USES

Chloroquine is still one of the most commonly used antimalarial drugs world-wide, *but increasing resistance (especially* P. falciparum*) has reduced its efficacy*. It is used in the treatment of the following:

1. acute malaria – chloroquine is effective in terminating an acute attack of benign vivax malaria, but is not radically curative because it does not eradicate the latent hepatic forms of the parasite, and relapses can occur subsequently. The routine course of chloroquine for malaria treatment is a total dose of 1.5 g (or 30 mg/kg) orally, given in divided doses (600 mg initially, 300 mg after 6 h and then 300 mg daily for 2 days). Children receive a smaller dose of 20 mg/kg. In babies the dose is 5.0 mg/kg by intramuscular injection. If given intravenously, chloroquine can cause encephalopathy. Following a course of chloroquine, primaquine (15 mg, daily) may be given for 14–21 days to achieve a radical cure (i.e. to eliminate hepatic forms and prevent relapse). Before initiating therapy, the possibility of causing haemolysis related to glucose-6–phosphate dehydrogenase deficiency (see Chapter 14) should be considered;
2. malaria prophylaxis (see above).
3. rheumatoid arthritis and systemic lupus erythematosus – chloroquine and hydroxychloroquine (see Chapter 25).

ANTIMALARIAL MECHANISM OF ACTION

The erythrocyte stages of *Plasmodium* are sensitive to chloroquine. At this stage of its life-cycle the parasite digests haemoglobin in a food vacuole to provide energy for the parasite. The food vacuole is acidic, and chloroquine (a weak base) is concentrated within it by diffusion ion-trapping. Chloroquine and other 4–aminoquinolines are believed to inhibit the malarial haem polymerase within the food vacuole of the plasmodial parasite, thereby inhibiting the conversion of toxic haemin (ferriprotoporphyrin IX) to haemozoin (a pigment which accumulates in infected cells and is not toxic to the parasite). Ferriprotoporphyrin IX accumulates in the presence of chloroquine and is toxic to the parasite, which is killed by the waste product of its own appetite ('hoist with its own petard').

ADVERSE EFFECTS

Short-term therapy These include the following:

1. mild headache and visual disturbances.
2. gastrointestinal upsets.
3. pruritus.

Prolonged therapy These include the following:

1. retinopathy, characterized by loss of central visual acuity, macular pigmentation ('bull's-eye' macula) and retinal artery constriction. Progressive visual loss is halted by stopping the drug, but is not reversible;
2. lichenoid skin eruption;
3. bleaching of hair;
4. weight loss;
5. ototoxicity;
6. cochleovestibular paresis in fetal life.

PHARMACOKINETICS

Chloroquine is rapidly and almost completely absorbed from the intestine. It is approximately 50% bound to plasma proteins. About 70% of a dose is excreted unchanged in the urine, and the main metabolite is desethylchloroquine. The mean $t_{\frac{1}{2}}$ is 120 h. High concentrations (relative to plasma) are found in all tissues, especially those containing melanin, notably the retina.

DRUG INTERACTIONS

Chloroquine and quinine are antagonistic and should not be used together.

Arylaminoalcohols (4-aminoquinoline derivatives)

This group consists of the quinoline methanols (**quinine**, **quinidine** and **mefloquine**) and the phenanthrene methanol (**halofantrine**).

Quinine

USES

Quinine is the main alkaloid of cinchona bark. The mechanism of its antimalarial activity remains unclear, but may be similar to that of chloroquine. In animal tissues it has local anaesthetic and irritant effects.

1. Quinine sulphate is the drug of choice in the treatment of an acute attack of falciparum malaria in areas where the parasite is known to be resistant to chloroquine. The usual course is 600 mg three times daily (children 10 mg/kg) for 7 days. Initially the drug is given intravenously as a slow infusion over 4 h, and orally when the patient improves. The mean $t_{\frac{1}{2}}$ is quite long, and in patients with renal or hepatic dysfunction dosing should be reduced to once or twice daily. To eradicate malaria, if quinine resistance is possible, quinine therapy should be followed by pyrimethamine, 75 mg and sulphadoxine, 1.5 g (fansidar three tablets) given as a single dose. The plasma $t_{\frac{1}{2}}$ of both of these drugs is long (96 h for pyrimethamine and 200 h for sulphadoxine. In combination they inhibit folate metabolism synergistically at two sites in the pathway. Both drugs are excreted in the urine, pyrimethamine being excreted mainly as metabolites. Fansidar occasionally causes the Stevens–Johnson syndrome, which limits its use. Pyrimethamine causes gastrointestinal upsets, megaloblastic anaemia, ataxia and fits. If the organism is known or suspected to be fansidar resistant, then doxycycline, 200 mg once daily then 100 mg daily, is substituted for 6 days (not for children under 8 years of age or pregnant women, because of its effects on developing bones and teeth).
2. Nocturnal cramps are sometimes treated with quinine, 200–300 mg given orally before going to bed. However, such treatment is without documented benefit when compared to placebo. As this is such a benign condition, which usually responds to simple measures such as plantar flexion of the foot against pressure, having first excluded iatrogenic causes (e.g. diuretics or β_2-agonists), the use of quinine is not justified.

ADVERSE EFFECTS

These include the following:

1. large therapeutic doses of quinine give rise to cinchonism, which consists of tinnitus, deafness, headaches, nausea and visual disturbances;
2. abdominal pain and diarrhoea;
3. rashes, fever, delirium, stimulation followed by depression of respiration, renal failure, haemolytic anaemia, thrombocytopenic purpura and hypoprothrombinaemia;
4. intravenous quinine can produce neurotoxicity such as tremor of the lips and limbs, and (more seriously) delirium, fits and coma.

PHARMACOKINETICS

Because quinine is almost completely absorbed in the upper part of the small intestine, peak concentrations are similar following oral or intravenous administration. Peak concentrations occur 1–3 h after ingestion. The mean $t_{\frac{1}{2}}$ is 10 h, but is longer in severe falciparum malaria. Around 95% or more of a single dose is metabolized in the liver, principally to inactive hydroxy derivatives, with less than 5% being excreted unaltered in the urine. The uses and properties of the arylaminoalcohols are listed in Table 46.1

8-Aminoquinolines – primaquine

Primaquine is used to eradicate gametocytes and the hepatic forms of *P.vivax* or *P.malariae* after standard chloroquine therapy, provided that the risk of re-exposure is low. It may also be used prophylactically with chloroquine. It interferes with the organism's mitochondrial electron transport chain. Gastrointestinal absorption is good, and it is rapidly metabolized, with a mean $t_{\frac{1}{2}}$ of 6 h. Its major adverse effects are gastrointestinal upsets, methaemoglobinaemia and haemolytic anaemia (which can be explosive and profound) in glucose-6–phosphate dehydrogenase-deficient individuals.

Table 46.1 Uses and properties of other arylaminoalcohols

Drug	Use and pharmacodynamics	Dosing and pharmacokinetics	Side-effects	Precautions/comments
Mefloquine	Used for prophylaxis and acute treatment of drug-resistant malaria (especially *P.falciparum*)	Prophylaxis: oral 250 mg weekly for 3 months	Gastrointestinal disturbances are common (up to 50% of cases)	Not used in pregnancy or in patients with neuropsychiatric disorders or epilepsy
	Schizonticidal in the blood	Acute treatment: oral dosing (20 mg/kg), two doses 6 h apart Maximum 1500 mg	CNS – hallucinations, psychosis, fits	Do not use in patients with renal or hepatic dysfunction
		Hepatic metabolism with enterohepatic circulation $t_{\frac{1}{2}}$ is 14–22 days		Potentiates bradycardia of beta-blockers and quinine potentiates its toxicity
Halofantrine	Used for only uncomplicated chloroquine-resistant *P.falciparum*	Acute treatment: oral dosing 500 mg 6-hourly for three doses, repeated in 1 week	Gastrointestinal disturbances; less common than with mefloquine Pruritus	Embryotoxic in animals – not used in pregnancy
	Schizonticidal in the blood	Food improves absorption. $t_{\frac{1}{2}}$ is 1–2 days. Hepatic metabolism to an active metabolite	Prolongs the QTc Hepatitis CNS – neuromuscular spasm	Cross-resistance with mefloquine may occur

Key points

Treatment of acute malaria

- If the infective species is not known, or is mixed, initial therapy is with intravenous quinine or mefloquine.
- *P.falciparum* is mainly resistant to chloroquine; treat with quinine, mefloquine or halofantrine.
- Benign malaria (caused by *P.malariae*) is treated with chloroquine alone.
- Benign malaria due to *P.ovale* or *P.vivax* requires chloroquine therapy plus primaquine to achieve a radical cure and prevent relapse.
- Careful attention to hydration and blood glucose is necessary.
- Anticipate complications and monitor the patient frequently.

Anti-folates (sulphadoxine, dapsone, proguanil, pyrimethamine)

Combinations of these drugs are taken orally on a daily or weekly basis (e.g. Maloprim – dapsone and pyrimethamine) in malaria prophylaxis, but their efficacy in acute malaria treatment is limited by the development of resistance. These agents inhibit folate metabolism at all stages of the malaria parasite's life-cycle, acting as competitive inhibitors of the malarial dihydropteroate synthase (**sulphadoxine** and **dapsone**) or the malarial dihydrofolate reductase (**proguanil**, **cycloguanil** or **pyrimethamine**). They have long or very long half-lives (24–200 h), and exhibit the typical anti-folate adverse effect profile (gastrointestinal upsets, skin rashes, bone-marrow suppression). More detailed clinical pharmacology of these agents is described in Chapters 42 and 45.

Treatment of a malaria relapse

Plasmodium falciparum does not cause a relapsing illness after treating the acute attack with schizonticides, because there is no persistent liver stage of the parasite. Infections with *P.malariae* can cause recurrent attacks of fever for up to 30 years, but standard treatment with chloroquine eradicates the parasite. Following treatment of an acute attack of vivax malaria with schizonticides, or a period of protection with prophylactic drugs, febrile illness can recur due to the establishment of liver stages of the parasite. Such relapsing illness can be prevented (or treated) by eradicating the parasites in the liver with primaquine, as described above. Proguanil hydrochloride administered continuously (100 mg daily) for 3 years, in order to suppress the parasites and allow time for the hepatic stages to die out naturally, is a useful alternative for patients with glucose-6-phosphate dehydrogenase deficiency.

Prospectus

Since the development of malaria resistant to chloroquine in the late 1950s, resistance to this drug has become widespread. The emergence of organisms that are resistant to sulphadoxine – pyrimethamine and more recently to mefloquine has necessitated the development of alternative antimalarial drugs. Some of the recently developed drugs, and also those currently undergoing clinical investigation, are shown in Table 46.2.

Trypanosomal infection

African sleeping sickness is caused by *Trypanosoma gambiense* and *T.rhodesiense*. The insect vector is the *Glossina* (tsetse) fly. Drugs used in antitrypanosomal therapy (see Table 46.3) include:

1. those that are active in blood and peripheral tissues, including **suramin**, **pentamidine**, **melarsoprol** and **trimelarsan** (also **puromycin** and **nitrofurazone**);
2. those that are active in the central nervous system, including **tryparsamide**, melarsoprol and trimelarsan.

Scheme of treatment

1. Suramin and pentamidine are both successful in treating bloodstream infections (normal cerebrospinal fluid) of *T.gambiense*. In *T.rhodesiense* infections only suramin is effective. When central nervous system (CNS) involvement has occurred, arsenical drugs are used. Advanced CNS disease caused by either parasite may

Table 46.2 Recently developed antimalarial agents for drug-resistant *P.falciparum*

Drug	Use and pharmacodynamics	Dosing and pharmacokinetics	Side-effects	Precautions/comments
Artemesinin (Quinghaosu)	Rapidly schizonticidal in blood	Oral, IM or IV. Dosing regimens being determined	Minimal toxicity in humans to date	Effective against resistant *P.falciparum*; combination with mefloquine reduces relapses
Used as an anti-pyretic in China for centuries	Increases oxygen stresses in the plasmodium and inhibits cytochrome oxidase and RNA synthesis	Metabolized to the active dihydroartemisinin. Half-life is short	Has caused damage to brain-stem nuclei in animals – the relevance of this to human use is not yet known	No known hepatic drug–drug interactions
Atovaquone	Schizonticidal in blood	Oral dosing, 250 mg 8-hourly	Gastrointestinal disturbances, hepatitis, skin rashes	Clears resistant *P.falciparum*. High incidence of recrudescence; combining with proguanil may reduce this (See also Chapter 45)
	Inhibits mitochondrial electron transport	Hepatic metabolism		

Table 46.3 Drug therapy of protozoal infection

Protozoan species	Drug therapy	Additional comments
Trichomonas vaginalis	Metronidazole (7-day course or single 2-g dose) or tinidazole (single 2-g dose)	The commonest protozoan infection Treat the patient and their sexual partner
T. cruzi (American)	Benznidazole or nifurtimox	Effective in the early acute stages
T. gambiense and *T. rhodesiense* (African)	Pentamidine and suramin are effective in the early stages	Later neurological disease – melarsoprol or eflornithine or nifurtimox
Toxoplasma gondii	Pyrimethamine/sulphadiazine	Add folinic acid to reduce risk of bone-marrow suppression
Pneumocystis carinii	Sulphamethoxazole/trimethoprim – high dose	Alternatives – pentamidine, atovaquone see Chapter 45 on drugs and HIV infection
Leishmania (visceral)	Sodium stibogluconate or meglumine antimoniate	Resistant cases – add allopurinol plus pentamidine with or without amphotericin B
Leishmania (cutaneous)	Intralesional – antimonials	Lesions usually heal spontaneously
Giardia lamblia	Metronidazole or tinidazole	Treat family and institutional contacts

Case history

A 27-year-old student goes to West Africa for an elective attachment to a rural hospital. He is taking chemoprophylaxis with oral chloroquine, 300 mg weekly, and proguanil, 200 mg daily. Two weeks after arriving at his destination he complains of lethargy, breathlessness on exertion, ankle swelling and paraesthesiae in his hands. He is seen by a physician's assistant who gives him some iron tablets as he looks pale and has a haemoglobin level of 6.8g/dl with 5% reticulocytes.

Question

What is the underlying problem here that has not been completely defined? How should he be further managed?

Answer

This patient has a significant haemolytic anaemia, which is of recent onset and is thus most likely to be due to his recent ingestion of prophylactic antimalarial therapy. He was tested for glucose-6-phosphate dehydrogenase deficiency and found to have a low activity of this enzyme in his red cells. The lack of this enzyme often only becomes clinically manifest when the red cell is stressed, as in the presence of an oxidant such as chloroquine (other common drugs that precipitate haemolysis include primaquine, dapsone, sulphonamides, the 4-quinolones nalidixic acid and ciprofloxacin, nitrofurantoin, aspirin and quinidine). The patient's erythrocytes cannot handle the increased oxidation stress and cannot utilize the hexose monophosphate shunt to synthesize NAPDH in order to reduce oxidized glutathione (which is the only way to achieve this in red cells), and are thus damaged by excessive redox stress. The patient should be asked whether anyone in his family has ever experienced a similar condition, as it is transmitted as an X-linked defect. It is also important to establish his family ethnic backround (commoner in people whose ethnic origins are Africa, Asia, southern Europe (Mediterranean) and Oceania). Stopping the chloroquine and giving folate and iron should improve both his symptoms and his haematogical abnormalities. He should be warned about those drugs that can precipitate haemolysis, and advised to inform his physician that he has this condition. He should also consider carrying a card or bracelet that bears this information.

Table 46.4 Drug therapy for common helminthic infections

Helminthic species	Drug therapy	Further comment
Tapeworms		
Taenia saginata	Praziquantel or niclosamide or gastrograffin	A single dose of praziquantel is curative
Cysticercosis		
Taenia soleum	Praziquantel or gastrograffin	
Diphyllobothrium latum	Praziquantel or niclosamide or gastrograffin	
Hydatid disease		
Echinococcus granulosus	Albendazole or mebendazole	Surgery for operably treatable cysts
Hookworm		
Ancylostoma duodenale	Mebendazole/albendazole, bephenium or pyrantel pamoate	
Necator americanus		
Strongyloides stercoralis	Albendazole	
Threadworm		
Enterobius vermicularis	Mebendazole/albendazole, bephenium or pyrantel pamoate	
Whipworm		
Trichuris trichiuria	Thiabendazole	
Tissue nematodes		
Ancylostoma braziliensae	Thiabendazole	
Guinea worm		
Dracunculus medinensis	Metronidazole	Symptoms quickly relieved
Visceral larvae/roundworms		
Toxocara canis	Diethylcarbamazine	Progressively increasing dose, allergic reactions to dying larvae, corticosteroids required for ocular disease
Toxocara catis		
Lymphatic filariasis		
Wuchteria bancrofti	Diethylcarbamazine	
Onchocerciasis		
Onchocerca volvulus	Ivermectin	Single dose is curative
Schistosomiasis/blood flukes		
Schistosoma mansoni	Praziquantel	Oxamiquine (*S.mansoni*)
Schistosoma japonicum		
Schistosoma hematobium		Metriphonate (*S.hematobium*)
Liver flukes/fascioliasis		
Fasciola hepatica, etc.	Praziquantel	
Other gut nematodes		
Ascariasis		
Ascaris lumbricoides	Pyrantel pamoate or levamisole	
Trichinosis		
Trichinella spiralis	Mebendazole, albendazole or pyrantel pamoate	

respond to melarsoprol. Eflornithine is effective in CNS infection with *T.gambiense*.

2 For prophylaxis, a single 1 g injection of suramin protects an adult against both infections for 6–12 weeks. A single dose of pentamidine, 200–250 mg, protects against *T.gambiense* for 3–6 months.
3 Treatment of the early acute phase of *T. cruzi* infections (South American trypanosomiasis) is with Nifurtimox or benznidazole.

Table 46.3 outlines the major drugs used to treat protozoal infections.

HELMINTHIC INFECTION

Table 46.4 outlines the primary drug treatments for common helminthic infections.

FURTHER READING

Bradley D, Warhurst DC. 1995: Malaria prophylaxis: guidelines for travellers from Britain. Malaria reference laboratory. *British Medical Journal*. **310**, 709–14.

Liu LX, Weller P. F. 1996: Antiparasitic drugs. *New England Journal of Medicine* **334**, 1178–84.

Molyneux M, Fox R. 1993: Diagnosis and treatment of malaria in Britain. *British Medical Journal* **306**, 1175–80.

White NJ. 1996: The treatment of malaria. *New England Journal of Medicine*. **335**, 800–806.

World Health Organization. 1990: *WHO model prescribing information: drugs used in parasitic diseases*. Geneva: World Health Organization.

Zucker JR, Campbell CC. 1993: Malaria. Principles and prevention and treatment. *Infectious Disease Clinics of North America* **7**, 547–67.

CHAPTER FORTY-SEVEN

CANCER CHEMOTHERAPY

- Introduction
- Pathophysiology of neoplastic cell growth
- General principles of use of cytotoxic drugs
- Resistance to cytotoxic drugs
- Common complications of cancer chemotherapy
- Drugs used in cancer chemotherapy

INTRODUCTION

In the UK there are approximately 150 000 cancer deaths per year. The commonest cancers are those of the lung, breast, prostate, and large bowel. Patients with malignant disease require treatment with a multidisciplinary treatment team approach. In addition to the principal treatment modalities of surgery, radiotherapy and chemotherapy (including immunotherapy), the importance of attending to psychiatric and social factors is being increasingly recognized. Accurate staging (i.e. determining the extent of the cancer) is an essential prerequisite of optimal management, and in those cases where localized disease is confirmed, cure may be possible with surgery or radiotherapy. In some cases chemotherapy is given following surgery in the knowledge that widespread microscopic dissemination almost certainly has occurred (this is termed *adjuvant chemotherapy*). If the tumour is widespread at presentation, systemic chemotherapy is more likely to be effective than radiotherapy or surgery, although these may none the less be worthwhile to control local disease and to reduce the tumour load before potentially curative chemotherapy.

PATHOPHYSIOLOGY OF NEOPLASTIC CELL GROWTH

Clones of neoplastic cells expand, invade adjacent tissue and can spread (via the bloodstream or lymphatics) as metastases throughout the body. Pathogenesis depends on both *environmental* (e.g. exposure to carcinogens) and *genetic* factors which derange the molecular mechanisms that control cell replication. Such abnormalities are the hallmarks of malignant transformation, they are often multiple, and they arise in many different ways. In approximately 50% of human cancers genetic mutations contribute to the neoplastic process. In some cancer cells oncogenes (first identified in viruses that caused cancers in laboratory animals) are overexpressed. Oncogenes encode growth factors and mitogenic factors that regulate cell cycle progression and cell growth. Alternatively, neoplastic cells may overexpress certain growth factor receptors, or underexpress proteins that inhibit cellular proliferation (e.g. p53 and the retinoblastoma protein). The latter proteins are the so-called tumour suppressor genes. It is the overall effect of such genetic and environmental factors that shifts the normal balance to dysregulated cell proliferation. Propagation of neoplastic cells requires that normal DNA recognition and repair mechanisms for genomic mutations are defective. Individuals

Key points

Principal features of neoplastic cells

- Abnormal growth.
- Mutation or absence of regulatory proteins.
- DNA instability.
- Immortalization.

with defects in these DNA repair genes are prone to develop cancer.

Unlike normal adult somatic cells, neoplastic cells are immortal, and do not have a programmed finite number of cell divisions before they become senescent. The element of cell replication responsible for this programme is the telomere that is located at the end of each chromosome and must pair and align at mitosis. The telomere is produced and maintained by the enzyme telomerase in germ cells and embryonic cells. Telomerase loses its function in the course of normal cell development and differentiation. In normal cells a component of the telomere is lost with each cell division, and such telomeric shortening functions as an intrinsic cellular clock. Approximately 95% of cancer cells re-express telomerase, allowing them to proliferate endlessly, but providing a potential therapeutic target.

Most drugs used in cancer chemotherapy interfere with synthesis of DNA and/or RNA, or the synthesis and/or function of cell cycle regulatory molecules, resulting in cell death (due to direct cytotoxicity or probably more commonly to programmed cell death – *apoptosis*) or inhibition of cell proliferation. These drug effects are not confined to malignant cells, and most cytotoxic agents are also toxic to normal dividing cells, particularly those in the bone marrow, gastrointestinal tract, gonads, skin and hair follicles.

General principles of use of cytotoxic drugs

The number of cytotoxic drugs available has expanded rapidly, and their effects on the stages of the cell cycle are now better defined, facilitating rational drug combinations. This has been of

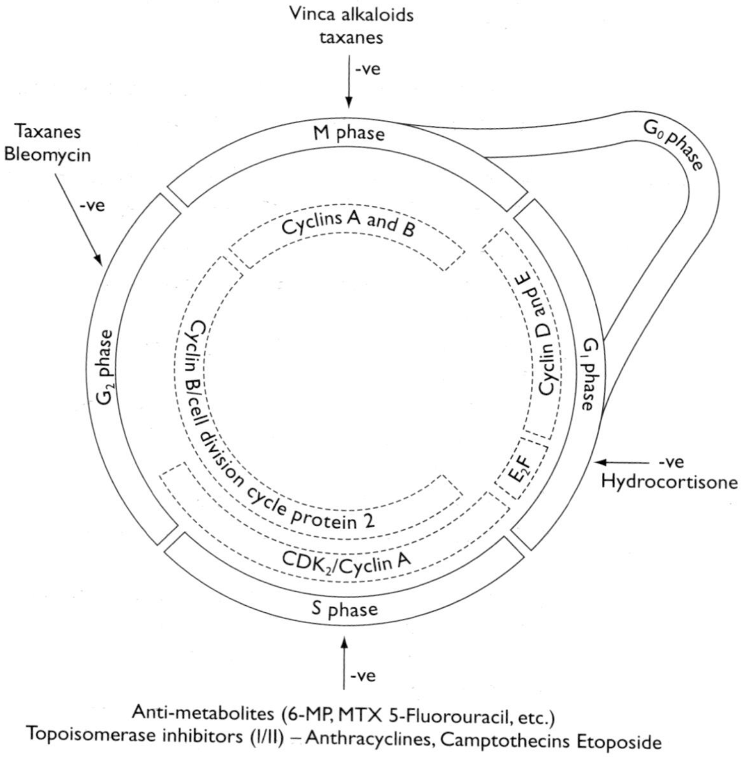

Figure 47.1 The cell cycle – regulatory systems and sites of drug actions.

crucial importance in achieving efficacy in several malignancies, especially lymphomas and leukaemias. The action of cytotoxic drugs on cell progression through the cell cycle (see Figure 47.1) can be broadly divided into two groups as follows.

Cell-cycle-non-specific drugs

These drugs act at all stages in the proliferating cell cycle (but not in the G_0-resting phase). Because of this, their dose–cytotoxicity relationships follow first-order kinetics (cells are killed exponentially with increasing dose). The linear relationship between dose and log cytotoxicity (Figure 47.2) is exploited in the use of high-dose chemotherapy. Cytotoxic drugs are given at very high doses over a short period, thus rendering the bone marrow aplastic, but at the same time achieving a very high tumour cell kill. Clinical efficacy has been established in haematological malignancies (e.g. leukaemias, lymphomas) using such agents. *Alkylating agents* are examples of cycle-non-specific drugs (e.g. **cyclophosphamide, melphalan** and nitrosoureas such as **cis-chloroethylnitrosourea** (**CCNU** – **lomustine**) and **bischloroethylnitrosourea** (**BCNU** – **carmustine**)).

Cell-cycle phase-specific drugs

These drugs act only at a specific phase in the cell cycle. Therefore the more rapid the cell turnover, the more effective they are. Their dose–cytotoxicity curve is initially exponential but at higher doses the response approaches a maximum (see Figure 47.3). Table 47.1 classifies the commonly used cytotoxic drugs according to their effect on the cell cycle, but until the kinetic behaviour of human tumours can be adequately characterized in individual patients, the value of this classification is somewhat limited. The distinction between cycle-non-specific and phase-specific drugs, although clear-cut in animal and *in vitro* experiments, is probably an over-simplification.

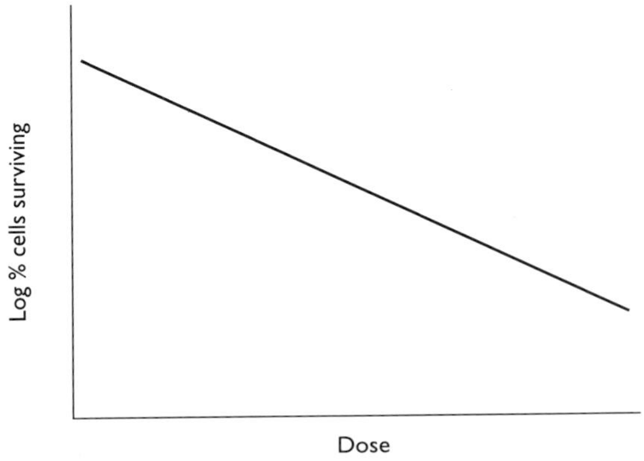

Figure 47.2 Dose–response relationship for a cycle-non-specific drug.

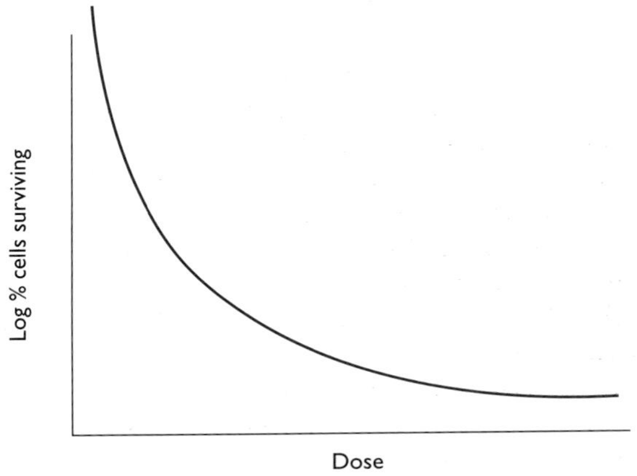

Figure 47.3 Dose–response relationship for a phase-specific drug.

Table 47.1 Classification of common cytotoxic drugs according to their effect on the cell cycle

Predominantly cycle-non-specific	Predominantly phase-specific
Nitrogen mustards	Methotrexate
Cyclophosphamide, ifosfamide	6-Mercaptopurine
Melphalan	6-Thioguanine
Busulphan	5-Fluorouracil
Chlorambucil	Cytosine arabinoside
Lomustine (CCNU), carmustine (BCNU)	Vinca alkaloids
Dacarbazine (DTIC)	Etoposide
Actinomycin D	Taxanes – paclitaxel/ docetaxel
Mitomycin C	Camptothecins – irinotecan
Mitozantrone	Gemcitabine
Doxorubicin, daunomycin	Capecitabune

CCNU *cis*-chloroethylnitrosurea, BCNu *bis*-chloroethyl-mitrosurea

Principles of cancer chemotherapy

Cancer chemotherapy is primarily used to induce and maintain a remission or response according to the following general principles.

1. Drugs are used in combination, to increase efficacy, inhibit the development of resistance and minimize overlapping toxicities.
2. Drugs that produce a high fraction cell kill are preferred.
3. Drugs are usually given intermittently, but in high doses. This is less immunosuppressive and generally more effective than continuous low-dose regimens.
4. Toxicity is considerable, and therefore frequent blood counts and intensive clinical support are essential.
5. Treatment usually needs to be prolonged (for 6 months or longer).
6. The earlier treatment is initiated, the better the prognosis.

Key points

Principles of cytotoxic chemotherapy

- Cytotoxic drugs kill a constant percentage of cells – not a constant number.
- Cells have discrete periods of time during which they are sensitive to cytotoxic drugs.
- Cancer chemotherapy slows progression through the cell cycle.
- Cytotoxic drugs are not totally selective in their toxicity to cancer cells.
- Cell cytotoxicity is proportional to total drug exposure.
- Cytotoxic drugs should be used in combination.

Key points

Combination chemotherapy

- Develop combinations in which the drugs have:
  - individual antineoplastic actions;
  - non-overlapping toxicities;
  - different mechanisms of cytotoxic effects.
- The dose and schedule used must be optimized.
- Combination therapy is better than single drug therapy because:
  - there is improved cell cytotoxicity;
  - heterogeneous tumour cell populations are killed;
  - it reduces the development of resistance.

Resistance to cytotoxic drugs

Resistance may be primary (i.e. a non-responsive tumour) or acquired. Acquired resistance results from the selection of resistant cells as a result of killing of susceptible tumour cells, or from an adaptive change in the neoplastic cell. The primary mechanisms of human tumour resistance are summarized in Table 47.2. The ability to predict the sensitivity of bacterial pathogens to antimicrobial substances *in vitro* produced a profound change in the efficacy of treatment of infectious diseases. The development of analogous predictive tests has long been a priority in cancer research. They would be particularly desirable because, in contrast to antimicrobial drugs, cytotoxic agents are administered in doses that produce toxic effects in most patients. Predictive toxicity tests could provide a considerable improvement in therapy, as patients with non-responsive tumours could be spared the toxic effects of inactive drugs. Unfortunately, clinically useful tests do not yet exist. It is possible that with advances in cell-culture techniques and understanding of tumour biology, *in vitro* tumour colony sensitivity assays may be validated in the future.

Common complications of cancer chemotherapy

Chemotherapeutic drugs vary in their potential to cause adverse effects, and there is considerable inter-individual variation in patient susceptibility. The common adverse effects of chemotherapy are summarized in Table 47.3.

Nausea and vomiting

Cytotoxic drugs cause nausea and vomiting to varying degrees (see Table 47.4). This is usually delayed for 1–2 h after drug administration, and may last for 24–48 h or even be delayed for 48–96 h

Table 47.2 Acquired tumour resistance to cytotoxic agents

Mechanism	Examples
1 Reduced intracellular drug concentration	
(i) increased drug efflux (MDR-1, Pgp and related proteins)	Anthracyclines (e.g. doxorubicin), vinca alkaloids (e.g. vincristine), taxanes (paclitaxel), podophyllotoxins (etoposide)
(ii) decreased inward transport	Antimetabolites – methotrexate, nitrogen mustards
2 Deletion of enzyme to activate drug	Cytosine arabinoside; 5-fluorouracil
3 Increased detoxification of drug	6-Mercaptopurine, alkylating agents
4 Increased concentration of target enzyme	Methotrexate, hydroxyurea
5 Decreased requirement for specific metabolic product	L-Asparaginase
6 Increased utilization of alternative pathway	Antimetabolites (e.g. 5-fluorouracil)
7 Rapid repair of drug-induced lesion	Alkylating agents (e.g. mustine, cyclophosphamide and cisplatinum)
8 Decreased number of receptors for drug	Hormones, glucocorticosteroids

Table 47.3 Common toxic effects of cytotoxic chemotherapy

Immediate	Delayed
1 Nausea and vomiting	1 Bone-marrow suppression predisposing to infection, bleeding and anaemia
2 Extravasation with tissue necrosis	2 Alopecia
	3 Infertility/teratogenicity
	4 Agent-specific organ toxicity (e.g. CNS – peripheral neuropathy with vincristine)
	5 Psychiatric morbidity
	6 Second malignancy

Table 47.4 Emetogenic potential of commonly used cytotoxic drugs

Severe	Moderate	Low
Doxorubicin	Lomustine, carmustine	Bleomycin
Cyclophosphamide (high dose)	Mitomycin C	Cytarabine
Dacarbazine	Procarbazine	Vinca alkaloids
Mustine	Etoposide	Methotrexate
Cisplatin	Ifosfamide	5–Fluorouracil
	Taxanes	Chlorambucil
		Mitozantrone

after therapy. The mechanisms by which such drugs induce vomiting include stimulation of the chemoreceptor trigger zone (in the floor of the fourth ventricle) and of peripheral receptors mediating gastric atony and cessation of peristalsis, and stimulation of gastro-intestinal 5-HT_3 receptors which stimulate vagal afferents.

Sometimes vomiting may be anticipatory, and it is normal to use prophylactic anti-emetics (see Chapter 33) before treatment, and to give the patient a supply of medication to take as needed over the ensuing days. No treatment is 100% effective, especially for cisplatin-induced vomiting.

Extravasation with tissue necrosis

Tissue necrosis, which is sometimes severe enough to require skin grafting, occurs with extravasation of the following drugs: **doxorubicin**, **BCNU**, **mustine**, **vinca alkaloids** and **paclitaxel**. Expert attention to vascular access for intravenous cytotoxic drug administration is mandatory.

Bone-marrow suppression

There are two patterns of bone-marrow recovery after suppression (see Figure 47.4), namely rapid and delayed. The usual pattern is of rapid recovery, but **chlorambucil**, BCNU, CCNU, melphalan and **mitomycin** can cause prolonged myelosuppression (up to 8 weeks). The recent advent of recombinant haematopoietic growth factors (erythropoietin, granulocyte colony-stimulating factor (G-CSF), granulocyte macrophage colony-stimulating factor (GM-CSF), interleukin-3 (IL-3), thrombopoietin (Tpo) and IL-11) and their use to minimize the bone-marrow suppression caused by various chemotherapeutic regimens holds great promise (see Chapter 48). **Vincristine**, **bleomycin** and glucocorticosteroids seldom cause myelosuppression.

Infection

Infection is the commonest life-threatening complication of chemotherapy. It is often acquired from the patient's own gastrointestinal tract flora. Effective isolation is achieved in purpose-built laminar-airflow units, but this does not solve the problem of the patient's own bacterial flora. Classical signs of infection – other than pyrexia – are often absent in neutropenic patients, and constant vigilance is required to detect and treat septicaemia early. Broad-spectrum antibiotic treatment must be started empirically in febrile neutropenic patients before the results of blood and other cultures are available. Combination therapy with an aminoglycoside active against *Pseudomonas* and other Gram-negative organisms (e.g. **amikacin**) plus a penicillin (e.g. **piperacillin**) is often appropriate. Alternatively, monotherapy with a third-generation cephalosporin active against β-lactamase-producing organisms (e.g. **ceftazidime**, **cefotaxime**) can provide suitable empirical cover in most instances. Therapeutic decisions need to be guided by knowledge of local organisms, the patient's previous antimicrobial therapy and culture results (see Chapter 42). Opportunistic infections with fungi or protozoa (e.g. *Pneumocystis carinii*) occur (see Chapters 44 and 45 for details of treatment).

Alopecia

Doxorubicin, **ifosfamide**, parenteral **etoposide**, vinca alkaloids, and taxanes all cause alopecia. This may be alleviated in the case of doxorubicin by cooling the scalp using ice-cold gel packs or ice-cooled water caps. Some hair loss occurs with almost all cytotoxic agents.

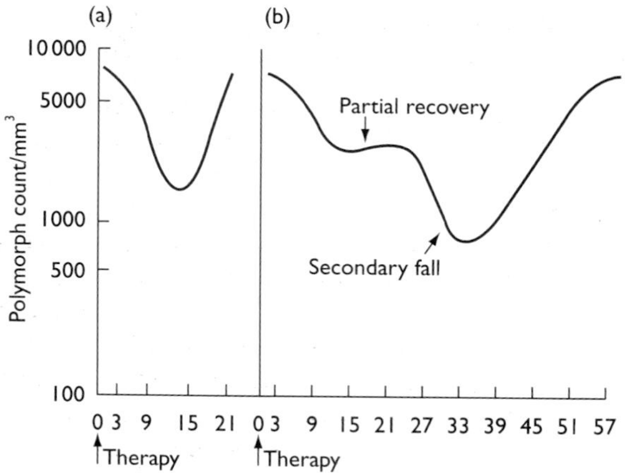

Figure 47.4 Patterns of bone-marrow recovery following cytotoxic therapy: (a) rapid (17–21 days) and (b) delayed (initial fall 8–10 days, secondary nadir at 27–32 days, recovery 42–50 days) (after D.E. Bergasagel).

INFERTILITY AND TERATOGENESIS

Cytotoxic drugs predictably impair fertility and increase the incidence of fetal abnormalities. Most women develop amenorrhoea if treated with cytotoxic drugs. However, many resume normal menstruation when treatment is stopped, and pregnancy is then possible, especially in younger women who are treated with lower total doses of cytotoxic drugs. Amenorrhoea is associated with low plasma oestrogen levels and high follicle-stimulating hormone (FSH) and luteinizing hormone (LH) levels, indicating a primary effect on the ovary. In men, a full course of cytotoxic drugs usually produces azoospermia due to direct damage to the germinal epithelium of the testis. Alkylating agents are particularly harmful. Recovery can occur, but is delayed for up to several years. The re-establishment of normal spermatogenesis is most common after a short course of treatment with a single agent. Cytotoxic drugs cause testicular damage in prepubertal boys, but the long-term reproductive outcome is unclear. Prepubertal girls are probably less prone to cytotoxic-induced ovarian damage. *Sperm storage* before chemotherapy can be considered for males who wish to have children in the future. Both men and women must be strongly advised to use contraceptives during chemotherapy, as a reduction in fertility with these drugs is not universal, and fetal malformations could ensue. It is best to avoid conception for at least 6 months after completion of chemotherapy.

SECOND MALIGNANCY

Up to 3-10% of patients treated for Hodgkin's disease (particularly those who received both chemotherapy and radiotherapy) develop a second malignancy, usually acute non-lymphocytic leukaemia. This malignancy is also approximately 20 times more likely to develop in patients with ovarian carcinoma treated with alkylating agents with or without radiotherapy. This complication of treatment will probably become more commonly recognized as the number of patients who survive after successful cancer chemotherapy increases.

Key points

Adverse effects of cytotoxic chemotherapy

- *Immediate effects:*
  - drug extravasation (e.g. vinca alkaloids, doxorubicin);
  - nausea and vomiting (e.g. cisplatin.)
- *Delayed effects:*
  - bone-marrow suppression – all drugs;
  - infection;
  - alopecia;
  - drug-specific organ toxicities (e.g. skin and pulmonary – bleomycin; cardiotoxicity – doxorubicin);
  - psychiatric morbidity;
  - teratogenesis.
- *Late effects:*
  - gonadal failure/dysfunction;
  - leukaemogenesis/myelodysplasia;
  - development of secondary cancer.

DRUGS USED IN CANCER CHEMOTHERAPY

These include the following:

1 alkylating agents;
2 antimetabolites;
3 DNA-binding agents;
4 topoisomerase inhibitors;
5 microtubular inhibitors (vinca alkaloids and taxanes);
6 hormones;
7 biological response modifiers.

ALKYLATING AGENTS

Alkylating agents are particularly effective when cells are dividing rapidly, but they are not phase-specific. They combine with DNA of both malignant and normal cells and thus damage not only malignant cells but also dividing normal cells, especially those of the bone marrow and the gastrointestinal tract (see Table 47.5). The alkyl groupings on these drugs are highly reactive, so although their most important effect is on DNA synthesis, they also combine with susceptible groups in cells and tissue fluids. If a tumour is

Table 47.5 Comparative pharmacology of classical alkylating agents

Drug	Route of administration	Nausea and vomiting	Granulo-cytopenia	Thrombo-cytopenia	Special toxicity
Mustine	IV	+++	+++	++++	Tissue necrosis if extravasated
Cyclophosphamide	Oral/IV	++	+++	+	Alopecia (10–20%) Chemical cystitis (reduced by mesna) Mucosal ulceration Impaired water excretion Interstitial pulmonary fibrosis
Ifosfamide	IV	++	++	+	Chemical cystitis (reduced by mesna) Alopecia Hypotension (if rapidly infused)
Chlorambucil	Oral	+	++	++++	Bone-marrow suppression
Melphalan	Oral	0	+++	+++	Chemical cystitis (very rare)
Busulphan	Oral	0	++++	+++	Skin pigmentation Interstitial pulmonary fibrosis Amenorrhoea Gynaecomastia (rare)

sensitive to one alkylating agent it is usually sensitive to another, but cross-resistance within the group does not necessarily occur. The pharmacokinetic properties of the different drugs are probably important in this respect. For example, although most alkylating agents diffuse passively into cells, mustine is actively transported by some cells.

Mustine

USES

Mustine is unstable in solution, and is given immediately after it has been made up. It is given slowly (over 2–3 min) via a rapidly running well-flushed proximal intravenous line. This minimizes the risk of local thrombosis and highly irritant extravasation into the surrounding tissues. The dose and frequency depend on the schedule being used. Mustine is usually combined with other cytotoxic drugs (e.g. **vinblastine**, **procarbazine** and **prednisolone** – 'MOPP'). It is used to treat Hodgkin's disease.

MECHANISM OF ACTION

In solution, mustine forms highly reactive ethylene-imine ions that alkylate macromolecules, cross-linking mainly the guanine bases on opposing strands of DNA (Figure 47.5). The tightly bound DNA strands are then unable to separate and cannot act as templates for RNA production or form new DNA. Mustine probably alkylates other cellular components such as enzymes and membranes – effects that contribute to its cytotoxicity.

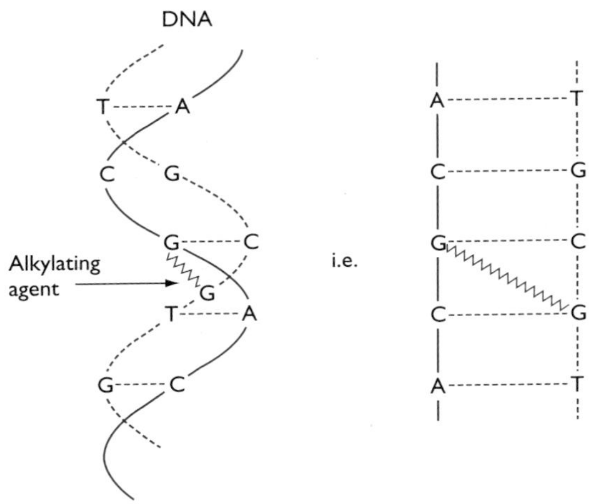

Figure 47.5 Mechanism of intramolecular bridging of DNA by alkylating agents. A = adenine, C = cytosine, G = guanine, T = thymidine.

ADVERSE EFFECTS

See Table 47.5.

PHARMACOKINETICS

Mustine must be given intravenously. The reactive ethylene-imine ion forms spontaneously due to cyclization in solution. The plasma $t_{\frac{1}{2}}$ is short (probably about 30 min).

Cyclophosphamide

USES

Cyclophosphamide is an oxazaphosphorine alkylating agent (**ifosfamide** is another member of this group). It is an inactive prodrug and so can be given orally (unlike mustine) or intravenously. Large doses are nauseating, and are given intravenously. Several combination regimens in current use include cyclophosphamide; rarely it may be used as the sole therapeutic agent at a dose of 50–150 mg orally daily. In combinations, doses of 400–600 mg/m^2 are commonly used, while in high-dose chemotherapy (e.g. to prepare patients with acute leukaemia and aplastic anaemia for allogeneic bone-marrow transplantation), doses of 45–60 mg/kg/day for 2–3 days are employed. Cyclophosphamide is most useful in the treatment of various *lymphomas* and *leukaemias* and in *myeloma*, but it also has some effect in other malignancies. In addition, cyclophosphamide is an effective immunosuppressant (see Chapter 49).

ADVERSE EFFECTS

See Table 47.5.

PHARMACOKINETICS

Cyclophosphamide is 80–90% metabolized and activated in the liver by cytochrome P_{450}, with the production of a number of cytotoxic alkylating metabolites, the most potent of which is phosphoramide mustard. Cyclophosphamide can be given intravenously or orally, and is almost completely absorbed from the intestine. The elimination $t_{\frac{1}{2}}$ of cyclophosphamide is in the range 3–12 h. When given repeatedly, the $t_{\frac{1}{2}}$ becomes progressively shorter. The half-life of the active species (phosphoramide mustard) is probably of the order of only minutes. Cyclophosphamide and its metabolites are excreted in the urine. Renal excretion of the metabolite acrolein is believed to cause the chemical haemorrhagic cystitis that accompanies cyclophosphamide administration.

Mesna (uroprotection agent)

USE

Mesna is an acronym for **2-mercaptoethane sulphonate sodium (Na)**, and is used to protect the urinary tract against the irritant effects of the toxic metabolites (especially *acrolein*) of cyclophosphamide and ifosfamide. Mesna is given by intravenous injection or by mouth. Because it is excreted more rapidly ($t_{\frac{1}{2}}$ < 30 min) than cyclophosphamide and ifosfamide, it is essential that mesna is given at the commencement of treatment, and that the maximum interval between doses is not more than 4 h. The dose of mesna is usually 20% of the dose of the cytotoxic agent given immediately; this mesna dosage is then repeated 4 and 8 h later. Higher doses (e.g. 40%), given four times at 3–hourly intervals, are used for patients at higher risk and for children. Urine is monitored for output, proteinuria and haematuria. The side-effects of mesna include headache and somnolence and rarely rashes.

MECHANISM OF ACTION

Mesna protects the uro-epithelium by providing sulphydryl groups to form a stable thioether with acrolein. It also reduces the decomposition rate of the 4–hydroxy metabolites of these drugs to acrolein by combining to form relatively stable compounds that are not toxic to the urinary tract. This interaction with cyclophosphamide and ifosfamide metabolites occurs almost exclusively in the kidney, where dimesna (the oxidation product of mesna formed in the blood *in vivo*) is excreted and then reduced back to active mesna.

OTHER ALKLATING AGENTS

Procarbazine

USES

Procarbazine is a hydrazine which is highly effective in Hodgkin's disease but less so in non-Hodgkins lymphoma. It forms part of the MOPP and MVPP regimens mentioned above. These treatments produce complete remission in about 65% of Hodgkins patients. Procarbazine is given daily by mouth.

MECHANISM OF ACTION

The cytotoxic effect depends on activation in the liver by cytochrome P_{450} enzymes to azoxy compounds which alkylate DNA. In addition, it causes DNA methylation, free-radical-mediated damage and inhibition of DNA synthesis and protein synthesis.

ADVERSE EFFECTS

These include the following:

1 dose-related haemopoietic suppression, leukopenia and thrombocytopenia occur after 10–14 days;
2 nausea and vomiting;
3 neurotoxicity – with high-dose intravenous therapy.

PHARMACOKINETICS

Procarbazine is rapidly and almost completely absorbed from the intestine, peak concentrations being obtained within 30–60 min. The $t_{\frac{1}{2}}$ of the parent compound in plasma is about 10 min. It is metabolized to a number of compounds that are excreted by the kidneys. Some of these, particularly the hydrazines, have cytotoxic activity. Procarbazine and its metabolites penetrate the blood–brain barrier.

DRUG INTERACTIONS

Procarbazine blocks aldehyde dehydrogenase (cf. **disulfiram**, see Chapter 52) and consequently causes flushing and tachycardia if ethanol is taken. It is also a weak *monoamine–oxidase inhibitor* and can potentially precipitate a hypertensive crisis with tyramine containing foods (see Chapter 19).

PLATINUM COMPOUNDS

Cisplatin

USES

Cisplatin (*cis*-diaminedichloroplatinum) is an inorganic platinum (II) co-ordination complex in which two amine (NH_3) and two chlorine ligands occupy *cis* positions (the *trans* compound is inactive). Cisplatin is the most effective single agent in testicular teratomas, but is usually given in combination with various other cytotoxic drugs. When combined with high-dose bleomycin and vinblastine, a remission rate of 70% is achievable. Platinum compounds are also combined with other agents to treat a number of solid tumours, including carcinoma of the ovary, lung, head and neck, and bladder. Cisplatin is given intravenously as either a bolus or an infusion in a number of regimes, often in combination with other cytotoxic agents. The usual dose is 50–100 mg/m^2 as a single dose or 15–20 mg/m^2 daily for 5 days every 3–4 weeks. Because of the efficacy of platinum compounds and the toxicity of cisplatin, there has been a search for less toxic analogues yielding, for example, **carboplatin** and oral platinum analogues (e.g. **JM-216**, which is currently undergoing phase III investigation).

MECHANISM OF ACTION

Cytotoxicity results from selective inhibition of tumour DNA synthesis by the formation of intra- and inter-strand cross-links at guanine residues in the nucleic acid backbone. This unwinds and shortens the DNA helix.

ADVERSE EFFECTS

These include the following:

1 severe nausea and vomiting;
2 nephrotoxicity, which is dose-related and dose limiting. It causes acute distal tubular necrosis. Prehydration and diuresis reduce the immediate effects but cumulative and permanent damage still occurs;
3 clinically significant hypomagnesaemia and hypokalemia. Magnesium and potassium supplements are usually given during the cisplatin infusion;
4 ototoxicity develops in up to 30% of patients, mostly in the frequency range above speech tones. Cisplatin irreversibly damages the organ of Corti, and this effect is related to cumulative dose. Audiometry should be carried out before, during and after treatment;
5 myelosuppression – usually thrombocytopenia;
6 nervous system effects – cerebellar syndrome and peripheral neuropathy can be disabling.

PHARMACOKINETICS

Cisplatin requires the replacement of the two chloride atoms with water to become active. This process is known as aquation and is slow (it takes 2.5 h). Plasma disappearance of cisplatin is multiphasic ($t_{\frac{1}{2}\alpha}$ is 25–50 min and $t_{\frac{1}{2}\beta}$ is 60–73 h). Although it is initially rapidly excreted, over 50% is retained by the body after 5 days, and low urinary concentrations are found up to 1 month after treatment.

DRUG INTERACTIONS

Because of the nephrotoxicity and ototoxicity of cisplatin, other agents such as aminoglycosides with similar toxicities should be avoided.

The comparative pharmacology of various platinum compounds is summarized in Table 47.6.

ANTIMETABOLITES

Antimetabolites are structural analogues of, and compete with, endogenous cellular metabolites. It was hoped that it would be possible to find and selectively block metabolic pathways that were unique to malignant cells. This hope has not been fulfilled, and the pathways blocked by antimetabolites are also important for normal cells. Thus their selectivity for malignant cells is only partial. Their action is usually confined to specific steps in the synthesis of nuclear material (i.e. the S-phase of the cell cycle).

Antifolate analogues

Methotrexate

USES

Methotrexate is the drug of choice for *choriocarcinoma*, it induces remission in acute lymphatic

Table 47.6 Comparative pharmacology of some platinum compounds

Drug	Standard dosing regimen	Side-effects	Pharmacokinetics	Additional comments
Carboplatin	IV dose is calculated based on the desired AUC by the Calvert formula	Like cisplatin, but less vomiting and nephrotoxicity Low potential for ototoxicity and neuropathy	Activation slower than cisplatin $t_{\frac{1}{2}}$ = 2–3 h 60–70% excreted in the urine in first 24 h	Anti-tumour spectrum similar to that of cisplatin
JM-216	Oral administration, 60–120 mg/m^2 daily for 5 days	Bone-marrow suppression Less nephro-, oto- and neurotoxicity than with cisplatin	Metabolized Non-linear kinetics at doses of > 120 mg/m^2	Phase-III development

leukaemia, and is effective against *breast cancer*, *osteogenic sarcoma* and *head and neck tumours*. It is also used as an immunosuppressant (see Chapters 25 and 49), and it reduces the rapid cellular proliferation in severe psoriasis (see Chapter 50). Methotrexate chemotherapy is administered by several different regimens. Conventional doses of up to $50\,mg/m^2$/week do not usually require folinic acid rescue. Intermediate doses of up to $150\,mg/m^2$ by intravenous bolus injection do not usually require folinic acid rescue unless the patient has renal impairment. However, massive doses of $1\text{–}30\,g/m^2$ routinely require folinic acid rescue, although the benefits of this dosing regimen are not yet clearly established.

MECHANISM OF ACTION

Folic acid is required in the synthesis of thymidylate (pyrimidine) and purine nucleotides, and thus for DNA synthesis (Figure 47.6). Methotrexate resembles folic acid and competes with it at the active site of the enzyme dihydrofolate reductase. The affinity of methotrexate for this site is 100 000 times greater than that of dihydrofolate. By blocking this step, methotrexate prevents nucleic acid synthesis and causes cell death. Folinic acid circumvents the block and thus non-competitively antagonizes the effect of methotrexate.

DETERMINANTS OF METHOTREXATE TOXICITY

These consist of:

1 a critical extracellular concentration for each target organ;
2 a critical duration of exposure that varies for each organ.

For bone marrow and gut, the critical plasma concentration is 2×10^{-8} M and the time factor is about 42 h. Both factors must be exceeded for toxicity to occur in these organs. The severity of toxicity is proportional to the length of time for which the critical concentration is exceeded, and is independent of the amount by which it is exceeded.

Folinic acid rescue bypasses the enzyme block and prevents methotrexate toxicity. Some malignant cells are less able to take up folinic acid than normal cells, thus introducing a degree of selectivity. Rescue is commenced 24 h after methotrexate administration with oral or intravenous doses of 10–15 mg given at 6-hourly intervals for 4–8 doses. Folinic acid administration is continued until the plasma methotrexate concentration falls below 5×10^{-8} M. Monitoring of the plasma methotrexate concentrations has improved the safety of this drug and allows identification of patients at high risk of toxicity. If a patient is at very high risk of toxicity, the metabolism of methotrexate can be rapidly increased by administering an inactivating enzyme, namely **carboxypeptidase-G2** (not routinely available in the UK), when methotrexate concentrations exceed 1×10^{-7} M.

ADVERSE EFFECTS

These include the following:

1 myelosuppression;
2 nausea and vomiting;
3 stomatitis;
4 diarrhoea;

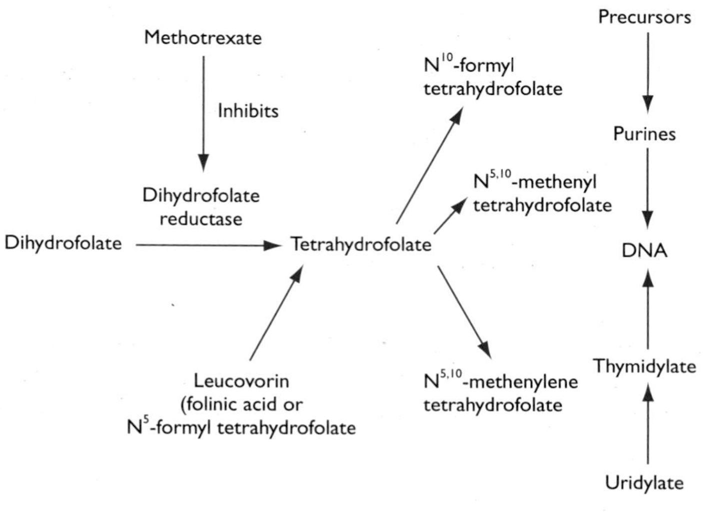

Figure 47.6 Folate metabolism: effects of methotrexate and leucovorin (folenic acid).

5 cirrhosis – chronic low-dose administration (as for psoriasis) can cause chronic active hepatitis and cirrhosis, interstitial pneumonitis and osteoporosis;
6 renal dysfunction and acute vasculitis (after high-dose treatment);
7 intrathecal administration also causes special problems, including convulsions, and chemical arachnoiditis leading to paraplegia, cerebellar dysfunction and cranial nerve palsies and a chronic demyelinating encephalitis.

Renal insufficiency poses special problems because it interferes with methotrexate elimination, and plasma methotrexate concentration monitoring is essential under these circumstances. Acute renal failure can be caused by tubular obstruction with crystals of methotrexate. Diuresis (>3 L/day) with alkalinization (pH >7) of the urine by intravenous administration of sodium bicarbonate reduces the incidence of nephrotoxicity. Renal damage is caused by the precipitation of methotrexate and 7-hydroxymethotrexate in the tubules, and these weak acids are more water soluble at an alkaline pH because this favours their charged (ionic) form rather than the free acid.

PHARMACOKINETICS

Methotrexate is given orally, intravenously or intrathecally. Absorption from the gut occurs via a saturable transport process, large doses of the order of 10 mg/kg being incompletely absorbed. After intravenous injection, methotrexate plasma concentrations decline over time in a triphasic manner. The $t_{\frac{1}{2}\alpha}$ is 0.75 h, $t_{\frac{1}{2}\beta}$ is 2–3.5 h (largely associated with renal elimination), and the final phase – which begins 6–24 h after conventional doses and 30–48 h after high doses – is prolonged due to enterohepatic circulation, with a $t_{\frac{1}{2}\gamma}$ of 10–12 h. This $t_{\frac{1}{2}\gamma}$ is important because toxicity is related to the plasma concentrations during this phase, as well as to the peak concentrations achieved. About 50–70% of methotrexate is bound to plasma protein (principally albumin), and alterations in plasma binding affect the pharmacokinetics of the drug. Methotrexate distributes in about 75% of body weight and penetrates transcellular water (e.g. the CNS) slowly by passive diffusion. Methotrexate plasma:CSF ratios are approximately 30:1, and the drug is injected directly into the CSF in order to prevent relapse in this site in appropriate cases.

Methotrexate enters normal and malignant cells via an energy-dependent carrier-mediated transport process, as does folate. About 80–95% of the drug finally undergoes renal excretion either unchanged or as metabolites. Methotrexate is both filtered and undergoes active tubular secretion into the urine. It is partly metabolized by the gut flora during enterohepatic circulation, and polyglutamate derivatives may be synthesized in the liver. These metabolites account for less than 10% of an intravenous dose, but if the same dose is given orally, 35% of the absorbed dose is excreted as metabolites, consistent with presystemic hepatic and gut metabolism. 7-Hydroxymethotrexate is produced in the liver, and is inactive but four times less soluble than methotrexate, and it contributes to renal toxicity by precipitation and crystalluria. Polyglutamate metabolites are potent inhibitors of the dihydrofolate reductase (DHFR) and accumulate within cells, persisting in the human liver for months after methotrexate administration.

DRUG INTERACTIONS

1 Probenecid and salicylate (and other NSAIDs) increase methotrexate toxicity by competing for renal tubular secretion, while simultaneously displacing it from plasma albumin-binding sites. Frusemide and high-dose vitamin C also block renal excretion.
2 Cellular uptake of methotrexate is decreased by cortisone and prednisone and enhanced by vincristine.
3 Methotrexate action is antagonized by triamterene (which increases intracellular dihydrofolate reductase) and allopurinol (which increases purine availability).
4 Gentamicin and cisplatin increase the toxicity of methotrexate by compromising renal excretion.

Pyrimidine antimetabolites

5-Fluorouracil

USES

5-Fluorouracil (**5FU**) is useful in the treatment of carcinomas of the breast, ovary, oesophagus, colon and skin. It is used to treat adenocarcinoma of the gastrointestinal tract, but even so the response rate is disappointing in these notoriously unresponsive tumours. Addition of the immunostimulant **levamisole** may be worthwhile in advanced colon cancers (see above and also Chapter 49). 5-Fluorouracil, 15 mg/kg administered by intravenous injection daily for 5 days is a typical regimen. Continuous infusions are an alternative, but a wide variety of dosage schedules are used. *Dose reduction is required for hepatic dysfunction, or if there is dihydropyridine dehydrogenase deficiency. An oral prodrug of 5-FU, capecitabune, is also now available.*

MECHANISM OF ACTION

5-Fluorouracil is a prodrug that is activated by anabolic phosphorylation (Figure. 47.7) to form:

1 5-fluorouridine monophosphate, which is incorporated into RNA, inhibiting its function and its polyadenylation;
2 5-fluorodeoxyuridylate, which binds strongly to thymidylate synthetase and inhibits DNA synthesis.

Incorporation of 5-fluorouracil itself into DNA causes mismatching and faulty mRNA transcripts.

ADVERSE EFFECTS

1 Oral ulceration and diarrhoea occur in about 20% of patients.
2 Bone-marrow suppression – megaloblastic anaemia usually occurs about 14 days after starting treatment.
3 Cerebellar ataxia (2% incidence) is attributed to fluorocitrate, a neurotoxic metabolite that inhibits the Krebs' cycle by lethal synthesis.
4 Patients with dihydropyridine dehydrogenase deficiency (enzyme activity $<5\%$ of normal) have an increased risk of severe or fatal toxicity from 5-FU.

PHARMACOKINETICS

5-Fluorouracil is usually given by injection because it is unreliably absorbed from the gut due to high hepatic first-pass metabolism. Deactivation occurs primarily in the liver, where the drug is reduced by the enzyme dihydropyridine dehydrogenase to inactive products that are excreted in the urine. It is rapidly cleared from plasma with a $t_{\frac{1}{2}}$ of 10–20 min. Only 20% is excreted unchanged in the urine, and the remainder is metabolized. 5-Fluorouracil distributes in total body water and readily penetrates the blood–

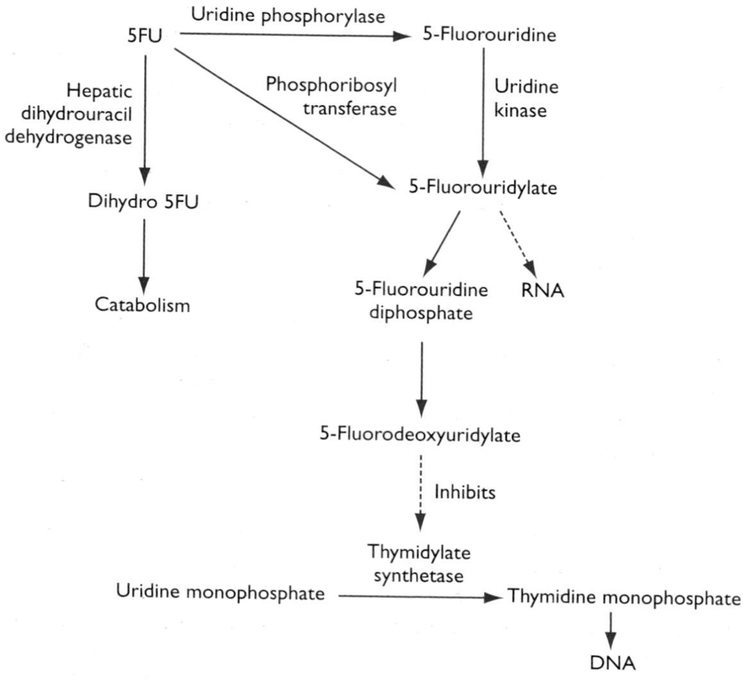

Figure 47.7 Metabolism and activation of 5-fluorouracil (5FU).

brain barrier. Intra-arterial administration to the liver allows selective administration to hepatic metastases.

Purine antimetabolites

6-Mercaptopurine (6-MP)

USES

6-Mercaptopurine (6-MP) is a purine antimetabolite. It is effective as part of combination therapy for acute leukaemias, especially in children, and is also used as an immunosuppressant (see Chapter 49). The usual oral dose of 6-MP is 2.5 mg/kg/day. Administration is continued for several weeks, and if after 4 weeks there has been no response, the dose is increased to 5 mg/kg/day. Other purine antimetabolites that are used clinically include **thioguanine**, **fludaribine** and **2-chlorodeoxyadenosine** (see Table 47.7).

MECHANISM OF ACTION

6-MP requires transformation by intracellular enzyme pathways involving hypoxanthine-guanine phosphoribosyltransferase to 6-thioguanine nucleotides which are active. These nucleotides inhibit the enzyme glutamine-5-phosphoribosyl pyrophosphate aminotransferase, the first step in *de novo* purine synthesis by negative feedback through mimicking purine nucleosides and thus impairing DNA synthesis. 6-MP also interferes with purine interconversions.

ADVERSE EFFECTS

These include the following:

Table 47.7 Other cytotoxic antimetabolites

Drug	Use	Mechanism	Side-effects	Additional comments
Cytosine arabinoside (cytarabine)	Acute leukaemia – AML	Inhibits pyrimidine synthesis and in its triphosphate form inhibits DNA polymerase	Nausea and vomiting Bone-marrow suppression Mucositis Cerebellar syndrome	Short half-life Continuous infusions or daily doses intravenously or subcutaneously Dose reduced in renal dysfunction
Fludrarabine	Chronic lymphatic leukaemia (CLL)	Inhibits purine synthesis	Myelosuppression Pulmonary toxicity CNS toxicity	Daily IV dosing Reduce dose in renal failure
2-Chlorodeoxy adenosine	CLL and acute leukaemia (ANLL)	Converted to triphosphate and inhibits purine synthesis	Severe neutropenia	IV infusion
Gemcitabine	Pancreatic and lung cancer	Cytidine analogue – triphosphate form incorporated into DNA, blocking replication	Haematopoietic suppression Mucositis Rashes	Inactivated by cytidine deaminase Active throughout the cell cycle Dose reduced in renal failure
Hydroxyurea	CML and myelo-proliferative disorders	Inhibits ribonucleotide reductase, affecting DNA and RNA synthesis	Neutropenia Nausea Skin reactions	Oral dosing Short half-life Rapidly reversible toxicity

1 bone-marrow suppression; leukopenia and thrombocytopenia;
2 mucositis;
3 nausea, vomiting and mild diarrhoea are uncommon, but occur with high doses;
4 reversible cholestatic jaundice.

Thiopurine-S-methyltransferase catalyses the S-methylation and deactivation of thiopurines such as 6–MP, **azathioprine** (a 6-MP prodrug) and **6-thioguanine**. It is deficient in 1 in 300 individuals, who are at very high risk of haematopoietic suppression with standard doses of 6-MP because of the accumulation of thiopurines.

PHARMACOKINETICS

Only about 15% of 6-MP is absorbed when given orally. The plasma $t_{\frac{1}{2}}$ in children is about 20 min, but it is double this in adults. It is only 20% bound to plasma protein, but cerebrospinal fluid concentrations are only 20% of those in plasma. 6-MP is eliminated mainly by hepatic metabolism via xanthine oxidase and thiopurinemethyltransferase. Approximately 20% of an intravenous dose of 6-MP is excreted in the urine within 6 h, and renal impairment may therefore enhance its toxicity.

DRUG INTERACTIONS

Allopurinol inhibits xanthine oxidase (see Chapter 25). The dose of 6-MP should be reduced to one-quarter to avoid toxicity in patients who are receiving allopurinol. This is important because allopurinol pretreatment is used to reduce the risk of acute uric acid nephropathy due to rapid tumour kill in patients with leukaemia.

ANTIBIOTICS

Several antibiotics (e.g. anthracyclines, anthracenediones – **mitozantrone**) have proved to be clinically useful antineoplastic agents. Other similar anti-tumour antibiotic agents (e.g. mitomycin C and bleomycin) are listed in Table 47.8.

Anthracyclines

Anthracyclines are widely used in the treatment of malignant disease. **Doxorubicin** and **daunorubicin** are the most widely used drugs in this group, but newer analogues (e.g. **epirubicin**, **idarubicin**) have reduced hepatic and cardiac toxicity, and idarubicin may be administered orally.

Doxorubicin

USES

Doxorubicin is a red antibiotic produced by *Streptomyces peucetius*. It is the most widely used drug of the anthracycline group, with proven activity in acute leukaemia, lymphomas, sarcomas and a wide range of carcinomas. Liposomal formulations of doxorubicin are used to treat Kaposi's sarcoma in AIDS patients. The usual dose is 30–60 mg/m^2 given intravenously (depending on the other drugs being administered concurrently) every 21 or 28 days.

MECHANISM OF ACTION

There are three main components of the cytotoxic mechanism of action:

1 intercalation between adjacent base pairs in DNA, thus inhibiting further nucleic acid synthesis and leading to fragmentation of DNA and inhibition of DNA repair, which is further enhanced by DNA topoisomerase II inhibition;
2 membrane binding alters membrane function – this alters sodium and calcium concentrations seen in the myocardium, and could be involved in the development of cardiomyopathy;
3 free-radical formation, which causes cardiotoxicity.

ADVERSE EFFECTS

These include the following:

1 cardiotoxicity – this is the major dose-limiting factor in long-term administration; there are two forms, namely acute and chronic (see below).
2 bone-marrow suppression with neutropenia and thrombocytopenia;
3 alopecia – occurs almost invariably, but may be mitigated by scalp cooling;
4 nausea and vomiting;
5 'radiation recall' reaction – this refers to the ability of anthracyclines to exacerbate or reactivate dormant radiation dermatitis or pneumonitis weeks or months after cessation of radiotherapy;
6 extravasation causes severe tissue necrosis – doxorubucin should never be injected into the

Table 47.8 Clinical pharmacology of other antitumour antibiotics

Drug	Indications and route of administration	Side-effects	Pharmacokinetics	Additional comments
Daunorubicin	Acute leukaemia IV dosing (total dose not to exceed 500 mg/m^2)	Vesicant Cardiotoxic Myelosuppression	Hepatic metabolism (cytochrome P_{3A4}) to a less active metabolite $t_{\frac{1}{2}} = 24$ h	Penetrates peripheral tissues less well than doxorubicin
Mitoxantrone	Advanced breast cancer; leukaemia and lymphoma IV dosing (12–14 mg/m^2 over 3 weeks)	Nausea and vomiting Stomatitis Low incidence of cardiotoxicity (< 3%)	Hepatic metabolism, extensively bound to tissues $t_{\frac{1}{2}} = 20$–40 h	Intercalates into DNA and inhibits DNA topoisomerase II
Mitomycin C	Gastrointestinal tumours, advanced breast cancer, head and neck tumours Intravenous infusions – 5–10 mg/m^2 per cycle	Vesicant Cumulative toxicity Myelosuppression Interstitial alveolitis Haemolytic-uraemic syndrome	Pharmacokinetics not affected by renal or hepatic function	It is a prodrug – transformed to an alkylating intermediate Alkylates guanine residues (10% of its adducts form inter-strand breaks) Synergistic with 5-FU and radiotherapy
Bleomycin	Lymphomas, testicular carcinoma and squamous-cell tumours IV dosing (5–15 units/week)	Fever, shivering, mouth ulcers Skin erythema – pigmentation Interstitial lung disease if dose > 300 units	50–70% of a dose is excreted in the urine $t_{\frac{1}{2}} = 9$ h; prolonged in renal dysfunction Also metabolized by peptidases; skin and lung have high drug concentrations as they lack peptidases	It causes single- and double-strand breaks in DNA Arrests cells in G_2/M phase

veins on the back of the hand, as severe damage to nerves and tendons may result.

ANTHRACYCLINE CARDIOTOXICITY

Acute This occurs shortly after administration, with the development of various arrhythmias that are occasionally life-threatening (e.g. ventricular tachycardia, heart block). These acute effects do not predict chronic toxicity.

Chronic Cardiomyopathy occurs, leading to death in up to 60% of those who develop signs of congestive cardiac failure. It is determined by the cumulative dose of doxorubicin administered with an incidence of less than 2% at total doses less than 400 mg/m^2, rising to over 20% at cumulative doses greater than 700 mg/m^2. Risk factors for cardiomyopathy (and that lower the cumulative dose at which this occurs) include prior mediastinal irradiation, age over 70 years, and pre-existing cardiovascular disease (including coronary artery disease and hypertension). A number of agents (e.g. probucol – a second-line cholesterol-lowering drug which is also an antioxidant; see Chapter 26), are showing promise in protecting against anthracycline cardiomyopathy and allowing dose intensification.

PHARMACOKINETICS

Doxorubicin is given intravenously. The plasma concentration–time profile shows a triphasic decline with half-lives of 2–6 min, 0.5–2.5 h and 15–50 h for the three phases, respectively. The volume of distribution is large (reflecting extensive tissue uptake), most of the drug being located in cell nuclei. Doxorubicin does not enter the CNS. The rate of hepatic extraction is high, with 40% appearing in the bile (40% unchanged, 20% as doxorubicinol and the remainder as other metabolites). Renal excretion accounts for less than 15%. The major metabolite, doxorubicinol, has some antitumour activity. Dose reduction is recommended in patients with liver disease.

TOPOISOMERASE INHIBITORS

DNA topoisomersase II inhibitors

A component of the cytotoxic action of anthracyclines (e.g. doxorubicin) is due to inhibition of DNA topoisomerase II. **Etoposide** and **teniposide** synthetic derivatives of podophyllotoxin (which is extracted from the American mandrake or May apple, and is topically effective against warts) are also reversible inhibitors of topoisomerase II.

Etoposide

USES

Etoposide is one of the most active drugs against small-cell lung cancer, and is used in combination therapy. It is also used to treat lymphomas, testicular teratomas and trophoblastic tumours. The usual dose is 60–120 mg/m^2 intravenously (or, 120–240 mg/m^2 orally) given daily for 5 days, every 21–28 days.

MECHANISM OF ACTION

DNA topoisomerase II is a nuclear enzyme that binds to and cleaves both strands of DNA. It is needed for DNA unwinding and to remove torsional stress, and it is necessary for DNA replication and RNA transcription. Topoisomerases form a covalent bond with DNA through a tyrosine–transester link. Etoposide stabilizes the topoisomerase II–DNA intermediate complex, preventing religation of the DNA strands. The exact cytotoxic mechanism is unclear, but possible terminal effects include inappropriate recombination of topisomerase-bound DNA strands or the induction of apoptosis (programmed cell death).

ADVERSE EFFECTS

These include the following:

1. nausea and vomiting are common, especially after oral administration;
2. alopecia;
3. bone-marrow suppression is dose-dependent and reversible.

PHARMACOKINETICS

Etoposide is given by intravenous injection or orally (bioavailability is 50%). It undergoes hepatic metabolism and a small amount is eliminated in the urine. The $t_{\frac{1}{2}}$ is approximately 12 h.

DNA topoisomerase I inhibitors

Camptothecins

Camptothecin is a plant alkaloid derived from the Chinese tree *Camptotheca accuminata*. **Irinotecan (CPT-11)** and **topotecan** are available for clinical use.

USES

The camptothecins are active against a broad range of epithelial tumours, including those of the lung, colon, cervix and ovary. Their current primary use is in refractory colon or ovarian cancer. Ongoing studies are defining their potential role in combination therapy. They are given intravenously either as a continuous infusion over 5 days every 3 weeks or in weekly schedules for 3 weeks. Doses of topotecan are given intravenously 1.5 mg/m^2 daily for 5 days, and for irinotecan 100–150 mg/m^2 weekly for 3 weeks.

MECHANISM OF ACTION

Camptothecins are effective against cells in the S-phase of the cell cycle. DNA topoisomerase I is a nuclear enzyme that binds to and cleaves a single strand of DNA. It is necessary for unwinding DNA for replication and RNA transcription. Topoisomerase I binds to DNA via a covalent tyrosine–transester link, and camptothecins stabilize the DNA topoisomerase I–DNA intermediate complex, preventing religation of the DNA strands. The potential cytotoxic mechanisms are as described previously for the podophyllotoxins.

PHARMACOKINETICS

Irinotecan undergoes metabolism by a carboxylesterase enzyme to a more potent cytotoxic (100 to 1000-fold) active metabolite SN38, which is hepatically glucuronidated. The concentrations of the parent compound and its metabolite decay with a $t_{\frac{1}{2}}$ of 5–20 h The clearance of irinotecan and SN-38 is not fully understood. Topotecan is hydrolysed in the blood, has a $t_{\frac{1}{2}}$ of 3 h and is excreted in the urine, thus requiring dose reduction in renal failure. They are both highly bound (>80 %) to plasma albumin.

ADVERSE EFFECTS

The principal adverse effects of these agents are myelosuppression, acute and delayed diarrhoea (especially with irinotecan), which can be dose limiting and require prophylactic therapy with, for example, loperamide, or treatment with octreotide. Other less severe side-effects include alopecia and fatigue.

MICROTUBULAR INHIBITORS – VINCA ALKALOIDS

This group consists of several agents, namely vincristine, **vinblastine** and the synthetic derivatives **vindesine** and **vinorelbine**. Despite their close structural relationship, they differ in their clinical spectrum of activity and toxicity. Vinblastine is used in the treatment of testicular cancer and Hodgkin's disease. It is given in combination with other drugs (e.g. mustine, prednisolone and procarbazine) at weekly intervals. Vincristine is used in breast cancer, lymphomas and the initial treatment of acute lymphoblastic leukaemia. Vinorelbine has activity against advanced breast cancer and non-small-cell lung cancer. It is often combined with platinum compounds.

MECHANISM OF ACTION

Vinca alkaloids bind to tubulin, a protein that forms the microtubules which are essential for the formation of the spindle that separates the chromosomes during mitosis. They cause 'crystallization' of free tubulin dimers, thus halting mitosis. Binding to microtubules concerned with neuronal growth and axonal transport accounts for their neurotoxicity. Vinca alkaloids have other actions on cell metabolism, including inhibition of nucleic acid and protein synthesis.

The clinical pharmacology of the vinca alkaloids is summarized in Table 47.9.

MICROTUBULAR INHIBITORS – TAXANES

Paclitaxel and docetaxel

These agents were only introduced relatively recently (paclitaxel is derived from the pacific Yew tree). They are used to treat solid tumours such as carcinoma of the lung, breast, ovary and cervix and head and neck tumours, as well as having activity in lymphomas. These drugs act by binding to the β-subunit of tubulin and stabilizing it in its polymeric form (microtubules), thus blocking its depolymerization and halting mitosis. Paclitaxel and docetaxel are given as intravenous infusions (135–275 mg/m^2 over 1–3 h for paclitaxel and 60–100 mg/m^2 over 1 h for docetaxel) every 3 weeks. They are both hepatically cleared by metabolism by cytochrome P_{2C8} and cytochrome P_{3A4} (paclitaxel) and cytochrome P_{3A4} (docetaxel) to inactive metabolites. They are highly protein bound, with elimination half-lives of 11–15 h. Less than 5% of the parent drug is excreted in the urine. They differ slightly in their side-effect profiles. Paclitaxel causes myelosuppression, hypersensitivity reactions, cardiac arrhythmias, alopecia,

> **Key points**
>
> Practical 'dos and don'ts' of cytotoxic therapy
>
> - Patients should have recovered fully from the toxic effects of previous cytotoxic administration before starting the next treatment cycle.
> - Ensure that the dose and schedule of certain drugs is adjusted for comorbid renal and hepatic impairment.
> - Avoid the concomitant use of platelet-inhibiting drugs.
> - Haematopoietic growth factors (for myelosuppression) have not been demonstrated to improve outcome, and should not be prescribed routinely.

Table 47.9 Summary of the clinical pharmacology of the vinca alkaloids

Drug	Route and typical dosing regimen	Side-effects	Pharmacokinetics	Additional comments
Vincristine	IV 1–2 mg/m^2 weekly	Vesicant if extravasated Reversible peripheral neuropathy, alopecia, SIADH*	Hepatic metabolism (cytochrome P_{3A4}). $t_{\frac{1}{2}} = 85$ h Non-linear kinetics	
Vinblastine	IV 8 mg/m^2 weekly	Less neurotoxic but more myelo-suppressive than vincristine SIADH*	Hepatic metabolism – active metabolite $t_{\frac{1}{2}} = 24$ h	
Vindesine	IV 3–5 mg/m^2 weekly	As for vincristine, except for less severe neuropathy SIADH*	Hepatic metabolism $t_{\frac{1}{2}} = 24$ h	
Vinorelbine	IV injection or infusion, 15–30 mg/m^2 weekly Oral dose, 100 mg/m^2 per week	Bone-marrow suppression SIADH*	Hepatic metabolism cytochrome P_{3A4} $t_{\frac{1}{2}} = 30$–40 h	Refractory breast cancer and advanced lung cancer Oral use currently being investigated

* SIADH = syndrome of inappropriate antidiuretic hormone.

mucositis and peripheral neuropathy, whereas docetaxel is also dose limited by myelosuppression, but causes fewer cardiac problems and less neurotoxicity, although it does induce peripheral fluid retention on cumulative dosing.

HORMONES

Hormones can cause remission of sensitive tumours (e.g. lymphomas), but do not eradicate the disease. They often alleviate symptoms over a long period, and they do not cause bone-marrow suppression. Sex hormones or their antagonists (see Chapter 40) are effective in tumours arising from cells that are normally hormone dependent, namely those of the breast and the prostate. There are several ways in which hormones can affect malignant cells.

1. A hormone may have a direct cytotoxic action on the malignant cell. For example, cells of the prostate are testosterone dependent, and if a carcinoma arises from these cells, the opposing action of oestrogens in large doses is cytotoxic to prostate carcinoma cells.
2. A hormone may suppress the production of other hormones by a feedback mechanism. This will change the hormonal milieu surrounding the malignant cells, and may suppress their proliferation. In breast cancer, patients who respond to one form of endocrine therapy are more likely to respond to subsequent hormone treatment than those who fail to respond initially.

Oestrogens

Oestrogens are now much less widely used than formerly in the management of prostatic carcinoma, because of the availability of gonadotrophin-releasing hormone (GnRH) analogues.

Progestogens

Endometrial cells normally mature under the influence of progestogens, and some malignant cells that arise from the endometrium respond in the same way. About 30% of patients with disseminated adenocarcinoma of the body of the uterus respond to a progestogen such as **megestrol**, 20 mg twice daily. Progestogen bound to its receptor impairs the regeneration of oestrogen receptors and also stimulates 17-β-oestradiol dehydrogenase, the enzyme that metabolizes intracellular oestrogen. These actions may deprive cancer cells of their oestrogen effects. There is also a direct cytotoxic effect at very high doses. In addition, progestogens may be used in carcinoma of the kidney. Here most experience has been obtained with **medroxyprogesterone acetate** given in daily oral doses of 100–300 mg, where responses are rare. Larger doses (1500 mg/day) have produced responses in over 40% of patients. Other progestogens that are used include **megestrol acetate**, **norethisterone acetate** and **hydroxyprogesterone**. There are no important toxic effects of progestogens that are relevant to cancer chemotherapy (see Chapter 40).

Glucocorticosteroids

Glucocorticosteroids (see Chapter 39) are cytotoxic to lymphoid cells and are combined with other cytotoxic agents to treat lymphomas and myeloma, and to induce remission in acute lymphoblastic leukaemia.

Hormonal manipulation therapy in advanced prostate cancer

In advanced prostate cancer patients, several treatments utilize manipulation of the androgen dependence of the tumour cells as their mechanism affecting cellular proliferation/cytotoxicity and control of the disease.

INHIBITION OF FSH AND LH RELEASE FROM THE PITUITARY

1 Gonadotrophin-releasing hormone (GnRH) analogues – drugs such as **leuprorelin** (see

Table 47.10 Selected examples of biological response modifier treatments for cancer (see also Chapter 44)

Drug	Therapeutic use	Side-effects	Additional comments
Interferon-α	Hairy cell leukaemia; metastatic melanoma (high dose); Kaposi's sarcoma, low-grade non-Hodgkin's lymphoma, CML	Fatigue, flu-like symptoms. Haematopoietic suppression	Combinations with conventional chemotherapy under investigation
Interleukin-2	Advanced renal-cell carcinoma, and melanoma	Cytokine related Fluid leak syndrome with pulmonary oedema, haematopoietic suppression	See Chapter 49 Not shown to increase survival
Monoclonal antibodies			
Anti-CD-20	Lymphoma	Flu-like syndrome	Investigational agents in phase-III development
Anti-Her-2 neu	Solid tumours (e.g. ovary or breast) expressing Her-2 neu	Bone-marrow suppression Development of neutralizing antibodies	

Chapter 41) stimulate and then reduce pituitary FSH/LH release.
2 Oestrogens such as **diethylstilboestrol** inhibit the release of GnRH from the hypothalamus by feedback suppression.

DIHYDROTESTOSTERONE SYNTHESIS INHIBITORS AND RECEPTOR BLOCKADE

1 **Aminogluthethimide** (an aromatase inhibitor) and high-dose **ketoconazole** (see Chapter 44) block the synthesis of testicular testosterone, adrenal androgens and other steroids. They are given orally to patients with refractory prostate cancer. Occasionally aminogluthethimide is used in the treatment of refractory breast cancer.
2 5-α-Reductase inhibitors (e.g. **finasteride**) inhibit the conversion of testosterone to the active hormone-dihydrotestosterone.
3 DHT-receptor-blockers (e.g. **flutamide**, **bicalutamide**, **cyproterone actetate**) block the intracellular receptors for dihydrotestosterone.

BIOLOGICAL RESPONSE MODIFIERS

These agents stimulate the immune response against the transformed neoplastic cells. They include **levamisole** (see Chapter 49), and other examples are shown in Table 47.10.

FUTURE DIRECTIONS IN CANCER CHEMOTHERAPY

Potential new agents in cancer therapy are being discovered at a prolific rate, commensurate with advances in tumour biology. Therapies in the early phases of development include angiogenesis inhibitors, protein-kinase C inhibitors, metalloproteinase inhibitors, farnesyl transferase inhibitors and cancer vaccines (for melanoma and renal-cell carcinoma). Other agents specifically generated from advances in the field of molecular biology include anti-sense oligonucleotides to gene products (e.g. Bcl-2) which prevent apoptosis, and gene therapy, inserting missing/mutated cell-cycle-regulatory proteins, or enzymes that increase drug sensitivity (see Chapter 16).

Case history

A 48-year-old man presented with cervical lymphadenopathy and night sweats, and was diagnosed with stage III Hodgkin's disease. Initial therapy with mustine, vincristine, prednisolone and procarbazine (MVPP) failed, and his chemotherapy was changed to doxorubicin 60 mg/m^2, bleomycin 15 units, vinblastine 5 mg/m^2 and dacarbazine 100 mg (ABVD). During the fifth cycle of ABVD he underwent an appendicectomy for acute appendicitis. Following his sixth cycle of ABVD he became dyspnoeic on exertion, and this progressed rapidly to dyspnoea at rest. Physical examination revealed cyanosis, no cervical lymphadenopathy, sinus tachycardia and bilateral basal and mid-zone late inspiratory crackles. Further investigations revealed normal haemoglobin, white blood count and platelets, normal coagulation screen, pO_2 on air 50 mmHg, and fluffy interstitial infiltrates in both lower- and mid-lung fields. Pulmonary function tests showed a restrictive pattern with a DL_{CO} of 25% of the predicted value. Bronchoalveolar lavage fluid was negative for pathogens, including *Pneumocystis carinii*.

Question

What was the cause of this patient's respiratory problems? How should he be treated?

Answer

In this patient the possible causes of such pulmonary symptoms and radiographic findings include opportunistic infection, haemorrhage into the lung, progression of disease, drug-induced interstitial alveolitis or pulmonary oedema due to fluid overload. Here, with the exclusion of haemorrhagic diasthesis and pulmonary infection, no fluid overload and apparent regression of his cervical disease, the probable diagnosis is bleomycin-induced interstitial pneumonitis. Although the patient had not received more than 300 units of bleomycin, it is likely that during his operation he received high inspired oxygen concentrations, and this could have put him at higher risk of developing 'bleomycin lung'. Currently he should receive the lowest inspired oxygen concentration that will yield a pO_2 of > 60 mmHg. Glucocorticosteroid therapy may be of benefit, but the syndrome may not be fully reversible. Bleomycin, other cytotoxic agents which cause a pneumonitis (e.g. cyclophosphamide, busulphan, carmustine, methotrexate and mitomycin) and radiation therapy (which can exacerbate bleomycin pulmonary toxicity) should not be used for this patient's future therapy.

Further reading

Baker SD, Grochow LB. 1997: Pharmacology of cancer chemotherapy in the older person. *Clinics in Geriatric Medicine* **13**, 169–83.

Chabner BA, Longo DL. 1996: *Cancer chemotherapy and biotherapy*, 2nd edn. Philadelphia, PA: Lippincott-Raven.

Ford JM, Yang JM, Hait WN. 1996: P-glycoprotein-mediated multidrug resistance: experimental and clinical strategies for its reversal. *Cancer Treatment and Research* **87**, 3–38.

Frei E. 1985: Curative cancer chemotherapy. *Cancer Research* **45**, 6523–37.

Lutzker SG, Levine AJ. 1996: Apoptosis and cancer chemotherapy. *Cancer Treatment and Research* **87**, 345–56.

Moorman DW, Culver KW. 1995: Gene transfer and cancer chemotherapy. *Molecular and Cell Biology of Human Diseases Series* **5**, 125–39.

PART X

HAEMATOLOGY

CHAPTER FORTY-EIGHT

ANAEMIA *and* OTHER HAEMATOLOGICAL DISORDERS

- Haematinics – iron, vitamin B_{12} and folate
- Haematopoietic growth factors
- Coagulation factors and haemophilia A and B
- Aplastic anaemia
- Idiopathic thrombocytopenic purpura
- Drug-induced haematological toxicity

HAEMATINICS – IRON, VITAMIN B_{12} AND FOLATE

IRON

PHYSIOLOGY AND BIOCHEMISTRY

Although iron is abundant in the earth's crust, anaemia due to iron deficiency is prevalent throughout the world. Iron plays a vital role in the body in several transport proteins and enzymes, including haemoglobin, myoglobin, cytochromes (e.g. cytochrome 450's), catalase, peroxidase, guanylyl cyclase and many others. It is stored in the reticulo-endothelial system and bone marrow. The total body iron content is 3.5–4.5 g in an adult, of which some 70% is incorporated in haemoglobin, 5% in myoglobin and 0.2% in enzymes. Most of the remaining iron (approximately 25%) is stored as ferritin or haemosiderin. About 2% (80 mg) comprises the 'labile iron pool' and about 0.08% (3 mg) is bound to transferrin (a specific iron-binding protein).

PHARMACOKINETICS

Absorption is the main mechanism controlling total body iron levels. This remains remarkably constant in healthy individuals despite variations in diet, erythropoietic activity and iron stores. Iron absorption occurs in the small intestine and is influenced by several factors.

Form of iron

1 Inorganic ferrous iron is better absorbed than ferric iron.
2 Absorption of iron from the diet depends on the source of the iron. Most dietary iron exists as non-haem iron and is poorly absorbed (approximately 5%) mainly because it is combined with phosphates and phytates (in cereals). Haem iron is well absorbed (20–40%) but is often deficient in the diet of poorer people and vegetarians.
3 Absorption of iron from orally administered iron salts is approximately 10%.

Factors increasing absorption

1 Vitamin C (ascorbic acid) facilitates iron absorption, and iron deficiency anaemia commonly accompanies vitamin C deficiency.
2 Alcohol increases ferric but not ferrous iron absorption and there is an association, between alcohol abuse and iron overload (haemosiderosis).

Gastrointestinal tract Gastric acid enhances the absorption of iron from food, and iron deficiency is actually more common than vitamin B12 deficiency following partial gastrectomy. Iron is absorbed in the jejunum and upper ileum, and malabsorption of iron can occur in coeliac disease.

Drugs Tetracycline chelates iron causing malabsorption of both iron, and tetracycline. Biphosphonates and magnesium trisilicate also reduce iron absorption from the gastrointestinal tract.

DISPOSITION OF IRON

Iron in the gut becomes bound to mucosal transferrin for transport across the mucosa. Iron is also transported in the plasma by transferrin (a protein of molecular weight 76 000–80 000), each molecule of which binds two atoms of iron. Transferrin gives up its iron to red-cell precursors in the bone marrow. When red cells reach the end of their lifespan, macrophages bind the iron atoms released, which are taken up again by transferrin. About 80% of total body iron exchange normally takes place via this cycle (Figure 48.1). Ferritin is the main storage form of iron. It is a roughly spherical protein with deeply located iron-binding sites, and is found principally in the liver. Aggregates of ferritin form haemosiderin, which accumulates when levels of hepatic iron stores are high.

IRON DEFICIENCY

In iron-deficient states, the serum iron concentration (normally 14–31 μmol/L in men and 11–29 μmol/L in women) falls only when stores have become considerably depleted. The total amount of transferrin determines the total iron-binding capacity (TIBC) of plasma, and is normally 54–80 μmol/L. Transferrin saturation (i.e. plasma iron divided by TIBC) is normally 20–50% and provides a clinically useful index of iron status. In iron-deficiency states, TIBC rises in addition to the fall in plasma iron, and when transferrin saturation falls to less than 16%, erythropoiesis starts to decline. Iron deficiency is the commonest cause of anaemia, and although it is commonest and most severe in Third World countries, it is also prevalent in developed countries. In one study, 8% of menstruating women in north-west America were found to have mild iron-deficiency anaemia. The cause of iron deficiency is most often multifactorial, e.g. poor diet combined with excessive demands on stores (pregnancy, chronic blood loss, lactation), reduced stores (premature birth) or defective absorption (achlorhydria, surgery to the gastrointestinal tract). Although treatment of iron deficiency is straightforward, its cause should be determined so that the underlying condition can be treated. Iron-deficiency anaemia in men or postmenopausal women is seldom due solely to dietary deficiency, and a thorough search for other causes (notably colon cancer) should be undertaken.

IRON PREPARATIONS

Oral iron

Most patients with iron deficiency respond to simple oral preparations. A total daily dose of 100–200 mg of elemental iron should stimulate a reticulocyte response, which begins after 5 days and lasts for about 10 days. The haemoglobin concentration will start to rise at 0.1–0.2 g/dL/day. Treatment is continued for 3–6 months after haemoglobin levels have entered the normal range, in order to

Dose 100–200 mg
Hb ↑ 0.1 – 0.2 gm/dL/day.
Reticulocyte response in 5/7.
Treatment for 3–6/12

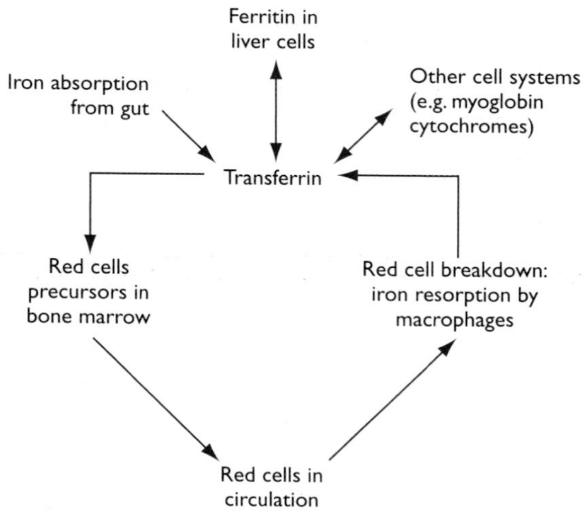

Figure 48.1: Iron metabolism.

replace iron stores. Failure to respond may be due to the following:

1 wrong diagnosis (i.e. iron deficiency is not the primary cause of the anaemia);
2 non-compliance;
3 continued blood loss;
4 malabsorption (e.g. coeliac disease, post-gastrectomy).

There are over 70 iron-containing oral preparations available, but many of them are combined preparations containing vitamins as well as iron. None of these combinations carries an advantage over iron salts alone, except for those containing folic acid, which are used prophylactically in pregnancy. Modified-release preparations of iron are unreliably absorbed from the upper small intestine (where iron uptake is at its most efficient), and are not recommended. Treatment should start with a simple preparation such as ferrous sulphate (200 mg three times daily), ferrous fumarate (200 mg three times daily) or ferrous gluconate (600 mg three times daily). These and other preparations are listed in Table 48.1.

Iron preparations for children

Liquid preparations are used in paediatrics. Such preparations should be sugar free and not stain the teeth (e.g. sodium ironedetate). The dose is calculated in terms of the amount of elemental iron.

ADVERSE EFFECTS

Gastrointestinal side-effects, including nausea, heartburn, constipation or diarrhoea, are common. Patients with ulcerative colitis and those with colostomies suffer particularly severely from these side-effects. No one preparation is universally better tolerated than any other, but individual patients often find that one salt suits them better than another. Ferrous sulphate is least expensive, but if it is not tolerated it is worth trying an organic salt such as the fumarate. Although iron is best absorbed in the fasting state, gastric irritation is reduced if it is taken after food. *Accidental overdose* with iron is common among toddlers and is extremely serious, with gastrointestinal haemorrage and hepatic and neurotoxicity. It is treated with an iron-chelating agent (**desferrioxamine**) which is administered both orally (to prevent further absorption) and parenterally.

Parenteral iron

Oral iron is effective, easily administered and cheap. Parenteral iron (formulated with sorbitol and citric acid) is also effective, but can cause anaphylactoid reactions and is expensive. The rate of rise in haemoglobin concentration is no faster than after oral iron, because the rate-limiting factor is the capacity of the bone marrow to produce red see Figure 48.2). The only advantages of parenteral iron are that:

1 iron stores are rapidly and completely replenished;
2 there is no doubt about compliance;
3 it is effective in patients with malabsorption.

Parenteral iron should therefore be considered in the following situations:

1 malabsorption;
2 genuine intolerance of oral iron preparations;
3 when continued blood loss is not preventable and large doses of iron cannot be readily given by mouth;
4 failure of patient compliance;
5 when great demands are to be made on a patient's iron stores - (e.g. in an anaemic pregnant woman just before term).

Table 48.1: Ferrous iron content and relative cost of available iron formulations

Iron formulation	Dose	Ferrous iron content	Approximate ratio of cost
Ferrous sulphate	200 mg	60 mg	1
Ferrous fumarate	200 mg	65 mg	2
Ferrous gluconate	300 mg	35 mg	2.6
Ferrous succinate	100 mg	35 mg	3
Sodium ironedetate	5–10 mL	27.5–55 mg	6
Polysaccharide iron complex	2.5–5 mL	50–100 mg	11

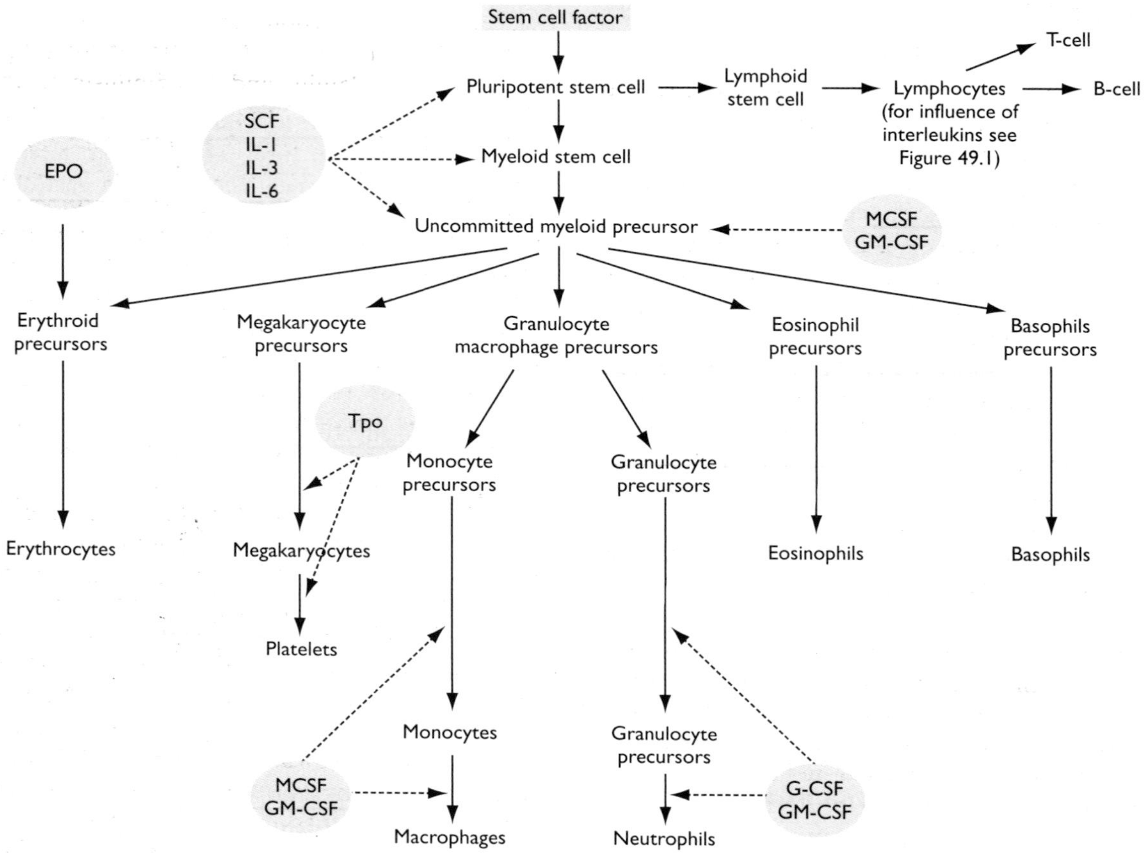

Figure 48.2: Haematopoiesis and haematopoietic growth factors. EPO = erythropoietin, IL = interleukin, G-CSF = granulocyte colony-stimulating factor, MCSF = macrophage colony-stimulating factor, GM-CSF = granulocyte macrophage colony-stimulating factor, SCF = stem-cell factor, Tpo = thrombopoietin.

Iron sorbitol injection

USE

This is administered by deep intramuscular injection to minimize staining of the skin. Peak concentrations, often with complete transferrin saturation, occur at 2–8 h. Of the retained iron, 30% is immediately available for haem synthesis and the rest is stored. Oral iron should be stopped 24 h before starting parenteral iron therapy.

ADVERSE EFFECTS

These include the following:

1 metallic taste in the mouth;
2 anaphylactoid reactions resulting in cardiovascular collapse;
3 a tendency to exacerbate pre-existing urinary tract infections (probably related to high concentrations in the urine).

Vitamin B_{12}

Vitamin B_{12} consists of a nucleotide linked to four pyrrole rings (similar to a porphyrin) with a cobalt atom attached. Linked to the cobalt atom may be a cyanide (cyanocobalamin), hydroxyl (hydroxocobalamin), methyl (methylcobalamin) or a 5′-deoxyadenosyl group. These forms are interconvertible, cyanocobalamin spontaneously forming hydroxocobalamin on exposure to light. Liver, kidney and heart are rich sources of vitamin B_{12}, and moderate amounts are found in other meats, fish and eggs. Vitamin B_{12} is absorbed in the terminal ileum, and absorption is dependent

Key points

Iron replacement therapy

- In health, normal iron losses require absorbed iron to be 0.5–1 mg (in males) and 0.7–2 mg (in menstruating females).
- Ferrous iron is best absorbed from the small intestine.
- Iron deficiency is the commonest cause of anaemia (e.g. malabsorption, menstrual, occult or gastrointestinal blood loss – the cause must be determined).
- For iron deficiency, 100–200 mg of elemental iron are given orally per day and continued until iron stores are replete, usually within 3–6 months.
- Parenteral iron use is restricted to cases of non-compliance or non-tolerance of oral preparations, or malabsorption states.
- During erythropoietin therapy, supplemental iron is given to support increased haem synthesis.

on the presence of 'intrinsic factor' secreted by the parietal cells of the stomach. Patients with Addisonian pernicious anaemia have antibodies both to intrinsic factor and to parietal cells. These cause atrophic gastritis and achlorhydria with failure of intrinsic factor production and consequent malabsorption of vitamin B_{12}. Vitamin B_{12} deficiency is diagnosed by measuring serum B_{12} concentrations and assessing its absorption from the intestine by the Schilling test.

USE

Replacement therapy is required in Vitamin B_{12} deficiency which may be due to the following:

1. malabsorption secondary to gastric pathology (pernicious anaemia, gastrectomy);
2. intestinal malabsorption (Crohn's disease or surgical resection of the terminal ileum, irradiation damage);
3. competition for vitamin B_{12} absorption by gut organisms (e.g. blind loop syndrome due to a jejunal diverticulum or other cause of bacterial overgrowth, infestation with the fish tapeworm *Diphyllobothrium latum*);
4. nutritional deficiency – this is rare and is limited to strict vegans. The few such individuals who do develop megaloblastic anaemia often have some coexisting deficiency of intrinsic factor.

Vitamin B_{12} replacement therapy is given by intramuscular injection. Hydroxocobalamin is preferred in the UK, as it is retained for longer than cyanocobalamin, and is administered initially as five doses of 1 mg given every 2–3 days, followed by 1 mg every 3 months for maintenance. A peak in the reticulocyte response (which may be massive, 25% or more reticulocytes) occurs 5 days after starting treatment. There is an alarmingly high incidence (up to 10%) of sudden death in the early treatment phase of patients with severe pernicious anaemia. This has been attributed to abrupt hypokalaemia during the early haematological response, which may provoke fatal cardiac arrhythmias. Maintaining plasma potassium is especially important if **digoxin** is being administered, because of the increased risk of digoxin toxicity associated with hypokalaemia (see Chapter 30). Transfusion is seldom necessary, and can precipitate pulmonary oedema. Iron and folate deficiency are often unmasked by with vitamin B_{12} treatment of megaloblastic or mixed anaemias, and iron and folate therapy can be initiated concomitantly. It is essential not to administer folate *before* vitamin B_{12}, because this can precipitate neurological consequences of B_{12} deficiency which may not be reversible (subacute combined degeneration of the spinal cord). Patients with vitamin B_{12} deficiency due to malabsorption (Addisonian pernicious anaemia) require lifelong replacement therapy, and they should be given an adequate explanation of this, as should family members, in view of the forgetfulness that occurs insidiously in vitamin B_{12} deficiency. Patients should carry a card with an up-to-date record of their B_{12} therapy.

CELLULAR MECHANISM OF ACTION

Vitamin B_{12} is needed for normal erythropoiesis and for the maturation of other cell types, and to maintain neuronal integrity. It is required for the isomerization of methylmalonyl coenzyme A to succinyl coenzyme A, and for the conversion of homocysteine into methionine (which also utilizes 5-methyltetrahydrofolate). Vitamin B_{12} is also involved in the control of active folate metabolism, and both of these vitamins are required for intracellular nucleoside synthesis. Deficiency of vitamin B_{12} leads to a macrocytic anaemia with megaloblastic erythropoiesis in the bone marrow, and may be accompanied by neurological disorders that include peripheral neuropathy, subacute combined degeneration of the spinal cord, dementia and optic neuritis.

PHARMACOKINETICS

Normal total body stores of vitamin B_{12} are about 3 mg. Following total gastrectomy these stores are adequate for 3–5 years, following which there is an increasing incidence of vitamin B_{12} deficiency. Thus the daily vitamin B_{12} loss is 0.5–3 μg, which results mainly from metabolic breakdown. Normally absorption from the diet is very efficient and the daily requirement is 3–5 μg. Absorption of vitamin B_{12} requires secretion of intrinsic factor from gastric parietal cells. Intrinsic factor is a glycoprotein of molecular weight approximately 55 000 which forms a stable complex with vitamin B_{12} in the presence of acid. The complex passes down the small intestine and is absorbed at specific receptor sites in the terminal ileum, in the presence of a neutral pH and calcium ions. Absorption is slow, starting 4 h after ingestion, with a peak at 8–12 h and continuing for up to 24 h. Very small amounts (approximately 1%) of an oral dose are absorbed by passive diffusion, and although vitamin B_{12} is synthesized by colonic bacteria, it is not appreciably absorbed in the colon, because this is distal to the primary absorptive site in the terminal ileum. Parietal cells are destroyed by an autoimmune reaction, so intrinsic factor is not produced in pernicious anaemia, resulting in vitamin B_{12} deficiency.

Vitamin B_{12} is transported by two plasma proteins, namely transcobalamins I and II (TC I and TC II). TC II is a β-globulin and acts as a transport protein collecting vitamin B_{12} from ileal cells and transporting it to the liver. TC I is an α-globulin that carries most of the body's vitamin B_{12} and this complex is probably the storage form of the vitamin. The normal range of plasma vitamin B_{12} concentration is 170–900 ng/L. High vitamin B_{12} concentrations occur in the plasma in hepatic necrosis, because of the release of stored vitamin B_{12}.

Vitamin B_{12} is secreted into the bile, but enterohepatic circulation results in most of this being reabsorbed via the intrinsic factor mechanism. Unbound vitamin B_{12} is excreted by glomerular filtration, but this is of minor importance.

Folic acid

USES

Folic acid is given to correct or prevent deficiency states. It consists of a pteridine linked to glutamic acid via *p*-aminobenzoic acid (PABA). It is present in a wide variety of plant and animal tissues, the richest dietary sources being liver, yeast and green vegetables.

Folate deficiency may be due to any of the following:

1 poor nutrition – in children, the elderly or those with alcoholism;
2 malabsorption – caused by coeliac disease, sprue or diseases of the small intestine;
3 excessive utilization – in pregnancy, chronic haemolytic anaemias (e.g. sickle cell disease) and leukaemias;
4 anti-epileptic drugs (e.g. phenytoin).

The normal requirement for folic acid is about 200 μg daily. In established folate deficiency large doses (5–15 mg orally per day) are given. If the patient is unable to take folate by mouth, it may be given intravenously. Patients with severe malabsorption may be deficient in both folic acid and vitamin B_{12}, and administration of folic acid alone may precipitate acute vitamin B_{12} deficiency. These patients require careful evaluation and replacement of both vitamins concurrently. Patients who are taking long-term anticonvulsants commonly have macrocytic red cells, but the majority have no detectable folate deficiency. However, few patients, develop a megaloblastic anaemia due to folate deficiency, the cause of which is complex. It is partly due to interference with DNA synthesis and partly to decreased absorption and increased metabolism of folate. Treatment is by the addition of folic acid, 5 mg daily, to the anticonvulsant regimen.

CELLULAR MECHANISM OF ACTION

Folic acid is required for normal erythropoiesis. As with vitamin B_{12}, a deficiency of folic acid results in a megaloblastic anaemia and abnormalities in other cell types. The role of folate in cell metabolism results from its ability to transfer groups containing single carbon atoms in biochemical reactions. These include the methylation of deoxyuridylic acid to form thymidylic acid, as well as other reactions in purine and pyrimidine synthesis. A key reaction in folate metabolism is its reduction to various forms of tetrahydrofolate by dihydrofolate reductase. It is this enzyme that is inhibited by methotrexate (see Chapters 25 and 47), pyrimethamine (see Chapter 46) and trimethoprim (chapter 42).

PHARMACOKINETICS

Folate is absorbed in the proximal small intestine within 5–20 min of ingestion. There is a specific absorptive mechanism. During absorption, folic acid is formylated and then methylated before it enters the portal blood. About one-third of total body folate (70 mg) is stored in the liver. This is only about 4 months' supply, and thus folate deficiency develops more rapidly than vitamin B_{12} deficiency. As with vitamin B_{12}, the faeces contain folate that has been synthesized by colonic bacteria, but this occurs too low in the gut for folate absorption to occur. The normal range for serum folate levels is 4–20 μg/L.

Key points

Vitamin B_{12} and folate therapy

- Healthy subjects require 3–5 μg of vitamin B_{12} and 200 μg of folate daily.
- Body stores of vitamin B_{12} are 3 mg; folate stores are approximately 200 mg.
- Vitamin B_{12} and folate are absorbed from the small intestine, and vitamin B_{12} is specifically absorbed from the terminal ileum.
- Vitamin B_{12} deficiency must not be incorrectly treated with folate alone, as any associated neurological damage may be irreversible.
- Oral folate replacement is adequate at 5–15 mg per day. Vitamin B_{12} replacement should be given parenterally as 5 × 1 mg every 2–3 days, and then given every 3 months for maintenance therapy.
- Drugs may cause folate (e.g. phenytoin) or vitamin B_{12} (e.g. metformin) deficiency.

Iron and folic acid therapy in pregnancy

Pregnancy imposes a substantial increase in demand on maternal stores of iron and folic acid. The average daily net flow of iron across the placenta from mother to fetus at term is 4.5 mg. At this stage of pregnancy, 90% of maternal plasma iron turnover is directed towards the fetus. A pregnant woman during the last trimester therefore requires approximately 5 mg of iron daily. A net gain of around 500–600 mg of elemental iron is required for each pregnancy to accommodate the requirements of the growing fetus together with expansion of the maternal red-cell mass, and most women are iron-depleted by the end of the pregnancy if they do not receive supplements.

Requirements for folic acid also increase by two to threefold in pregnancy. Deficiency is associated with prematurity, low birth weight for gestational age, and neural-tube defects (see Chapter 9). In the UK the usual practice is to give iron and folic acid supplements throughout pregnancy. Tablets containing 100 mg of elemental iron and 200–500 μg folic acid are available to be taken once daily. Folate supplementation (400–800 μg/day) should be given before conception to women who are attempting to become pregnant, in order to reduce the incidence of neural-tube defects. Higher-dose prophylaxis (folate, 5 mg daily) is advised for women who have previously given birth to a child with a neural-tube defect.

HAEMATOPOIETIC GROWTH FACTORS

Gene identification, cloning and recombinant DNA technology have been utilized to synthesize several human haematopoietic growth factors (see Figure 48.2 for an outline of haematopoiesis). Haematopoietic growth factors now have a clear role in the treatment of many forms of bone-marrow dysfunction.

Recombinant human erythropoietin (epoetin)

Erythropoietin is a protein consisting of 165 amino acids, four of which are glycosylated, with a molecular weight of 34 000. About 90% of endogenous erythropoietin is produced by interstitial cells of the renal cortex adjacent to the proximal tubules, and 10% by the liver. Biosynthesis is stimulated by tissue hypoxia. The production and actions of erythropoietin are linked in a negative feedback loop that maintains red-cell mass at an optimal level for oxygen transport. It is the only haematopoietic growth factor that is a hormone. **Epoetin**, the recombinant form of erythropoietin, is available in two forms with minor structural differences. Epoetin-α is available as 1-mL ampoules of 2000 units and epoetin-β containing 1000, 2000 and 25 000 units is available as a powder to be reconstituted with water. Therapeutically the actions of the α- and β-forms are indistinguishable.

USES

Epoetin is used to treat the anaemia of chronic renal failure. It is normally given by either intravenous or subcutaneous injection, initially at a dose of 50 IU/kg three times a week (this is a convenient schedule for patients on three times weekly haemodialysis, but is otherwise arbitrary), increasing according to response by 25 IU/kg at 4–weekly intervals. The maximum dose is 600 IU/kg in three divided doses per week. The usual maintenance dose is 100–300 IU/kg week. Other causes of anaemia (iron or folate deficiency) should be excluded. Aluminum toxicity, concurrent infection and other inflammatory diseases impair the response.

Epoetin has been used with some benefit in other various conditions:

1 anaemia of drug-induced bone-marrow suppression (e.g. cancer chemotherapy or ZDV therapy, if pretreatment erythropoietin is < 500 IU/L);
2 anaemia of myelodysplastic syndromes;
3 myeloma;
4 anaemia of rheumatoid arthritis;
5 autologous blood harvesting for transfusion during elective surgery;
6 prevention of anaemia in premature babies of low birthweight.

MECHANISM OF ACTION

Epoetin binds to a membrane receptor on erythroid cell precursors in the bone marrow. The epoetin–receptor complex promotes phosphorylation of a tyrosine kinase, and this increases transcription of the genes for δ-aminolevulinic acid synthetase and porphobilinogen decarboxylase, which are key haem biosynthetic enzymes. Thus epoetin increases haem biosynthesis and causes differentiation of erythroid precursors into mature erythroid cells.

PHARMACOKINETICS

Epoetin has a mean $t_{\frac{1}{2}}$ of 5 h with a volume of distribution of 50 mL/kg. After subcutaneous injection, its systemic bioavailability is about 40%. Elimination occurs by catabolism in the erythroid cells in the marrow following internalization, by hepatic metabolism and by urinary excretion.

ADVERSE EFFECTS

These include the following:

1 hypertension – blood pressure should be monitored weekly until a plateau is reached, and thereafter should be monitored 6-weekly. Severe hypertension with headaches and fits can occur. Epoetin is contraindicated in patients with severe uncontrolled hypertension;
2 thrombosis, for example of shunts, or causing a cardiovascular/cerebrovascular accident;
3 influenza-like symptoms;
4 Iron deficiency may be unmasked. Many physicians start iron prophylactically with the use of epoetin.

Human granulocyte colony-stimulating factor (filgrastim,lenograstim)

Granulocyte colony-stimulating factor (G-CSF) is a glycoprotein consisting of 174 amino acids that are variably glycosylated (molecular weight 18 000–22 000). The varying degree of glycosylation is not a factor in therapeutic efficacy, but may be important in making recombinant G-CSF more antigenic. G-CSF has been produced in both bacterial and mammalian systems. **Filgrastim** is unglycosylated rhG-CSF, and **lenograstim** is glycosylated rhG-CSF.

USES

Indications for G-CSF include the following:

1 to prevent and treat the neutropenia induced by cancer chemotherapy;
2 congenital neutropenia and cyclical neutropenia;
3 myelo-ablative therapy followed by bone-marrow transplantation;
4 mobilization of peripheral blood-cell progenitors and subsequent harvesting for transplant;
5 aplastic anaemia;

Table 48.2: Comparison of the effects of granulocyte colony-stimulating factor (G-CSF) and granulocyte-macrophage colony-stimulating factor (GM-CSF)

	G-CSF	GM-CSF	G-CSF and GM-CSF
Bone marrow	Marked increase in neutrophils (9.4-fold)	Mild increase in neutrophils (1.5-fold)	Increased cellularity and M/E ratio
Bone marrow	Increased promyelocytes	Increased eosinophils and cycling progenitors	Increased promyelocytes and myelocytes
Peripheral blood	Normal neutrophil survival Macropolycytes	Increased neutrophil survival Increased eosinophils and monocytes	Increased neutrophil count with young cells (left shift) Increased numbers of circulating immune cells
Leucocyte function	Normal surface markers and motility	Decreased motility and chemotaxis Monocytes: increased cytotoxicity	Increased stimulated superoxide production
Biochemistry	Increased urate, lysozyme and IL-2 receptor	Increased AST/ALT; decreased albumin	Increased LDH, alkaline phosphatase and cholesterol

M/E ratio = ratio of myeloid cells/erythroid cells, IL-2 = interleukin-2, AST = aspartate transaminase, ALT = alanine transaminase, LDH = lactate dehydrogenase.

6 human immunodeficiency virus (HIV)-related AZT-induced neutropenia.

G-CSF is usually self-administered by subcutaneous injection. If intravenous dosing is necessary, it is given as a 15–20 to-min infusion. The dose varies from 1 to 20 μg/kg/day (1 μg = 100 000 units) for a course of up to 14 days. Therapy is monitored by performing blood counts twice weekly. Table 48.2 compares the effects of G-CSF and granulocyte monocyte colony-stimulating factor (GM-CSF). G-CSF is primarily used to reduce neutropenia after cancer chemotherapy. It causes an immediate transient neutropenia and monocytopenia 5–15 min and 30–60 min after intravenous and subcutaneous administration, respectively. This is followed by a sustained dose-dependent increase in white blood cell count in 5–6 days. Elevated neutrophil counts stabilize in the second week of a 2–week course of treatment. After cessation of therapy, neutrophil counts return to baseline after 4–7 days.

MECHANISM OF ACTION

G-CSF stimulates the proliferation and differentiation of progenitor cells of the myelogranulocyte lineage. It binds to a specific receptor on myelogranulocyte precursors, enhancing cell replication and differentation. Once bound to its receptor, G-CSF is internalized. At a subcellular level its actions are complex, and signal transduction to the nucleus involves a number of tyrosine kinase proteins including p21/MAP kinase (for proliferation) and JAK and STAT kinases, which then induce the synthesis of proteins which up-regulate cell-cycle and differentiation processes.

ADVERSE EFFECTS

These include the following:

1 bone pain;
2 myalgia;
3 fever;
4 splenomegaly;
5 thrombocytopenia;
6 abnormal liver enzymes.

Contraindications

G-CSF should not be given to patients with myeloid or myelomonocytic leukaemia, because it increases proliferation of the malignant clone.

PHARMACOKINETICS

The bioavailability of subcutaneously administered G-CSF is 54%, and it yields plasma concentrations higher than 10 ng/mL for 10–16 h. The plasma $t_{\frac{1}{2}}$ of G-CSF ranges from 1.3 to 7.2 h. Clearance of G-CSF is complex, and increases as the granulocyte count rises, suggesting that granulocytes are themselves involved. In addition, G-CSF is metabolized in the kidney and liver to its component amino acids. Little or no unchanged G-CSF is found in the urine. In humans there is evidence of zero-order pharmacokinetics at doses of >10 μg/kg.

Granulocyte-macrophage colony-stimulating factor molgramostim

GM-CSF is a glycoprotein consisting of 127 amino acids. It is variably glycosylated (molecular weight 14 000–35 000). Glycosylation is not a factor in therapeutic efficacy, but may be important in making recombinant GM-CSF more antigenic, and possibly in influencing its plasma half-life. It is produced in yeast, bacterial or mammalian systems.

USES

GM-CSF has been used in bone-marrow transplantation, neutropenia secondary to chemotherapy, myelodysplastic syndromes and aplastic anaemia, and in bone-marrow failure of HIV patients whether due to the virus or to drug therapy (with AZT/ganciclovir). There are theoretical concerns that GM-CSF could stimulate HIV replication, which at present have neither been confirmed nor refuted *in vivo*. *In vitro* it potentiates the efficacy of AZT against HIV. GM-CSF is self-administered by subcutaneous injection. The dose ranges from 0.3 to 10 μg/kg/day (60 000–110 000 units/kg/day) for 7–10 days, usually starting 24 h after chemotherapy. In bone-marrow-transplant therapy, GM-CSF is given intravenously by two 2 to 4-h infusions daily (110 000 units/kg/day) for a maximum of 30 days. Therapy is monitored by performing blood counts and serum albumin estimation once or twice weekly. GM-CSF does not increase neutrophil numbers as potently as G-CSF. Each dose of GM-CSF causes a transient leukopenia (neutrophils, eosinophils and monocytes), followed by an increase in white blood cell count. Fifty-fold increases in circulating leukocytes can occur after doses of 20 μg/kg.

MECHANISM OF ACTION

GM-CSF binds to specific receptors on myeloid cells and stimulates proliferation and differentiation of progenitor cells of all haematopoietic lineages, and increases peripheral white blood cell numbers. GM-CSF does not shorten the time for neutrophil precursors to mature. It increases the neutrophil production rate by 50%, and the circulating half-life of neutrophils is prolonged from 8 to 48 h. GM-CSF binds to its receptor and by a variety of pathways probably involving p21/mitogen-activated protein (MAP) kinase and Janus kinase (JAK) and signal transducers and activators of transcription (STAT) kinases, brings about specific protein synthesis to upregulate the cell cycle and differentiation processes.

ADVERSE EFFECTS

These include the following:

1. first-dose reaction – muscle pain, hypotension, dyspnoea, nausea and vomiting. These reactions are probably due to cytokine-related capillary leakage, at high doses;
2. fluid retention;
3. fever, chills and anorexia;
4. lethargy and myalgia;
5. bone pain and arthralgia;
6. skin eruptions (both generalized and at the injection site);
7. pericarditis and pericardial effusion;
8. pleural effusion;
9. eosinophilia;
10. abnormal liver function tests: hepatitis.

Several of these adverse effects are mediated by cytokine release.

PHARMACOKINETICS

Intravenous administration is followed by a bi-exponential decay in plasma concentration. The elimination $t_{\frac{1}{2}}\beta$ varies considerably (0.8–9 h). After subcutaneous administration, maximum plasma concentrations are only achieved after 15–20 h, and plasma GM-CSF concentrations return to baseline by 48 h. GM-CSF clearance is via the reticulo-endothelial system and liver.

Interleukin-3 (IL-3)

This is a glycoprotein of molecular weight 14 000–280 000 produced by T-lymphocytes. It is not yet generally available in the UK, but may be effective in a rare congenital red cell aplasia called Diamond–Blackfan syndrome. Adverse effects include fever, headache, rashes, nausea, influenza-like syndrome and eosinophilia.

Other Haematopoietic growth factors

Other haematopoietic growth factors currently undergoing clinical investigation include interleukins 6, 11 and Flt3–ligand (which may well replace the excessively toxic stem-cell factor). Thrombopoietin, a recombinant protein which binds to the mpl-proto-oncogene, stimulates megakaryocyte proliferation and differentiation in humans and appears to synergize with G-CSF in promoting bone-marrow production of granulocytes. Thrombopoietin will no doubt come to play a role in therapy for drug-induced thrombocytopenia, and in bone-marrow transplantation.

Key points

Haematopoietic growth factors

- The clinically used haematopoietic growth factors are recombinant DNA products of the endogenous glycoprotein.
- Erythropoietin (Epo):
  - stimulates proliferation of erythroid (red cell) precursors;
  - is used in the treatment of the anaemia of renal failure (myelodysplasia);
  - is given parenterally; its toxicities include hypertension and thrombotic episodes.
- Granulocyte colony-stimulating factor (G-CSF):
  - stimulates proliferation of myeloid precursors;
  - is used in the treatment of neutropenia of chemotherapy, aplastic anaemia and bone-marrow transplant;
  - is given parenterally; its toxicities include myalgias, bone pain, fever, thrombocytopenia and hepatitis.
- Granulocyte-macrophage colony-stimulating (GM-CSF):
  - stimulates proliferation of myelo-monocyte precursors;
  - is used in the treatment of bone-marrow transplant, aplastic anaemia and myelodysplastic syndromes;
  - is given parenterally; its toxicities include pulmonary capillary leakage syndrome bone pain, fluid retention and rashes.

COAGULATION FACTORS AND HAEMOPHILIAS A AND B

PATHOPHYSIOLOGY

Haemophilia A is an X-linked recessive disease where there is a deficiency of factor VIII in the blood. Haemophilia B is also an X-linked recessive disorder in which there is a deficiency of factor IX. Haemophilia B has an incidence one-sixth that of haemophilia A. Both types of haemophilia present with identical clinical symptoms of excessive bleeding in response to trauma, e.g. muscle haematoma, haemarthrosis, haemorrhage after minor (e.g. dental) or major surgery, and intracranial bleeding following minor head injury.

THERAPEUTIC PRINCIPLES

The extent of haemorrhage depends on the severity of the factor VIII or IX deficiency and the severity of the trauma. Therapy consists of reducing haemorrhage by temporarily raising the concentration of the deficient factor, appropriate supportive measures, analgesia and graded physiotherapy. In minor trauma in mild haemophilia A, infusions of a synthetic vasopressin analogue (desmopressin, DDAVP; see Chapter 35), 0.4 μg/kg, produces a short-term two- to fourfold increase in factor VIII. Fluid overload due to the antidiuretic hormone action of DDAVP must be prevented by limiting water intake. DDAVP also stimulates release of plasminogen activator, and is therefore given with an inhibitor of fibrinolysis such as tranexamic acid. If the haemophilia and/or trauma is severe, then infusions of factor VIII or IX are required. The amount required and the number of infusions depend on the severity of the trauma. For minor haemarthrosis, a level of 15% of the deficient factor is targeted and is usually achieved by a single infusion. In cases with muscle bleeding or major haemarthrosis, a level of 25% is targeted, which may require repeated infusions for several days over a week. In patients with head injury, major trauma or surgery, a minimum level of 50% is targeted and maintained by repeated infusions.

Patients and their parents or other carers are taught to administer these factors at home in order to minimize delay in therapy.

Factor VIII

Factor VIII is a protein cofactor in the intrinsic pathway of blood coagulation which is deficient in patients with haemophilia A and von Willebrand disease. It is used in the treatment and prophylaxis of haemorrhage in patients with factor VIII deficiency. It is a single-chain protein of molecular weight 330 000. It circulates as a procofactor bound to von Willebrand factor. It is obtained from purified pooled plasma of blood donors, or more recently, from micro-organisms by recombinant DNA techniques. Recombinant preparations are free of all potential viral pathogens, including hepatitis B, hepatitis C, HIV and cytomegalovirus (CMV). These are inactivated by heat or chemical treatment of pooled human plasma preparations to give highly purified factor VIII. The latter is given as an intravenous infusion over several hours and has a mean $t_{\frac{1}{2}}$ of 10 h. It is highly bound to von Willebrand factor (> 95%) and has a small volume of distribution and is degraded by reticulo-endothelial cells in the liver. The dose of factor VIII is calculated on the basis of the severity of the injury and the required increase in plasma factor VIII concentration. The main adverse effects are due to impurities or contaminants in the pooled plasma-derived preparations. Anaphylactic reactions are rare, and transmission of HIV, hepatitis B and hepatitis C viruses should not occur with current methods, but recent tragedies provide a grim warning of potential future dangers. In low-purity factor VIII, fibrinogen can accumulate and promote abnormal haemostasis when it has initially been corrected. Transient reactions to infusions (e.g. urticaria, flushing and headache) occur, but they respond to antihistamines. Repeated infusions of non-recombinant factor VIII may induce allo-antibodies to factor VIII, and to certain impurities, in the recipient.

Factor IX

Factor IX is a protein cofactor in the intrinsic pathway of blood coagulation which is deficient in patients with haemophilia B. It is used in the treatment and prophylaxis of haemorrhage in patients with factor IX deficiency. It acts as a cofactor for factor VIII, and is currently available as a dried fraction from pooled plasma concentrates, which also contains the other vitamin K-dependent coagulation factors (II, VII and X; see Chapter 29) and is therefore sometimes used to treat life-threatening bleeding in patients who have been overtreated with warfarin. Recombinant factor IX will soon be available for patients with haemophilia B which will not contain these other factors or potential pathogens. Factor IX is given as an intravenous infusion over several hours, and has a mean plasma $t_{\frac{1}{2}}$ of 18 h. Otherwise its use and adverse effects are similar to those described for factor VIII.

Key points

Coagulation factor therapy

- Factor VIII is used to treat haemophilia A (factor IX is used for haemophilia B) when patients present with severe bleeding.
- These factors are given intravenously, and the dose is based on the level of factor deficiency and blood loss.
- Recombinant coagulation factors are free from the risk of contamination with infectious agents such as HIV and hepatitis C, and cause less antibody production.

Aplastic anaemia

Aplastic anaemia is characterized by pancytopenia associated with the replacement of normal cellular bone marrow by fat, without evidence of malignancy or proliferation of reticulin. Some cases are congenital (e.g. Fanconi's anaemia), but many are acquired, and in 50% of these an aetiological agent (a virus, chemical or drug) can be implicated. Certain drugs have a particularly strong association with aplastic anaemia. These include *alkylating agents*, as well as phenylbutazone, chloramphenicol, and zidovudine. They should be avoided unless there is a specific indication, because although aplastic anaemia is rare, it is often fatal.

Treatment

Support is provided with transfusions (of red cells and platelets) and appropriate antibiotics. Successful bone-marrow transplantation is curative, and has become the therapy of choice for young patients. For those who are unsuitable for this treatment, or in cases where there is no available histocompatible donor, anabolic steroids may reduce the requirement for transfusions. Two 17–α-alkyl derivatives of testosterone have been used, namely oxymetholone and stanozolol (see Chapter 40). The effiecacy of erythropoietin, G-CSF and GM-CSF (see above) is now also established.

Idiopathic thrombocytopenic purpura

It is important to exclude other causes of thrombocytopenia, including drugs. Platelet transfusions are required to control active bleeding or to cover operations. Other treatment options include the following:

1 glucocorticosteroids – prednisolone 1 mg/kg daily and slowly reduced; a response (rising platelet count) may take 1–2 weeks to occur. If these fail, or the disease relapses rapidly on reducing the steroid dose, splenectomy should be considered. If splenectomy is performed, the patient should be immunized against pneumococcal infection several weeks pre-operatively if possible, as there is a risk of overwhelming pneumococcal sepsis following splenectomy. Glucocorticosteroids should be continued after the operation until the platelet count rises;
2 immunosuppressive drugs (see Chapters 47 and 49), especially vincristine, can be used in refractory cases. Alternative therapies include danazol, intravenous immunoglobulin and cyclosporin;
3 thrombopoietin (megakaryocyte growth and differentiation factor; see above) enhances platelet production. It will soon become generally available.

Drug-induced haematological caltoxicity

Haematological toxicity, which is often severe, is often drug induced. Drugs commonly associated with haematolgical toxicity are described in Chapter 12 (p.92–3). Table 48.3 lists some common drugs which produce haemolysis in patients with glucose 6-phosphate dehydrogenase (G-6-PDH) deficiency.

Table 48.3: Drugs that are contraindicated in patients with glucose-6-phosphate dehydrogenase deficiency

Drug or drug class	Likelihood of causing haemolysis in glucose-6-phosphate dehydrogenase-deficient patient
Dapsone and other sulphones Methylene blue Nitrofurantoin Primaquine 4-Quinolones (ciprofloxacin, etc.) Sulphonamides	All these drugs have a definite risk of causing haemolysis
Aspirin (doses of > 1g /day) Chloroquine (acceptable in acute malaria) Probenacid Quinidine (acceptable in acute malaria) Quinine (acceptable in acute malaria)	All of these drugs have a possible risk of causing haemolysis

Key points

Drug-related haematological toxicity

- Cancer chemotherapy can cause suppression of all bone-marrow cell lines.
- Drugs that cause aplastic anaemia include chloramphenicol indomethacin and carbimazole.
- Drugs that cause agranulocytosis include, for example, carbamazepine, propylthiouracil, NSAIDs, H_2 antagonists and antipsychotics (e.g. chlorpromazine, clozapine).
- Drugs that cause thrombocytopenia include, for example, heparin, azathioprine, quinidine and thiazides.
- Drugs that cause haemolytic anaemia include, for example, methyldopa, β-lactams (penicillins and cephalosporins).

Further reading

Cook JD. 1994: Iron deficiency anaemia. *Baillieres Clinical Haematology*. 7, 787–84.

Fisher JW. 1997: Erythropoietin: physiologic and pharmacologic aspects. *Proceedings of the Society of Experimental Biology and Medicine* **216**, 358–69.

Kaushansky K. 1994:The mpl ligand, molecular and cellular biology of the critical regulator of megakaryocyte development. *Stem Cells* **12** (**Suppl. 1**) 91–7.

Kaushansky K. 1997: Thrombopoietin; more than a lineage-specific megakaryocyte growth factor. *Stem Cells* **15** (**Suppl. 1**) 97–102.

Limentani SA, Roth DA, Furie BC, Furie B. 1993: Recombinant blood clotting proteins for haemophilia therapy. *Seminars in Thrombosis and Hemostasis* **19**, 62–7

McGrath K. 1989: Treatment of anaemia caused by iron, vitamin B_{12} or folate deficiency. *Medical Journal of Australia*. **157**, 693–7.

Nemunatis J. 1997 A comparative review of colony-stimulating factors. *Drugs* **54**, 709–29.

Scott J, Weir D. 1994: Folate/vitamin B_{12} inter-relationships. *Essays in Biochemistry* **28**, 63–72.

Case history

A 65-year-old woman presents to the medical outpatient department with a history of fatigue. She has rheumatoid arthritis and has been taking naproxen for many years. Recently she was started on omeprazole, 20 mg once a day, because of symptoms of reflux oesophagitis, and since then these symptoms have improved. Clinical examination shows quiescent rheumatoid arthritis. The patient is pale, but no other abnormalities are noted. Her full blood count shows a haemoglobin level of 9.5 g/dL with a mean corpusular volume of 90 fL; other haematological indices and serum transferrin are normal. Her faecal occult blood is negative × 3. She is started on oral iron sulphate and given three times weekly injections of erythropoietin 300 IU / kg subcutaneously. Three months later her haemoglobin level has risen to 13 g/dL, but she presents with acute-onset dysphasia and loss of the use of her right arm. Her supine blood pressure is 198/122 mmHg. Her neurological deficit resolves over 24 h, and her blood pressure settles to 170/96 mmHg. She has no evidence of cardiac arrhythmias or of carotid disease on ultrasonic duplex angiography, and her serum cholesterol concentration is 4.2 mmol/L.

Question

What led to this patient's acute neurological episode? Does she require further therapy?

Answer

Her mild normochromic-normocytic anaemia of chronic disease (rheumatoid arthritis) could have contributed to her initial symptom of fatigue. There was no evidence of gastrointestinal blood loss, despite prolonged NSAID use. Treatment with iron and erythropoietin was not rational. She was not iron deficient, and using iron and erythropoietin in combination for a haemoglobin level of 9.5 g/dL is unjustified. The most common dose-limiting side-effects of epoetin administration are hypertension and thrombosis, which are implicated in the left middle cerebral TIA.

Treatment with erythropoetin and iron should be stopped, and her blood pressure monitored over 8–12 weeks. If hypertension is solely related to the erythropoetin therapy, her blood pressure should normalize and no further treatment will be indicated.

PART XI

IMMUNOPHARMACOLOGY

CHAPTER FORTY-NINE

CLINICAL IMMUNOPHARMACOLOGY

- Introduction
- Immunosuppressive agents
- General adverse effects of immunosuppression
- Chemical mediators of the immune response and drugs that block their actions
- Drugs that enhance immune system function
- Vaccines
- Immunoglobulins as therapy

INTRODUCTION

The introduction of a foreign antigen into the body may provoke an immune reaction, but for this to occur the body must recognize the antigen as foreign. Antigens are usually large molecules with a molecular weight of over 5000 daltons. They are often multivalent and have a consistent charge and molecular profile, being proteins, glycoproteins or high-molecular-weight carbohydrates. Most antigens are initially processed by macrophages before being presented to T-lymphocytes. The immune response is initiated by the interaction of antigen with receptors on the surface of the lymphocytes, and the response may be one of two types, namely *humoral* or *cellular* immunity.

HUMORAL IMMUNITY

This is the production of circulating immunoglobulin by plasma cells that are derived from B-lymphocytes. In humans these lymphocytes arise largely from lymphoid tissue of the gastrointestinal tract. The humoral response occurs in two stages as follows:

1. *primary reactions* – these occur with the first exposure to the antigen. There is a small and short-lived rise in antibody titre which consists largely of IgM;
2. *secondary reactions* – these occur with subsequent exposure to the antigen. The rise in antibody titre is greater and persists for a long period. The antibody consists mainly of IgG. The reaction requires the interaction of helper T-cells and B-lymphocytes.

CELLULAR IMMUNITY

This is mediated by sensitized T-lymphocytes which recognize and bind the antigen and subsequently release a cascade of lymphokines which are vital in orchestrating the response. The immune response is an essential defence against invasion of the body by bacteria, viruses and other foreign materials. However, it may be defective, disorganized or overactive, and can produce a wide variety of diseases. The body has the potential to stimulate its own immune system so that antibodies are produced against itself. Normally this situation is prevented by a number of autoregulatory mechanisms, but if these fail then autoimmune disease results. Deficiencies in the immune system may be congenital or result from the use of certain drugs, particularly cytotoxic agents, glucocorticosteroids, and cyclosporin and its analogues.

Table 49.1: Summary of the role of selected cytokines in the immune system

Cytokine	Cellular source(s)	Primary target and major action
Interleukin-1 (IL-1)	Macrophages	T- and B-cell activation
Interleukin-2 (IL-2)	T-cells	T-cell activation and proliferation
Interleukin-3 (IL-3)	T-cells	CD38 positive cell (stem-cell) proliferation and differentiation
Interleukin-4 (IL-4)	T-cells	B-cell differentiation and IgE class switch TH_2 cell differentiation
Interleukin-5 (IL-5)	T-cells	Eosinophil activation and differentiation
Interleukin-6 (IL-6)	T-cells	B-cell differentiation
Interleukin-7 (IL-7)	Stromal cells	B-cell proliferation and differentiation
Interleukin-8 (IL-8)	Macrophages	Granulocyte chemotaxis
Interleukin-10 (IL-10)	T-cells	Inhibition of TH_1-cells
Interleukin-11 (IL-11)	Stromal cells	Stem-cell proliferation and differentiation
Interleukin-12 (IL-12)	Macrophages	TH_1-cell differentiation
Interferon-α (IFN-α)	Macrophages	NK-cell activation, and MHC class I induction
Interferon-γ (IFN-γ)	T-cells, NK cells	Inhibition of TH_2 cells, macrophage activation and MHC Class I and II receptor induction
GM-CSF	T-cells	Eosinophil activation
Tumour necrosis factor (TNF-α)	Macrophages	Activation of macrophages, granulocytes and cytotoxic T-cells
Transforming growth factor-β (TGF-β)	Macrophages	Activation of macrophages, granulocytes and cytotoxic T-cells

NK cells = natural-killer cells, TH cells = T-helper cells, MHC = major histocompatibility complex,
GM-CSF = granulocyte-monocyte colony-stimulating factor.

Active immunity

This consists of immunity that is developed either in response to infection or following innoculation with an attenuated strain of organism, or with a structural protein or toxic protein to which the host produces protective antibodies.

Passive immunity

This is immunity that is transferred by the administration of preformed antibodies (e.g. immune globulin/serum) either from another host or from recombinant techniques *in vitro.*

Hypersensitivity

Sometimes the immune response to an antigen results in damage to the tissue; this is known as *hypersensitivity*. There are four types of hypersensitivity which are categorized according to their pathophysiology.

Type-I hypersensitivity

This reaction results from the combination of antigen with high-affinity IgE (reaginic) antibody on the surface of tissue mast cells and/or blood basophils releasing potently vasoactive and pro-inflammatory mediators. These mediators include histamine, leukotrienes C_4, D_4 and E_4 (previously known as SRS-A), eosinophil chemotactic factor (ECF), serotonin, tachykinins and prostaglandins. The combined effects of the release of these mediators can lead to anaphylaxis, allergic asthma, hay fever and some types of urticaria.

Type-II hypersensitivity

These reactions occur when antibody combines with antigenic components on a cell or tissue surface. This leads to cell lysis or tissue damage as a result of antibody-directed cell-mediated cytotoxicity (ADCC) by macrophages and NK cells through Fc receptors or by activation of complement. This reaction may form the basis of a drug reaction (e.g. penicillin- or quinidine-induced haemolytic anaemia or thrombocytopenia). Another example of this type of reaction is haemolytic disease of the newborn, when antibodies produced by a rhesus-negative mother against the rhesus factor on the red cells of the fetus cross the placental barrier and cause haemolysis. Such reactions may be mediated by IgM or IgG antibodies.

Type-III hypersensitivity (Arthus reaction – immune complex mediated)

This is the result of the deposition of soluble antigen–antibody complexes (formed in conditions of antigen excess) in vessels or other tissues. The immune complex deposition activates complement components and initiates a sequence which results in chemotaxis of polymorphs, tissue injury and vasculitis. This reaction is delayed and is maximal a few hours after exposure to the antigen. Serum sickness is a result of this type of response. It is mediated by IgM or IgG antibodies.

Type-IV (delayed or cell-mediated hypersensitivity)

This is mediated by sensitized CD4+ circulating T-lymphocytes reacting to antigen. Circulating antibodies are not involved in the reaction. The activation of these primed CD4+ T-cells causes their proliferation and the release of cytokines which produce local inflammation, attracting and activating non-killer (NK) cells, macrophages and granulocytes. This type of reaction takes place 1–2 days after secondary antigen exposure, and is exemplified by contact dermatitis and organ transplant rejection.

Immune responses are essential for health. Suppression of an unwanted component poses difficult problems. Ideally, immunosuppressant therapy should be highly selective and leave the rest of the immune system intact.

IMMUNOSUPPRESSIVE AGENTS

See Figure 49.1 for sites of action of agents.

Azathioprine

See also Chapter 25.

Azathioprine is closely related to 6-mercaptopurine (6-MP), to which it is metabolized, differing only in having an imidazole group added to the molecule.

USES

Azathioprine is used to prevent transplant rejection, the usual dose being 1–4 mg/kg/day administered orally. It has also been used with some success in the treatment of autoimmune diseases (e.g. systemic lupus erythematosus, rheumatoid arthritis, chronic active hepatitis and some cases of glomerulonephritis). Owing to its potential toxicity, it is usually reserved for situations in which glucocorticosteroids alone are inadequate.

MECHANISM OF ACTION

Azathioprine is an antimetabolite, and is therefore most effective on proliferating cells. It is metabolized to 6-MP *in vivo*. The latter has no intrinsic activity, but requires transformation by intracellular enzyme pathways involving hypoxanthine-guanine phosphoribosyltransferase to 6-thioguanine nucleotides. These interfere with purine synthesis and are incorporated into DNA. Azathioprine causes immunosuppression by inhibiting lymphocytes which would normally proliferate in response to stimulation by an antigen. It inhibits delayed hypersensitivity (cell-mediated immunity) and those aspects of inflammation that depend on cell division.

PHARMACOKINETICS

The drug is variably but well absorbed. It is 98% cleared by hepatic metabolism to its active metabolite 6-MP. This is further detoxified by xanthine oxidase and thiopurinemethyl-transferase. The mean elimination $t_{\frac{1}{2}}$ of azathioprine is approximately 12 min.

ADVERSE EFFECTS

These include the following:

1 bone-marrow suppression, particularly granulocytopenia and thrombocytopenia. Azathio-

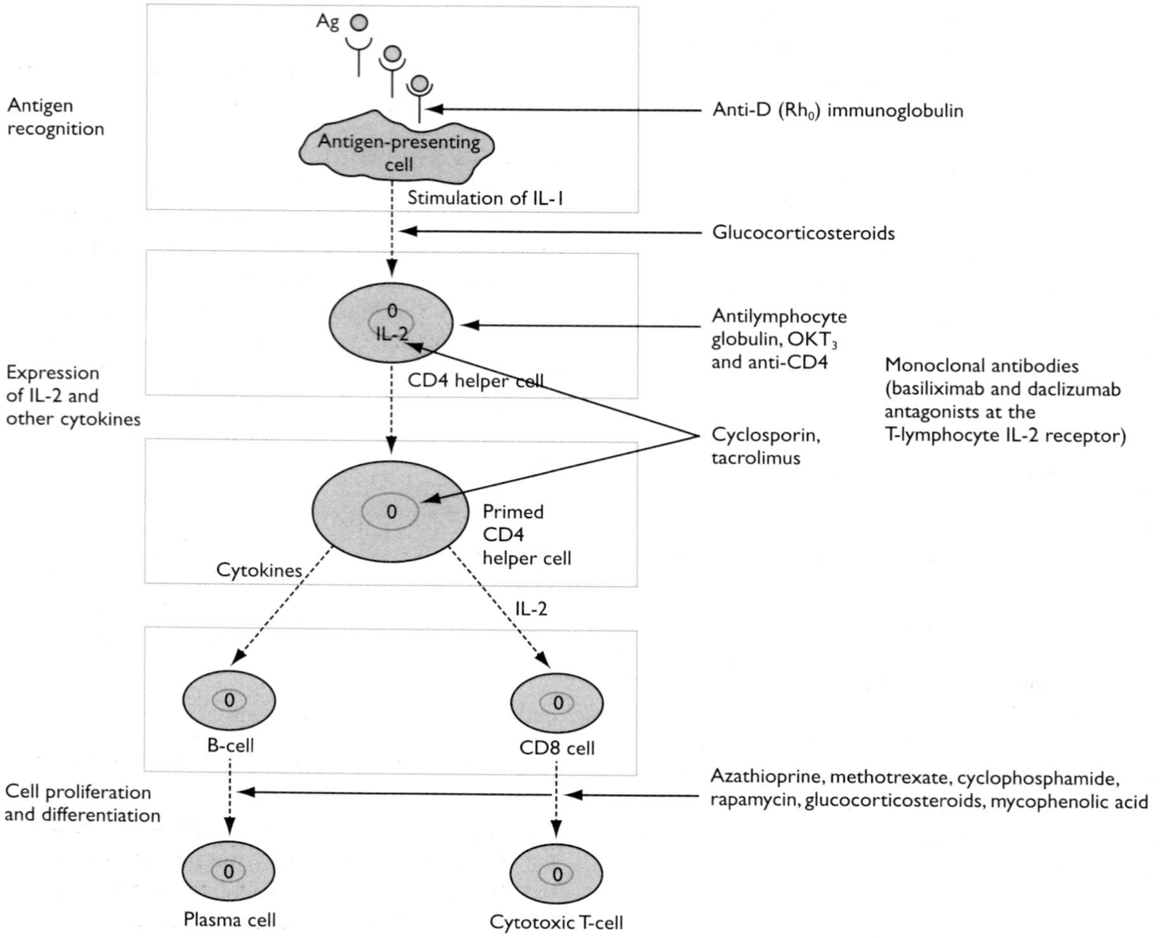

Figure 49.1 Sites of action of certain immunosuppressive agents.

prine therapy requires regular monitoring of bone-marrow function;

2 diarrhoea.

DRUG INTERACTIONS

If azathioprine is given with a xanthine oxidase inhibitor (e.g. allopurinol), accumulation and toxicity will occur unless the dose is reduced by approximately 30%.

Methotrexate

See Chapters 25 and 47.

Methotrexate is an immunosuppressive agent which acts by inhibiting replication of rapidly dividing cells. It is used as low-dose oral (5–10 mg) weekly therapy to treat rheumatoid arthritis as a second-line agent, and has limited usefulness as adjunctive therapy in the treatment of chronic steroid-dependent asthma. The major dose-limiting toxicities when used chronically in low dose are hepatic cirrhosis and bone-marrow suppression.

Cyclophosphamide

See also Chapter 47.

USES

Cyclophosphamide can be used to prevent solid-organ transplant rejection and as an immunosuppressant in a variety of autoimmune disorders. Perhaps its most important role in this context is in the treatment of nephrotic syndrome with minimal change in the glomeruli on microscopy, particularly in patients who are resistant to glucocorticosteroids, or when toxicity is troublesome. It appears to be superior to azathioprine in treatment of this type of disease. The cyclophosphamide dose is 3 mg/kg/day orally for 8 weeks. It is also used in the treatment of nephritis due to systemic lupus, Wegener's granulomatosis and (rarely) in severe rheumatoid disease.

MECHANISM OF ACTION

Cyclophosphamide inhibits lymphocyte proliferation by alkylating DNA. It is most effective if given after antigenic stimulation, and it reduces B-cell antibody production more than it depresses T-cell-mediated immunity.

Mycophenolate mofetil

USES

Mycophenolate mofetil is an ester of a product of the *Penicillium* mould. It is used in combination with cyclosporin and glucocorticosteroids in solid-organ (e.g. renal, cardiac) transplantation, and is a more effective alternative than azathioprine. Mycophenolate mofetil may also be effective in the treatment of other autoimmune disorders such as rheumatoid arthritis and psoriasis, and possibly as an anti-cancer agent. Drug toxicity at a dose of 3 g/day is considerably greater than at the now recommended oral dose of 1 g twice daily.

MECHANISM OF ACTION

In vivo the active entity, **mycophenolic acid**, inhibits inosine monophosphate dehydrogenase (a pivotal enzyme in purine synthesis), depleting guanine nucleotides and impairing RNA-primed DNA synthesis. It therefore selectively suppresses proliferation of both T- and B-lymphocytes, as they depend more on *de novo* purine synthesis than on the salvage pathway, while neutrophils rely more on the salvage pathway. In addition, mycophenolic acid may have an inhibitory effect on the production of pro-inflammatory cytokines.

ADVERSE EFFECTS

These include the following:

1 gastrotintestinal disturbances – diarrhoea (more commonly than with azathioprine) and haemorrhage;
2 bone-marrow suppression, especially leukopenia and anaemia (again more common than with azathiprine);
3 deep-seated CMV infection;
4 increased incidence of lymphomas, as with other immunosuppressants.

PHARMACOKINETICS

Mycophenolate mofetil is a prodrug ester of mycophenolic acid, and esterification improves absorption. After oral administration in humans the ester is rapidly and completely cleaved to mycophenolic acid. The bioavailability of mycophenolic acid from the mofetil ester is 94%. Mycophenolic acid undergoes hepatic elimination to its inactive glucuronide metabolite, with a terminal $t_{\frac{1}{2}}$ of 18 h and a volume of distribution of 4 L/kg.

DRUG INTERACTIONS

Antacids may decrease the absorption of this drug, while cholestyramine and other agents which interfere with enterohepatic recirculation may impair the bioavailability of mycophenolic acid.

Key points

Cytotoxic agents used as immunosuppressive therapy

- These include azathioprine (6-MP), methotrexate, cyclophosphamide and mycophenolate mofetil.
- They are used as components of combination therapy with cyclosporin and/or steroids.
- Their severe toxicities are the major limitation of their use.

Glucocorticosteroids

See also Chapter 39.

USES

1 Glucocorticosteroids are used in the treatment of allergic rhinitis, atopic dermatitis, acute severe asthma, chronic asthma and anaphylaxis. In allergic rhinitis and atopic dermatitis (type-I reactions) the principal benefit probably arises from their non-specific anti-inflammatory effects, including vasoconstriction and decreased vascular permeability, mediated in part by decreased histamine and leukotriene release and facilitation of β_2-adrenergic stimulation.

2 The normal humoral immune response is not usually inhibited by glucocorticosteroids, but they are often effective in treating type-II autoimmune diseases. They are the drugs of choice for pemphigus vulgaris and autoimmune haemolytic anaemia, and are often effective in idiopathic thrombocytopenic purpura (ITP). Glucocorticoids induce remission in about 80% of cases of immune haemolytic anaemia where warm-reacting antibodies are involved, and about 50% of these will remain in long-term or permanent remission. In pemphigus vulgaris there is a strong correlation between depression of autoantibody production and clinical response, but this does not appear to be so clear-cut in other diseases, such as ITP.

3 Immune complex disease (type-III hypersensitivity) may also be successfully treated with glucocorticosteroids, and they often produce symptomatic relief without necessarily altering the fundamental disease process. Thus in rheumatoid arthritis, although they are effective in controlling some features of the disease, the natural course of the disease is not improved. However, in systemic lupus erythematosus, glucorticosteroid therapy is often associated with decreases in antinuclear autoantibody titre, and there is limited evidence that high doses may improve renal function and prolong survival in some patients with renal involvement.

4 Glucocorticosteroids are potent inhibitors of the cell-mediated hypersensitivity (type-IV) reactions. Clinically they are used to prevent acute graft rejection and improve severe contact dermatitis.

Key points

Glucocorticosteroids as immunosuppressants

- Topical (e.g. beclomethasone) or systemic (e.g. prednisolone) glucocorticosteroids are very effective immunosuppressants.
- Appropriate dosing schedules of glucocorticoids are effective in diseases due to all types of hypersensitivity.
- Cellular pharmacodynamics:
  inhibits expression of pro-inflammatory cytokines-IL-2,3 and 6, TNF, GM-CSF and IFN-γ;
  inhibits production of adhesion molecules – ICAM-1, E-selectin and vascortin – leading to reduced vascular permeability;
  reduces synthesis of arachidonic acid metabolites (prostaglandins, leukotrienes) and reduces histamine release;
  reduces synthesis of Fc and C3 receptors.
- Hepatic metabolism (cytochrome P_{3A4}), dosed to minimize HPA suppression – lowest dose, once a day.
- Adverse effects include:
  acute-effects – metabolic disturbances (glucose/hypokalaemia), CNS (mood disorders, insomnia);
  chronic-effects – features of Cushing's syndrome; immunosuppression, risk of infection, and HPA axis suppression.

Antilymphocyte globulin

Antilymphocyte globulin (**ALG**, also known as antithymocyte globulin) is prepared by injecting human T-lymphocytes into animals (e.g. horses) to raise antibodies. The active immunoglobulin is largely in the IgG fraction, and ALG is a polyclonal antilymphocyte antibody with inherent variability from batch to batch. The major effect is probably to prevent antigen from accessing the antigen-recognition site on the T-helper cells. It is given intravenously for acute organ rejection and in patients who are at high risk of rejecting their transplant. Adverse effects include anaphylaxis and serum sickness, and production of anti-animal (horse) IgG is common (50%), as well as toxicity to tissues such as red blood cells and the kidneys.

Anti-CD3 antibodies (anti-CD3 receptor monoclonal antibodies)

USES

These monoclonal antibodies are used as adjuvant (often as second-line) immunosuppressive therapy in patients with acute transplant rejection. They are IgG2a antibodies produced from murine hybridoma cells, and are given as an intravenous bolus, 5 mg/day for 10–14 days. After a 10- to 14-day course patients develop neutralizing antibodies to the therapeutic **anti-CD3 antibodies**.

MECHANISM OF ACTION

These antibodies are targeted specifically at the T-lymphocyte CD3 protein (receptor), and when they bind to CD3, antigen is blocked from binding to the T-cell antigen-recognition complex adjacent to the CD3 protein. Anti-CD3 antibody also causes a decrease in number of CD3 (T3) positive lymphocytes in the blood. In addition, binding of anti-CD3 to its receptor causes cytokine release (see section below on adverse effects). The overall effect is to reduce T-cell participation in acute solid-organ graft rejection.

ADVERSE EFFECTS

These include the following:

1 hypersensitivity reactions ranging from anaphylaxis to an acute influenza-like syndrome (pretreatment with glucocorticosteroids may reduce this);
2 chest pain, wheezing and dyspnoea (pulmonary oedema occurs after the first dose in 1% of patients);
3 CNS effects – seizures, reversible meningo-encephalitis and cerebral oedema.

Cyclosporin (and its congeners)

Cyclosporin is a cyclic hydrophobic decapeptide that was originally extracted from fungal cultures.

USES

The main use of cyclosporin is in immunosuppression for solid-organ transplantation, but it is also effective in refractory psoriasis. A high dose of cyclosporin is given 4–12 h before transplantation, if possible. It may be given in doses of 4 mg/kg/day intravenously, but this is liable to produce renal failure, and it is safer to start with 14 mg/kg/day orally, reducing over a period of 3 months to a maintenance dose of around 6 mg/kg/day. Measurement of trough plasma concentrations of cyclosporin A is essential, and the dose should be adjusted to keep this in the range 60–300 μg/L. Opinions vary as to whether cyclosporin needs to be combined with steroids. In graft-versus-host disease and bone-marrow transplantation, intravenous treatment (3–5 mg/kg/day) is used initially, followed by oral administration for 6–9 months. The oral maintenance dose of cyclosporin is 5–10 mg/kg in divided doses, sometimes given with glucocorticosteroids.

MECHANISM OF ACTION

Cyclosporin is a specific T-lymphocyte suppressor, primarily acting on the T-helper (Th) cells, with a unique effect on the primary but not the secondary immune response. It inhibits the production of interleukin-2 (IL-2) and other cytokines by activated lymphocytes. At a cellular level this is due to cyclosporin A binding to its transport protein cyclophilin. This conjugate subsequently interacts with a Ca^{2+}-calmodulin-dependent calcineurin complex and inhibits its phosphorylase activity. This impairs access to the nucleus of the cytosolic component of the transcription promoter nuclear factor of activated T-cells (NF-ATc), which in turn reduces the transcription of messenger RNA for IL-2, other pro-inflammatory lymphokines and IL-2 receptor expression.

ADVERSE EFFECTS

These include the following:

1 nephrotoxicity is a serious problem (affecting 75% of patients). Serum creatinine and urea levels are increased in patients who are receiving cyclosporin. Nephrotoxicity may be minimized by calcium-channel blockade (e.g. with nifedipine);
2 hyperkalaemia;
3 nausea and gastrointestinal disturbances in up to 20% of patients;
4 hypertension;
5 hirsutism;
6 gingival hypertrophy;
7 tremor (which can be an early sign of increasing plasma concentrations), paraesthesia and fits;
8 hepatotoxicity, but this is not dose limiting;
9 anaphylaxis may occur with intravenous administration;
10 although it was originally feared that the use of cyclosporin would result in a serious number of malignancies (mainly lymphoma) developing, careful control of dosage and the avoidance of undue immunosuppression has considerably reduced this risk.

PHARMACOKINETICS

Cyclosporin is variably absorbed after oral administration (35–45%), but micro-emulsion formulations seem to be less variable. It undergoes variable presystemic metabolism (its bioavailability is approximately 30%) probably due to the gastrointestinal cytochrome $P_{450\,3A4}$ and P-glycoprotein content. Peak plasma concentrations occur within 1–4 h. The plasma log concentration–time relationship is biphasic with a $t_{\frac{1}{2}\alpha}$ of 1.2 h and $t_{\frac{1}{2}\beta}$ of 27 h. Because of its lipid solubility it has a large volume of distribution (3.5 L/kg). It is highly protein bound (90–95%). The major route of clearance is metabolism via the hepatic cytochrome $P_{450\,3A4}$ isoenzyme, and more than 30 metabolites have been identified. Renal dysfunction does not affect cyclosporin clearance, but caution is needed because of its nephrotoxicity. Dose reduction is required in patients with hepatic impairment.

THERAPEUTIC DRUG MONITORING

Cyclosporin is assayed by radioimmunoassay (RIA) or high-performance liquid chromatography (HPLC). Radioimmunoassay is preferred for clinical monitoring despite cross-reactions with several cyclic metabolites. Trough plasma concentrations of 100–300 μg/L are satisfactory when the drug is given by intravenous infusion. Effective immunosuppression occurs at trough concentrations of 60–300 μg/L when the drug is given orally. Careful monitoring of plasma concentrations is required for all patients, but especially if there is gastrointestinal disturbance, hepatic impairment, or the patient is concomitantly receiving other nephrotoxic drugs, or drugs that are known to interact with cyclosporin.

DRUG INTERACTIONS

These are numerous and include allopurinol, cimetidine, ketoconazole (and other azoles), erythromycin, diltiazem (and other calcium-channel blockers), anabolic steroids and norethisterone and other inhibitors of cytochrome $P_{450\,3A4}$, which reduce the hepatic clearance of cyclosporin by enzyme inhibition, leading to increased toxicity. Phenytoin, phenobarbitone and rifampicin increase hepatic clearance (phenytoin reduces absorption, while phenobarbitone and rifampicin enzyme induce cytochrome $P_{450\,3A4}$ activity), thus reducing plasma concentrations. Concomitant use of nephrotoxic agents such as aminoglycosides, vancomycin and amphotericin B may lead to cumulative nephrotoxicity with high plasma concentrations. ACE inhibitors increase the risk of hyperkalaemia. Renal function and plasma drug concentration should be monitored carefully in patients who are treated with these agents. The combined use of cyclosporin and steroids in bone-marrow-transplant patients has led to an increase in hypertension and convulsions, perhaps due to increased fluid retention.

In view of the toxic effects of cyclosporin a number of related alternative immunosuppressives are currently being evaluated (e.g. staurosporin, anti-CD4 antibodies, deoxyspergualin).

Key points

Cyclosporin

- First-line immunosuppressive agent in solid-organ transplant immunosuppression.
- Used in severe refractory psoriasis.
- Inhibits transcription of IL-2 and other pro-inflammatory cytokines by T-lymphocytes.
- Given orally or intravenously, shows variable absorption and hepatic metabolism (cytochrome $P_{450\,3A4}$) to many inactive metabolites.
- Toxicity – nephrotoxicity, nausea, hypertension, CNS effects (tremor and fits).
- Many drug interactions – toxicity potentiated by azoles, macrolides and diltiazem.
- New agents include tacrolimus (more potent) and sirolimus (potentiates cyclosporin).

GENERAL ADVERSE EFFECTS OF IMMUNOSUPPRESSION

Prolonged use of non-specific immunosuppressive drugs is associated with an appreciable incidence of adverse effects due to reduced immunity or drug-induced damage to the nuclear structure of the cell.

Increased susceptibility to infection Bacterial infections are common, and require prompt treatment with appropriate antibiotics. Tuberculosis may also occur, and sometimes takes unusual forms. Viral infections may be more severe than usual, and include the common herpes infection, but occasionally also such rarities as multifocal leukoencephalopathy. Fungal infections are also common, including

Table 49.2: Cyclosporin-like agents

Drug	Standard dosing regimen	Side-effects	Pharmacokinetics	Additional comments
Tacrolimus (FK 506)	Usually for patients who are refractory to cyclosporin – given intravenously or orally	Same as those of cyclosporine	Variable absorption (5–56% bioavailable) Elimination $t_{\frac{1}{2}}$ is 12–21 h	More potent than cyclosporin Better for liver transplant
	Intravenous dose, 25–50 μg/kg/day in two doses for adults	More neurotoxic and nephrotoxic than cyclosporin	Hepatic metabolism by cytochrome P_{3A4} (<1% excreted unchanged in urine)	Drug interactions likely to be as for cyclosporin
	Oral dose 150–200 μg/day in two doses for adults	May cause HOCM in children	Therapeutic drug monitoring available	
Sacrolimus (rapamycin)	Currently being determined	Mild gastrointestinal disturbances	Well absorbed Elimination $t_{\frac{1}{2}}$ is 57 h	Phase II/III development
	Oral doses studied are in the range 3–15 mg/m^2	Thrombocytopenia	Hepatic metabolism by cytochrome P_{3A4} Linear kinetics	Possible use in conjunction with cyclosporin Sirolimus AUC increased if given with cyclosporin

Candida albicans (which may be local or systemic), and protozoal infections (e.g. *Pneumocystis carinii*) can also occur.

Sterility Azoospermia in men is particularly common with alkylating agents (e.g cyclophosphamide). In women, hormone failure leading to amenorrhoea is common.

Teratogenicity This is less common than might be anticipated. However, it is, prudent to recommend to patients that they avoid conception while on these drugs, and men should wait 12 weeks (the time required to clear abnormal sperm) after stopping treatment.

Carcinogenicity Immunosuppression is associated with an increased incidence of malignant disease. Large-cell diffuse lymphoma can present early in treatment, but with prolonged treatment other types of malignancy may arise. The incidence in transplant patients is about 1%.

Other drugs that attenuate the immune response include penicillamine, gold and chloroquine. These drugs are used in an attempt to modify disease progression in patients with severe rheumatoid arthritis (see Chapter 25).

CHEMICAL MEDIATORS OF THE IMMUNE RESPONSE AND DRUGS THAT BLOCK THEIR ACTIONS

An alternative method of modifying the immune response is to block the release or action of chemical mediators that play an important part in certain immune reactions, especially type-I hypersensitivity. There are several pharmacologically active mediators, and their relative importance differs between species. In humans, histamine is important, although not exclusively so.

HISTAMINE

Histamine is widely distributed in the body and is derived from the decarboxylation of histidine. It is concentrated in mast-cell and basophil granules. The highest concentrations are found in the lung, nasal mucous membrane, skin, stomach and duodenum (i.e. at interfaces between the body and the outside environment). Histamine is liberated by several basic drugs (usually when these are given in large quantities intravenously), including tubocurarine, morphine, codeine, pethidine, vancomycin and suramin. The physiological role of this potent amine is uncertain. It may function as a local controller of vascular responses, particularly in the skin, where it is concerned with response to injury. There is also evidence of its involvement in neuronal transmission in the brain. Its main functions appear to be the release of gastric acid (see Chapter 33) and as part mediator of the allergic response. There are two main types of histamine receptors, namely H_1 and H_2.

H_1-RECEPTORS

In humans, stimulation of H_1-receptors causes dilatation of small arteries and capillaries, together with increased permeability, which leads to formation of oedema. Histamine induces vascular endothelium to release nitric oxide, which stimulates guanylate cyclase to produce cGMP which in turn causes vasodilatation. Inhaled histamine induces bronchospasm (causing smooth muscle contraction, via H_1-receptors) in sensitive individuals, and helps to assess the efficacy of drugs used for bronchodilatation and prophylaxis in asthmatics. In fetal vessels (e.g. the umbilical artery) histamine causes vasoconstriction. If it is injected into the skin, histamine produces the characteristic triple response which consists, in order of appearance, of a *localized red spot* (due to capillary dilatation), then a *larger flush or flare* (due to arteriolar dilatation via an axon-reflex mechanism), and finally a *wheal* (localized oedema subsequent to increased vessel permeability). Local injection of histamine causes itching and sometimes pain due to stimulation of peripheral nerves.

H_2- AND H_3-RECEPTORS

H_2-receptors are principally concerned with the stimulation of gastric acid release (see Chapter 33). Their contribution to most vascular responses is minor, but some (e.g. in the pulmonary vasculature) are H_2-receptor mediated. H_3-receptors may have negative modulatory effects on gastric secretions and be involved in neurotransmission.

Hypersensitivity reactions involving histamine release

ANAPHYLACTIC SHOCK (ACUTE ANAPHYLAXIS)

In certain circumstances, injection of an antigen is followed by the production of reaginic IgE antibodies. These coat mast cells and basophils, and further exposure to the antigen results in rapid degranulation with release of histamine and other mediators, including tachykinins, prostaglandin D_2 and leukotrienes. Clinically the patient presents a picture of shock and collapse with hypotension, bronchospasm and oropharyngeal-laryngeal oedema, often accompanied by urticaria and flushing. A similar so-called 'anaphylactoid reaction' may occur after the non-immune-generated release of mediators by X-ray contrast media.

ATOPY

Some individuals with a hereditary atopic diathesis have a propensity to develop local allergic reactions if exposed to appropriate antigens, causing hay fever, allergic asthma or urticaria. This is due to antigen combining with mast-cell-associated IgE in the mucosa of the respiratory tract or the skin.

SERUM SICKNESS

See section on type-III hypersensitivity reaction above.

DRUGS THAT BLOCK THE EFFECTS OF MEDIATORS OF ALLERGY

Possible therapeutic approaches to the management of allergic disease produced by mediators include the following:

1 inhibition of their biosynthesis;
2 blocking of their release;
3 antagonism of their effects.

(A) INHIBITION OF BIOSYNTHESIS OF MEDIATORS

Intranasal and topical glucocorticosteroids

See Chapters 32 and 39.

USES

These preparations are used in the therapy of allergic rhinitis, and they are very effective in reducing the symptoms of nasal itching, sneezing, rhinorrhoea and nasal obstruction (they are more effective than cromoglycate or its analogues). Common agents used to treat hay fever include the following:

1 **beclomethasone diproprionate** – dose 50–100 μg to each nostril twice daily;
2 **budesonide** – dose 200 μg to each nostril once daily;
3 **flunisolide** – dose 50 μg to each nostril tds;
4 **fluticasone diproprionate** – 100 μg to each nostril once daily (50 μg for children).

ADVERSE EFFECTS

The adverse effects of all these preparations are similar, namely sneezing, and dryness and irritation of the nose and throat. Occasionally epistaxis is a problem. It is claimed that the systemic absorption of **fluticasone** is least, and therefore that the likelihood of systemic side-effects is lowest with this drug. However, this has not yet been clearly proven for the intranasal route.

(B) BLOCKADE OF RELEASE OF MEDIATORS

Sodium cromoglycate and nedocromil sodium

See Chapter 32.

USES

Sodium cromoglycate and nedocromil are effective in preventing attacks of asthma, and are also effective in preventing hay fever and its symptoms. Cromoglycate is used as 2% nasal or eye drops for allergic rhinitis and conjunctivitis. Local adverse effects include occasional nasal irritation or transient stinging in the eye.

(c) Antagonism of the effects of mediators

Antihistamines

There are a large number of antihistamines (H_1-receptor antagonists) available, several of which are available without prescription. Some of those in common use are listed in Table 49.3. Their antihistaminic actions are similar when used in clinically appropriate dosage, but their major differences are in duration of effect, degree of sedation and anti-emetic potential.

USES

Antihistamines are widely used to treat hypersensitivity reactions, and are most effective in some types of urticaria and hay fever. They are less useful for treating anaphylactic shock. They help to reduce laryngeal oedema, which is occasionally dangerous in anaphylaxis, but their onset of action is slow, so **epinephrine** (**adrenaline**), which is more rapidly effective, is used as the first-line drug. Antihistamines are useful if given promptly and systemically in preventing excessive reactions to bee and wasp stings, which both contain histamine and trigger its release. The older antihistamines, combined with sympathomimetics, have been available in non-prescription formulations for treating nasal stuffiness associated with viral upper respiratory tract infections for many years. Local application as a cream is liable to lead to contact dermatitis.

Antihistamines have not proved to be clinically useful in the treatment of asthma, probably because other mediators are overridingly important in this disease. Antihistamines are used for their central sedative actions, particularly in the prevention of motion sickness (e.g. **cyclizine**). Antihistamines are also used, despite lack of evidence of their efficacy, in the symptomatic treatment of the common cold and viral sinusitis. They are used in various cough mixtures, where their sedative action plays a role. Sedation is often a problem with the older (first-generation) antihistamines, particularly if they are taken regularly. Several antihistamines have been introduced with little if any central effect (e.g. **astemizole**, **cetirizine**; see Table 49.3). They are more expensive, but are indicated in patients who find sedation a problem. *Some of these agents are available over the*

Table 49.3: Properties of some commonly used H_1-antagonists

Drug	Duration of effect (h)	Degree of sedation	Anti-emetic action	Usual dose (mg)	Risk of ventricular tachycardia when prescribed with other drugs inhibiting their metabolism
First generation					
Promethazine	20	Marked	Some	10–25	?
Diphenhydramine	6	Some	Little	50	?
Chlorpheniramine	4–6	Moderate	Little	4	?
Cyclizine	6	Some	Marked	50	?
Triprolidine (slow release)	24	Moderate	Little	10	?
Second generation					
Acrivastine	6–8	Nil	Little	8	None
Terfenadine	12	Nil	Little	60	High – now prescription only
Fexofenadine	12	Nil	Little	60	None (active metabolite of terfenadine)
Astemizole	24	Nil	Little	10	High
Cetirizine	24	Nil	Little	10	None
Loratidine	24	Nil	Little	10	None

counter, but there is concern that certain agents (e.g. terfenadine is now not available but astemizole is) may produce an unusual form of ventricular tachycardia (torsades de pointes) *in patients who overdose on them, who take other drugs concomitantly that inhibit their metabolism (macrolides, azoles, etc.), or who are predisposed by virtue of a long QT interval.* This can be inherited (Ward–Romano syndrome, a rare disorder) or acquired with the use of class III anti-arrhythmic drugs such as amiodarone or sotalol (see Chapter 31) and some other drugs (e.g. probucol; see Chapter 26).

MECHANISM OF ACTION

Antihistamines are competitive antagonists of histamine at H_1-receptors. They are effective in blocking the oedema and vascular response to histamine, but not in improving a shocked state. Although they block bronchoconstrictor responses to histamine *in vitro*, they have little effect on bronchoconstriction in asthmatics *in vivo*. *Most of the first generation H_1-antagonists have some central sedative action. Their use with alcohol, benzodiazepines or other central depressant drugs produces additive or synergistic CNS depressant effects.* Most of these drugs also have some anti-emetic effects, which may be clinically useful (see Chapter 33). Additional antimuscarinic effects result in drying of secretions (cf. atropine), which may contribute to their efficacy in allergic rhinitis.

PHARMACOKINETICS

Antihistamines are rapidly absorbed from the intestine, and are effective within about 30 min. They generally undergo hepatic metabolism. Newer agents such as **fexofenadine**, **cetirizine** and **loratidine** have half-lives of 12–24 h. **Astemizole** has a $t_{\frac{1}{2}}$ of 19 h, a slow onset of action and binds almost irreversibly to H_1-receptors. These newer agents do not penetrate the blood–brain barrier very well, and so cause less psychomotor impairment than earlier antihistamines.

ADVERSE EFFECTS

These include the following:

1 sedation and psychomotor impairment, especially with older (first-generation) agents;
2 nausea;
3 photosensitivity rashes;
4 antimuscarinic effects – dry mouth, blurred vision, etc.; (first generation agents)
5 *prolongation of the QT interval, which may in overdose or when given with another drug that blocks metabolism (e.g. ketoconazole, erythromycin) cause* torsades de pointes.

CONTRAINDICATIONS

Antihistamines should be avoided in porphyria and in the Ward–Romano syndrome (congenital long-QT syndrome).

Key points

Antihistamines and therapy of allergic disorders

- Antagonists at H_1-receptors; widely available agents, often without prescription (e.g. chlorpheniramine).
- Used to treat hay fever and urticaria, and also used as therapy for motion sickness.
- Should not be applied topically for skin irritation, as they cause dermatitis.
- Hepatically metabolized (cytochrome $P_{450\ 3A4}$ – long- and shorter-acting drugs.
- Duration of effects often outlasts their presence in the blood.
- First-generation agents are shorter acting (e.g. chlorpheniramine), sedating and anticholinergic, better anti-emetics, and have some 5HT and α-adrenoreceptor antagonist activity.
- Second-generation agents have few or no sedative or ancilliary properties, and are longer acting (e.g. cetirizine).
- Astemizole, if prescribed with erythromycin or ketoconazole, causes prolonged QTc which can lead to ventricular tachycardia.
- Newer agents (e.g. **cetirizine**, **loratidine**) are safe (i.e. ventricular tachycardia is not a risk) if co-prescribed with macrolides or azoles.

Epinephrine (adrenaline)

Epinephrine (adrenaline) is uniquely valuable therapeutically as an effective antagonist of the acute anaphylactic reaction. Its rapid action may be life-saving in general anaphylaxis due to insect venom allergy and reaction to drugs. The usual dose is 0.5–1.0 mL of a 1:1000 solution (0.5–1.0 mg), repeated after 10 min if necessary, given intramuscularly or if necessary intravenously. It is effective by virtue of its α-agonist activity which reverses vascular dilatation and oedema, and its

β_2-agonist activity which produces bronchodilatation. It also reduces the release of pro-inflammatory mediators and cytokines.

Treatment of anaphylactic shock

1 Stop any drug or blood that is being administered intravenously, and lay the patient flat.
2 Give epinephrine (adrenaline), 0.5–1.0 mg intramuscularly (it may have to be given intravenously, with appropriate monitoring, if the patient has a blood pressure of <70 mmHg), and repeat after 10 min if there is no improvement.
3 Give intravenous colloid.
4 Administer 100% oxygen (i.e. an inspired oxygen concentration of 40–60%).
5 Give hydrocortisone, 100–200mg intravenously.
6 Give antihistamine intravenously (e.g. chlorpheniramine 12.5 mg).
7 Consider giving nebulized salbutamol, 5 mg, or intravenous aminophylline, 250 mg over 20–30 min, for residual bronchospasm.

Key points

Treatment of anaphylactic shock

Anaphylactic shock is a medical emergency, and its treatment is as follows.

- Stop the offending drug or blood/blood-product infusion.
- Check the patient's blood pressure (lie them flat) and check for the presence of stridor/bronchospasm.
- Administer oxygen (FiO_2 40–60%).
- Administer epinephrine (adrenaline) 0.5–1 mg intramuscularly, and repeat after 10 min if necessary.
- Give intravenous colloids for refractory hypotension.
- Administer hydrocortisone, 100–200 mg IV.
- Administer chlonpheniramine, 12.5 mg IV.
- Give nebulized salbutamol, 5 mg (or IV aminophylline) for refractory bronchospasm.

Therapy of allergic rhinitis (hay fever)

The patient who presents with symptoms of allergic rhinitis should be assessed to ensure that infection is not the primary problem. If infection is the cause, the presence of a foreign body should be excluded and appropriate antibacterial therapy prescribed. If the symptoms are due to allergy, the first step in therapy is allergen avoidance and minimization of exposure (e.g. to ragweed pollen). However, complete avoidance is difficult to achieve. For patients with mild intermittent symptoms, either intranasal antihistamine (e.g. azelastine 0.1% 1–2 sprays per nostril twice a day or intranasal 2% cromoglycate, 1 spray 3–4 times a day) or a shorter-acting non-sedating antihistamine (e.g. **acrivastine** or **fexofenadine**) is effective. Short-term use of a nasal decongestant such as pseudoephedrine is effective, but if used for longer periods causes rebound vasomotor rhinitis. **Ipratropium bromide** (20–40 μg applied to each nostril three times a day) is added if rhinorrhoea is the predominant symptom. If symptoms are more chronic, the first-line therapy is intranasal glucocorticosteroids because these are effective against all symptoms, and are more effective than antihistamines or cromoglycate. In children, topical cromoglycate given by insufflator (10 mg into each nostril qds) or nasal spray (one spray – 2.6 mg per nostril two to four times a day) is useful. If rhinorrhoea is the main problem, ipratropium bromide may be added with or without a long-acting antihistamine (e.g. cetirizine 10 mg daily). If these measures are ineffective, consider low-dose

Key points

Anaphylaxis and anaphylactoid reactions

- Anaphylaxis:
  - is IgE-mediated hypersensitivity (type-1) that occurs in a previously sensitized individual;
  - its pathophysiology is major cardiovascular and respiratory dysfunction due to vasoactive mediator release from mast cells;
  - common causes are penicillins, cephalosporins and many other drugs, insect stings and food allergies (e.g. strawberries, fish).
- Anaphylactoid reactions:
  - are due to dose-related pharmacologically induced mediator release from mast cells and basophils;
  - common causes include aspirin, NSAIDs and radiographic contrast media.

intranasal steroids, or immunotherapy or surgery if there is evidence of sinusitis.

DRUGS THAT ENHANCE IMMUNE SYSTEM FUNCTION

ADJUVANTS

Adjuvants non-specifically augment the immune response when mixed with antigen or injected into the same site. This is achieved in the following ways:

1 release of the antigen is slowed and exposure to it is prolonged;
2 various immune cells are attracted to the site of injection, and the interaction between such cells is important in antibody formation.

There are a number of such substances, usually given as mixtures and often containing lipids, extracts of inactivated tubercle bacilli and various mineral salts.

IMMUNOSTIMULANTS

Immunostimulants non-specifically enhance immune responses, examples including Bacille Calmette-Guérin (BCG) or killed *Corynebacterium parvum*.

Levamisole

Originally developed as an anthelminthic, **levamisole** stimulates immune responses against infection and neoplasia in animal models. However its clinical efficacy in humans has not been clearly proven, but it is used in combination chemotherapy for some tumours, (e.g. with 5-fluorouracil in colonic carcinoma). It is given orally at 2.5 mg/kg daily for 3 days every 2 weeks. Levamisole is thought to stimulate macrophages and T-helper lymphocytes and restore depressed lymphocyte function. The oral absorption of levamisole is good (> 95%), and its plasma $t_{\frac{1}{2}}$ is 4–6 h. The major route of clearance is via extensive and rapid hepatic metabolism. The major adverse effects are agranulocytosis (particularly if given to patients with ankylosing spondylitis (i.e. HLA-B27 genotype), rashes, and disturbances of taste and smell.

Interleukin-2

Interleukin-2 (IL-2) is a 15 420-dalton peptide with 133 amino acids that is normally produced by T- helper lymphocytes. Human recombinant IL-2 is now available. IL-2 stimulates T-cells and cytotoxic lymphocytes to proliferate. It has activity against renal carcinoma, and has been used *ex vivo* to stimulate lymphocytes into lymphokine-activated killer cells which, when injected back into the patient, lyse tumours in a non-antigen-specific manner. IL-2 can be administered by intravenous bolus or continuous infusion, the latter resulting in less toxicity. It disappears from the plasma in a biphasic manner with a $t_{\frac{1}{2}\alpha}$ of 6–7 min, during which phase most of the IL-2 is cleared, and a $t_{\frac{1}{2}\beta}$ of approximately 70 min. Its major adverse effects are fluid overload and fluid retention due to cytokine-mediated vascular leakage. This can cause life-threatening pulmonary oedema (the mechanism underlying this may be the effect of IL-2 on activating endothelial cells), fever and chills.

VACCINES

IMMUNOLOGY AND GENERAL USE

Vaccines stimulate the production of protective antibodies and other full medicated components of the immune response. They consist of the following:

1 either an attenuated form of the infectious agent, such as the live vaccines used against some viral infections (e.g. rubella, measles, polio), or BCG used against tuberculosis;
2 inactivated preparations of the virus (e.g influenza virus) or bacteria (e.g. typhoid vaccine);
3 extracts of or detoxified exotoxins produced by a micro-organism (e.g. tetanus vaccine).

Live vaccine immunization is generally achieved with a single dose, but three doses are required for oral polio (which has different strains). Live vaccine replicates while in the body and produces protracted immunity, albeit not as long as that acquired after natural infection. When two live vaccines are required (and are not in a combined preparation) they may be given at different sites simultaneously or at an interval of at least 3 weeks. Inactivated vaccines usually require a primary series of doses of vaccine to produce an adequate antibody response. Booster injections are required at intervals. The duration of immunity acquired with the use of inactivated vaccines ranges from months to years. The vaccination programmes recommended by the UK Department of Social Security (the DSS in the UK) are described in detail in a memorandum entitled *Immunization against Infectious Disease*, available to doctors from the DSS.

Contraindications

Postpone vaccination if the patient is suffering from acute illness. Ensure that the patient is not sensitive to antibiotics used in the preparation of the vaccine (e.g. neomycin and polymyxin). Egg sensitivity excludes the administration of influenza vaccine (also measles, mumps and rubella (MMR) and yellow fever vaccine) if evidence of previous anaphylaxis is obtained . Live vaccines should not be given to pregnant women, nor should they be given to patients who are immunosuppressed (whether due to drugs, radiotherapy or human immunodeficiency virus-1 (HIV-1) infection). Live vaccines should be postponed until at least 3 months after stopping corticosteroids and 6 months after chemotherapy. Yellow fever, BCG and typhoid (oral) vaccines should not be administered to HIV-1-positive individuals.

> **Key points:**
>
> Vaccine therapy
>
> - Vaccines generally stimulate the production of protective antibodies or activated T-cells.
> - Vaccines consist of:
>   attenuated infectious agents – antiviral vaccines (e.g. mumps, rubella, etc.).
>   inactivated viral/bacterial preparations (e.g. influenza virus or typhoid vaccine).
>   extracts of detoxified toxins (e.g. tetanus toxin).
> - Live vaccines produce protracted immunity, and some (e.g. measles and mumps vaccines) have a low risk of causing a mild form of the disease.
> - Different countries have different vaccination schedules based on the prevalence of the disease in the population and the level of herd immunity.
> - Research into anti-HIV and anti-cancer vaccines continues to make progress.

Immunoglobulins as therapy

Immunoglobulin injection gives immediate passive protection for 4–6 weeks. Recombinant technology will yield a greater source of antibodies of consistent quality in the future, so their importance may increase. Currently there are two types of immunoglobulin, namely normal immunoglobulin and specific immunoglobulin.

Human normal immunoglobulin

Human normal immunoglobulin (HNIG) is prepared from pooled donations of human plasma. It contains antibodies to measles, mumps, varicella and hepatitis A, and other viruses.

Uses

HNIG is used to protect susceptible subjects from infection with hepatitis A and measles and, to a lesser extent, to protect the fetus against rubella in pregnancy when termination is not an option. It is given intramuscularly at doses in the range 0.02–0.12 mL/kg for hepatitis A. For measles, 0.2 mL/kg is given, and for prevention of a clinical attack of rubella in pregnancy 20 mL are used (serological follow-up for rubella prophylaxis is essential). Special formulations for intravenous administration are available for replacement therapy in agammaglobulinaemia, hypogammaglobulinaemia and IgG subclass deficiency (e.g. Bruton's agammaglobulinaemia, Wiskott–Aldrich syndrome), idiopathic thrombocytopenic purpura and for prophylaxis of infection in bone-marrow-transplant patients.

Adverse effects

The commonest adverse effects occur during the first infusion and are dependent on the antigenic load (dose) given. They include the following:

Table 49.4: Common vaccines, their dose regimens and major adverse effects

Vaccine	Dose and regimen	Use	Adverse effects
BCG vaccine Live attenuated *Mycobacterium bovis*	0.1 mL intradermal injection for at-risk groups; 80% effective in providing immunity	Exposed patients: children entering school who are Heaf negative	Ulceration to subcutaneous abscess due to poor injection technique
Cholera vaccine Heat-killed *Vibrio cholerae*	0.5 mL by deep intramuscular or subcutaneous injection	Individuals due to travel in endemic countries	–
DTP vaccine Diphtheria formol toxoid, tetanus formol toxoid and live attenuated pertussis vaccine (DTP)	0.5 mL by deep intramuscular or subcutaneous injection at 3 and 6 months	Childhood vaccination schedule	Adverse reaction to pertussis, local induration/inflammation at site. Fever, convulsions, anaphylaxis, wheeze, laryngeal oedema, collapse within 48 h of injection
Haemophilus b vaccine A conjugated bacterial polysaccharide	Given as a 0.5 mL deep subcutaneous or intramuscular injection. For primary immunity it is given as three doses at monthly intervals	Children who are less than 2 months old or 2–14 months of age	–
Hepatitis A vaccine Formaldehyde inactivated hepatitis virus	Two 1-mL intramuscular injections 1 month apart	Vaccination should be considered for those travelling to endemic areas	Transient soreness, erythema at the injection site. Rarely an influenza-like syndrome
Hepatitis B vaccine Recombinant Hb, Ag made biosynthetically	Three 1-mL doses given intramuscularly into the deltoid; the second dose is 1 month after the first, and the third dose 3 months later	High-risk groups (e.g. health personnel, haemophiliacs)	–
Influenza vaccine Inactivated influenza vaccine of surface antigen or split virion (always N and H antigens of prevalent strain)	0.5 mL deep subcutaneous or intra-muscular injection. In children repeated once in 4–6 weeks	Patients with chronic cardiac, renal and pulmonary conditions, diabetics, immunosuppressed and the elderly	Contraindicated in individuals allergic to eggs

Table 49.4: Continued

Vaccine	Dose and regimen	Use	Adverse effects
MMR vaccine			
Live mumps, measles and rubella	0.5 mL by deep subcutaneous or intramuscular injection	All children before entry to primary school, and rubella for females <13 years of age if seronegative	Fever and rash, parotid swelling. Contraindicated in egg-allergic patients and the immunosuppressed
Meningoccal polysaccharide vaccine			
From groups A and C	0.5 mL by deep subcutaneous or intramuscular injection	Adults and children aged over 2 months during epidemics, and travellers going to areas with high incidence of meningococcal carriage	–
Pneumococcal vaccine			
23 subtypes of pneumococcal capsule	0.5 mL by subcutaneous or intramuscular injection	Patients, e.g. splenectomized, at risk of pneumococcal infection	Hypersensitivity reactions may occur
Poliomyelitis vaccine			
Live attenuated virus (Sabin) or inactivated (Salk)	Live vaccine of attenuated strains 1, 2 and 3 as oral suspension. Inactivated suspension as 0.5 mL injection. Three doses are required for primary immunization	Childhood immunization schedule	Rarely (1 per 2×10^6 doses) the subject or a contact of a vaccinee develops a mild form of the disease
Smallpox vaccine			
Live vaccine attenuated	0.5 mL injected subcutaneously	Workers with smallpox virus. Travellers do not need it as it has been eradicated globally	–
Typhoid vaccine			
Whole live vaccine (killed bacteria), polysaccharide vaccine and oral attenuated vaccine	0.5 mL by deep subcutaneous or intramuscular injection. Oral – three capsules on alternate days	Travellers and during epidemics. Oral vaccine inactivated by sulphonamides, which must be avoided	Local reactions, fever, malaise, headache

Case history

A 35-year-old woman had a cadaveric renal transplant for polycystic kidneys 2 years previously and was stable on her immunosuppressive regimen of cyclosporin, 300 mg bd, and mycophenolate mofetil, 1 g bd. Her usual trough cyclosporin concentrations were 200–250 μg/L and her hepatic and liver function was normal. She went on holiday to San Diego in Southern California for 10 days, where she was well, but drank plenty of fluids (but no alcohol) as she was warned about the dangers of dehydration. By the end of her visit she noted some nausea and a mild tremor. Following a long return flight she went to her local hospital and sustained a spontaneously remitting epileptic fit in the out-patient department where she was having her blood cyclosporin concentration checked. The fit lasted about 1 min and she was taken to casualty. Examination revealed no abnormalities apart from slight tremor which she said she had noticed for the last 48 h. Her cyclosporin concentration was 550 μg /L. All other medical biochemistry was normal, including liver function tests and renal function. She adamantly denied taking any prescribed medications or over-the-counter drugs.

Questions

What caused this patient's seizures? How can you explain the markedly toxic trough cyclosporin concentration?

Answer:

In this patient the development of an acute epileptic seizure in the context of a very high cyclosporin trough concentration suggests that her acute CNS dysfunction is most probably due to cyclosporin toxicity; epilepsy is a well-recognized toxic effect of high cyclosporin concentrations. The difficult issue in the case is why she developed high cyclosporin blood concentrations (in the face of normal renal and hepatic function) when she was adamant that there had been no alteration in the daily dose of cyclosporin she was taking, nor had she started any other agents (prescribed or over-the-counter-drugs). When questioned more closely about what she had been drinking in California, she said mainly fruit juices and bottled water. When asked more specifically about this, she admitted that she was drinking about 1 L/day of grapefruit juice – a taste she had acquired while on holiday! Here was the answer – grapefruit juice contains psoralens and flavones such as navingenin which inhibit the drug-metabolizing cytochrome $P_{450\ 3A4}$ enzyme (gastrointestinal and hepatic) and increase the bioavailability of cyclosporin by 19–60%, thus leading to higher concentrations without a change in dose. (Vitamin E – α-tocopherol – can also increase cyclosporin AUC by 30%, although the mechanism involved is still unclear). The patient had her cyclosporin dosing withheld until the concentration was < 300 μg/L. She had no further fits, her nausea and tremor subsided, and she was then restarted on her normal dose *with clear instructions not to drink grapefruit juice.*

Other drugs whose metabolism is reduced and or/bioavailability increased in humans with co-ingestion of *grapefruit juice* include midazolam, oestrogens, testosterone, felodipine, nifedipine (*but not diltiazem*), terfenadine (no longer OTC) and some anti-HIV protease inhibitors. Patients who are taking these agents or other drugs metabolized by cytochrome $P_{450\ 3A4}$, should be warned *not to ingest even single cupfuls of grapefruit juice*, as this may precipitate toxic drug concentrations.

1 Fever, chills and rarely anaphylaxis – most commonly seen with the first dose, and reduced by slow administration and premedication with antihistamines and glucocorticosteroids;
2 increased plasma viscosity – caution is needed in patients with ischaemic heart disease;
3 aseptic meningitis (high dose).

CONTRAINDICATIONS

Normal immunoglobulin is contraindicated in patients with known class-specific antibody to IgA.

DRUG INTERACTIONS

Live virus vaccinations may be rendered less effective.

Specific immunoglobulins

These antibodies are prepared by pooling the plasma of selected donors with high levels of the specific antibody required. The following are currently available and effective: rabies immunoglobulin; tetanus immunoglobulin (human origin – **HTIG**); varicella zoster immunoglobulin (**VZIG**) (limited supply); **anti-CMV** immunoglobulin (on a named patient basis).

Anti-D (rho) immunoglobulin

This immunoglobulin is used to prevent a rhesus-negative mother from forming antibodies to fetal rhesus-positive cells that enter the maternal circulation during childbirth or abortion. An intramuscular injection of 500–5000 units is given to rhesus-negative mothers up to 72 h after the birth/abortion. This prevents a subsequent child from developing haemolytic disease of the newborn.

Further reading

de Mattos AM, Olyaei AJ, Bennett WM. 1996: Pharmacology of immunosuppressive medications used in renal disease and transplantation. *American Journal of Kidney Diseases* **28**, 631–7.

Dertzbaugh MT. 1998: Genetically engineered vaccines: an overview. *Plasmid* **39,** 100–13.

Heilman CA, Baltimore D. 1998: HIV vaccines – where are we going? *Nature Medicine* **4, (Suppl. 5**) 532–4.

Lipsky JJ. 1996: Drug profile. Mycophenolate mofetil. *Lancet* **348**, 1357–9.

Simons ERF, Simons KJ. 1994: Drug therapy: the pharmacology and use of H_1-receptor antagonist drugs. *New England Journal of Medicine* **330**, 1663–70.

PART XII

THE SKIN

CHAPTER FIFTY

DRUGS *and the* SKIN

- Introduction
- Acne
- Alopecia and hirsutism
- Dermatitis
- Psoriasis
- Urticaria
- Superficial bacterial skin infections
- Fungal skin and nail infections
- Viral skin infections
- Treatment of other skin infections (lice, scabies)
- Adverse drug reactions involving the skin
- Prospects for skin therapy

INTRODUCTION

Skin conditions account for up to 2% of consultations in general practice. The ability of the practitioner to make a correct diagnosis is paramount, and is aided by the ease of biopsy of the abnormal tissue. The non-specific use of drugs which can modify the appearance of skin lesions (e.g. potent topical corticosteroids) should be avoided in the absence of a diagnosis. Adverse reactions to topical or systemic drugs produce a wide variety of skin lesions. Drugs applied topically to the skin may act locally and/or enter the systemic circulation and produce either a harmful or beneficial systemic pharmacological effect. Further details of transdermal drug absorption/delivery are discussed in Chapter 4.

ACNE

INCIDENCE AND PATHOPHYSIOLOGY

Acne vulgaris is one of the commonest skin disorders seen by physicians, occurring in 80–90% of adolescents. It is associated with *Propionibacterium acnes* infection of the sebaceous glands of the skin, and causes inflammatory papules, pustules, nodules, cysts and scarring, mainly on the face, chest, back and arms.

PRINCIPLES OF TREATMENT

The efficacy of abrasive agents is uncertain, but the topical use of keratolytic (peeling) agents such as **benzoyl peroxide** (2–5% solution applied twice daily) or **retinoic acid** (tretinoin) on a regular basis in conjunction with systemic antibiotic therapy is successful in the majority of cases. The main side-effect of keratolytic agents is skin irritation. Because of the powerful teratogenic effects of oral vitamin A analogues, there has been concern about the safety of topical retinoic acid derivatives in the first trimester of pregnancy. However, a large study from the USA has shown that topical retinoic acid is not associated with an increased risk of major congenital abnormalities. Suitable antibiotic treatment (see Chapter 42) includes **oxytetracycline** (250 mg three times a day for 1–4 weeks, reducing to twice daily until improvement occurs, which may take several months), **minocycline** (50 mg twice daily for 6 weeks) or **erythromycin** (250 mg three times a day for 1-4 weeks, reducing to twice daily until improvement occurs, which may take several months). Oxytetracycline and minocycline should not be used until the secondary dentition is established (i.e. after the age of 12 years). Pseudomembranous colitis has occurred in patients on long-term tetracyclines for acne, as has the development of microbial resistance. Minocycline can cause cerebellar ataxia and may rarely cause fever, joint pain and hepatic dysfunction. Topical antibiotic preparations (e.g. **tetracycline** or **clindamycin**) are less effective than systemic therapy, but may help those who are intolerant of peeling agents. **Azelaic acid** (20% cream applied twice daily) is a natural product of *Pityrosporum ovale*, and has both antibacterial and anti-keratinizing activity. When compared to other topical therapies for treating mild acne it was found to be equi-effective, but not as effective as oral isotretinoin for severe acne. Side-effects include skin irritation and photosensitivity. The treatment period should not exceed 6 months.

For patients with disease that is refractory to these therapies, the use of either low-dose anti-androgens or isotretinoin (see below) should be considered, but only under the supervision of a consultant dermatologist.

Hormonal therapy of acne

Acne depends on the actions of androgens on the sebaceous glands. Hormone manipulation is often successful in women with acne that is refractory to antibiotics, and is useful in patients who require contraception, which is essential because of the potential for feminizing a male fetus. **Cyproterone acetate**, 2 mg daily is an anti-androgen with central and peripheral activity, and is combined with low-dose oestrogen, **ethinylestradiol**. Therapies currently undergoing investigation include synthetic peptide analogues of gonadotrophin-releasing hormone (e.g. goserelin see Chapter 41).

Retinoid therapy in acne

The management of severe acne has changed dramatically with the advent of the synthetic vitamin A analogues.

Isotretinoin

USES

Isotretinoin is the D-isomer of tretinoin, another vitamin A analogue. It is used for severe acne or rosacea, and should only be prescribed under hospital supervision. The usual dose is 0.5-1 mg/kg in one or two divided doses with food. Topical isoretinoin (0.05% gel) or tretinoin (0.025% gel or lotion) applied twice daily are effective alternatives. The usual course is 4 months, with 80% improvement. Clinical benefit continues after discontinuation of therapy.

MECHANISM OF ACTION

The primary action of retinoids is inhibition of sebum production, reducing the size of the sebaceous glands by 90% in the first month. These drugs also inhibit keratinization of the hair follicle, resulting in reduced comedones.

ADVERSE EFFECTS

These include the following:

1. teratogenic effects;
2. mucocutaneous effects – cheilitis, dry mouth, epistaxis, dermatitis, desquamation, hair and nail loss;
3. CNS effects – ocular (papilloedema, night blindness), raised intracranial pressure;
4. musculoskeletal effects – arthralgia, muscle stiffness, skeletal hyperostosis, premature fusion of epiphyses;
5. hepatotoxic effects;
6. hypertriglyceridaemia.

CONTRAINDICATIONS

Systemic use of any vitamin A analogue is contraindicated in pregnant or breast-feeding women.

PHARMACOKINETICS

Isotretinoin is well absorbed (> 90%), and its bioavailability is increased by taking it with meals. The plasma $t_{\frac{1}{2}}$ is 10–20 h. It has a large volume of distribution and is highly bound (99.5%) to plasma protein. Tissue binding is high, and it is eliminated over a period of at least 1 month after treatment has been discontinued. This explains the ongoing clinical benefit after stopping drug therapy, and also the persistent risk of teratogenicity after a course of treatment. Isotretinoin is almost totally cleared from the body by hepatic metabolism.

DRUG INTERACTIONS

There is an increased incidence of raised intracranial pressure if isotretinoin is prescribed with tetracyclines.

Key points

Acne

- Common in adolescence; the face, back, chest and arms are mainly affected.
- Keratolytics (peeling agents) are first-line therapy (e.g. 2–6% salicylic acid or azelaic acid (20%) creams).
- If systemic antibiotics are indicated, use oral oxytetracycline or erythromycin.
- Do not use tetracyclines in children under 12 years of age (adverse effects on maturing dentition).
- In adults, tetracyclines are preferred to erythromycin (they reduce developing resistance to macrolides).
- *Propionibacterium acnes* drug resistance is developing (possibly up to 40% in hospital patients).
- Vitamin A analogues (topical or systemic isotretinoin) should only used in refractory cases.

Alopecia and hirsutism

In androgenic baldness it is possible to promote hair growth by twice daily topical application of **minoxidil sulphate** (the active metabolite of minoxidil) as a 2% solution to the scalp. This is believed to have a mitogenic effect on the hair follicles. Adverse effects include local itching and dermatitis. Approximately 30% of subjects respond within 4–12 months, but hair loss recurs once therapy is discontinued. In women, cyproterone acetate combined with ethinyl oestradiol prevents the progression of androgenic alopecia.

The anti-androgen activity (both central and peripheral) of cyproterone acetate makes it the systemic drug of choice for female hirsutism, if topical depilation has failed or the hirsutism is too general. It is given as a single 2 mg daily dose with ethinyloestradiol to prevent pregnancy (feminization of the fetus). Clinical improvement may take 6–12 months.

Dermatitis

Principles of treatment

The most common forms of dermatitis that present to physicians are atopic dermatitis, synonymous with atopic eczema, seborrhoeic dermatitis and contact dermatitis.

Management of atopic eczema should include both avoidance of trigger factors and the use of emollients. Dry skin is a major factor, and emollients should be used when bathing and applied as often as necessary. Aqueous cream or emulsifying ointment are usually all that is necessary for dry, fissured scaly lesions. Inflammation should be treated with short courses of mild to moderate topical corticosteroids. A more potent corticosteroid may be required for particularly severely affected areas or for more general flare-ups. Oral antihistamines are often effective in reducing pruritus. Ichthammol and zinc cream may be used in chronic lichenified forms of eczema. Weeping eczema requires topical corticosteroids and often antibiotics to treat secondary infection. There is little evidence that the essential fatty acid, gamolenic acid, is of value. Immunosuppressant therapy such as cyclosporin is sometimes effective in severe, resistant eczema. Ultraviolet B or psoralens plus ultraviolet A, or azathioprine are also sometimes used in these patients.

Seborrhoeic dermatitis may respond to a mild topical corticosteroid or to a topical antifungal cream (e.g. ketoconazole). Lithium succinate and zinc sulphate ointment may also be of benefit, whilst scalp seborrhoeic dermatitis is often improved by cold tar, salicylic acid and sulphur preparations.

Contact dermatitis is caused by external agents (e.g. detergents, solvents, dusts and friction) but often complicates a pre-existing dermatitis. Avoidance of precipitating factors, and the use of protective clothing, emollients and topical corticosteroids are the most common forms of treatment.

Corticosteroids

Topical corticosteroids act as anti-inflammatory vasoconstrictors and reduce keratinocyte proliferation. They include **hydrocortisone** and its fluorinated semi-synthetic derivatives, which have increased anti-inflammatory potency compared to hydrocortisone (see Chapter 39).

USES

The use of systemic corticosteroids (e.g. oral prednisolone, 60 mg daily) in the treatment of skin diseases is limited to serious disorders such as pemphigus or refractory exfoliative dermatitis (e.g. Stevens–Johnson syndrome). Topical corticosteroids are widely used and effective in treating eczema, lichen planus, discoid lupus erythematosus, lichen simplex chronicus and palmar plantar pustulosis, but rarely in psoriasis. Corticosteroids applied topically to the skin effectively suppress inflammation, cause vasoconstriction and reduce epidermal cell proliferation. The symptoms of eczema are rapidly suppressed, but these drugs do not treat the cause, and are contraindicated in the presence of infection unless they are combined with an appropriate antimicrobial agent. Practitioners should always attempt to use the lowest potency corticosteroid preparation that will control the disease. The formulation is applied sparingly two to three times daily. Quantities appropriate to the area of skin involved should be prescribed. Occlusive dressings should only be used on a short-term basis (2–3 days). In resistant disease, a high-potency steroid should ideally be used for no more than 4 weeks to control the condition before changing to a less potent drug. Potent fluorinated corticosteroids should not be used on the face because they cause dermatitis medicamentosa.

Many preparations are available, some of which are listed in descending order of anti-inflammatory potency in Table 50.1.

ADVERSE EFFECTS OF CUTANEOUSLY APPLIED CORTICOSTEROIDS

These include the following:

1 hypothalamic–pituitary adrenal suppression where very potent drugs are used long term on large areas of skin or when systemic absorption is increased under occlusive dressing;
2 spread of local infection – bacterial or fungal;
3 irreversible striae atrophicae;
4 mild depigmentation and vellus hair formation;
5 perioral dermatitis when applied to the face;
6 rebound exacerbation of disease (e.g. pustular psoriasis);
7 exacerbation of glaucoma if applied to the eyelids;
8 contact dermatitis (rare);
9 hirsutism and acne if systemic absorption is very high.

Key points

Eczema

- Identify the causal agent and minimize/eradicate exposure if possible.
- For dry, scaly eczema, use emollients (e.g. E45 or liquid paraffin mixture creams) plus a keratolytic.
- For wet eczema use drying lotions (e.g. aluminium acetate or calamine) or zinc-medicated bandages.
- Topical corticosteroids are often required, but do not use high-potency corticosteroids on the face.
- Systemic toxicity from topical corticosteroids (especially fluorinated analogues) can be problematic. Therefore use the lowest potency steroid for the shortest time possible required to produce clinical benefit
- Be cognizant that occlusive dressings enhance systemic drug absorption by up to 10-fold; in wet eczema this is already high because of the eroded stratum corneum.

PSORIASIS

Psoriasis occurs in approximately 2% of the population. Its cause is unknown and no treatment is curative. The skin lesions are characterized by epidermal thickening and scaling due to increased epidermal undifferentiated cell proliferation with abnormal keratin. Therapy in mild cases consists of reassurance and a simple emollient cream (e.g. E45, Alpha Keri cream) or oil applied frequently to moisturize the skin. Such preparations should be continued even after improvement is observed. More resistant cases are treated with salicylic acid, coal tar or dithranol applied accurately to the lesions. Topical steroids are reserved for cases that do not respond to these simple remedies, and their use should be monitored by a specialist, as they can worsen the disease in some patients (notably

Table 50.1: Topical corticosteroids and their anti-inflammatory potency

Potency	Drug and strength
Extremely potent	Clobetasol (0.05%) Halcinonide (0.1%) Diflucortolone (0.3%)
Potent	Beclomethasone (0.025%) Budesonide (0.025%) Fluocinolone (0.025%) Fluocinonide (0.05%)
Moderately potent	Clobetasone (0.05%) Flurandrenolone (0.0125%)
Mild	Hydrocortisone (0.5–2.5%) Alclomethasone (0.05%) Methylprednisolone (0.25%)

precipitation of pustular psoriasis on stopping treatment). Calcitriol (a vitamin D analogue) is effective topically. In some cases, therapy with psoralens and ultraviolet A (UV-A) light (PUVA) (see below) is used in combination with good effect. Refractory cases are treated with oral retinoids (e.g. acetretin 25–50 mg/day).

Occasionally refractory cases justify immunosuppression with methotrexate (10–25 mg weekly; see Chapters 25 and 49), but chronic use can cause liver damage, leading insidiously to cirrhosis. Potential recipients need to be warned about this and their liver function must be monitored meticulously. Cyclosporin (see Chapter 49), 3 mg/kg/day, is an alternative, but causes hypertension and nephrotoxicity. Regular monitoring of blood pressure and plasma cyclosporin concentrations is essential. Second-line therapies (phototherapy or systemic drugs) should only be used under the supervision of a dermatologist.

Keratolytics

Keratolytics such as salicylic acid may be helpful. Preparations of 2% salicylate are used initially, applied to the plaque, increasing gradually to 3–6% if necessary. Salicylic acid increases the rate of loss of surface epithelium. Side-effects are few and include excessive drying, irritation, allergic contact sensitivity and, if used on large areas of skin, salicylism.

Dithranol

Dithranol is the most potent coal tar preparation for use against psoriasis. It may usefully be combined with ultraviolet B phototherapy. Short-contact dithranol therapy is effective, and the use of high-concentration dithranol (3–4%) formulated in a cream base and applied to lesions for 1 h and then washed off is more acceptable than older regimens. It is convenient for use at home, is not so messy, is less irritant and produces less staining on the skin and clothes than longer contact therapy.

Calcipotriol or talcalcitol (1-α, 24-dihydroxyvitamin D_3

These analogues of vitamin D_3 (calcitriol) are used as a cream applied to mild to moderate psoriasis. Calcipotriol is applied twice daily and tacalcitol is applied once daily up to a maximum of 100 g weekly for up to 6 weeks. Vitamin D receptors are present in increased numbers in skin keratinocytes, T- and B-lymphocytes and dermal fibroblasts of psoriatics, and the stimulation of vitamin D receptors on keratinocytes inhibits proliferation and differentiation. The adverse effects of these analogues include local irritation, facial and perioral dermatitis (especially with calcipotriol, but less so with talcalcitol), and possible hypercalcaemia and hypertriglyceridaemia if they are used too extensively. They should not be used in pregnancy, and are currently undergoing investigation as combination therapy with other therapies.

Photochemotherapy with UVA and psoralens

Oral psoralen (usually 8-methoxypsoralen) and ultraviolet A light (PUVA) is now a well-established and effective but somewhat inconvenient therapy for chronic plaque psoriasis. Psoralens intercalate DNA bases and, when activated by light, produce highly reactive oxygen species which sensitize the skin to the cytotoxic effects of long-wave UVA (320–400 nm wavelength) radiation. Psoralen is taken 2 h before phototherapy and the usual course lasts for 4–6 weeks. Skin burning and ageing, cataracts and skin cancer are potential complications, especially with the higher total doses of UVA. Sun-glasses are worn during UVA exposure in order to reduce the risk of cataract formation. Technological advances in psoralens and UVA light, notably optimization of the dose regimen, have reduced the risk of carcinogenicity. Combination therapy with retinoids or methotrexate, together with psoralens and UVA, is widely used. In Scandinavia, bathing with psoralens and UVA light has been in regular use for years. Photosensitivity is maximal immediately after the bath, and is about 15 times greater than with oral psoralens; it remains high for 15 min and then declines rapidly. Doses of UVA must be reduced accordingly and the minimum phototoxic dose assessed. Absorption of psoralen from the bath is low, thus obviating the need to wear sun-glasses.

The use of UVB (300–320 nm wavelength) together with coal tar is long established for patients with moderate to severe disease, but has lost favour due to its inconvenience, cost and high relapse rates. The emergence of narrow-band UVB (311-nm) therapy, with early data showing improved efficacy and reduced relapse rates is encouraging.

Retinoids in psoriasis

Acitretin

USES

Acitretin is the active carboxylated metabolite of etretinate. It is given orally for the treatment of severe resistant or complicated psoriasis and other disorders of keratinization. It should only be given under hospital supervision. A therapeutic effect occurs after 2–4 weeks, with maximal benefit after 6 weeks. Because it is highly teratogenic, women must take adequate contraceptive precautions for 1 month prior to and during therapy, and for 2 years after stopping the drug.

MECHANISM OF ACTION

The precise cellular mechanism of action of retinoids is currently being elucidated. Retinoids bind to specific retinoic acid receptors (RARs) in the nucleus. RARs have many actions, one of which is to inhibit AP-1 (transcription factor) activity.

ADVERSE EFFECTS AND CONTRAINDICATIONS

See section on isotretinoin (p. 610).

Acitretin is contraindicated in the presence of hepatic and renal impairment.

PHARMACOKINETICS

Acitretin is well absorbed orally (20–90%), and fatty food enhances its absorption. Unlike its parent compound, etrenitate, acetretin is not highly bound to adipose tissue. Its elimination $t_{\frac{1}{2}}$ is between 2–4 days (shorter than that of its parent drug, etretinate). Hepatic metabolism to etretinate (see Table 50.2) and 13-*cis*-acetretin is the major route of elimination.

DRUG INTERACTIONS

1. Concomitant therapy with tetracycline and corticosteroids increases the risk of raised intracranial pressure.
2. Caution should be exercised when prescribing other drugs that increase serum lipids (e.g. corticosteroids, thiazide diuretics).
3. It increases methotrexate plasma concentrations and the risk of heptotoxicity.
4. It possibly antagonizes the action of warfarin.

Key points

Psoriasis

- Occurs in 1–2% of the population.
- Simple emollients (e.g. E45, Alpha Keri creams or oil applied to the lesions) should be used to treat mild cases.
- Keratolytics such as salicylic acid, dithranol or propylene glycol may be used in moderate cases.
- Additional therapies for such patients or for more severe cases include:
  - topical vitamin D analogues (calcipotriol or tacalcitol (1–α 24–dihydroxy vitamin D_3);
  - narrow-band UV light plus dithranol or psoralens.
- Oral etretinate and acitretin may benefit severe psoriatics, but therapy requires careful supervision.
- Corticosteroids are effective, but tachyphylaxis occurs; on withdrawal, pustular psoriasis may appear.
- In completely refractory psoriasis, methotrexate, cyclosporin, tacrolimus (FK506) and cytokines are very toxic treatments and should only be prescribed by hospital dermatologists.

Table 50.2: Other retinoids currently in use or being developed for the treatment of severe psoriasis

Vitamin A analogue	Major use	Dosing regimen	Pharmacokinetics	Adverse effects and contraindications	Drug interactions
Etretinate	Not available now in the UK, but used in USA for oral therapy for psoriasis	20–50 mg/day	Well absorbed, absorption increased by fat. Hepatic metabolism 80–90% Plasma $t_{\frac{1}{2}}$ 6–13 h, tissue $t_{\frac{1}{2}}$ 80–170 days	See section on isotretinoin	Many (see section on acitretin, plus impaired metabolism of phenobarbitone and phenytoin
Tazarotene	Psoriasis – topical	Once daily application of 0.05–0.1% gels to no more than 20% of the body surface area	Very poorly absorbed via skin, converted to active tazoretinic acid *in vivo*. No tachyphylaxis to its effects	Skin irritation, pruritus, erythema. Not recommended in pregnant women	–

5 If taken with alcohol it is metabolized to etretinate.

Table 50.2 summarizes the data for other retinoids used clinically for the treatment of severe psoriasis.

TOPICAL AND SYSTEMIC CORTICOSTEROIDS

Topical and systemic steroids should only be used in psoriasis under specialist supervision. Although corticosteroids may be effective, subsequent therapy becomes more difficult due to tachyphylaxis, and severe refractory pustular psoriasis may occur during steroid withdrawal.

URTICARIA

Acute urticaria is usually due to a type-1 allergic reaction to an allergen. It may need therapy with adrenaline if associated with anaphylactic shock or laryngeal oedema, but less severe cases respond to an oral antihistamine (e.g. chlorpheniramine or cetirizine). Systemic corticosteroids are needed in severe or refractory cases. Chronic urticaria usually responds to the combination of an oral antihistamine plus an oral β_2-agonist such as salbutamol, 4–8 mg, or terbutaline, 8–16 mg (see Chapter 32), or an H_2-blocker (cimetidine, 200 mg, or ranitidine, 150 mg, twice daily). Cold-induced urticaria, in which low temperatures release histamine and cause local biosynthesis of prostaglandin D_2, usually responds to a combination of H_1- and H_2-blockers, and sometimes also to a cyclo-oxygenase inhibitor given prophylactically.

SUPERFICIAL BACTERIAL SKIN INFECTIONS

Skin infections are commonly due to staphylococci or streptococci. Impetigo or infected eczema

Table 50.3: Drug therapy of fungal skin and nail infections

Fungal skin infection	Drug therapy	Comment
Candida infection of the skin, vulvovaginitis or balanitis	Topical antifungal therapy with nystatin cream (100 000 units/g) or ketoconazole 2%, clotrimazole 1% or miconazole 2% cream	Alternative topical agents are terbinafine 1% or amorolfine 0.25% creams. Systemic therapy may be necessary in refractory cases. Consider underlying diabetes mellitus
Fungal nail infections, onchomycosis dermatophytes	Griseofulvin, 10 mg/kg daily for 6–12 months, or alternatively fluconazole, 200 mg daily for 6–12 months	If systemic therapy is not tolerated, tioconazole 28% is applied daily for 6 months. Topical amorolfine 5% is an alternative
Pityriasis capitis, seborrhoeic dermatitis (dandruff)	Topical steroids – clobetasol propionate 0.05%, or betamethasone valerate 0.1%, with cetrimide shampoo	Severe cases may require additional topical ketoconazole 2% or clotrimazole 1%
Tinea capitis	Systemic therapy with fluconazole, itraconazole, miconazole or clotrimazole	–
Tinea corporis	Topical therapy with, for example, ketoconazole 2% or clotrimazole 1% applied for 2–3 weeks	Systemic therapy is only necessary in refractory cases
Tinea pedis	As above	As above

Table 50.4: Summary of drug therapy of viral skin infections

Viral skin infection	Drug therapy	Comment
Initial or recurrent genital, labial, herpes simplex	Topical 5% acyclovir cream applied, 4-hourly for 5 days is used, but is of questionable benefit. Systemic acyclovir therapy is required for buccal and vaginal herpes simplex	Topical penciclovir (2% cream) is an alternative for recurrent orolabial herpes Systemic valcyclovir or famciclovir are new alternatives to acyclovir
Skin warts, papilloma virus infections	All treatments are destructive Cryotherapy (solid carbon dioxide, liquid nitrogen) Daily keratolytics such as 12% salicylic acid	For plantar warts use 1.5% formaldehyde or 10% glutaraldehyde. For anal warts use podophyllin resin 15% or podophyllotoxin 0.5% solution applied precisely on the lesions once or twice weekly

is treated topically for no more than 2 weeks with antimicrobial agents. Suitable preparations include **mupirocin** and **lucidin**.

Fungal skin and nail infections

See Table 50.3 for a summary of the drug therapy of fungal skin and nail infections, and Chapter 44 for a more detailed account of the clinical pharmacology of antifungal drugs.

Viral skin infections

See Chapter 44 for a detailed account of the pharmacology of antiviral drugs, and Table 50.4 for a summary of the drug therapy of viral skin infections.

Treatment of other skin infections (lice, scabies)

Table 50.5: Summary of the treatments for other common dermatological infections

Disease	Causal agent	Treatment	Toxicity of therapy	Additional comments
Lice	Caused by *Pediculus humanus capitis*	0.5% malathion or carbamyl are recommended – leave in contact for 12 h	Use aqueous rather than alcohol preparations in asthmatic and small children	Apply to affected area and repeat in 7 days to kill lice that have just emerged from eggs
Scabies	Caused by transmission of *Sarcoptes scabei* during sexual intercourse	Lindane 1% (apply topically and leave for 24 h then repeat after 7 days if needed *or* Malathion 0.5% applied to hair and left for 12 h (if on whole body leave for 24 h) omit face and neck	Major toxicity is skin irritation	Do not use lindane or malathion during pregnancy or in children. Permethrin is an effective alternative pyrethroid

Table 50.6: Adverse effects of drugs on the skin

Cutaneous eruption	Drugs commonly associated	Comment
Acne	Corticosteroids, androgens, anabolic steroids, phenytoin	
Alopecia	Cytotoxic chemotherapy, etretinate, gold, long-term heparin, oral contraceptives, sodium valproate	
Eczema	β-Lactams, phenothiazines	
Erythema multiforme	Sulphonamides, penicillins (β-lactams), barbiturates, allopurinol, rifampicin, all NSAIDs, phenytoin, carbamazepine and lamotrigine	Inclusive of Stevens–Johnson syndrome
Erythema nodosum	Sulphonamides, antimicrobials (especially β-lactams), oral contraceptives	
Exfoliative dermatitis	Allopurinol, carbamazepine, gold, penicillins, phenothiazines and erythroderma	
Fixed eruptions	Barbiturates, laxatives, phenolphthalein, naproxen, nifedipine, penicillins, sulphonamides, tetracyclines, quinidine	These eruptions recur at the same site (often circumorally) with each administration of the drug and may be purpuric or bullous
Lichenoid eruptions	Captopril, chloroquine, frusemide, gold, phenothiazines, thiazides	
Lupus erythematosus with butterfly rash	Hydralazine, isoniazid, phenytoin, procainamide	
Photosensitivity		
Systemic drugs	Amiodarone, chlorodiazepoxide, frusemide, griseofulvin, nalidixic acid, thiazides, tetracyclines, piroxicam	
Topical drugs	Coal tar, hexachlorophane, *p*-aminobenzoic acid and its esters	
Pigmentation	Amiodarone, chloroquine, oral contraceptives, phenothiazines	AZT causes grey nails; oral chloroquine causes hair and skin depigmentation
Pruritus	Oral contraceptives, phenothiazines, rifampicin	Without any rashes – rifampicin causes biliary stasis
Purpura	Thiazides, phenylbutazone, sulphonamides, sulphonylureas, quinine	May be thrombocytopenic or vasculitic
Toxic epidermal necrolysis	NSAIDs, penicillins (β-lactams), phenytoin, sulphonamides	

Table 50.6: Continued

Cutaneous eruption		Drugs commonly associated	Comment
Toxic erythema		Ampicillin, sulphonamides, sulphonylureas, frusemide, thiazides	Usually occurs after 7–9 days of therapy or after 2–3 days in those previously exposed
Urticaria	Acute	Radiocontrast media	
	Acute/chronic	Aspirin (NSAIDs), ACE inhibitors, gold, penicillins	
Vasculitis – allergic		NSAIDs, phenytoin, sulphonamides, thiazides, penicillins and retinoids	

NSAIDs = non-steroidal anti-inflammatory drugs, ACE = angiotensin-converting enzyme.

Adverse drug reactions involving the skin

Cutaneous adverse drug reactions can arise from topically or systemically administered drugs (see Chapter 12). The clinical presentation of an adverse cutaneous drug reaction is seldom pathognomonic and may vary from an erythematous, macular or morbilliform rash to erythema multiforme. Such reactions generally occur within the first 1–2 weeks of therapy. However, immunologically mediated reactions may take months to become clinically manifest. Contact dermatitis is usually eczematous and is most commonly seen with antimicrobial drugs or antihistamines, but the possibility that the vehicle in which the drug is formulated could be the cause of such a reaction should always be considered.

The diagnosis of a drug-induced cutaneous reaction requires an accurate drug history from the patient, especially defining the temporal relationship of the skin disorder to any and all concomitant drug therapy. In milder cases and fixed drug eruptions, re-administration (rechallenge) with the suspect agent may be justified. Patch testing is useful for contact dermatitis, reproducing the exposure and the causative process. Intradermal testing has little or no role. The treatment of drug-induced skin disorders involves removing the cause, applying cooling creams and antipruritics, and reserving topical steroids only for the most severe cases.

Table 50.6 lists some of the commonest drug-related cutaneous reactions.

Photosensitivity

The term 'photosensitivity' combines both phototoxicity and photoallergy. Phototoxicity (like drug toxicity) is a predictable effect of too high a dose of UVB in a subject who has been exposed to a drug. The reaction is like severe sunburn, and the threshold returns to normal when the drug is discontinued. Photoallergy (like drug allergy) is a cell-mediated immune reaction that only occurs in certain individuals, is not dose related and may be severe. It is due to a photochemical reaction caused by UVA where the drug combines with a tissue protein to form an antigen. These reactions are usually eczematous, and may persist for months or years after withdrawal of the drug. Some agents that commonly cause photosensitivity are shown in Table 50.6.

Prospects for skin therapy

The definition of the role of a number of cytokines in the pathogenesis of eczema has led an intensive effort to develop new therapeutic strategies that use cytokines or cytokine antagonists. Preliminary evidence of the beneficial effects of interferon-γ in patients with eczema is encouraging. Other novel therapies currently being investigated include interleukin-2 and soluble interleukin 1R and thymopentin (a pentapeptide derived from the thymic hormone thymopoietin, which suppresses the Th-2-cell-derived cytokines (e.g. IL-4). The role of specific phosphodiesterase inhibitors is also under investigation, as is a resurgence of interest in hyposensitization.

In psoriasis, leukotrienes play a major role in the pathogenesis of the disease. The lipoxygenase product LTB_4 (a powerful neutrophil chemotaxin) has been found in psoriatic lesions, and probably synergizes with other inflammatory mediators. Fish-oil concentrates that are rich in eicosapentaenoic acid and docosahexanoic acid alter the pathway of leukotriene biosynthesis, reducing LTB_4 and increasing LTB_5. There is some evidence of modest efficacy of fish oil consumption in psoriasis. Topical application of a selective inhibitor of 5-lipoxygenase reduces LTB_4 in chronic plaque psoriasis with an associated clinical improvement. Skin irritation is the major adverse effect. Prospects for other 5-lipoxygenase inhibitors that cause less topical irritation are promising.

Case history

A 45-year-old white woman with a prior history of one culture-positive urinary tract infection (UTI) presents with a 3-day history of dysuria and frequency of micturition. Her urinalysis shows moderate blood and protein and is positive for nitrates. She is started on a 7-day course of co-trimoxazole, two tablets twice a day, as she has a history of penicillin allergy with urticaria and wheezing. In the early morning of the last day of therapy she develops a generalized rash on her body, which is itchy and worsens, despite the fact that she has not taken the last two doses of her antibiotic, her UTI symptoms having resolved. By the following morning she feels much worse, with itchy eyes, has had fevers overnight and is complaining of arthralgia and buccal soreness, and is seen by her community physician. He notes conjunctivitis, with swollen eyelids, soreness and ulceration on her lips and buccal and vaginal mucosa. She has a generalized macular-papular rash which involves her face and has become confluent in areas on her abdomen and chest, and there is evidence of skin blistering and desquamation on her chest.

Question

What is the most likely diagnosis here? What is the probable cause, and how should this patient be managed?

Answer

The most likely diagnosis of a rapidly progressive generalized body rash involving the eyes, mouth and genitalia with systemic fever and early desquamation is erythema multiforme – major (Stevens–Johnson syndrome). The commonest causes of this syndrome are viral infections, especially herpes virus, drugs and (less frequently) systemic bacterial infections such as meningitis, nephritis and streptoccocal infection. Many drugs can cause this adverse reaction, but the most commonly incriminated classes of drugs are antibacterial agents such as sulphonamides, β-lactams (especially aminopenicillins), vancomycin and rifampicin, anticonvulsants, salicylates and other NSAIDs, and allopurinol. In this patient the most likely aetiology is that she is taking co-trimoxazole, which contains 400 mg of sulphamethoxazole and 80 mg of trimethoprim per tablet. Stopping the offending agent is the most important part of her initial management. Her further management should include admission to hospital for intravenous fluids to maintain hydration, supportive care for the skin in order to minimize further desquamation and secondary infection with sterile wet dressings and an aseptic environment, analgesia if necessary, and maintenance and monitoring of her hepatic and renal function. If her condition is very severe, the patient may need to be transferred to a burns unit. Short courses of high-dose corticosteroids early in the disease have been recommended, but controlled clinical studies have not demonstrated the benefit of corticosteroids in this condition. The disease may progress for up to 4–5 days and recovery may take from one to several weeks. The mortality rate for Stevens-Johnson syndrome is $< 5\%$, but increases to about 30% if the diagnosis is toxic epidermal necrolysis with more extensive desquamation.

Further reading

Brehler R, Hildebrand A, Luger T. 1997: Recent advances in the treatment of atopic eczema. *Journal of the American Academy of Dermatology* **36**, 983–94.

Guzzo C. 1997: Recent advances in the treatment of psoriasis. *Dermatologic Clinics.* **15**, 59–68.

Leppard I, Ashton R. 1993: *Treatment in dermatology.* Oxford: Radcliffe Medical Press.

Leyden JJ. 1997: Therapy for acne vulgaris. *New England Journal of Medicine* **336**, 1156–62.

Roujeau JC, Stern RS. 1994: Severe adverse cutaneous reactions to drugs. *New England Journal of Medicine.* **331**, 1272–85.

PART XIII

THE EYE

CHAPTER FIFTY-ONE

DRUGS AND THE EYE

- Introduction
- Ocular anatomy, physiology and biochemistry
- General pharmacokinetics of intra-ocular drug administration
- Drugs used to dilate the pupil
- Drugs used to constrict the pupil and to treat glaucoma
- Drugs used to treat eye infections
- Local anaesthetics and the eye
- Adverse effects on the eye of systemic drug therapy
- Contact lens wearers

INTRODUCTION

The eye is the window of the soul. More prosaically, it also provides a unique opportunity to monitor the effects of drugs, especially those that act on the autonomic nervous system. The eye is protected by a series of barriers, namely the blood–retinal, blood–aqueous and blood–vitreous barriers, and so represents both an opportunity for localized drug administration and also a challenge to drug delivery.

OCULAR ANATOMY, PHYSIOLOGY AND BIOCHEMISTRY

See figure 51.1 for a cross-sectional view.

The globe is protected by the eyelids and by the bony orbit. The structures of the eye itself are divided into the anterior and posterior segments. The anterior segment includes the cornea, limbus, anterior and posterior chambers, trabecular meshwork, Schlemm's canal, the iris lens and the ciliary body. The posterior segment consists of the sclera, choroid, retina, vitreous and optic nerve. The anterior surface of the eye is covered by the conjunctiva. At the reflection of the palpebral and bulbar conjunctiva is a space called the fornix located superiorly and inferiorly behind the upper and lower eyelids. Topical medications are usually placed in the lower fornix. The lacrimal system consists of secretory glandular and excretory ducts. The ocular secretory system is composed of the main lacrimal gland located in the upper outer orbit, and accessory glands located in the conjunctiva. The lacrimal gland has both sympathetic and parasympathetic innervation. Parasympathetic innervation is relevant in that many drugs with anticholinergic side-effects cause the symptom of dry eyes (see Table 51.1). Tear drainage starts through small puncta located in the medial aspects of the eyelids. Blinking causes tears to enter the puncta and drain through the canaliculi, lacrimal sac and nasolacrimal duct into the nose. The nose is lined with highly vascular epithelium which permits direct access of absorbed drugs to the systemic circulation. Consequently, even though the dose administered as eye drops is much smaller than the usual dose of the same drug (e.g. **timolol**) administered by mouth, the lack of first-pass metabolism may none the less lead to unwanted systemic effects.

THE IRIS AND CILIARY BODY

The *iris* is the most anterior portion of the uveal tract that also includes the ciliary body and choroid. Dilator smooth muscle is orientated

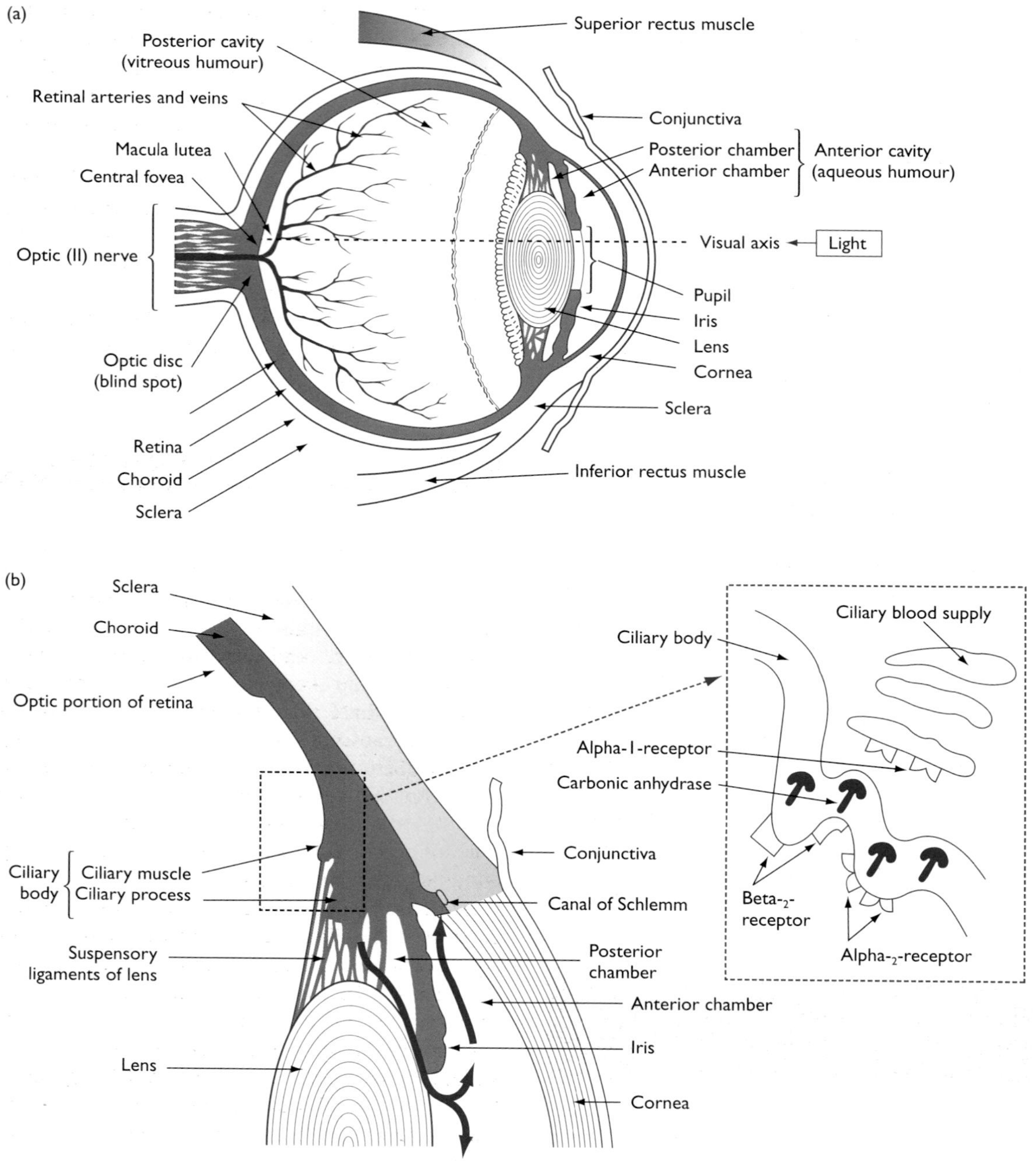

Figure 51.1 The eye. (a) General features and the visual axis. (b) Enlargement to show features of the ciliary body and the circulation of aqueous humour and high magnification area detailing the distribution of adrenergic receptor and carbonic anhydrase location. (Reproduced from Clancy J, McVicar AJ. 1995: *Physiology and anatomy*, with the permission of Edward Arnold, London.)

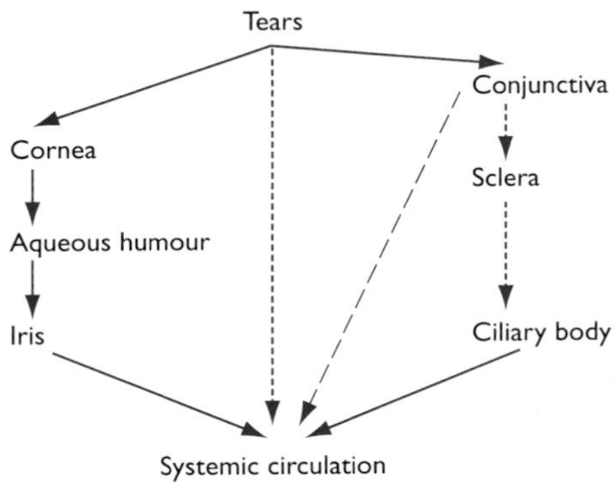

Figure 51.2 Potential absorption pathways for drugs applied to the eye.

radially and innervated by the sympathetic system, which produces dilatation (mydriasis). At the pupillary margin, the sphincter smooth muscle is organized in a circular orientation with parasympathetic innervation which, when stimulated, leads to pupillary constriction (miosis) (see Table 51.1 for a summary of the autonomic pharmacology of the eye).

The *ciliary body* serves two specialized functions, namely secretion of the aqueous humour and accommodation. Parasympathetic stimulation contracts the ciliary muscle and allows the lens to become more convex, focusing on near objects. Contraction of this muscle also widens the spaces in the trabecular meshwork and this also explains, in part, the effect of parasympathomimetics in lowering intra-ocular pressure.

General pharmacokinetics of intra-ocular drug administration

The bioavailability of intra-ocularly administered drugs depends on pH and other pharmaceutical properties of the vehicle. Specialized ocular routes of administration that are used by opthalmic surgeons are listed in Table 51.2 and we shall not deal further with these in the present chapter. Most ophthalmic drugs in general use are delivered as drops, usually in aqueous solution. Formulations which prolong the time for which a drug remains in contact with the eye surface include gels, ointments, solid inserts, soft contact lenses and collagen shields. Drug penetration into the eye itself is approximately linearly related to the concentration of drug applied. Membrane-controlled delivery systems have theoretical advantages, but many patients have difficulty placing them and retaining them *in situ*.

Nasolachrymal drainage plays a key role in the systemic absorption of drugs administered to the eye, and drugs absorbed via this route circumvent hepatic first-pass metabolism. Thus ocular drugs such as β-adrenergic antagonists can cause wheezing in asthmatic patients. Table 51.3 shows the plasma concentrations that are achieved with some commonly administered eye drops.

Drugs used to dilate the pupil

Mydriasis (pupillary dilatation) is often required for detailed examination of the retina. Two major groups of drugs are used to cause pupillary dilatation, namely *muscarinic antagonists* (anticholinergics) and *sympathomimetics*. Short-acting relatively weak mydriatics such as **tropicamide** facilitate retinal examination. **Cyclopentolate** and **atropine** are preferred for producing cycloplegia (paralysis of the ciliary muscle) for refraction in young children. Atropine is also used for the treatment of iridocyclitis mainly to prevent posterior synechiae, when it is often combined with **phenylephrine**.

Table 51.4 shows some commonly used agents, their receptor effects, dose schedule and toxicity. Agents that dilate the pupil may abruptly increase the intra-ocular pressure in closed-angle glaucoma by causing obstruction to the outflow tract, and are contraindicated in this condition. Patients should be asked whether they are driving before having their pupils dilated, and should be warned not to drive afterwards until their vision has returned to normal.

Table 51.1: Autonomic pharmacology/physiology of the eye and associated structures

Tissue	Adrenergic receptor and subtype	Response	Cholinergic receptor and subtype	Response
Iris radial muscle	α_1	Mydriasis		
Iris sphincter muscle	–	–	M_3	Miosis
Ciliary epithelium	α_2/β_2	Aqueous humour production		
Ciliary muscle	β_2	Relaxation	M_3	Accommodation
Lacrimal gland	α_1	Secretion	M_2/M_3	Secretion

Table 51.2: Characteristics of ocular routes of drug administration

Route	Absorption profile	Benefits and uses	Problems
Topical	Fairly rapid; varies with formulation	Convenient, economical and safe	Compliance, side-effects
Subconjunctival, sub-Tenon's and retrobulbar injections	Sustained – slow release	Anterior segment infection and surgical anaesthesia	Local toxicity and tissue injury
Intra-ocular injection	Rapid	Anterior segment injury	Local toxicity
Intravitreal injection/device	Absorption phase bypassed and immediate local effect	Endophthalmitis, retinitis	Local toxicity and surgical use

DRUGS USED TO CONSTRICT THE PUPIL AND TO TREAT GLAUCOMA

PHYSIOLOGY OF AQUEOUS HUMOUR DYNAMICS AND REGULATION OF INTRA-OCULAR PRESSURE

Aqueous humour is produced at a rate of 2–2.5 μL/min and flows from the posterior chamber through the pupil into the anterior chamber. Around 80–95% of it exits via the trabecular meshwork and into the canal of Schlemm and subsequently into the episcleral venous plexus and eventually into the systemic circulation. Fluid can also flow via the ciliary muscles into the suprachoroidal space. The geometry of the anterior chamber differentiates the two forms of glaucoma, namely open-angle glaucoma (the commoner form) and angle-closure glaucoma (closed-angle glaucoma). Open-angle glaucoma is usually treated medically in the first instance, by reducing aqueous humour flow and/or production. Closed-angle glaucoma is treated by iridectomy following urgent medical treatment to reduce the intra-ocular pressure in preparation for surgery.

PRINCIPLES OF THERAPY FOR GLAUCOMA

Acute glaucoma is a medical emergency. Mannitol can reduce the intra-ocular pressure acutely by its osmotic effect. In addition, therapy with a carbonic anhydrase inhibitor (intravenous acetazolamide or topical dorzolamide) may be required. This is then supplemented with either a topical β-adrenergic antagonist (e.g. timolol) or cholinergic agonists (e.g. **pilocarpine**), or both.

Chronic simple glaucoma is due to a limitation of flow through the trabecular meshwork. Initial treatment is with a topical beta-blocker. Other drugs (e.g. **dipivefrine**, a prodrug of adrenaline designed to penetrate the cornea readily, or pilocarpine) are added as necessary. Disappointingly, visual impairment may progress despite adequate control of intra-ocular pressure, and surgery has a place in this as well as in the acute form of glaucoma.

DRUGS USED TO TREAT GLAUCOMA

Mannitol

Mannitol is an osmotic diuretic. It is used in an emergency or before surgery, and is given as an intravenous infusion (e.g. 100–200 mL of a 20% solution) over 30–60 min. It shifts water from intracellular and transcellular compartments (including the eye) into the plasma, and promotes loss of fluid by its diuretic action on the kidney. Its major adverse effect is dehydration.

Carbonic anhydrase inhibitors

Acetazolamide is used in acute and chronic glaucoma, and it also has highly specialized uses in

Table 51.3: Plasma concentrations achieved with some commonly administered eye drops

Drug	Dose (μg)	Plasma concentration (ng/ml) (time post dose)
Timolol	100	0.7 (30 min)
Levobunolol	500	0.5 (60 min)
Atropine	400	0.9 (8 min)
Cyclopentolate	600	8.3 (5–15 min)
Phenylephrine	5000	10.2 (10 min)
Betamethasone	50	0.5 (30 min)

certain seizure disorders in babies, and in adapting to altitude. It was previously used as a diuretic. It is a sulphonamide.

MECHANISM

Acetazolamide is a competitive inhibitor of carbonic anhydrase, the enzyme that converts CO_2 and H_20 into H_2CO_3. Carbonic anhydrase is present in many tissues, including the proximal renal tubules (where it is involved in the reabsorption of bicarbonate ions; see Chapter 35) and choroid plexuses (where it is involved in the secretion of cerebrospinal fluid). Inhibition of this enzyme in the eye reduces aqueous humour production by the ciliary body.

ADVERSE EFFECTS

These include the following:

1 paraesthesiae and tingling;
2 nausea, vomiting and loss of taste;
3 metabolic acidosis;
4 polyuria due to its mild diuretic properties;
5 hypersensitivity reactions – particularly of the skin;
6 bone-marrow suppression (rare).

Acetazolamide is poorly tolerated orally, although its formulation as a slow-release preparation has reduced the incidence of side-effects. The recent development and use of the topically

Table 51.4: Drugs commonly used to dilate the pupil

Drug	Receptor	Dose, onset of mydriasis and schedule	Toxicity and other comments
Anticholinergics			
Tropicamide		Single drop of 0.5% solution, maximum onset of effect is in 20–40 min and lasts 3–6 h	Photosensitivity, blurred vision and systemic absorption can occur
Cyclopentolate	All anticholinergics are antagonists at the M_3 – receptor on the ciliary muscle	Single drops of 0.5 or 1.0% solution, maximum onset of effect is in 30–60 min and lasts 24 h	As for tropicamide
Atropine		Single drop of 0.5 or 1.0% solution, maximum onset of effect is 30–40 min, and lasts 7–10 days	As for tropicamide
Sympathomimetics			
Adrenaline	All of these agents are agonists at the α_1-receptor on the radial muscle of the iris	One or two drops of 1% solution, lasts 12–24 h	All agents can cause photosensitivity, conjunctival hyperaemia and hypersensitivity
Phenylephrine		One of two drops of 10% solution, lasts up to 12 h	Systemic absorption can occur (*avoid in patients with CAD or hypertension*)
Dipivefrin		One drop of 0.3% solution, lasts up to 12 h	Dipivefrin is a prodrug of adrenalin, designed for improved ocular penetration

applied carbonic anhydrase inhibitor **dorzolamide** may reduce the need for systemic acetazolamide therapy.

PHARMACOKINETICS

Acetazolamide is well absorbed, with high bioavailability and low plasma protein binding. It has a $t_{\frac{1}{2}}$ of 8 h and is cleared from the body by renal excretion. The availability of a slow-release preparation has enabled twice daily dosing.

CONTRAINDICATIONS

Acetazolamide should not be used in patients with renal failure, renal stones or known hypersensitivity to sulphonamides, or in pregnant women.

TOPICAL AGENTS FOR GLAUCOMA

Dorzolamide

This is another sulphonamide derivative which acts as a topically applied carbonic anhydrase inhibitor. It may be used either alone or as an adjunct to a β-antagonist. Systemic absorption does occur, and systemic side-effects (e.g. rashes, urolithiasis) may require drug withdrawal. Typical adverse effects include local irritation of the eye and eyelid with burning, stinging and visual blurring, and a bitter taste. The usual dose is one drop of a 2% solution three times a day, or twice daily if used with a β-antagonist.

Latanoprost

Latanoprost is a prostaglandin $F_{2\alpha}$ analogue. It can be used in patients who are intolerant of β-antagonists or as add-on therapy when the response to the first drug has been inadequate. The usual dose is one drop of a 0.005% solution once a day. Latanoprost is an inactive prodrug which readily penetrates the cornea and is hydrolysed to the free acid. The free acid diffuses out of the cornea into the aqueous humour and reaches peak concentrations in this compartment within about 2 h. It lowers the intra-ocular pressure by increasing uveoscleral outflow. It is eliminated from the eye with a $t_{\frac{1}{2}}$ of about 2 h. Systemic absorption does occur via conjunctivae and mucous membranes. Latanoprost is cleared from the body by hepatic metabolism. The main side-effects are local irritation with stinging, burning and blurred vision. Punctate keratopathy has occurred, and it increases the amount of brown pigment in the iris in patients with mixed-coloured eyes, which may be a cosmetic problem, especially if treatment is only needed for one eye.

α_2-Agonists

Brimonidine is a selective α_2- agonist. It was introduced recently for chronic open-angle glaucoma when other drugs are unsatisfactory. It is used alone or as an adjunct to β-antagonist therapy in chronic glaucoma. It decreases aqueous humour production and increases uveoscleral flow. Trace amounts do get into the circulation and undergo hepatic metabolism. One drop of a 0.2% solution is administered twice a day. The major toxicities include - local ocular irritation and occasional corneal staining, and systemic adverse effects include dry mouth (25% of cases), headache, fatigue, drowsiness and allergic reactions. It is contraindicated in patients taking monoamine oxidase inhibitors (MAOIs), and should be used with caution in those with severe coronary artery disease (CAD) or taking tricyclic antidepressants.

Apraclonidine (a derivative of clonidine) is another selective α_2-agonist which is formulated for ophthalmic use.

Key points

Drugs and the pupil

- Miosis (pupillary constriction)
  - Parasympathetic stimulation:
    - muscarinic agonists (e.g. carbachol, pilocarpine);
    - cholinesterase inhibitors (e.g. neostigmine, physostigmine).
  - Sympathetic blockade:
    - α_1–antagonists (e.g. phentolamine).
- Mydriasis (pupillary dilatation)
  - Parasympathetic blockade:
    - muscarinic antagonists (e.g. atropine, tropicamide).
  - Sympathetic stimulation:
    - α_1-agonists (e.g. phenylephrine).

Key points

Drugs used to lower intra-ocular pressure

- Systemic administration of:
  - osmotic agents (e.g. mannitol);
  - acetazolamide (carbonic anhydrase inhibitor).
- Topical administration of:
  - pilocarpine (muscarinic agonist);
  - timolol (β-adrenoceptor antagonist);
  - dorzolamide (carbonic anhydrase inhibitor);
  - latanoprost ($PGF_{2\alpha}$ analogue);
  - brimonidine (α_2–agonist).

Drugs used to treat eye infections

Several antimicrobial agents (see Chapters 42 and 44) are formulated for ophthalmic use. (see Tables 51.5, 51.6 and 51.7). Appropriate selection of an antibacterial agent and the route of administration depend on the clinical findings and culture and sensitivity results. Acute bacterial conjunctivitis is usually due to *Staphylococcus aureus* or *Streptococcus*. Chloramphenicol, gentamicin, fusidic acid or one of the fluoroquinolones (e.g. ciprofloxacin, ofloxacin), all of which are available as eye drops, may be appropriate.

Drugs used to treat inflammatory disorders in the eye

Post surgery

Non-steroidal anti-inflammatory drugs (NSAIDs) are used to reduce post-operative inflammation. Several such ophthalmic preparations are available, including **diclofenac**, **flurbiprofen** and **ketorolac**.

Other anti-inflammatory ocular drug therapies

Corticosteroids

Topical ocular corticosteroids should only be used under specialist supervision to treat uveitis and scleritis, and sometimes in the post-operative set-

Table 51.5: Antibacterial agents used to treat conjunctivitis and blepharitis

Drug class or drug	Indication and use	Toxicity
Chloramphenicol Fluoroquinolones (e.g. norfloxacin, ofloxacin, ciprofloxacin) Framycetin sulphate Aminoglycosides (e.g. gentamicin sulphate, neomycin sulphate)	Broad-spectrum antibacterials	Local irritation and hypersensitivity reactions
Ciprofloxacin hydrochloride	Corneal ulceration	Causes local burning and itching; best avoided in children
Chlortetracycline	Chlamydial infections	Local irritation and hypersensitivity reactions
Gentamicin sulphate Tobramycin	*Pseudomonas aeroginosa* infections	Local irritation and hypersensitivity reactions
Sodium fusidate	Staphylococcal infections	Hypersensitivity reactions

Table 51.6: Antiviral agents for eye infections

Drug	Route	Indication for use	Toxicity
Idoxuridine	Topical	*Herpes simplex* keratitis	Punctate keratopathy and hypersensitivity
Acyclovir	Topical (3%) Oral/intravenous	*Herpes simplex* keratitis *Herpes zoster* ophthalmicus	
Foscarnet	Intravenous/intravitreal	CMV retinitis	
Ganciclovir	Intravenous/intravitreal	CMV retinitis	

Table 51.7: Antifungal agents used to treat fungal keratitis, blepharitis and conjunctivitis

Drug class or drug	Route	Indication for use
Polyenes (e.g. amphotericin)	Topical	Fungal keratitis, endophthalmitis
Imidazoles (e.g. clotrimazole, miconazole)	Topical Topical and intravitreal	Fungal keratitis Fungal keratitis and endophthalmitis
Pyrimidines (e.g. flucytosine)	Topical	Fungal keratitis

ting. They should never be used to treat the undiagnosed 'red-eye' which could be due to a herpes infection, which is aggravated by corticosteroids and may progress to visual loss or even loss of the eye. Furthermore, topical steroids produce or exacerbate glaucoma in genetically predisposed individuals (see Chapter 14). Thinning of the cornea or perforation of the sclera may occur in susceptible patients. Ocular steroid therapy therefore requires special care and ophthalmological expertise. A number of preparations are available (e.g. **hydrocortisone** or **betamethasone** – both available as drops or ointment – or **clobetasone** drops).

Antihistamines and mast cell stabilizers

These agents are used to treat allergic or seasonal conjunctivitis. Topical *antihistamines* for ophthalmic use include **antazoline** and **levocabastine**. Ocular irritation, oedema of the eyelids or blurred vision can occur, as can systemic effects (e.g. drowsiness).

Sodium **cromoglycate** or **nedocromil** (see also Chapter 32) drops are widely used in the longer-term treatment of allergic conjunctivitis. These agents are instilled four times a day. Sodium cromoglycate in particular is very safe and only causes local stinging as its main side-effect. Lodoxamide has been reported to cause itching, lacrimation and flushing. Olopatadine (available as 0.1% drops), a new topical agent with combined anti-H_1 and mast-cell-stabilizing activity, is currently being compared with other more traditional agents for treatment of allergic conjunctivitis.

Local anaesthetics and the eye

Oxybuprocaine and **amethocaine** are widely used in the eye as topical local anaesthetics. **Proxymetacaine** causes less initial stinging and is useful in paediatric patients. Amethocaine causes more profound anaesthesia and is suitable for minor surgical procedures. Oxybuprocaine or a

Table 51.8: Adverse ocular effects of drugs

Drug class or drug	Ocular structure affected	Adverse ocular effects
Anticholinergic drugs (antispasmodics; tricyclic antidepressants, phenothiazines, first-generation antihistamines	Lacrimal apparatus	Dry secretions, ocular irritation and burning
Cholinergic agents (methacholine, neostigmine)	Lacrimal apparatus	Increased tear secretions
Amiodarone Amodiaquone Phenothiazine Gold	Corneal – microdeposits	Few symptoms, but reduced vision and ocular discomfort
Corticosteroids and antimitotics (e.g. busulphan, nitrogen mustards)	Lens	Cataract formation
Anticholinergics	Lens	Impaired accommodation – blurred vision
Oral contraceptives, sulphonamides, tetracyclines	Lens	Lens hydration increased – blurred vision
Anticholinergics in people with glaucoma; systemic and topical corticosteroids	Intra-ocular pressure is increased	Reduced visual acuity
Chloroquine Ethambutol Chloramphenicol	Optic nerve	Retrobulbar neuritis, optic atrophy; permanent visual loss may occur
Digoxin	Retina	Impaired yellow–green vision
Sildenafil (viagra)	Retina	Blue-vision

combination of lignocaine and fluorescein is used for tonometry. Lignocaine with or without adrenaline is often injected into the eyelids for minor surgery. Lignocaine is also often injected for surgical procedures on the globe of the eye.

Adverse effects on the eye of systemic drug therapy

One of the most devastating ocular complications of systemic drug therapy is the Stevens–Johnson syndrome (erythema multiforme major; – see Chapter 50). Ocular involvement occurs in up to two-thirds of patients, of whom approximately one-third suffer permanent visual sequelae. Table 51.8 illustrates the diversity of adverse ocular effects of drugs.

Contact lens wearers

As the number of patients who wear contact lenses increases, an awareness has developed that these patients represent a special subgroup in which particular care is needed when prescribing, as they may develop specific additional problems related to commonly prescribed drugs. A summary of such agents is given in Table 51.9.

Key points

Adverse effects of drugs on the eye

- Many systemically administered agents can adversely affect the eye.
- Stevens–Johnson syndrome commonly involves the eye.
- Loss of accommodation and visual blurring may be caused by any drug with anticholinergic properties.
- Cataracts are caused by corticosteroids, phenothiazines and cytotoxic agents.
- Retinopathy is caused by chloroquine and oxygen (in neonates from high concentrations).
- Optic neuropathy may be caused by ethambutol and methanol (toxic).
- Glaucoma may be caused by steroids in genetically predisposed individuals, and mydriatics can precipitate acute-angle closure glaucoma.

FURTHER READING

Harrison RJ. 1996: Ocular adverse reactions to systemic drug therapy. *Adverse Drug Reaction Bulletin* **180**, 683–6.

Salminen L. 1990: Review: systemic absorption of topically applied ocular drugs in humans. *Journal of Ocular Pharmacology* **6**, 243–9.

Schoenwald RD. 1990: Ocular drug delivery. Pharmacokinetic considerations. *Clinical Pharmacokinetics* **4**, 255–69.

Case history

A 68-year-old man has hypertension and ischaemic heart disease. His angina and blood pressure are well controlled while taking oral therapy with bendrofluazide, 2.5 mg daily, and slow-release, diltiazem 120 mg daily. His visual acuity gradually declines and he is diagnosed as having simple open-angle glaucoma. His ophthalmologist starts therapy with pilocarpine 2% eye drops, one drop four times a day, and carteolol drops, two drops twice a day. A week after starting to see his ophthalmologist he attends his GP's surgery complaining of shortness of breath on exertion, paroxysmal nocturnal dyspnoea and othopnoea. Clinical examination reveals a regular pulse of 35 beats/min, blood pressure of 158/74 mmHg, and signs of mild left ventricular failure. His ECG shows sinus bradycardia with no evidence of acute myocardial infarction.

Question

How can you explain this problem, and what should your management be?

Answer

Carteolol is a non-selective β-adrenergic antagonist that can gain access to the systemic circulation via the nasolachrymal apparatus and avoid heptic first - pass metabolism. It can thus act (especially in conjunction with a calcium antagonist – diltiazem in this case) on the cardiac conducting system and on the working myocardium. Discontinuing the ocular carteolol should resolve the problem.

Table 51.9: Common drug-induced problems in patients with contact lenses

Drug	Adverse effects	Comment
Oral contraceptives (high oestrogen)	Swelling of the corneal surface – poorly fitting lenses	Visual acuity deterioration
Anxiolytics, hypnotics, first-generation antihistamines (e.g. diphenhydramine, etc.)	Reduced rate of blinking	Dry eyes and higher risk of infections
Antihistamines, anticholinergics, phenothazines, diuretics and tricyclic antidepressants	Reduced lacrimation	Dry eyes – irritation and burning
Hydralazine and ephedrine	Increased lacrimation	
Isotretinoin, aspirin	Conjunctival inflammation and irritation	
Rifampin and sulphasalazine	Discolour lenses	

PART XIV

CLINICAL TOXICOLOGY

CHAPTER FIFTY-TWO

DRUG *and* ALCOHOL ABUSE

- Introduction
- Pathophysiology of drug dependence
- General principles of treating addictions
- Opioid/narcotic analgesics
- Drugs that alter perception
- Central stimulants
- Central depressants
- Miscellaneous

INTRODUCTION

The World Health Organization (WHO) definition of drug *dependence* is 'a state, psychic and sometimes physical, resulting from the interaction between a living organism and a drug characterized by behavioural and other responses that always include a compulsion to take the drug on a continuous or periodic basis in order to experience its psychic effects and sometimes to avoid the discomfort of its absence'. More recent definitions include the WHO's ICD-10 and the American Psychiatric Association's DSM-IV diagnostic criteria for Substance-Related Disorders, which emphasize the importance of loss of control over drug use and its consequences in limiting other, non-drug-related activities, in addition to tolerance and physical dependence.

In the above definitions, a distinction is made between physical and psychological dependence. Although psychological dependence has not been shown to produce gross physical or structural changes in the body, it must be assumed that changes have occurred in the brain at a molecular or receptor level. Central to the definition of psychological dependence is the compulsion or craving to take a drug repeatedly. In contrast, physical dependence is seen in the absence of a drug, when a range of physical and psychic symptoms – a withdrawal state – is present. The ease and degree to which withdrawal symptoms develop defines the liability of a particular drug to produce physical dependence. As a generalization, the withdrawal syndrome seen after cessation of a drug tends to be the opposite of the symptoms produced by acute administration of that drug (e.g. anxiety, insomnia and arousal seen after withdrawal of alcohol or benzodiazepines, or depression and lethargy seen after withdrawal of stimulants). Physical and psychological dependence may be distinguished clinically. For instance, abrupt cessation of tricyclic antidepressants produces a hyperautonomic state, with no

Key points

Features of drug dependence

- A subjective awareness or compulsion to use a drug, often related to unsuccessful efforts to reduce drug intake.
- Continued drug use despite awareness of its harmful effects on physical health, social functioning, etc.
- Priority of drug-taking or obtaining drugs over other activities, limiting normal social or work roles.
- The development of tolerance and withdrawal symptoms.
- After abstinence, dependence may recur rapidly with reuse of the drug.

evidence of psychological dependence, whereas nicotine withdrawal produces predominantly psychological changes, with minimal physical symptoms. The major difference between drug *abuse* and drug *dependence* is quantitative.

Tolerance is another important concept. It occurs when repeated exposure to a drug produces diminshed effects compared to those produced after initial drug administration. It may be caused by changes in the rate at which the drug is distributed or metabolized in the body, or by adaptive processes occurring in the brain. Another feature of tolerance is that of cross-tolerance. If tolerance to one type of drug occurs, tolerance to other, chemically dissimilar drugs may also be present. This has been clearly demonstrated for alcohol, benzodiazepines, barbiturates and other hypnosedative drugs, and forms the basis for substitution treatment of dependency.

PATHOPHYSIOLOGY OF DRUG DEPENDENCE

The majority of people who are exposed to drugs do not become dependent on them. Factors that may increase the likelihood that a particular individual may become addicted to a drug include the following.

Genetic factors Twin and family studies have shown that alcoholism has a strong genetic component, especially among males. Phenotypically this may be manifested as a diminished sensitivity to the intoxicating effects of alcohol. Genetic factors may also protect against alcoholism (e.g. defective alcohol and aldehyde dehydrogenase genes in Orientals produce an unpleasant flushing response after drinking alcohol). The role of genetic influences is not known for other drugs of dependence.

Personality factors/diagnosis Two broad personality groups have been associated with drug dependency. The first type has antisocial personality features (drug dependence being part of a general antisocial picture), and the second is characterized by traits of personal anxiety (where drugs may be used to self-medicate anxiety, leading to dependence). Associations have also been made for adult addiction and childhood conduct disorder. For alcoholics, aggressive and impulsive personality characteristics during childhood are associated with early onset of alcoholism. Smokers tend to have stronger neuroticism or anxiety-related traits than non-smokers.

Family/social environmental factors An individual's drinking or drug-taking behaviour may be influenced by the example set by his or her family or peer group, or by cultural norms.

Drug availability and economic factors Rates of dependence are increased in a population if a drug is easily available. This may explain why dependence on nicotine and alcohol is a much greater public health problem than dependence on illegal drugs, because of their greater availability than the latter. Also, drug use is very sensitive to price (e.g. rates of alcoholism are reduced by increasing alcohol prices).

Biochemical reinforcement Drugs of abuse and dependence have a common biochemical pathway in that they all increase dopamine concentrations in areas of the nucleus accumbens. Symptomatically, increased dopamine concentrations appear to be associated with mood elevation and euphoria, and behaviourally they appear to be linked, with reinforcement of drug-taking. Liability to and speed of onset of dependence differs between drugs, and may be due to different potencies in releasing dopamine (cocaine is most potent), as well as to the speed with which this effect occurs (smoked and intravenous drugs give a more rapid effect than oral drugs).

The contribution of one or several of these factors to the development of dependence will vary from one individual to another. For example, in countries where alcohol intoxication is culturally acceptable and alcohol is widely available (e.g. France, Germany), it is possible to find large numbers of patients with alcohol dependence who have few or no antisocial personality features, whereas in countries where intoxication is not culturally accepted or alcohol availability is more restricted (e.g. Taiwan, Israel), antisocial personality traits are much more common among alcoholics.

General principles of treating addictions

Earlier approaches to treating drug dependence involved stopping drug use and employing some form of psychological or social therapy to encourage patients to remain drug-free. The emphasis of these approaches was non-medical, and pharmacological treatment tended to be restricted to management of withdrawal symptoms. While this approach may have been successful for some patients, overall success rates were modest, and there was little opportunity to assess and treat patients' coexisting medical and psychiatric disorders, the rates of which are extremely high in this population.

By the time an addicted patient appears for assessment and treatment, he or she is likely to have major problems in a number of areas. There may be physical or mental illness present, or emotional or attitudinal problems, which may have contributed to the addiction and/or resulted from it. The patient's financial or living circumstances may have been adversely affected by their drug habit, and they may have legal problems relating to drug possession, intoxication (e.g. drink-driving offences), or criminal activities carried out to finance drug purchases. Attitudes to drug use may be unrealistic (e.g. denial). The best chance of a successful treatment outcome requires that all of these factors are considered in assessment and treatment, and the use of a wide range of treatment options is likely to be more successful than a narrow repertoire.

Treatment objectives regarding drug use in modern drug addiction treatment programmes vary, depending on the type of drug. The need for complete abstinence is almost always emphasized for nicotine, alcohol or cocaine addiction, whereas for heroin addiction the majority of patients will require methadone maintenance treatment. Other objectives are to improve the health and social functioning of addicted patients. Treatment success can only be determined over a long period of time, and should be based on reduction in drug use or improvements in health and social functioning, rather than on rates of abstinence (complete abstinence after a single course of treatment is rare). Therefore the components of a treatment programme should include medical and psychiatric assessment, some form of psychological counselling or support, and social support. While it is possible for non-specialists to provide some of these treatments, ideally the addicted patient should be referred to specialist services. Other services based in the voluntary sector (e.g. alcohol and narcotic support groups such as Alcoholics Anonymous and Narcanon) are also valuable and complementary resources. Medical and psychiatric assessment may need to be repeated once the patient is abstinent, as it is often difficult to diagnose accurately certain disorders in the presence of withdrawal symptoms (e.g. anxiety, depression and hypertension are features of alcohol withdrawal, but are also common in abstinent alcoholics).

The pharmacological treatment of addictions, which includes treatment of intoxication, detoxification (removal of the drug from the body, including management of withdrawal symptoms), and treatment to prevent relapse, is discussed below.

Opioid/narcotic analgesics

The estimated number of opioid addicts in the UK is at least 120 000 and increasing. Although this is a relatively minor problem compared to that in the USA, it is a major cause of crime and spread of the human immunodeficiency virus (HIV) infection in the UK. Addicts may need more than £400 per week to supply their addiction from the black market. Intake of 0.25 g of pure heroin daily (contained in 1 g of black-market 'heroin') is not uncommon in a dependent addict. Often multiple drugs are used. Heroin (diamorphine) is the drug of preference. It is often adulterated with other white powders such as quinine (which is bitter, like opiates), caffeine, lactose and even chalks, starch and talc. Due to the variable purity, the dose of black-market heroin is always uncertain. The drug is taken intravenously, subcutaneously, orally or by inhalation of smoked heroin ('chasing the dragon'). The latter method of use is more common among the 15–25 years age group. In addition to the illegal supply of heroin from the Middle East and the Far East, opioids are obtained from pharmacy thefts and the legal prescription of

Table 52.1 Opioid drugs that are commonly abused

Drugs	Comment
Diamorphine*	Mainly obtained on the black market. It is of variable purity and cut with quinine, talc, lactose, etc. It is usually mixed with water, heated until dissolved, and sometimes strained through cotton. It may be used intravenously (mainlining), subcutaneously (skin popping) or inhaled ('snorted'/'chasing the dragon', by heating up on foil and inhaling the smoke) ($t_{\frac{1}{2}}$ = 60–90 min)
Methadone	This is the mainstay of drug addiction clinics, and is usually given as an elixir (long ($t_{\frac{1}{2}}$ of 15–55 h). It is very difficult to use elixir for injection
Dipipanone* (+ cyclizine = 'diconal'®)	Previously much used by non-clinic doctors treating addicts. It is easily crushed up and dissolved for intravenous use
Dextromoramide ('palfium')	Similar in its abuse potential to dipipanone
Other opoids	All opioids, including mixed agonists/antagonists (e.g. buprenorphine) have the potential to cause dependence

* Diamorphine, dipipanone and cocaine (not an opioid) can only be prescribed to addicts for treatment of their addiction by doctors with a special license.

Table 52.2: Central nervous system effects of opioids

Analgesia
Euphoria
Drowsiness → sleep → coma
Decrease in sensitivity of respiratory centre to CO_2
Depression of cough centre
Stimulation of chemoreceptor trigger zone (vomiting in 15% of cases)
Release of antidiuretic hormone

drugs for treatment of the addiction. Some of the drugs used are listed in Table 52.1.

The pharmacological actions of opioids are described in Chapter 24, and their effects on the central nervous system (CNS) are summarized in Table 52.2.

Medical complications

Medical complications of opioid addiction are common, and some of them are listed in Table 52.3. The majority of these relate to use of infected needles, the effects of contaminating substances used to cut supplies, or the life-style of opioid addicts. These are the principal reasons for the development of methadone clinics and needle-exchange programmes as a way of minimizing medical complications of opioid dependence.

Intoxication and overdose

For several seconds following intravenous injection, heroin produces an intense euphoria (rush) which may be accompanied by nausea and vomiting, but is nevertheless pleasurable. Over the next few hours the user may describe a warm sensation in the abdomen and chest. However, chronic users often state that the only effect they obtain is remission from abstinence symptoms. On examination the patient may appear to be alternately dozing and waking. The patient may be hypotensive with a slow respiratory rate, the pin-point pupils and infrequent and slurred speech. These signs can be reversed with naloxone. Hypothermia may be severe in a cold environment.

Overdose is commonly accidental due to unexpectedly potent heroin or waning tolerance (e.g. after release from prison). Severe overdose may cause immediate apnoea, circulatory collapse, convulsions and cardiopulmonary arrest. Alternatively, death may occur over a longer period of time, usually due to hypoxia from direct respiratory centre depression with mechanical asphyxia (tongue and/or vomit blocking airway).

Table 52.3: Medical complications of opioid addiction

Infection	Endocarditis – bacterial, often tricuspid valve, staphyloccocal, fungal (e.g. *Candida*) HIV/hepatitis B virus (HBV) /hepatitis C virus (HCV) Abscesses Tetanus Septicaemia Hepatitis
Pulmonary	Pneumonia – bacterial, fungal, aspiration Pulmonary oedema – 'heroin lung' Embolism Atelectasis Fibrosis/granulomas
Skin	Injection scars Abscesses Cellulitis Lymphangitis Phlebitis Gangrene
Neurological	Cerebral oedema Transverse myelitis Horner's syndrome Polyneuritis Crush injury Myopathy
Hepatic	Cirrhosis
Renal	Nephrotic syndrome with proliferative glomerulonephritis
Musculoskeletal	Osteomyelitis (usually lumbar vertebrae, *Pseudomonas*, *Staphylococcus*, *Candida*), crush injury, myoglobinuria, rhabdomyolysis

A common complication of opioid poisoning is non-cardiogenic pulmonary oedema. This is usually rapid in onset, but may be delayed. Therefore any patient who is admitted following heroin overdose should be hospitalized for at least 24 h.

Table 52.4 Symptoms of the opioid abstinence syndrome

Early	Intermediate	Late
Yawning	Mydriasis	Involuntary muscle spasm
Lacrimation	Piloerection	Fever
Rhinorrhoea	Flushing	Nausea and vomiting
Perspiration	Tachycardia Twitching Tremor Restlessness	Abdominal cramps Diarrhoea

Naloxone reverses opioid poisoning. It is important to look for an increase in pupil diameter, respiratory rate and depth of respiration during the intravenous injection. It may precipitate an acute abstinence syndrome in addicts and (very rarely) convulsions. This does *not* contraindicate its use in opioid overdoses in addicts. Severe hypoxia causes mydriasis.

TOLERANCE AND WITHDRAWAL

This occurs when increasingly larger doses of opioid (or any other drug) must be administered in order to obtain the effects of the original dose. Tolerance affects the euphoric and analgesic effects, so the addict requires more and more opioid for his or her 'buzz'. Changes in tolerance are much less apparent in the therapeutic use of opioids for the treatment of pain.

Withdrawal symptoms usually start at the time when the next dose would normally be given, and their intensity is related to the usual dose. For heroin, symptoms usually reach a maximum at 36–72 h and gradually subside over the next 5–10 days. Table 52.4 lists the features of the opioid abstinence syndrome.

Withdrawal symptoms can be treated acutely by substitution with another opioid agonist (e.g. **methadone**), the dose of which can be reduced and stopped over 1–2 weeks. Alternatively, the majority of withdrawal symptoms can be effectively treated with **lofexidine** (an α_2-antagonist with less marked hypotensive effects than clonidine), and an antidiarrhoeal agent such as loperamide, administered over 48–72 h.

MANAGEMENT OF OPIOID ADDICTS

Because of the complicated issues which can arise during the treatment of opioid addicts, these patients should be managed by specialized addiction clinics. General practitioners rarely like to manage addicts themselves, although some doctors treat addicts privately. A grossly simplified outline of the management is summarized in the Key points below. Both pharmacological and psychosocial management approaches will be needed for almost all opioid addicts. The morbidity of opioid dependence is related not only to the drug effects but also to the use of infected needles, injection of unsterile material, or opioids which are cut with unsafe substances, and the daily need to obtain large amounts of money to pay for these drugs (e.g. the need to steal or to work as a prostitute, etc.). In specialist clinics addicts may be switched from illicit opioids to prescription opioids (e.g. methadone or **buprenorphine**), thus diminishing the medical risk to addicts, and reducing the need for them to engage in risky or illegal activity to finance their drug habits. A detoxification regime (e.g. lofexidine and **loperamide**) combined with psychological support is of value in some cases. Although these clinics have the objective of weaning addicts off therapeutic opioids, in practice many patients require long-term maintenance therapy.

An alternative approach is to use an orally available opioid antagonist drug such as **naltrexone**. These drugs have no intrinsic agonist effects, but will antagonize the effects of opioid agonists. Compared to methadone maintenance, very few opioid addicts (<10% of those who enter treatment) choose to remain on long-term antagonist therapy. This may be due to the lack of intrinsic 'reward' associated with antagonists compared to opioid agonists.

Opioid addicts rarely present to hospital asking for treatment of their addiction, but more commonly present to physicians during routine medical or surgical treatment for a condition which may or may not be related to their addiction. Some patients will deny drug abuse, and clinical examination should always include a search for signs of needle-tracking and withdrawal. Acute abstinence in a casualty/general hospital setting is uncomfortable for the patient but most unlikely to be dangerous. Physicians are not allowed to pre-

Key points

Management of opioid dependence

- Refer to specialized addiction clinic.
- Conduct assessment (to include two urine samples positive for opioids).
- Give maintenance treatment (e.g. full agonists such as methadone, or partial agonists such as buprenorphine).
- Give antagonist treatment (e.g. naltrexone).
- Provide detoxification regimens (e.g. lofexidine plus loperamide).
- Glve counselling/social support.
- Repeat urine testing to confirm use of methadone and not other drugs.
- Contract system.
- Avoid prescriptions of other opioids/sedatives.
- Special 'drug-free' centres – concentrate on psychological and social support through the acute and chronic abstinence phases, and are successful in some patients.

Key points

Management of opioid addicts in hospital

1. Attempt to confirm addiction by telephoning prescriber. Confirm dosing regimen.
2. Obtain urine screen for a full drug misuse screen.
3. Look for evidence of needle marks.
4. Look for signs of opioid withdrawal.
5. Contact psychiatric liaison team.
6. In Accident and Emergency departments it is rarely appropriate to prescribe methadone. If clear withdrawal signs are evident, treat symptomatcially (e.g. with antidiarrhoeal agent); discuss with psychiatric liaison team regarding dose titration.
7. For in-patients, methadone may be appropriate – consult with psychiatric liaison regarding dose titration.
8. Analgesia – address needs as for other patients, but note the effects of tolerance.
9. On discharge, contact the patient's usual prescriber, or if this is a new presentation make arrangements through psychiatric team.

scribe diamorphine, cocaine or dipipanone to addicts for treatment of their addiction or abstinence unless they hold a special license. It is reasonable to treat a genuine opioid withdrawal syndrome with a low dose of opioid (e.g. oral **codeine phosphate**) which will reduce some of the symptoms as well as being an effective antidiarrhoeal agent. If the patient requires an opioid for treatment of pain (e.g. myocardial infarction), then an opioid such as **diamorphine** may be administered. It is almost certain that an opioid addict will require a larger dose than a non-addict patient because of the tolerance that has developed. If a patient says that they are being treated for their addiction it is always wise to confirm this by telephoning their usual prescriber and/or the supplying pharmacist. If the patient is admitted to hospital, expert advice must be obtained. Knowledge of local policies towards drug addicts is essential for anyone working in the accident and emergency department or who comes into contact with drug addicts. Newborn children of addicted mothers may be born with an abstinence syndrome or, less commonly, with features of drug overdose. Assisted ventilation is preferred to naloxone if apnoeic at birth in this situation.

There are legal requirements for the prescription of controlled drugs (Misuse of Drugs Regulations 1985) distinguished in the *British National Formulary* by the symbol CD (e.g. diamorphine, morphine, injectable dihydrocodeine, dipipanone, fentanyl, buprenorphine, dexamphetamine, methylphenidate, Ritalin®, barbituates, temazepam). Among the requirements are that the prescription must be written by hand by the prescriber, in ink, with the dose and quantity of dose units stated in both figures and words (see *British National Formulary*). There is a relaxation of requirements for phenobarbitone and temazepam. *Diamorphine, dipipanone and cocaine may only be prescribed to an addict* ***for their addiction*** *by doctors with a special licence.* Doctors are expected to continue to report the treatment demands of all drug misusers by returning the local drug misuse database reporting forms, which provide anonymized data to the appropriate national or regional Drug Misuse Database (DMD). Information in the database is not limited (as is the Addicts Index), to opioid and cocaine misuse, but includes any misused drug that generates treatment demand.

Key points

Prescription of controlled drugs

Preparations which are subject to the prescription requirements of the Misuse of Drugs Regulations 1985 are labelled CD. The principal legal requirements are as follows:

Prescriptions ordering Controlled Drugs subject to prescription requirements must be *signed* and *dated* by the prescriber and specify the prescriber's address. The prescription must always *state in the prescriber's own handwriting* in ink or otherwise so as to be indelible:

1 the name and address of the patient;
2 in the case of a preparation, the form and, where appropriate, the strength of the preparation;
3 the total quantity of the preparation, or the number of dose units, in both words and figures;
4 the dose.

Prescriptions ordering 'repeats' on the same form are not permitted.
It is an offence for a doctor to issue an incomplete prescription (see the *British National Formularly* for full details).

DRUGS THAT ALTER PERCEPTION

Cannabis

Cannabis (Indian hemp, marijuana) is the most widely used illicit drug in the UK. The most active constituent is Δ-9-tetrahydrocannabinol, which produces its effects through actions at specific cannabinoid receptors in the brain. It is most commonly mixed with tobacco and smoked, but it may be brewed into a drink or added to food. The pleasurable effects of cannabis include a sensation of relaxation, heightened perception of all the senses and euphoria. The nature and intensity of the effects varies between individuals, and is related to dose (the purity is often variable), and to the motivation and mood of the subject. The effects usually occur within minutes and last for 1–2 h. Conjunctival suffusion is common. **Tetrahydrocannabinol** and other cannabinoids are extremely lipid soluble and are only slowly released from body fat. Although the acute effects wear off within hours of inhalation, cannabinoids are eliminated in the urine for weeks following ingestion. It is claimed that cannabis may be of value in the symptomatic management of multiple sclerosis, particularly if nausea is a prominent symptom. It has no approved medicinal use in the UK.

Acute adverse effects include dysphoric reactions such as anxiety or panic attacks, the impairment of performance of skilled tasks, and sedation. This may lead to road traffic accidents. Chronic use has been associated with personality changes, including 'amotivational syndrome' which is characterized by extreme lethargy. The association of chronic cannabis use with onset of schizophrenia is unproven. A physical dependence syndrome has been reported for cannabis, but only after extremely heavy and frequent intake. Dependence on cannabis as a primary problem is clinically extremely rare, and there are no specific treatments for cannabis dependence. Similarly, there are no treatments for cannabis intoxication, although dysphoric reactions may require brief symptomatic treatment (e.g. with benzodiazepines).

LSD and other psychedelics

Psychedelics are drugs which produce hallucinations and other alterations of perception. Hallucinations may involve multiple modalities (e.g. visual, somatic, olfactory), and other changes in perception may include feelings of dissociation, alteration of perception of time, etc.). Psychedelics can be divided into two chemical groups, namely serotonin- or indoleamine-like psychedelics (e.g. **lysergic acid diethylamide** (**LSD**) and **psilocybin**) and phenethylamines (e.g. **mescaline**, **phencyclidine** (angel dust) and **methylenedioxymethylamphetamine** (**MDMA** or **ecstasy**)). All of these compounds are agonists at the serotonin 5-HT_2-receptor, and their potency as hallucinogens is closely correlated with their affinity for this receptor. Some phenethylamine psychedelics such as MDMA/ecstasy have mixed hallucinogenic and stimulant properties and may also produce feelings of increased energy and euphoria and heightened perception. In extreme cases, usually after extremely high doses, hyperpyrexia, dehydration, hyponatraemia, rhabdomyolysis, coma, hepatic damage and death have been reported. Interactions with antidepressants may be life-threatening. The principal, lasting psychological sequelae associated with recreational use of 'ecstasy' are elevated impulsivity and impaired memory. Ominously, chronic MDMA usage has been shown to produce degeneration of serotonergic neurones.

When first discovered, psychedelics were used experimentally as adjunctive treatment in psychotherapy, but were subsequently found to be of no benefit. Although of considerable academic interest to psychopharmacologists, this class of drugs has no demonstrated clinical or therapeutic role. Almost all psychedelics are taken orally, and the onset of perceptual changes occurs approximately 1 h later. The duration of effects is dependent on the dose taken and the rate of clearance of the drug ingested, but is generally more than several hours but less than a day. Clinically, it is extremely uncommon to find patients who show compulsive use of psychedelic drugs, and while tolerance of some of their behavioural effects may develop, no withdrawal syndrome has yet been demonstrated.

Physicians are most likely to come into contact with psychedelic drug abusers when they contact emergency services as a result of dysphoric reactions or 'bad trips' (usually in response to frightening hallucinations or perceptual or mood changes). These symptoms can respond to reassurance and quiet surroundings, although low doses of chlorpromazine (which has 5-HT_2-antagonist effects) or diazepam may also be of benefit. Evidence of more severe reactions to phenethylamines, such as hyperpyrexia, requires in-patient supportive care.

Phencyclidine

Phencyclidine (PCP, angel dust) was originally developed as an injectable anaesthetic. It binds to a specific receptor in the glutamate ion channel and antagonizes cation flow through the channel. Its therapeutic use in humans was stopped after early clinical studies showed that it produced confusion, delirium and hallucinations. However, it is still used for anaesthetic purposes by veterinarians. Its use has increased over the last 20 years, mainly in the USA, where it is used alone or combined with other drugs such as cannabis or crack cocaine. Patients may show extreme changes in behaviour and mood (e.g. rage and aggression, lethargy and negativism, euphoria), hallucinations, autonomic arousal (hypertension, hyperthermia) and, in extreme cases, coma and seizures. Symptoms of PCP intoxication should be treated symptomatically. PCP abuse is rare in the UK.

CENTRAL STIMULANTS

Amphetamines

Amphetamines are abused for their stimulant properties, which are related acutely to the release of dopamine and noradrenaline. Their therapeutic use is limited to specialist treatment of narcolepsy and hyperactivity in children. They should not be prescribed in the management of depression or obesity. Acutely they may alleviate tiredness and induce a feeling of cheerfulness and confidence, and because of their sympathomimetic effects they raise blood pressure and heart rate. With high doses, particularly after intravenous use, a sensation of intense exhilaration may occur. Users tend to become hyperactive at high doses, especially if these are repeated over several days. Repeated use of amphetamines can produce 'amphetamine psychosis', which is characterized by delirium, panic, hallucinations and feelings of persecution, and can be difficult to distinguish from acute schizophrenia. Anxiety, irritability and restlessness are also common. Prolonged use leads to psychological dependence, tolerance and hostility as well as irritation due to lack of sleep and food. The most commonly used amphetamine is amphetamine sulphate in oral or injectable forms, which are only available illegally. More recently, free-base amphetamine has become available ('Ice'), which can be smoked, and this has pharmacokinetic and subjective effects similar to those of injected amphetamine sulphate. There are no specific drug treatments for amphetamine dependence, and the mainstay of therapy involves counselling and social management.

Cocaine

Cocaine is derived from the Andean coca shrub. It has powerful stimulant properties which are related to its action in blocking synaptic reuptake of dopamine, and to a lesser extent noradrenaline and serotonin. In the UK, cocaine is relatively expensive; regular users might consume 1–2 g a day and the cost can be £100 a gram for the hydrochloride salt. As the salt it is most commonly sniffed up the nose, although it can also be injected. In the USA, the free base of cocaine ('Crack') is most widely available. The pharmacokinetics of smoked crack cocaine are almost identical to those of intravenous cocaine.

Acutely cocaine causes arousal, exhilaration, euphoria, indifference to pain and fatigue, and the sensation of having great physical strength and mental capacity. Repeated large doses commonly precipitate an extreme surge of agitation and anxiety. In contrast to alcohol and opioids, which addicts tend to use on a regular basis, cocaine is used in binges, where doses may be taken several times an hour over a day or several days until exhaustion or lack of money prevents this. Tolerance of the euphoric effects of cocaine occurs. However, upon stopping a cocaine binge, withdrawal symptoms including excessive sleep, fatigue and mild depression, may occur. Repeated cocaine use may produce adverse effects including anorexia, confusion, exhaustion, palpitations, damage to the membranes lining the nostrils and, if injected, blood-borne infections. Use of cocaine in pregnancy is associated with damage to the central nervous system of the fetus. 'Crack babies' can usually be cured of their 'addiction' by abstinence over a few weeks. Despite some initial promising reports that antidepressants such as desipramine might be of benefit in cocaine addiction, these have not shown activity in controlled studies, so that currently there are no specific drug treatments for cocaine dependence. Counselling and social management of patients have been shown to be of only modest benefit in maintaining abstinence.

Nicotine

Nicotine is an alkaloid present in the leaves of the tobacco plant, *Nicotiana tabacum*. There are no medical uses of nicotine, but it is of very great importance in medicine because of its addictive properties and its presence in tobacco. The percentage of nicotine in tobacco varies, but the smoke of a completely burned cigarette usually contains 1–6 mg and that of a cigar contains 15–40 mg of nicotine. Acute administration of 60 mg of nicotine orally by ingestion may be fatal. In low concentrations, nicotine stimulates the nicotinic receptors of autonomic ganglia, and in higher concentrations it is a ganglion blocker. Thus smoking can accelerate the heart via sympathetic stimulation, or slow it by sympathetic block or parasympathetic stimulation. There is usually cutaneous and splanchnic vasoconstriction with an increased peripheral vascular resistance. Respiration is stimulated, partly via stimulation of chemoreceptors in the carotid body. Adrenaline and noradrenaline are secreted from the adrenal medulla. The motor end-plate acetylcholine receptors are initially stimulated and then blocked, producing a paralysis of voluntary muscle. The results of extensive central stimulation include wakefulness, tremor, fits, anorexia, nausea, vomiting, tachypnoea and secretion of antidiuretic hormone (ADH).

ADVERSE EFFECTS OF SMOKING

In men under 70 years of age, the ratio of the death rate among cigarette smokers to that among non-smokers is 2:1. Above the age of 70 years this ratio falls to 1.5:1. The harmful effects are related to nicotine, carcinogenic tars and carbon monoxide. Some of the specific causes of death which are positively related to smoking are listed in Table 52.5.

Cigarette smoking is a major risk factor for peptic ulcer recurrence. H_2-blockers appear to be less effective in smokers, whilst sucralfate produces similar healing rates in smokers and non-smokers.

Some of the metabolic disturbances of smoking, such as the release of catecholamines and other amines from the adrenal glands, heart and platelets, and increases in blood fatty acids and glucose, predispose to cardiac arrhythmias, thrombosis and atherosclerosis. Further serious hazards from other products in smoke, particularly carbon monoxide, may also act as cardiotoxins and endanger ischaemic tissues.

Buerger's disease (thromboangitis obliterans) is a disease of unknown aetiology, but is severely aggravated by smoking. The coronary vessels may show other changes in addition to atherosclerosis. Hyaline thickening in the arterioles occurs almost exclusively in heavy smokers, and fibrous intimal thickening of the coronary arteries is also characteristic of 'smoker's heart'. Although smoking usually increases the cardiac output, in patients with impaired cardiac function a fall in cardiac output can result.

Smoking accelerates ageing-related changes in the lungs. These processes include increased residual volume, decreased vital capacity, increased closing volume and a progressive fall in arterial oxygen tension. The underlying degenerative changes appear to be loss of lung elasticity and loss of compliance of the chest wall. In addition, chronic obstructive airways disease and bronchitis are associated with smoking. The development of emphysema is markedly accelerated in cigarette smokers who have homozygous α_1-antitrypsin deficiency.

Smoking during pregnancy is associated with spontaneous abortion, premature delivery, small babies, increased perinatal mortality and an increased incidence of sudden infant death syndrome (cot death). In households where the parents smoke, there is an increased risk of pneumonia and bronchitis in preschool and school-age children, which is most marked during the first year of life.

PHARMACOKINETICS

Large amounts of tobacco taken by mouth result in delayed gastric emptying, and the nicotine may provoke vomiting. About 90% of nicotine from inhaled smoke is absorbed, while smoke taken into the mouth results in only 25–50% absorption. As well as being absorbed via the gastrointestinal, buccal and respiratory epithelium, nicotine is

Table 52.5 Principal causes of death associated with smoking

- Ischaemic heart disease (strongest correlation)
- Cancers of the lung, other respiratory sites and the oesophagus, lip and tongue
- Chronic bronchitis and emphysema, respiratory tuberculosis
- Pulmonary heart disease
- Aortic aneurysm

absorbed through the skin. A high concentration of nicotine may be present in the breast milk of smokers. Around 80–90% of circulating nicotine is metabolized in the liver, kidneys and lungs. Nicotine and its metabolites are excreted in the urine, and acidification of the urine accelerates excretion.

Each puff of cigarette smoke which is inhaled results in the absorption of 50–150 μg of nicotine. Smoking cigarette butts results in a much higher yield per inhalation. Thus each inhalation is equivalent to an intravenous injection of 1–2 μg/kg of nicotine. Smokers usually absorb 20–25% of the total nicotine in a cigarette. There is a rough correlation between the nicotine content of cigarettes and the peak plasma concentration of nicotine. The plasma elimination $t_{\frac{1}{2}}$ is 25–40 min.

Peak plasma levels after smoking cigarettes (typically containing 1.2 mg nicotine) are similar to those observed after chewing gum containing 4 mg of nicotine. However, the rate of increase is much slower after chewing gum or applying transdermal patches. The use of such gums to wean smokers off cigarettes has had only limited success, perhaps because of this inability to mimic the nicotine pharmacokinetics of smoking.

EFFECT OF SMOKING ON DRUG DISPOSITION AND EFFECTS

The commonest effect of tobacco smoking on drug disposition is an increase in elimination consistent with induction of drug-metabolizing enzymes. Nicotine itself is metabolized more extensively by smokers than by non-smokers, and this is associated with an alteration in the rate of elimination of a number of other drugs. In general, substrates for cytochrome P_{450} 1A2 (e.g. theophylline, caffeine, imipramine) are metabolized more rapidly in smokers than in non-smokers.

DRUG TREATMENT FOR NICOTINE DEPENDENCE

Smoking is pleasurable for confirmed smokers, and once the habit is established it is very difficult to eradicate. Even though the rituals of smoking can enhance sociability and provide tactile, gustatory and oro-labial gratification, it is clear that nicotine is active as a drug of dependence. Withdrawal can lead to an abstinence syndrome consisting of craving, irritability and sometimes physical features (e.g. alimentary disturbances). The appetite for sugar is often increased during the withdrawal state.

There are two pharmacological approaches to the treatment of nicotine dependence – first, the substitution of nicotine via skin patches or nicotine gum, and secondly, the antidepressant **buproprion** (unlicensed in the UK). The mechanism by which buproprion works is unknown, but it appears to reduce the desire to smoke. Neither treatment is particularly effective, and both require ongoing counselling and support to maximize abstinence.

Xanthines

This group of compounds includes caffeine (present in the seeds of the coffee plant, *Coffea arabica*, tea leaves from *Thea sinensis*, cocoa from the seeds of *Theobroma cacao*, and in soft drinks derived from the cola nut of the *Cola acuminata* tree). Other members of the group include theobromine (found in tea, coffee, cocoa and cola beverages) and theophylline (see Chapter 32). Caffeine is undoubtedly the most widely ingested alkaloid – in the USA the average intake from coffee alone is about 200 mg/day for people over 10 years of age. In addition, caffeine is included in a number of proprietary and prescription medicines, particularly those which occur in analgesic combinations. The major effects of these compounds are mediated by inhibition of phosphodiesterase, resulting in a raised intracellular cyclic adenosine monophosphate (AMP) concentration.

ADVERSE EFFECTS

A very wide range of behaviour – from putting the shot to increased vigilance in boring tasks – has allegedly been enhanced by caffeine. These effects are less marked than those of amphetamine, and have been difficult to prove objectively. In large doses caffeine exerts an excitatory effect on the CNS that is manifested by tremor, anxiety, irritability and restlessness, and interference with sleep. The evidence that exists indicates that caffeine does not possess properties which lead to improved intellectual performance except perhaps when normal performance has been downgraded by fatigue or boredom. In animal experiments, caffeine excites the CNS at all levels, but the cerebral cortex is affected first, and then the medulla, while the spinal cord is only affected by very large doses. The medullary respiratory, vagal and cardiovascular centres are all stimulated. Toxic doses result in convulsions, but in humans the toxic dose (over 10 g) is so large that human fatality is unlikely. Theophylline shares these actions, but theobromine is virtually inactive in this respect.

Circulatory effects include direct myocardial stimulation producing tachycardia, increased cardiac output, ectopic beats and palpitations. A direct effect on the blood vessels results in dilatation of coronary, pulmonary and systemic vasculature, but stimulation of the medullary vasomotor centre tends to counter this, so that the effect on blood pressure is unpredictable. Recently it has been suggested that patients with hypertension may be susceptible to increased blood pressure following caffeine intake. The cerebral circulation responds differently, by constriction, – hence the use of caffeine in migraine. The bronchial smooth muscle relaxes, producing bronchodilatation. Respiration is also stimulated centrally. Mild diuresis occurs due to an increased glomerular filtration rate subsequent to dilatation of the afferent arterioles. Theophylline is the most powerful xanthine diuretic. Theobromine has a more sustained effect, but is less active, whilst caffeine is the least powerful diuretic. Caffeine increases gastric acid secretion via its action on cyclic AMP, and xanthines in general may cause gastric irritation.

PHARMACOKINETICS

Caffeine is rapidly and completely absorbed after oral administration. Xanthines undergo a complex series of hepatic metabolic transformations by demethylation and oxidation as well as eventual ring cleavage to produce a series of methylxanthines and methylurates. The plasma $t_{\frac{1}{2}}$ of caffeine is 2.5–12 h. The plasma protein binding of caffeine is about 15%. Only 1–10% is excreted unchanged in the urine.

CAFFEINE DEPENDENCE

It is difficult to establish that caffeine causes dependence, in that it does not cause clinically significant impairment that would be consistent with a dependence syndrome. Tolerance is low grade but it definitely exists, although it does not appear to develop uniformly to all the effects of caffeine. Heavy users are allegedly less sensitive than light users to the nervousness and wakefulness caused by coffee, but are more sensitive to the euphoriant and stimulant actions. A mild withdrawal syndrome manifested by headache (possibly due to withdrawal of caffeine's vasoconstrictor effect), lethargy, nervousness, irritability and inefficiency occurs 12–16 h after discontinuation, although again this is subjective and difficult to demonstrate under controlled conditions.

CENTRAL DEPRESSANTS

Alcohol

Ethyl alcohol (alcohol) has few clinical uses when given systemically, but is of great medical importance because of its pathological and psychological effects when used as a beverage. The alcohol content of drinks ranges from 3.5–6% in beer, through 10% in wine and 20% in port to 40–55% in spirits (100° proof is 57% vol./vol.). The maximum recommended weekly intake is 21 units for men and 14 units for women (1 unit is equal to 10 g of ethanol, which is equivalent to half a pint of normal strength beer, one glass of wine or one single measure of spirits). Alcohol is the most important drug of dependence, and in Western Europe and North America the incidence of alcoholism is about 5% among the adult population.

PHARMACOKINETICS

Ethyl alcohol is absorbed from the buccal, oesophageal, gastric and intestinal mucosae – approximately 80% is absorbed from the small intestine. Alcohol delays gastric emptying, and in high doses it delays its own absorption by a negative feedback mediated via duodenal osmoreceptors. Large amounts of alcohol taken in dilute solution are also absorbed relatively slowly, possibly as a result of a volume effect on the gastric emptying rate. Following oral administration, alcohol can usually be detected in the blood within 5 min. Peak concentrations occur between 0.5 and 2 h. Fats and carbohydrates delay absorption, which follows zero-order kinetics. Individuals show great variation in the speed of absorption, and those habituated to alcohol often show a steeper rise and a higher peak in blood concentration.

Alcohol is distributed throughout the body water. About 95% is metabolized (mainly in the liver), and the remainder is excreted unchanged in the breath, urine and sweat. Hepatic oxidation to acetaldehyde is catalysed by three parallel processes. The major pathway (Figure 52.1) is rate limited by cytoplasmic alcohol dehydrogenase using nicotinamide adenine dinucleotide (NAD) as coenzyme. Large amounts of fructose (1–2 g/kg) accelerate alcohol metabolism, but this is not of clinical significance.

Although nutritional deficiencies may contribute to the toxicity of ethanol, which is a source of calories but not of vitamins or protein, it is now thought that it is the altered intracellular redox balance, caused by an increased NADH/NAD$^+$ ratio, which is responsible for the biochemical effects of acute and chronic alcohol abuse. An increase in the relative concentration of NADH results in reduced metabolism and therefore accumulation of lactate, β-hydroxybutyrate, glutamate, malate, α-glycerophosphate and other substances that require NAD$^+$ for elimination. The net effect of such changes includes impaired gluconeogenesis resulting in alcohol-induced hypoglycaemia, and fatty infiltration of the liver due to impaired elimination of exogenous and endogenous fatty acids via the Krebs' cycle and enhanced triglyceride synthesis due to increased levels of α-glycerophosphate. Originally it was postulated that alcohol elimination obeyed zero-order kinetics, i.e. it was independent of the blood concentration above about 0.1 mg/mL. However, there is now substantial evidence that Michaelis–Menten kinetics more accurately describe the situation. The maximum reaction rate (V_m) and Michaelis–Menten constant (K_m) for the average man are approximately 25 mg/100 mL/h and 10.5 mg/100 mL, respectively (see Chapter 3). However, it is true to say that the average rate of alcohol elimination is approximately 10 mL/h, so that once an intoxicated state is reached, an intake of 10 mL/h will suffice to maintain it. The rate of metabolism is much more nearly the same in identical twins than in fraternal twins, and genetic factors rather than environmental differences appear to control the overall rate. The rate of metabolism is very similar in young and old subjects, although the elderly have a smaller apparent volume of distribution, probably due to decreased lean body mass, and so develop higher levels for a given dose. Similarly, women, who have relatively more

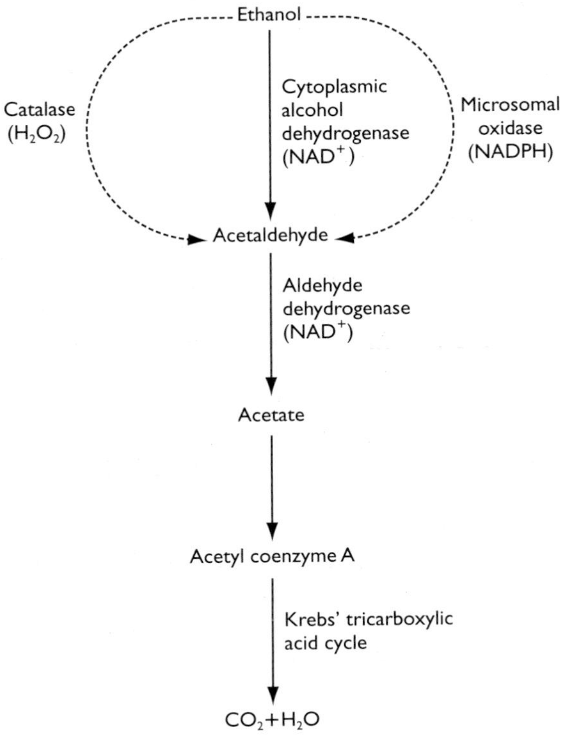

Figure 52.1 Pathways of ethanol oxidation. → major pathway. ---> minor pathways. NADP = nicotamide diphosphate.

subcutaneous fat than men, also develop higher blood levels, which accounts for their susceptibility to toxic damage from alcohol at lower levels of consumption.

ACUTE EFFECTS OF ALCOHOL

Nervous system Functionally, alcohol produces decreases in learning ability, association formation, attention span, concentration, versatility, judgement and discrimination, and reasoning. In individuals who are not heavy drinkers there is a rough correlation between blood alcohol concentration and acute central nervous system effects, and the rate at which alcohol concentrations rise is also important:

20 mg/100 mL	sensation of relaxation;
30 mg/100 mL	mild euphoria;
50 mg/100 mL	mild inco-ordination;
100 mg/100 mL	obvious ataxia;
300 mg/100 mL	stupor;
400 mg/100 mL	deep anaesthesia.

This list of blood alcohol concentrations is of no value in chronic alcoholics, in whom a level of 200 mg/100 mL may produce little effect, while at 400 mg/100 mL they may hold a coherent conversation. At high blood concentrations the gag reflex is impaired, vomiting may occur and death may result from aspiration of gastric contents. The importance of alcohol as a factor in road traffic accidents is well known (see Figure 52.2). At present in the UK the legal limit for alcohol in the blood is 80 mg/100 mL. At this level of intoxication serious personal injuries or fatalities occur in some 10% of road accidents, which is more than double the rate found in accidents involving sober drivers. The central depressant actions of alcohol greatly enhance the effects of other central depressant drugs. In patients with organic brain damage alcohol may induce unusual aggression and destructiveness known as pathological intoxication. Death may also result from direct respiratory depression.

Circulatory system Atrial fibrillation, cardiomyopathy, cutaneous vasodilatation, increased sweating (which can produce hypothermia) and splanchnic vasoconstriction occur. Increased myocardial excitability produces an increased heart rate, raised cardiac output, raised systolic blood pressure and increased pulse pressure.

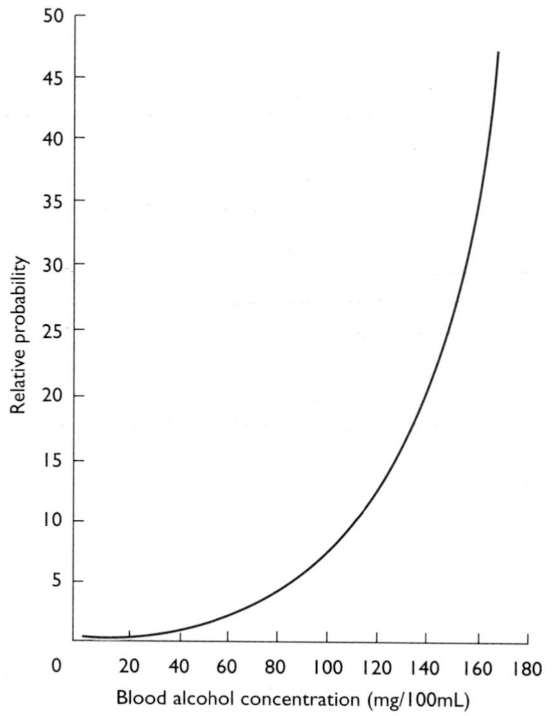

Figure 52.2 Relative probability of causing a road accident at various blood alcohol concentrations. (Reproduced from Harvard JDJ. 1975: *Hospital Update* **1**, 253.)

Other actions Low concentrations of alcohol in the stomach increase acid and mucous secretion and produce congestion of the gastric mucosa. This is followed by a decrease in acid secretion and acute gastritis. Alcohol suppresses ADH secretion, and this is one of the reasons why polyuria occurs following its ingestion. Reduced gluconeogenesis leading to hypoglycaemia may cause fits. The accumulation of lactate and other acids produces metabolic acidosis with excretion of an acidic urine and stimulation of the respiratory centre. In chronic alcoholics, severe thiamine deficiency may also precipitate lactic acidosis, and in such cases immediate treatment with intravenous thiamine is required. Hyperuricaemia may occur, resulting in acute gout in those who are predisposed to the condition, partly because of increased renal tubular excretion of organic acids, which compete with uric acid for secretion into the tubules.

Key points

Acute effects of alcohol

- Central effects include disinhibition, impaired judgement, inco-ordination, trauma (falls, road traffic accidents), violence and crime.
- Coma and impaired gag reflex; asphyxiation on vomit.
- Convulsions, enhancement of sedative drugs.
- Atrial fibrillation, vasodilation.
- Gastritis, nausea, vomiting, Mallory–Weiss syndrome.
- Hepatitis.
- Hypoglcycaemia, metabolic acidosis, etc.

CHRONIC EFFECTS OF ALCOHOL

Nervous system/alcohol withdrawal Behavioural changes occur, resulting in excessive alcohol intake with loss of control, i.e. the drinker can never be sure that they will be able to call a halt to their drinking once they have started to drink. This may lead to drinking with gradual loss of interest in normal activities, gradually resulting in social disintegration with loss of job, friends and family. Some alcoholics make repeated attempts at abstinence but then go on a binge. Others are unable to abstain and do not get drunk frequently, but top up intermittently day in, day out. In the confirmed alcoholic, periods of amnesia, emotional extremes (rage, depression, pathological jealousy), insomnia and seizures may occur.

After a period of chronic alcohol intake, a pattern of withdrawal symptoms develops. These may be seen after a brief period of abstinence or falling blood alcohol levels, and are frequently present when dependent patients wake in the morning. Classic features of acute withdrawal are due to autonomic overactivity, and include hypertension, sweating, tachycardia, tremor, anxiety, agitation, anorexia and insomnia. These are most severe 12–48 h after stopping drinking, and they then subside over 1–2 weeks. A small proportion of patients have evidence of additional neuronal excitation, and may have seizures (generally 12–48 h post abstinence). A third set of symptoms consists of alcohol withdrawal delirium or delirium tremens (acute disorientation, severe autonomic hyperactivity, and auditory and visual hallucinations). Delirium tremens is a medical emergency and, if untreated, death may occur as a result of respiratory or cardiovascular collapse.

Wernicke's encephalopathy (difficulty in concentrating, confusion, coma, nystagmus and ophthalmoplegia) and Korsakov's psychosis (gross memory defects with confabulation and disorientation in space and time) are mainly due to the nutritional deficiency of thiamine associated with alcoholism. Any evidence of Wernicke's encephalopathy should be immediately treated with intravenous thiamine (e.g. at least 100 mg daily for 3 days, followed by 100 mg orally for several months). Some individuals inherit an abnormal form of the enzyme transketolase with a reduced affinity for its coenzyme, thiamine. Thus if dietary thiamine intake falls, tissue transketolase activity is decreased, which may result in neurological damage. This explains why only some alcoholics experience these syndromes, and demonstrates the general principle of a genetically determined variant being disclosed by an environmental stress or drug. Similarly, peripheral neuropathy and retrobulbar neuritis are due to a lack of thiamine. A pellagra-like state may develop as a result of nicotinic acid deficiency.

Chronic alcoholism can also produce a range of neurological syndromes, including chronic cerebral degeneration (leading to dementia) with or without diffuse cerebral atrophy, Marchiafava–Bignami syndrome (symmetrical demyelination of the corpus callosum leading to dementia, fits, paralysis and disturbance of motor skills) and central pontine myelinolysis (producing quadriplegia and pseudobulbar palsy).

Alimentary system Chronic effects of alcohol include morning nausea and vomiting, abdominal pain, belching, gastritis, peptic ulceration and haematemesis (including the Mallory–Weiss syndrome, which is haematemesis due to oesophageal tearing during forceful vomiting). Liver pathology associated with chronic alcoholism includes enlargement of the liver due to fatty infiltration in 70–80% of alcoholics, which is reversible upon abstinence. Alcoholic hepatitis exhibits clinical features similar to those of other forms of toxic liver injury. The hypermetabolic state produced by alcohol produces maximal anoxia in the centrilobular hepatocytes, which become necrotic. Poor dietary intake does not appear to be as important as was once believed to be the case in the hepatotoxic effects of alcohol. A direct hepatotoxic role for alcohol implies that dietary supplements cannot counteract its effects on the liver, and that the only way to reduce its toxicity is by complete abstinence. Approximately 10% of chronic alcoholics develop cirrhosis of variable severity. The level of alcohol intake at which the risk of liver disease becomes significant is contentious. Probably less than 60 g per day in men is innocuous, but above this level of intake the risk of cirrhosis increases markedly. Predisposing factors for the development of cirrhosis include the female sex, histocompatibility antigens HLA B8, B13 and B40, and the presence of hepatitis B markers. The rate of development of cirrhosis is independent of the duration of alcohol abuse and the amount of alcohol consumed. Pancreatitis (acute, subacute and chronic) is also associated with chronic alcoholism. Alcohol stimulates secretin production, which increases the flow of pancreatic enzymes. If these are retained in the pancreas due to oedema of the sphincter of Oddi, then autodigestion can lead to pancreatic destruction and inflammation.

Cardiovascular system Alcoholism is occasionally complicated by a myopathy that affects cardiac and/or skeletal muscle. A negative association between moderate alcohol intake and coronary disease has been demonstrated in several epidemiological studies. There is evidence of a correlation between chronic alcohol consumption and hypertension.

Hematological effects Bone-marrow suppression occurs, with consequent thrombocytopenia and inability to counter infections, which are more common and serious in alcoholics. Macrocytic or hypochromic anaemias (probably nutritional in origin) may develop, and occasionally a haemolytic or sideroblastic anaemia occurs.

Metabolic effects Alcohol metabolism increases the intracellular NADH/NAD^+ ratio, which inhibits the pyruvate carboxylase step in gluconeogenesis, thus causing hypoglycaemia. Hypertriglyceridaemia may occur in alcoholics with liver complications, and also in those with normal liver function. Zieve's syndrome consists of jaundice, haemolytic anaemia and hyperlipidaemia. Some patients with types III and IV hyperlipoproteinaemia develop more severe triglyceridaemia after consuming alcohol. Hyperuricaemia, sometimes associated with acute gout, may occur.

In pregnancy Alcoholic mothers produce babies that exhibit features of intrauterine growth retardation and mental deficiency, sometimes associated with motor deficits and failure to thrive. There are characteristic facial features which include microcephaly, micrognathia and a short upturned nose. This so-called fetal alcohol syndrome is unlike that reported in severely undernourished women. Some obstetricians now recommend total abstinence during pregnancy.

> **Key points**
>
> Chronic effects of alcohol
>
> - Dependence.
> - Behavioural changes.
> - Encephalopathy (sometimes thiamine deficient), dementia, convulsions.
> - Cardiomyopathy.
> - Gastritis, nausea and vomiting; peptic ulceration.
> - Pancreatitis.
> - Cirrhosis.
> - Myopathy.
> - Bone-marrow suppression.
> - Gout.
> - Hypertension.
> - Fetal alcohol syndrome.

MEDICAL USES OF ALCOHOL

Apart from widespread use as a topical antiseptic and rubefacient, systemic alcohol has a number of therapeutic uses. In methanol poisoning, the administration of large amounts of ethanol competes for oxidation, slowing the rate of metabolism of methanol to toxic formaldehyde. An ethanol infusion is also useful in the management of ethylene glycol poisoning. Alcohol is also included in oral opioid mixtures (e.g. of heroin and cocaine – Brompton mixture) for administration to the terminally ill patient, and may improve appetite in such cases. Small quantities of alcohol may be of value in the prevention of ischaemic heart disease.

MANAGEMENT OF ALCOHOL WITHDRAWAL

Symptoms of autonomic overactivity Tremor, sweating and other classic symptoms can be managed with long-acting oral benzodiazepines (e.g.

diazepam, 10 mg orally as required until symptoms are diminished). The highest daily doses are administered over the first 24–36 h, when symptoms are most severe, and then the dose can be reduced and stopped over the next 2–3 days. If there are residual symptoms, these should be carefully reassessed, as they more likely to represent another disorder (e.g. anxiety) and not alcohol withdrawal. All patients should receive oral thiamine, 100 mg, for several months after withdrawal.

Seizures Seizures during alcohol withdrawal generally develop within 12–24 h of stopping drinking. They are usually generalized, and status epilepticus is rare. Benzodiazepines are effective.

Delirium tremens Delirium tremens is a medical emergency with a mortality of 5–10%. It rarely occurs, but it is critical to exclude it in every patient who presents with alcohol withdrawal. Management includes the following:

1 careful nursing in a quiet evenly illuminated room, if possible by the same staff on each shift;
2 symptomatic treatment of withdrawal symptoms (tremor, anxiety, sweating, hypertension) with a long-half-life benzodiazepine (e.g. diazepam). Large doses may be needed because of the cross-tolerance between these drugs and alcohol. Chlormethiazole was used extensively in the past for symptomatic treatment, but it may cause respiratory depression in overdose, and its pharmacokinetics are substantially altered in patients with cirrhosis. Therefore diazepam is preferred;
3 correction of fluid and electrolyte balance;
4 vitamin replacement with adequate thiamine (e.g. 100 mg parenterally daily for 3 days, followed by oral thiamine for 3 months);
5 psychiatric and medical assessment.

Key points

Delirium tremens

- Mortality is 5–10%.
- There is a state of acute confusion and disorientation associated with frightening hallucinations and sympathetic overactivity. Delirium tremens occurs in less than 10% of alcoholic patients withdrawing from alcohol.
- Management includes:
  nursing in a quiet, evenly illuminated room;
  sedation (either chlormethiazole or diazepam);
  vitamin replacement with adequate thiamine;
  correction of fluid and electrolyte balance;
  psychiatric referral.

LONG-TERM MANAGEMENT OF THE ALCOHOLIC

Psychological and social management Some form of psychological and social management is important to help the patient to remain abstinent. No clear advantage has been shown for one type of therapy compared to any other (e.g. in-patient vs. out-patient, individual vs. group treatment, dynamic psychotherapy vs. cognitive or behavioural methods), but any type of therapy is better than none. Whatever approach is used, the focus has to be on abstinence from alcohol. A very small minority of patients may be able to take up controlled drinking subsequently, but it is impossible to identify this group prospectively, and this should not be a goal of treatment. Voluntary agencies such as Alcoholics Anonymous (AA) are also important and complementary resources, and patients should be encouraged to attend them.

Naltrexone Alcoholics in treatment programmes who received the opioid antagonist naltrexone, 50 mg/day, had less craving for alcohol and fewer relapses than those who received placebo. Alcoholics on naltrexone who drank alcohol reported less of a 'high' compared to the effects of alcohol prior to treatment, suggesting that brain opioid sytems are involved in some of the rewarding or reinforcing effects of alcohol.

Alcohol-sensitizing drugs These produce an unpleasant reaction when taken with alcohol. The only drug of this type used to treat alcoholics is **disulfiram** (Antabuse), which inhibits aldehyde dehydrogenase, leading to acetaldehyde accumulation if alcohol is taken, causing flushing, sweating, nausea, headache, tachycardia and hypotension. Cardiac arrhythmias may occur if large amounts of alcohol are consumed. The small amounts of alcohol included in many medicines may be sufficient to produce a reaction, and it is advisable for the patient to carry a card warning of the danger of alcohol administration. Disulfiram also inhibits phenytoin metabolism and can lead to phenytoin intoxication. Unfortunately, there is only weak evidence that disulfiram has any benefit in the treatment of alcoholism. Its use should be limited to highly selected individuals in specialist clinics.

Acamprosate The structure of **acamprosate** resembles that of GABA and glutamate. It appears to reduce the effects of excitatory amino acids and, combined with counselling, it may help to maintain abstinence after alcohol withdrawal.

INTERACTIONS OF ALCOHOL WITH OTHER DRUGS

Alcohol can potentiate the effects of other CNS depressants (e.g. barbiturates, chloral, morphine, and benzodiazepines). Ethanol induces activity of cytochrome P_{450} 2E1 and 4E1, but in practice this is of little clinical importance. Increases in the rates of metabolism of warfarin, barbiturates, tolbutamide and phenytoin have been reported in alcoholics, although the mechanism for this is unclear. Alcohol may enhance the gastric irritation caused by aspirin, indomethacin and other gastric irritants. Alterations in ethanol metabolism by other drugs are relatively unusual since, unlike most drugs, alcohol is predominantly metabolized in the cytoplasm. Chlorpromazine inhibits ethanol metabolism by direct inhibition of the dehydrogenase, whilst phenobarbitone, clofibrate and fructose enhance its elimination. Disulfiram-type reactions (flushing of the face, tachycardia, sweating, breathlessness, vomiting and hypotension) have been reported with metronidazole, sulphonylureas and trichloroethylene (industrial exposure). Enhanced hypoglycaemia may occur following coadministration of alcohol with insulin and oral hypoglycaemic agents.

Barbiturates

With the significantly reduced prescription of barbiturates due to the introduction of the much safer benzodiazepines, the prevalence of barbiturate addiction has fallen dramatically. Barbiturates should *never* be used for patients with anxiety or insomnia, and their only uses today are for certain types of epilepsy or for anaesthetic pre-induction. Barbiturates are sedative and anxiolytic, with tolerance and marked physical and psychological dependence occurring after chronic administration. They have similar central effects to alcohol. However, during withdrawal, convulsions are more often seen in barbiturate-dependent patients than in those dependent on alcohol. Barbiturate overdoses are commonly fatal due to respiratory depression and/or asphyxia, and the risk of lethality may be increased if alcohol and barbiturates are co-administered. **Chloral hydrate** and **chlormethiazole** have similar potential for dependence, and their use is difficult to justify.

Benzodiazepines

See Chapter 17.

Solvents

Solvent abuse is common in certain groups, predominantly in adolescents aged between 12 and 16 years. It almost always occurs as part of a more widespread pattern of antisocial behaviour, and a dependence syndrome has not been identified. Solvents such as glues, paints, nail-varnish removers, dry-cleaning fluids and 'Tippex' are sniffed, often with the aid of a plastic bag to increase the concentration of vapour. Inhaled solvent rapidly reaches the brain. The effect may be enhanced by reduced oxygen. In contrast to drinking alcohol, the effects occur almost instantly (because of the rapid absorption of volatile hydrocarbons from the lungs) and usually resolve within 30 min. Disinhibition can lead to excessively gregarious, aggressive or emotional behaviour. Some sniffers just vomit. In a stupor accidents are common, and if overdose occurs, coma and asphyxiation may result. Some products may sensitize the heart and result in cardiac arrhythmias. Most deaths are associated with asphyxia as a result of aerosol inhalations or bags placed over the head. Excessive chronic use is rare, but may lead to major organ failure as well as permanent brain damage. There are no specific drug therapies for solvent abusers, and psychological and/or social management is required.

MISCELLANEOUS

Anabolic steroids

Anabolic steroids are abused by athletes in order to build up muscle tissue. Most synthetic anabolic steroids are derived from testosterone, and they are particularly popular among body builders. The prevalence of anabolic steroid abuse among athletes is uncertain. If given by injection using unsterile equipment, there is obviously a risk of blood-borne disease, as with other drugs of abuse. It is likely that chronic use is associated with hypertension, unusual hepatic and renal tumours, psychotic reactions and depression on withdrawal, and possibly sudden death from cardiac arrhythmias. Other 'performance-enhancing' drugs, usually of doubtful benefit but with side-effects, include human chorionic gonadotrophin, growth hormone, caffeine, amphetamines, beta-blockers and erythropoietin.

Case history

A 20-year-old man is brought by the police to the Accident and Emergency Department unconscious. The police believe that he ingested condoms full of diamorphine prior to his arrest following a drugs raid. He had been in police custody for approximately 1 h. On examination he is centrally cyanosed, breathing irregularly, with pinpoint pupils and no response to painful stimuli. There is bruising over many venepuncture sites.

Question 1
What is the immediate management?

Question 2
Abdominal radiography reveals six unbroken condoms in the patient's intestine. Is surgery indicated?

Answer 1
Give oxygen, maintain an airway, and give intravenous naloxone.

Answer 2
Since naloxone is an effective antidote to diamorphine poisoning, close observation with repeated injections or infusion of naloxone, inhaled oxygen and bulk laxatives should be sufficient.

Case history

A 70-year-old man is admitted with confusion, nystagmus and opthalmoplegia. His breath does not smell of alcohol. Laboratory tests reveal a raised mean corpuscular volume (MCV) and gamma-glutamyl transferase (GT), but were otherwise unremarkable.

Question 1
What is the likely diagnosis?

Question 2
What does the initial treatment involve?

Answer 1
Wernicke's encephalopathy.

Answer 2
Intravenous thiamine.

Amyl nitrate and butyl nitrate

These inhaled drugs cause almost instant vasodilatation, hypotension, tachycardia and a subjective 'rush'. They are claimed to enhance sexual pleasure and in addition dilate the anus. The hypotension can cause coma, and frequent use of these drugs is associated with methaemoglobinaemia.

FURTHER READING

Ferner RE. 1998: Interactions between alcohol and drugs. *Adverse Drug Reaction Bulletin* **189**, 719–22.

Meyer RE. 1996: The disease called addiction: emerging evidence in the 200–year debate. *Lancet* **347**, 162–6.

O'Conner PG, Schottenfield RS. 1998: Patients with alcohol problems. *New England Journal of Medicine* **338**, 592–602.

Vale A, Strang J (eds) 1999: Alcohol. *Medicine Journal* **27**, 1–28.

CHAPTER FIFTY-THREE

DRUG OVERDOSE *and* POISONING

- Intentional self-poisoning
- Accidental poisoning
- Criminal poisoning

INTENTIONAL SELF-POISONING

Self-poisoning remains one of the commoner causes of acute medical admission in the UK. Co-proxamol (dextropropoxyphene plus paracetamol), paracetamol alone and tricyclic antidepressants are the commonest drugs used in fatal overdose (see Table 53.1). Lithium, paraquat, salicylates, β-adrenoreceptor antagonists, digoxin and aminophylline continue to cause fatalities. This list of agents that cause death from overdose does not reflect the drugs on which individuals most commonly overdose. Benzodiazepines (often taken with alcohol) are commonly taken in an overdose, but are seldom fatal if taken in isolation. Around 80% of deaths from overdose occur outside hospital, with the mortality of those treated in hospital being less than 1%. The majority of cases of self-poisoning fall into the psychological classification of suicidal gestures (or a cry for help). However, the prescription of potent drugs with a low therapeutic ratio can cause death from an apparently trivial overdose.

Table 53.1: Top seven drugs implicated in fatal suicides

Agent	Number of deaths/year (1992)
1. Dextropropoxyphene-paracetamol (eg. co-proxamol, distalgesic)	148
2. Dothiepin	80
3. Paracetamol	80
4. Amitriptyline	67
5. Temazepam	26
6. Dextropropoxyphene	21
7. Aspirin	19

Source: *Mortality Statistics 1992*. The numbers shown exclude cases where more than one agent other than alcohol was taken.

Carbon monoxide from motor-vehicle exhaust fumes is still a frequent cause of suicide, although the number of cases has been falling since 1993, a trend which may be related to the introduction of catalytic converters and the increased popularity of diesel engines, which both result in lower carbon monoxide emissions.

DIAGNOSIS

History

Self-poisoning may present as an unconscious patient being delivered to casualty, or with a full history available from the patient or their companions. Following an immediate assessment of vital functions, as full a history as possible should be obtained from the patient, relatives, companions and ambulance drivers, as appropriate. A knowledge of the drugs or chemicals that were available to the patient is invaluable. Some patients in this situation give an unreliable history. A psychiatric history, particularly of depressive illness, previous suicide attempts or drug dependency, is relevant.

Examination

A meticulous, rapid but thorough clinical examination is essential not only to rule out other causes of coma or abnormal behaviour, (e.g. head injury, epilepsy, diabetes, hepatic encephalopathy), but also because the symptoms and signs may be characteristic of certain poisons. The clinical manifestations of some common poisons are summarized in Table 53.2.

Laboratory tests

Routine investigation of the comatose overdose patient should include blood glucose (rapidly determined by stick testing), and biochemical determination of plasma electrolytes, urea, creatinine and arterial blood gases. Drug screens are often requested, although they are rarely indicated as an emergency.

Table 53.3 lists those drugs where the clinical state of a patient may be unhelpful in determining the severity of the overdose in the acute stages. In each of these suspected overdoses, emergency measurement of the plasma concentration can lead to life-saving treatment. For example, in the early stages patients with paracetamol overdoses are often asymptomatic, and although it only

Table 53.2: Clinical manifestations of some common poisons

Symptoms/signs of acute overdose	Common poisons
Coma, hypotension, flaccidity	Benzodiazepines and other hypnosedatives, alcohol
Coma, pinpoint pupils, hypoventilation	Opioids
Coma, dilated pupils, hyper-reflexia, tachycardia	Tricyclic antidepressants, phenothiazines; other drugs with anticholinergic properties
Restlessness, hypertonia, hyper-reflexia, pyrexia	Amphetamines, MDMA, anticholinergic agents
Convulsions	Tricyclic antidepressants, phenothiazines, carbon monoxide, monoamine oxidase inhibitors, mefenamic acid, theophylline, hypoglycaemic agents, lithium, cyanide
Tinnitus, overbreathing, pyrexia, sweating, flushing, usually alert	Salicylates
Burns in mouth, dysphagia, abdominal pain	Corrosives, caustics, paraquat

MDMA = methylenedioxymethylamphetamine.

Table 53.3: Common indications for emergency measurement of drug concentration

Suspected overdose	Effect on management
Paracetamol	Administration of antidotes – acetylcysteine or methionine
Iron	Administration of antidote – desferrioxamine
Methanol/ethylene glycol	Administration of antidote – ethanol with or without dialysis
Lithium	Dialysis
Salicylates	Simple rehydration or alkaline diuresis or dialysis
Theophylline	Necessity for intensive-care unit (ITU) admission

rarely causes coma acutely, patients may have combined paracetamol with alcohol, a hypnosedative or an opioid. As such, an effective antidote (acetylcysteine) is available, and it is recommended that the paracetamol concentration should be measured in all unconscious patients who present as cases of drug overdose.

When there is doubt about the diagnosis, especially in coma, samples of blood, urine and (when available) gastric aspirate should be collected. Subsequent toxicological screening may be necessary if the cause of the coma does not become apparent or recovery does not occur. Avoidable morbidity is more commonly due to a missed diagnosis such as head injury than to failure to diagnose drug-induced coma.

Prevention of further absorption

Emesis can be achieved by stimulation of the pharynx (by the fingers or a blunt instrument such as a teaspoon) or oral syrup of ipecacuanha. The former may be useful as first aid in the home, but is often ineffective. The latter is very rarely recommended by Poison Centres in the UK although it is often used in the home in the USA. Syrup of ipecacuanha is a plant extract whose most active ingredients are emetine and cephalin. These act as direct irritants to the gastrointestinal tract and stimulate the medullary vomiting centre, possibly through central $5HT_3$-receptors (the effect can be blocked by ondansetron, a $5HT_3$-receptor antagonist; see Chapter 32). Syrup of ipecacuanha is effective in inducing vomiting in over 90% of patients within 30 min, although there is much less evidence of its ability to empty the stomach, and for this reason it is now very rarely recommended in the management of poisoning when more effective methods are available.

Gastric aspiration and lavage is the only acceptable method of emptying the stomach in a patient with impaired consciousness, having first secured the airway with a cuffed endotracheal tube. If there is *any* suppression of the gag reflex, a cuffed endotracheal tube is mandatory. Surprisingly, the aspiration of tablet residues is often incomplete. Although the beneficial effect on outcome is difficult to prove, it is still common practice to perform a stomach washout if the patient presents within 1–2 h of ingestion of a potentially toxic overdose. The sooner after ingestion this is performed, the more likely significant recovery of drugs will occur. After ingestion of drugs which delay gastric emptying (e.g. tricyclic antidepressants) or a large salicylate overdose, gastric lavage may be advised even later. However, there is little evidence that this is of benefit, and oral activated charcoal is recommended to reduce absorption. Gastric lavage may be unpleasant and is potentially hazardous. It should only be performed by experienced personnel with efficient suction apparatus close at hand (see Table 53.5).

If the patient is unco-operative and refuses to give consent, this procedure cannot be performed. Gastric lavage is usually contraindicated following ingestion of corrosives and acids, due to the risk of oesophageal perforation. Following petroleum distillate ingestion, the risk of aspiration pneumonia necessitates the use of a cuffed endotracheal tube.

Table 53.4: Methods of reducing absorption of poison

Emesis
Gastric aspiration and lavage
Oral activated charcoal
Gut lavage and cathartics

Table 53.5: Gastric aspiration and lavage

1. If the patient is unconscious, protect airway with cuffed endotracheal tube
   If semiconscious with effective gag reflex, place the patient in the head-down, left-lateral position. An anaesthetist with effective suction must be present
2. Place the patient's head over the end/side of the bed so that their mouth is below their larynx
3. Use a wide-bore lubricated orogastric tube
4. Confirm that the tube is in the stomach (not the trachea) by auscultation of blowing air into the stomach; save the first sample of aspirate for possible future toxicological analysis (and possible direct identification of tablets/capsules)
5. Use 300–600 mL of tap water for each wash, and repeat 3 to 4 times. Continue if ingested tablets/capsules are still present in the final aspirate
6. Unless an oral antidote is to be administered, leave 50 g of activated charcoal in the stomach

An increasingly popular method of reducing drug/toxin absorption either after or instead of gastric lavage is by means of oral activated charcoal, which adsorbs drug in the gut. To be effective, large amounts of charcoal are required, typically 10 times the amount of poison ingested, and again timing is critical, with maximum effectiveness being obtained soon after ingestion. Its effectiveness is due to its large surface area (> 1000 m^2/g). Binding of charcoal to the drug is by non-specific adsorption. Aspiration is a potential risk in a patient who subsequently loses consciousness or fits and vomits. Oral charcoal may also inactivate any oral antidote (e.g. methionine).

The use of repeated doses of activated charcoal may be indicated after ingestion of sustained-release medications or drugs with a small volume of distribution, low pk_a and prolonged elimination $t_{\frac{1}{2}}$ (e.g. salicylates, quinine, carbamazepine, barbiturates or theophylline). The rationale is that these drugs will diffuse passively from the bloodstream if charcoal is present in sufficient amounts in the gut.

Whole gut lavage using large amounts of electrolyte solutions may be useful when large amounts of sustained-release preparations, iron or lithium tablets or packets of smuggled narcotics have been taken. Bulk laxatives are also used in the latter situation.

SUPPORTIVE THERAPY

Patients are generally managed with intensive supportive therapy whilst the drug is eliminated naturally by the body. After an initial assessment of vital signs and instigation of appropriate resuscitation, repeated observations are necessary, as drugs may continue to be absorbed with a subsequent increase in plasma concentration after admission. In the unconscious patient, repeated measurements of cardiovascular function, including blood pressure, urine output and (if possible) continuous electrocardiographic (ECG) monitoring should be performed. Plasma electrolytes and acid–base balance should be measured. Hypotension is the commonest cardiovascular complication of poisoning. This is usually due to peripheral vasodilatation, but may be secondary to myocardial depression following, for example, β-blocker, tricyclic antidepressant or dextropropoxyphine poisoning. Hypotension can usually be managed with intravenous colloid. If this is inadequate, positive inotropic agents (e.g. dobutamine) may be necessary. If arrhythmias occur any hypoxia or hypokalaemia should be corrected, but anti-arrhythmic drugs should only be administered in life-threatening situations. Respiratory function is best monitored using blood gas analysis – a $PaCO_2$ of > 6.5 is usually an indication for assisted ventilation. Serial minute volume measurements or continuous measurement of oxygen saturation using a pulse oximeter are also helpful for monitoring deterioration or improvement in self-ventilation. Oxygen is not a substitute for inadequate ventilation. Respiratory stimulants increase mortality.

ENHANCEMENT OF ELIMINATION

Methods of increasing poison elimination are appropriate in less than 5% of overdose cases. Repeated oral doses of activated charcoal may enhance the elimination of a drug by 'gastrointestinal dialysis'. Several drugs are eliminated in the bile and then reabsorbed in the small intestine. Activated charcoal can interrupt this enterohepatic circulation by adsorbing drug in the gut lumen, thereby preventing reabsorption and enhancing faecal elimination. Cathartics such as magnesium sulphate can accelerate the intestinal transit time, which facilitates the process. Orally administered activated charcoal adsorbs drug in the gut lumen and effectively leaches drug from the intestinal circulation into the gut lumen down a diffusion gradient. Although studies in volunteers have shown that this method enhances the elimination of certain drugs, its effectiveness in reducing morbidity in overdose is generally unproven. However, it is extremely safe unless aspiration occurs. There are anecdotal reports of its value in the management of paracetamol, salicylate, digoxin, quinine, anticonvulsant and theophylline overdose. Forced diuresis is hazardous and is no longer recommended. Alkaline diuresis should be considered in cases of salicylate and phenobarbitone poisoning, and may be combined with repeated doses of oral activated charcoal. Acid diuresis may theoretically accelerate drug elimination in phencyclidine and amphetamine/'ecstasy' poisoning. However, it is not

Table 53.6: Methods and indications for enhancement of poison elimination

Method	Poison
Alkaline diuresis	Salicylates, phenobarbitone
Haemodialysis (peritoneal dialysis is also effective, but two to three times less efficient)	Salicylates, methanol, ethylene glycol, lithium, phenobarbitone
Charcoal haemoperfusion	Barbiturates, theophylline, disopyramide
'Gastrointestinal dialysis' via multiple-dose activated charcoal	Salicylates, theophylline, quinine, most anticonvulsants, digoxin

usually necessary, may be harmful and is almost never recommended.

Adjustment of urinary pH is much more effective than causing massive urine output. Alkaline diuresis is particularly hazardous in the elderly due to sodium and water overload. A forced alkaline diuresis is no longer recommended. Peritoneal dialysis, haemodialysis and, much less commonly, charcoal haemoperfusion are sometimes used to enhance drug elimination. Table 53.6 summarizes the most important indications and methods for such elimination techniques. In addition, exchange transfusion has been successfully used in the treatment of poisoning in some young children and infants. The risk of an elimination technique must be balanced against the possible benefit of enhanced elimination.

Specific antidotes

Antidotes are available for a small number of poisons, and the most important of these are summarized in Table 53.7.

Chelating agents

Chelating agents possess two or more electron donor groups in a molecule that can co-ordinate with a polyvalent metal. The resulting coordination metal complex has a ring structure. For use in medicine, the chelating agent and its metal complex must be non-toxic, soluble and readily excreted. Some recommended chelating agents are listed in Table 53.7.

Naloxone

Naloxone is a pure opioid antagonist at the μ-receptor with no intrinsic agonist activity (see Chapter 24). It rapidly reverses the effects of opioid drugs, including morphine, diamorphine, pethidine, dextropropoxyphene, codeine and dipipanone. When injected intravenously, naloxone acts within 2 min and the plasma $t_{\frac{1}{2}}$ is up to 1 h. The $t_{\frac{1}{2}}$ of most opioid drugs is longer (e.g. for dextropropoxyphene it is 12–24 h), and repeated doses or infusions of naloxone may be required. The usual dose is 0.8–1.2 mg, although much higher doses may be needed after massive opioid overdoses, which are common in addicts and especially after a partial agonist (e.g. buprenorphine) overdose, because partial agonists must occupy a relatively large fraction of the receptors compared to full agonists such as morphine in order to produce even modest effects. Naloxone is not itself sedating, does not depress respiration and, although it does not directly affect pupil size, it does dilate a pupil constricted by an opiate. It has been given intramuscularly to achieve a longer duration of action. Naloxone can precipitate withdrawal reactions in narcotic addicts. This is not a contraindication, but it is wise to ensure that patients are appropriately restrained before administering naloxone.

Management of specific overdoses

Paracetamol

This over-the-counter mild analgesic is commonly taken in overdose. Although remarkably safe in therapeutic doses, overdoses of 7.5 g or more may

Table 53.7: Antidotes and other specific measures

Overdose drug	Antidote/other specific measures
Paracetamol	Acetylcysteine IV Methionine p. o.
Iron	Desferrioxamine
Cyanide	Oxygen, amyl nitrate (inhalation), dicobalt edetate IV, sodium nitrite IV followed by sodium thiosulphate IV
Benzodiazepines	Flumazenil IV
Beta-blockers	Atropine Isoprenaline Glucagon
Carbon monoxide	Oxygen Hyperbaric oxygen
Methanol/ethylene glycol	Ethanol, 4-methyl-pyrazole*
Lead (inorganic)	Sodium EDTA IV Penicillamine p.o. Dimercaptosuccinic acid (DMSA*) IV or p.o.
Mercury	Dimercaptopropane sulphonate, (DMPS*) Dimercaptosuccinic acid, (DMSA*) Dimercaprol Penicillamine
Opioids	Naloxone
Organophosphorus insecticides	Atropine, pralidoxime
Digoxin	Digoxin-specific fab antibody fragments
Calcium-channel blockers	Calcium chloride or gluconate IV
Insulin	50% dextrose IV Glucagon IV or IM

* *Note*: DMSA, DMPS and 4-methyl-pyrazole are not licensed in the UK.

cause hepatic failure, less commonly renal failure, and death (for discussion of the mechanism involved see Chapter 5). The patient is usually asymptomatic at the time of presentation, but may complain of nausea and sweating. Right hypochondrial pain and anorexia may precede the development of hepatic failure. Coma is rare unless a hypnosedative or opioid (e.g. in the form of dextropropoxyphene in co-proxamol) has been taken as well.

If a potentially toxic overdose is suspected, the stomach should be emptied if within 1–2 h of ingestion. The antidote should be administered and blood taken for determination of paracetamol concentration, prothrombin time, creatinine and liver enzymes. The decision to stop or continue the antidote can be made at a later time. The plasma paracetamol concentration should be obtained urgently and related to the graph shown in Figure 53.1, which plots time from ingestion against plasma paracetamol concentration and probability of liver damage. A more precise treatment graph is printed in the *British National Formulary* (it is unreliable for staggered overdoses). If doubt exists concerning the time of ingestion it is better to err on the side of caution and give the antidote.

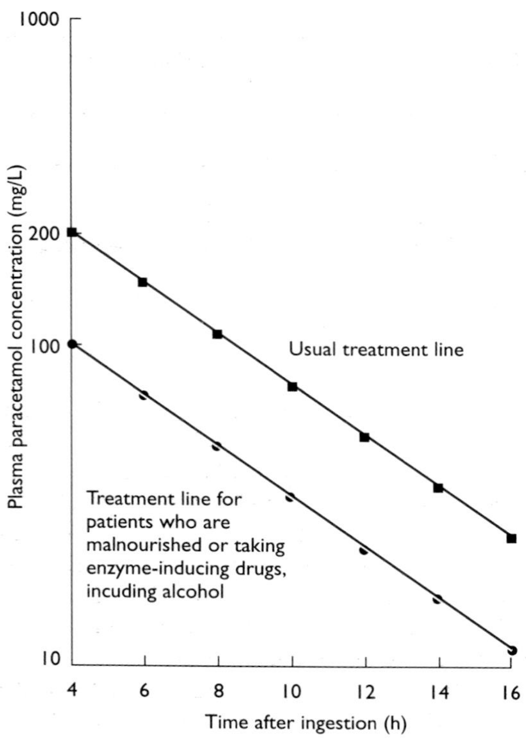

Figure 53.1: Treatment graph for paracetamol overdose. The graph provides guidance on the need for acetylcysteine treatment. The time (in hours) after ingestion is often uncertain. If in doubt – treat.

Intravenous acetylcysteine and/or oral methionine are potentially life-saving antidotes and are most effective if given within 12 h of ingestion, although benefit may be obtained from acetylcysteine up to 24 h after ingestion. Acetylcysteine is administered as an intravenous infusion. The standard regimen is described in Table 53.8. In approximately 5% of patients, pseudoallergic reactions occur, which are usually mild. If any hypotension or wheezing occurs, it is recommended that the infusion be stopped and an antihistamine administered parenterally. If the reaction has completely resolved, acetylcysteine may be restarted at a lower dose. Alternatively, methionine may be used (see below).

Patients who are taking enzyme-inducing drugs (e.g. phenytoin, carbamazepine) and chronic alcoholics are at a higher risk of hepatic necrosis following paracetamol overdose. The prothrombin time is the first indicator of hepatic damage. If the prothrombin time and serum creatinine level are normal when repeated at least 24 h after the overdose, significant hepatic or renal damage is unlikely.

Table 53.8: Administration of acetylcysteine (in 5% dextrose).

Dose	Diluent volume	Infusion period
150 mg/kg then	200 mL	15 min
50 mg/kg then	500 mL	4 h
100 mg/kg	1000 mL	16 h

Methionine is an effective oral antidote in paracetamol poisoning. It has the advantages that it is very safe and cheap, but has the disadvantage that absorption is delayed compared to intravenous acetylcysteine. Its efficacy has not been studied in late paracetamol overdoses. It may be particularly useful in remote areas where there will be a delay in reaching hospital.

Salicylate

Although also conscious, in contrast to the individual with paracetamol overdose, the patient usually feels ill after significant salicylate overdose, and presents with tinnitus and hyperventilation and is hot and sweating. Immediate management includes estimation of arterial blood gases, electrolytes, renal function and plasma salicylate concentration. The patient is usually dehydrated and requires intravenous fluids. A stomach washout is often performed, but objective evidence of benefit beyond 1 h is lacking. Activated charcoal should be administered. Blood gases and arterial pH normally reveal a mixed metabolic acidosis and respiratory alkalosis. Respiratory alkalosis frequently predominates, and is due to direct stimulation of the respiratory center. The metabolic acidosis is due to uncoupling of oxidative phosphorylation and lactic acidosis. If acidosis predominates, the prognosis is poor. Absorption may be delayed and the plasma salicylate concentration can increase over many hours after ingestion. Depending on the salicylate concentration (see Table 53.9) and the patient's clinical condition, an alkaline diuresis should be commenced

Table 53.9: Urinary alkalinization regimen for aspirin

Indicated in adults with a salicylate level in the range 600–800 mg/L and in elderly adults and children with levels in the range 450–750 mg/L
Adults: 1 L of 1.26% sodium bicarbonate (isotonic) + 40 mmol KCl IV over 4 h, and/or 50-ml IV boluses of 8.5% sodium bicarbonate (*note*: additional KCl will be required)
Children: 1 mL/kg of 8.4% sodium bicarbonate (= 1 mmol/kg) + 20 mmol KCl diluted in 0.5 L of dextrose saline infused at 2–3 mL/kg/h

Source: National Poisons Information Service, Guy's and St Thomas's Trust London Centre.

using sodium bicarbonate. However, this is particularly hazardous in the elderly. Children metabolize aspirin less effectively than adults, and are more likely to develop a metabolic acidosis and consequently are at higher risk of death. Plasma electrolytes, salicylate and arterial blood gases and pH must be measured regularly. Sodium bicarbonate may lead to hypokalaemia, which discourages formation of an alkaline urine. Hence supplemental intravenous potassium may have to be added to the bicarbonate. If the salicylate concentration reaches 800–1000 mg/L, haemodialysis is likely to be necessary. Haemodialysis may also be life-saving at lower salicylate concentrations if the patient's metabolic and clinical condition deteriorates.

Tricyclic antidepressants

Tricyclic antidepressants cause death by arrhythmias, myocardial depression, convulsions or asphyxia. If the patient reaches hospital alive they may be conscious, confused, aggressive or in deep coma. Clinical signs include dilated pupils, hyperreflexia and tachycardia. Following immediate assessment of the patient, including resuscitation and ECG monitoring as necessary, blood should be taken for determination of arterial blood gases and electrolytes. Gastric lavage should be performed up to 2 h after ingestion. The patient must continue to be ECG monitored during this procedure and for 24 h after clinical recovery.

The commonest arrhythmia is sinus tachycardia, predominantly due to anticholinergic effects, and does not require any intervention. Broadening of the QRS complex indicates a quinidine-like effect (unless pre-existing bundle branch block is present) and is associated with a poor prognosis. The only preventative anti-arrhythmic therapy should be correction of any metabolic abnormalities, especially hypokalaemia, hypoxia and acidosis. Intravenous sodium bicarbonate (1–2 mmol/kg body weight) is the most effective treatment for the severely ill patient, and its mode action may involve a redistribution of the drug within the tissues. Some centres recommend prophylactic bicarbonate and potassium to keep the pH in the range of 7.45–7.55 and the potassium concentration at the upper end of the normal range if the QRS duration is >100 ms or the patients is hypotensive despite intravenous colloid. In extreme cases prolonged chest compressions may be required to maintain cardiac output. If life-threatening ventricular arrhythmias occur, phenytoin may be effective. Anticholinergic drugs should be avoided. If resistant ventricular tachycardia occurs, intravenous magnesium, intravenous isoprenaline or overdrive pacing have been advocated. If ventricular tachycardia results in hypotension, DC shock is indicated. Convulsions should be treated with intravenous benzodiazepines.

Occasionally, assisted ventilation is necessary. The patient should be ECG monitored for at least 12 h after the overdose, and if arrhythmias occur then for longer.

Paracetamol/dextropropoxyphene compound preparations

It is usually the dextropropoxyphene that causes death from overdose with this mixture of dextropropoxyphene and paracetamol. The patient may present with coma, hypoventilation and pinpoint pupils. The cardiac toxicity includes negative inotropism and arrhythmias. Immediate cardiopulmonary resuscitation and intravenous naloxone are indicated. The plasma paracetamol concentration should be measured and acetylcysteine administered as shown in Figure 53.1.

Opioid overdose

See Chapter 24.

Carbon monoxide

This is a common cause of fatal poisoning. Carbon monoxide suicides are usually male and under 65 years of age, and die from carbon monoxide generated from car exhaust fumes (catalytic converters reduce the carbon monoxide emission, and this may have reduced the number of deaths.) Accidental carbon monoxide poisoning is also common, and should be considered in the differential diagnosis of confusional states, headache and vomiting, particularly in winter as a result of inefficient heaters and inadequate ventilation. Measurement of the carboxyhaemaglobin level in blood may be helpful. Carbon monoxide may also be present in survivors of fires. The immediate management consists of removal from exposure and administration of oxygen. *There is increasing evidence that hyperbaric oxygen speeds recovery and reduces neuropsychiatric complications.*

Non-drug poisons

A vast array of plants, garden preparations, pesticides, household products, cosmetics and industrial chemicals may be ingested. Some substances, such as paraquat and cyanides, are extremely toxic, whilst many substances are non-toxic unless enormous quantities are consumed. It is beyond the scope of this book to catalogue and summarize the treatment of all poisons and the reader is strongly advised to contact one of the poisons, information services (see Table 53.10 for telephone numbers) whenever any doubt exists as to toxicity management.

PSYCHIATRIC ASSESSMENT

It is important that selected overdose patients are reviewed by a psychiatrist. Although most patients take overdoses as a reaction to social or life events, some overdose, patients are pathologically depressed. Tricyclic antidepressant drugs are potentially very toxic in overdose so the decision to treat is a balance between the efficacy of the drug and the risk of further overdose. Safer alternatives such as selective serotonin reuptake inhibitors should be considered.

Table 53.10: Poisons information

Belfast	01232 240503
Birmingham	0121 507 5588/9
Cardiff	01222 709901
Dublin	Dublin 8379964
	or Dublin 8379966
Edinburgh	0131 536 2300
Leeds	0113 243 0715
	or 0113 292 3547
London	0171 635 9191
Newcastle	0191 232 5131

Note: Some of these centres also advise on laboratory analytical services which may be of help in the diagnosis and management of a small number of cases.

Key points

Diagnosis of acute self-poisoning in comatose patients

- History:
  from companions, ambulance staff, available drugs/poisons, suicide note.
- Examination:
  immediate vital signs;
  signs of non-poison causes of coma. (e.g. intracerebral haemorrhage);
  signs consistent with drug overdose (e.g. meiosis, depressed respiration due to opioid).
- Investigation:
  to determine severity. (e.g. blood gases. ECG);
  paracetamol level to determine whether acetylcysteine is appropriate;
  to exclude metabolic causes of coma (e.g. hypoglycaemia);
  to diagnose specific drug/poison levels if this will affect management.

Note: Acute overdose may mimic signs of brainstem death, yet the patient may recover if adequate supportive care is provided. Always measure the blood glucose concentration in an undiagnosed comatose patient.

Accidental poisoning

Accidental poisoning with drugs causes between 10 and 15 deaths per annum in children. Most commonly, tablets were prescribed to the parents and left insecure in the household or handbag. Unfortunately, many drugs resemble sweets. Tricyclic antidepressants are commonly implicated. The use of child-proof containers and patient education should reduce the incidence of these unnecessary deaths. Non-drug substances that cause significant poisoning in children include antifreeze, cleaning liquids and pesticides.

In adults, accidental poisoning most commonly occurs at work and usually involves inhalation of noxious fumes. Factory and farm workers are at particular risk. Carbon monoxide is associated with approximately 50 accidental deaths and seriously injures at least 200 individuals in the UK per year. The onset of symptoms is often insidious. There is particular concern in the UK about the effect of organophosphate pesticides, not only as a cause of acute poisoning, but also because it is possible that repeated exposure to relatively low doses may result in chronic neurological effects. Those working with sheep dip appear to be most at risk.

Key points

Symptoms of accidental carbon monoxide poisoning

■ Headache	90%
■ Nausea and vomiting	50%
■ Vertigo	50%
■ Alteration in consciousness	30%
■ Subjective weakness	20%

Source: the Chief Medical Officer.

Criminal poisoning

This is one mode of non-accidental injury of children. Homicidal poisoning is rare but possibly underdiagnosed. Suspicion is the key to diagnosis, and toxicological screens are invaluable.

Case history

A 21-year-old student is brought into your casualty department having been at a party with his girlfriend. She reports that he drank two non-alcoholic drinks but had also taken 'some tablets' that he had been given by a stranger at the party. Within about 1 h he started to act oddly, becoming unco-ordinated, belligerent and incoherent. When you examine him he is semiconscious, responding to verbal commands intermittently. During the period when you are interviewing/examining him he suddenly sustains a non-remitting grand-mal seizure.

Question 1

What are the agents he is most likely to have taken?

Question 2

How would you treat him?

Answer 1

The most likely agents that could have caused an altered mental status and then led to seizures are:

- sympathomimetics (e.g. amphetamines, cocaine, MDMA);
- hallucinogens LSD, phencyclidine (PCP) – (latter unusual in the UK).
- tricyclic antidepressants;
- selective serotonin reuptake inhibitors.

Much less likely causes are:

- antihistamines (especially first-generation antihistamines in high dose; these are available over the counter);
- theophylline;
- ethanol and ethylene glycol can also do this, but are unlikely in this case, because of the patient's girlfriend's account of events.

Answer 2

This patient should be treated as follows:

1. Ensure a clear airway with adequate oxygenation – avoid aspiration.
2. Ensure that other vital functions are adequate.
3. Prevent him from injuring himself (e.g. by falls (off a trolley) or flailing limbs).
4. Give therapy to stop the epileptic fit:
   diazepam, 10 mg IV and repeated if necessary;
   if the patient is refractory to this consider thiopentone anaesthesia and ventilation.
5. Monitor the patient closely, including ECG, and observe for respiratory depression and further seizures. Attempt to define more clearly which agent he ingested to allow further appropriate toxicological management.

Case history

A 20-year-old known heroin addict who is HIV, hepatitis C and hepatitis B positive is brought to the Accident and Emergency department. It is winter and there is a major flu epidemic in the area. He is certified dead on arrival.

Many old venepuncture sites and one recent one are visible on his arms. He does not appear cyanosed.

The history from his girlfriend, also a heroin addict, is that he was released from prison 1 week earlier and they moved into an old Victorian flat. They had tried to stay off heroin for 1 week (he had obtained a limited supply while in prison), but both had experienced headaches, nausea, vomiting, stomach cramps, tremor and diarrhoea.

The patient had told his girlfriend that he had to have some heroin. She left the flat for 6h to pick up her unemployment benefit, and returned home to find him prostrate on the floor with a syringe and needle beside him. She called an ambulance and attempted to resuscitate him with CPR and an amphetamine.

Question

Name two possible causes of death.

Answer

Carbon monoxide poisoning and heroin overdose.

Comment

Some of this patient's symptoms are not typical of heroin withdrawal, but are characteristics of carbon monoxide poisoning. His flatmate should be examined neurologically, a sample taken for carboxyhaemoglobin and the flat inspected. Oxygen is the antidote to carbon monoxide poisoning, and naloxone is the antidote to heroin poisoning.

Further reading

Ellenhorn MJ, Schonwald S, Ordog G. 1996: *Ellenhorn's medical toxicology: diagnosis and treatment of human poisoning*, 2nd edn. Baltimore, MD: Williams & Wilkins.

Henry J, Hoffman A. 1988: Gut decontamination–controversy continues. *Lancet* **352**, 420.

Vale JA. 1997: Position statement: gastric lavage. American Academy of Clinical Toxicology; European Association of Poisons Centres and Clinical Toxicologists. *Journal of Toxicology – Clinical Toxicology* **35**, 711–9.

INDEX

Note: page numbers in *italics* refer to figures and tables

Griseofulvin

effective against candida
Aspergillus

should not be given > 2/52

↑ Anticoagulant action
of warfarin

avoided in Renal failure

metronidazole

inhibits dihydrofolate metabolism ?

80 % bioavailability given rectally

Disulfiram like effect | alcohol

polyneuropathy

elimination unaltered in renal failure

prophyria ??

syringomyelia ??(?)

psychiatric disorders

HMG COA reductase inhibitors

↓ risk of reinfarction

↑ risk of non CVS deaths

slows progression of coronary atheroma

Regression of " "

recognized cause of rhabdomyolysis

Endocrine

- Control DM
- Malignancy bone [illegible]
- Hypoparathyroidism [illegible]
- [illegible]
- Hypopituitarism ? [illegible]

~~Crohn's~~

- Prednisolone in IBD.
- IV prednisolone
- [illegible]

Renal

Cholesterol emboli

Rhabdomyolysis
Haemochromatosis
2° polycythaemia
ITP
primary sclerosing cholangitis
pancreatic ca
- Asthma

Rheumatology

1) Osteoarthritis
2) psoriatic arthritis
3) Circinate Balanitis
4) Dermatomyositis
5) H-S purpura (steroids)
6) Systemic sclerosis
7) Osteoporosis skin & [illegible] necros

Overdoses

- Digoxin (charcoal)
- Opiate
- [illegible]
- MTX pneumonitis
- carbamazepine [illegible]
- chloroquine [illegible] in [illegible]
Amoebiasis
- TB

Nephrology

- [illegible]
- Antithrombin Def.
- IV iron.

- psychiatry
- psychiatric [illegible]
Reassurance.
[illegible]
Headings
[illegible]

Skin

- ~~[illegible]~~
- Epidermolysis bullosa
- Bullous pemphigoid
- fungal infection [illegible] (1)
- Anthrax Skin (2)
- tetracycline photosens
- [illegible]

Renal

- Membranous GN (CA)
- [illegible] Acc.
- [illegible]
- Myeloma Renal failure

CVS.

Aortic dissection

Urgent angiography MVP.

- non Q MI
- constrictive pericard
- Temporary pacing 2:1 block
- 2:1 block
- pericarditis
- [illegible]
- Bacterial endocarditis - Echo
- B bd.

Respiratory

- Ventilation
- PCP pneum
- Cryptogenic [illegible]
- pneumococcal pneum
- [illegible] Aspiration
- Anticoagulation
- VQ mismatch

Infections

Sarcoidosis

CNS

- Herpes Encephalitis
- Cryptococcal [illegible]
- Alzheimers
- [illegible]
- Motor neurone
- [illegible]

GB (1) (2)

Median (N)

[illegible]